Catheter Ablation

Kenzo Hirao
Editor

Catheter Ablation

A Current Approach on Cardiac Arrhythmias

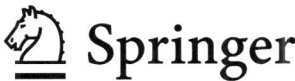

Editor
Kenzo Hirao
Cardiovascular Medicine
Tokyo Medical and Dental University
Tokyo
Japan

ISBN 978-981-10-4462-5   ISBN 978-981-10-4463-2 (eBook)
https://doi.org/10.1007/978-981-10-4463-2

Library of Congress Control Number: 2017962305

© Springer Nature Singapore Pte Ltd. 2018
This work is subject to copyright. All rights are reserved by the Publisher, whether the whole or part of the material is concerned, specifically the rights of translation, reprinting, reuse of illustrations, recitation, broadcasting, reproduction on microfilms or in any other physical way, and transmission or information storage and retrieval, electronic adaptation, computer software, or by similar or dissimilar methodology now known or hereafter developed.
The use of general descriptive names, registered names, trademarks, service marks, etc. in this publication does not imply, even in the absence of a specific statement, that such names are exempt from the relevant protective laws and regulations and therefore free for general use.
The publisher, the authors and the editors are safe to assume that the advice and information in this book are believed to be true and accurate at the date of publication. Neither the publisher nor the authors or the editors give a warranty, express or implied, with respect to the material contained herein or for any errors or omissions that may have been made. The publisher remains neutral with regard to jurisdictional claims in published maps and institutional affiliations.

Printed on acid-free paper

This Springer imprint is published by Springer Nature
The registered company is Springer Nature Singapore Pte Ltd.
The registered company address is: 152 Beach Road, #21-01/04 Gateway East, Singapore 189721, Singapore

Preface

"With the discovery of the conduction system of Tawara, heart research entered a new epoch."—Sir Arthur Keith [1].

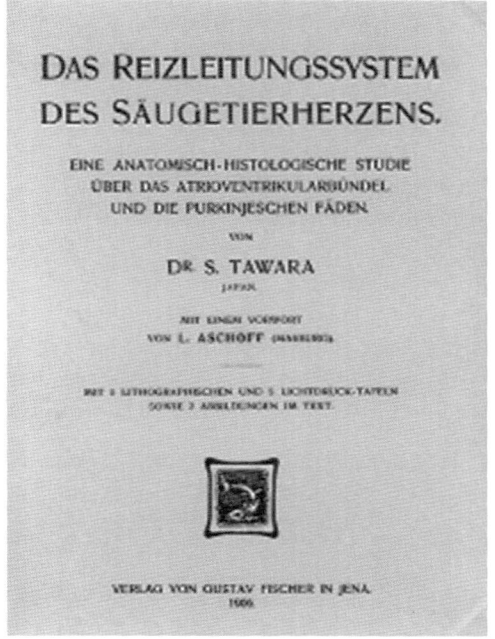
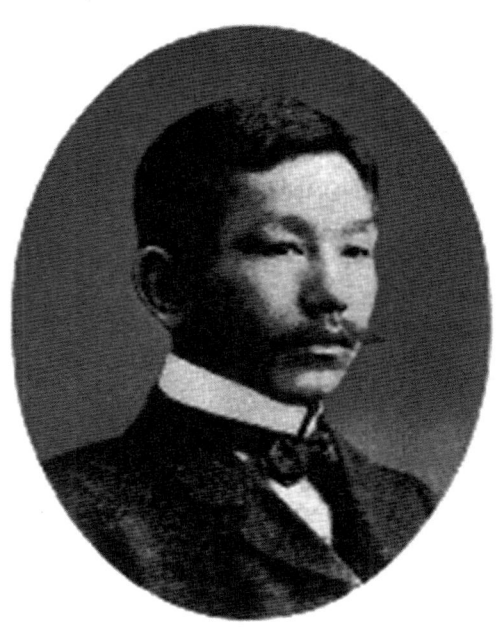

Tawara's monograph in 1906   Sunao Tawara, M.D.

   The atrio-ventricular conduction system is so wisely and efficiently created that the signals from the atria can travel slowly through the AV node and then be delivered at a high conduction velocity via both bundle branches to the ventricles, which eventually enable an effective pumping action of the whole heart. Professor Sunao Tawara discovered the AV conduction system, which was reported in a monograph in German in 1906 [2]. Tawara undertook his laborious work on the pathology and anatomy of the heart with Professor Ludwig Aschoff in Philipps University Marburg, Germany. His work covered the discovery of the AV node, connecting proximally to the His bundle with both bundles branches then connecting to the His bundle, and the accurate tracing of the Purkinje fibers from the bundle branches. Moreover, the interdigitating connections between the Purkinje fibers and ventricular myocardium were precisely drawn as well as the node and atrial myocardium. Thus, what he established and named was the "stimulus conduction system" of the heart, where he succeeded in identifying a complete discreet pathway starting from the atrial myocardium and ending in the ventricular myocardium. Of note, he predicted the conduction velocity of each component within the system as well as the precise description of the location of all the components of the AV conduction system. Thus, Tawara's discovery of the AV conduction system is regarded as having advanced cardiology, particularly cardiac electrophysiology and electrocardiology [3].

The ingenious work of Tawara on the anatomy of the AV conduction system and his extraordinary insight into the electrophysiological characteristics of each component of the system has allowed us to understand the critical factors for a successful catheter ablation. That is, it has provided us with an accurate knowledge of the cardiac anatomy, including the AV conduction system, as well as a full understanding of the normal electrophysiological properties of the whole heart.

From that perspective, the 39 chapters have been designed to progress from cardiac anatomy and a fundamental understanding of the techniques for diagnosing the tachycardia mechanism to practical and advanced techniques for catheter ablation of tachycardias. We have assembled a mostly Japanese team of experts to describe the up-to-date information, which is supplemented by extensive illustrations and images. These experts include some who have advocated new concepts of tachycardia circuits, new pacing diagnostic maneuvers, and new ablation methods, and others who have experienced a great number of cases with common tachycardias or rare cases such as inherited arrhythmogenic diseases. I hope that the information contained in each chapter will provide electrophysiologists with invaluable knowledge skills for this field and can help their understanding of catheter ablation.

I have been truly fortunate to have enlisted the superb support of my colleagues, Drs. Yagishita A. and Shirai Y., who have helped revise the entire text with great commitment and patience. It is thanks to the Springer Editorial Team's tireless efforts that it has been possible to publish this book within such a short period of time. For this, I would like to express my deepest appreciation. It is my great honor to have edited this book and to have invited the world-leading Japanese electrophysiologists as the authors for each chapter. Finally, it is my sincerest hope that this book will be a valuable part of every electrophysiology laboratory.

Tokyo, Japan   Kenzo Hirao, M.D.

References
1. Keith A. An autobiography. Watts & Co., London, 1950. p. 254–9.
2. Tawara S. Das Reizleitungssystem des Saugetierherzens. Verlag von Gustav Fische, Jena 1906.
3. Akiyama T. Sunao Tawara: Discover of the atrioventricular conduction system of the heart. Cardiol J. 2010; 17:428–33.

Contents

Part I Cardiac Anatomy for Catheter Ablation

1. **Atrial and Atrioventricular Junctional Anatomy: Myocardial Orientation and Its Heterogeneity** 3
   Shin Inoue, Genyo Ogawa, and Taka-Aki Matsuyama

2. **Anatomy of Aorta, Pulmonary Artery, and Ventricles** 11
   Osamu Igawa

Part II Techniques and Interpretation to Diagnose the Mechanism of Supraventricular Tachycardias

3. **Entrainment Pacing: A Diagnostic Tool for Reentrant Tachycardia and Its Application for Catheter Ablation** 23
   Ken Okumura and Hideharu Okamatsu

4. **Para-Hisian Pacing** 35
   Kenzo Hirao

5. **Entrainment Pacing for Differential Diagnosis of Supraventricular Tachycardias** 43
   Mitsunori Maruyama

Part III Special Sites for Ablation

6. **Aortic Sinus Cusps for Catheter Ablation of Supraventricular and Ventricular Arrhythmias** 53
   Takumi Yamada

7. **Coronary Sinus for Ablation of Ventricular Tachyarrhythmia and Supraventricular** 65
   Seiichiro Matsuo

8. **Vein of Marshall Chemical Ablation of Atrial Tachyarrhythmias** 73
   Kaoru Okishige

Part IV Catheter Ablation of Atrial Tachycardias and Flutter

9. **Cavo-tricuspid Isthmus-Dependent Atrial Flutter** 91
   Shinsuke Miyazaki

10. **Uncommon Atrial Flutter** 101
    Yasushi Miyauchi

11. **Adenosine-Sensitive Atrial Tachycardia** 109
    Hiroshige Yamabe

12	**Focal Atrial Tachycardia**	119
	Kazuhiro Satomi	
13	**Catheter Ablation of Atrial Tachycardia Following Catheter and Surgical Ablation of Atrial Fibrillation**	127
	Hiroshi Nakagawa and Warren M. Jackman	

Part V Catheter Ablation of Atrial Fibrillation

14	**Pulmonary Vein Isolation: Radiofrequency Energy**	137
	Teiichi Yamane	
15	**Pulmonary Vein Isolation: Cryoballoon Ablation**	145
	Kaoru Okishige	
16	**Radiofrequency HotBalloon Ablation**	157
	Hiroshi Sohara	
17	**Catheter Ablation of Posterior LA Isolation: Box Isolation**	169
	Koichiro Kumagai	
18	**Isolation of Superior Vena Cava**	175
	Koji Higuchi	
19	**Catheter Ablation of Non-pulmonary Vein Foci**	183
	Yoshihide Takahashi	
20	**Stepwise Ablation for Persistent Atrial Fibrillation**	189
	Yoshihide Takahashi	
21	**Substrate Ablation of Persistent AF**	199
	Takeshi Tsuchiya, Takanori Yamaguchi, and Akira Fukui	
22	**Autonomic Ganglionated Plexi Ablation in Patients with Atrial Fibrillation**	209
	Hiroshi Nakagawa, Benjamin J. Scherlag, Deborah Lockwood, and Warren M. Jackman	

Part VI Catheter Ablation of Atrio-ventricular Nodal Tachycardias

23	**Slow Pathway Ablation for Atrioventricular Nodal Reentrant Tachycardia**	221
	Kenichiro Otomo	
24	**Ablation of Superior Slow Pathway in Atypical Fast-Slow Atrioventricular Nodal Reentrant Tachycardia**	229
	Yoshiaki Kaneko	
25	**Retrograde Fast Pathway Ablation in Atrioventricular Nodal Reentrant Tachycardia**	237
	Yasuteru Yamauchi	

Part VII Catheter Ablation of Accessory Pathways

26	**Free Wall Atrioventricular Accessory Pathways**	247
	Seiji Takatsuki	
27	**Posteroseptal Atrioventricular Accessory Pathways**	257
	Junichi Nitta	

28 **Catheter Ablation of Antero-septal (Supero-paraseptal) and Mid-septal (True Septal) Accessory Pathways** 269
Takashi Kurita and Ryobun Yasuoka

29 **Atriofascicular Accessory Pathways** 283
Yukio Sekiguchi

30 **Nodofascicular/Nodoventricular Accessory Pathway** 291
Nitish Badhwar and Melvin M. Scheinman

Part VIII Catheter Ablation of Ventricular Tachycardias

31 **Outflow Tract Ventricular Tachycardias and Ventricular Premature Contractions: ECG-Based Prediction of Origin Sites** 299
Hitoshi Hachiya

32 **Idiopathic Left Fascicular Ventricular Tachycardia** 313
Akihiko Nogami

33 **Bundle Branch Reentrant Ventricular Tachycardia** 325
Mitsuhiro Nishizaki, Seiji Fukamizu, and Harumizu Sakurada

34 **Papillary Muscle Ventricular Tachycardia** 335
Hiroshi Tada

35 **Ventricular Tachycardia in Non-ischemic Cardiomyopathy** 341
Masahiko Goya

36 **Ventricular Tachycardia in Ischemic Heart Disease** 349
Kyoko Soejima and Akiko Ueda

37 **Ablation of Brugada Syndrome** 359
Yasuya Inden

38 **Ablation of Catecholaminergic Polymorphic Ventricular Tachycardia** .. 365
Keita Masuda, Takashi Kaneshiro, and Kazutaka Aonuma

39 **Epicardial Ablation for Ventricular Tachycardia** 371
Shiro Nakahara

40 **Ablation of Electrical Storm** 381
Yoshinori Kobayashi

Part I
Cardiac Anatomy for Catheter Ablation

Atrial and Atrioventricular Junctional Anatomy: Myocardial Orientation and Its Heterogeneity

Shin Inoue, Genyo Ogawa, and Taka-Aki Matsuyama

Keywords

Conduction system · Isthmus · Nodal extension · Anatomy · Retroaortic node

1.1 Anatomy of the Right Atrium

1.1.1 The Sinoatrial Node and Terminal Crest

One of the most important structures in the right atrium (RA) is the sinoatrial (SA) node, adjacent to prominent myocardial bundle named the terminal crest (TC) (Fig. 1.1a). The SA node distributes along the TC with several atrionodal connections as shown in Fig. 1.1b. In 1907, Keith and Flack first described the human SA node near the border between the right atrial appendage and the superior vena cava (SVC) [1]. Distribution of the SA node has considerable variation with the inferior extension near the orifice of the inferior vena cava (IVC) [2]. Since the SA nodal cell is very small in size (<10 μm), and the SA node contains a large amount of collagenous tissue in its body, detailed observation of the nodal structure is very difficult under light microscope [3]. The location and volume of the SA node are very diverse in each heart; the longitudinal length may exceed 30 mm and distributes inferiorly beyond the midline between the SVC and IVC orifices [4]. Elongated SA node, or discrepancy between the nodal morphology and function, seems to explain the widely distributed automaticity in wandering pacemaker [5] or AT in the vicinity of the TC [6]. As for the conduction block around the TC observed in atrial flutter, anisotropy of the TC musculature may attribute this phenomenon [7]. In addition, however, distribution of the SA node between the TC and vinous sinus may potentially affect conductivity in this area.

1.1.2 Pectinate Muscle and Septal Insertion to Bachmann's Bundle

In sinus rhythm, impulse propagates toward the atrial septum and the Bachmann's bundle and finally reaches the compact AV node through the peak of Koch's triangle (Fig. 1.1c). In the opposite direction, impulse propagates through the TC and pectinate muscle to the vestibule of the tricuspid valve and finally enters the bottom of Koch's triangle.

1.1.3 The Venous Sinus

In describing the anatomy of the posterior right atrial wall, Papez [8] detailed the orientation of several bundles of the atrial musculature. He referred to the musculature running through the venous sinus as "the intercaval bundle." This musculature was recently referred to by Ho et al. as the interatrial muscular bridge [9] (Fig. 1.1a). The age-related fibrosis of the venous sinus may be relevant to atrial flutter. In our experience, muscular volume of the TC did not change with age, but fibro-fatty change was more conspicuous in the venous sinus in elder hearts [4].

S. Inoue (✉) · G. Ogawa
Division of General Medicine, Department of Perioperative Medicine, Showa University Dental Hospital Medical Clinic, Showa University School of Dentistry, 2-1-1 Kitasenzoku, Ota-ku, Tokyo 145-8515, Japan
e-mail: inoues@med.showa-u.ac.jp

T.-A. Matsuyama
Department of Legal Medicine, Showa University School of Medicine, 1-5-8 Hatanodai, Shinagawa-ku, Tokyo 142-8555, Japan

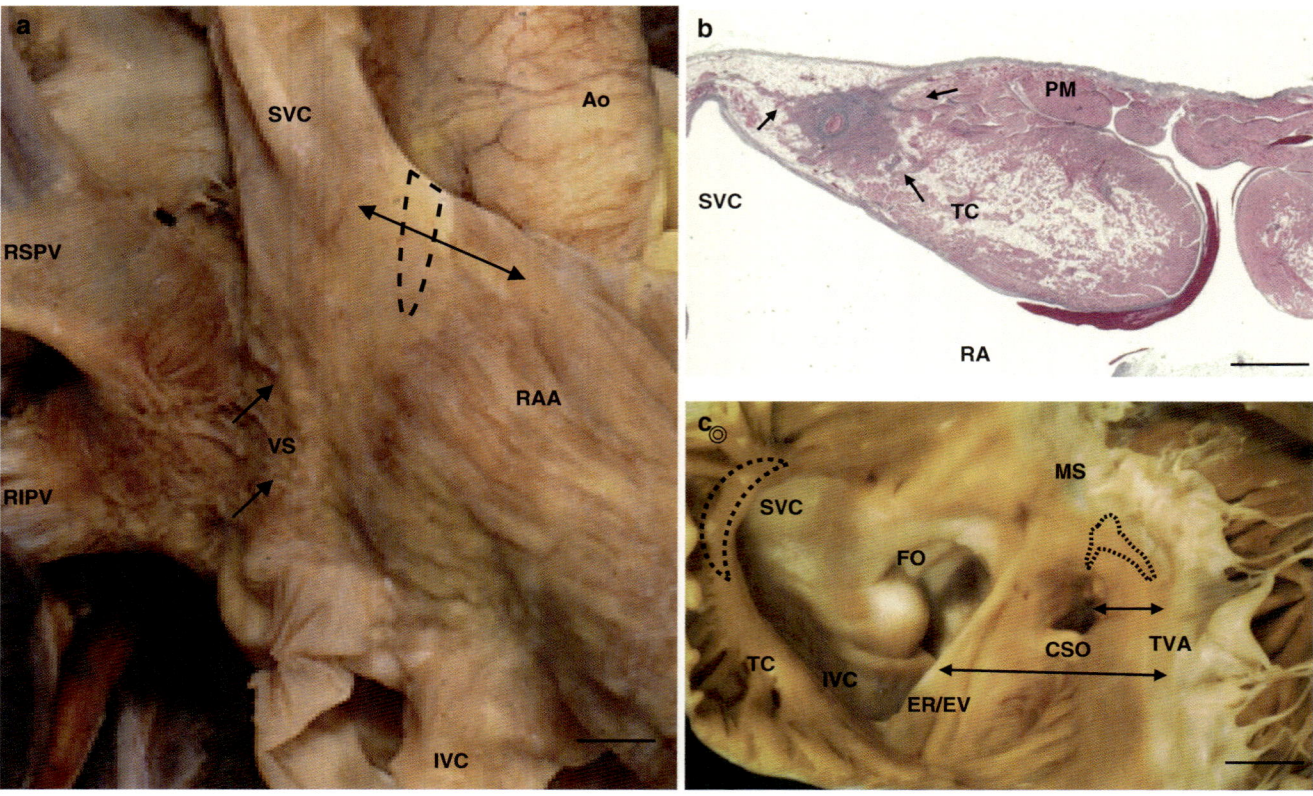

Fig. 1.1 Composite photograph of RA. (**a**) A pericardial aspect of the sinoatrial junction from the right anterior oblique view (RAO). The SA node is indicated by *dotted line*. Free wall of the right atrium mainly composes of the right atrial appendage, lining with pectinate muscle shown in (**c**). Single-*headed arrowheads* indicate the intercaval bundle or possible myocardial connection between the right pulmonary vein musculature and right atrial musculature by Ho et al. [9]. *Double-headed arrow* indicates the area for tissue preparation shown in (**b**). Bar = 1 cm. (**b**) Histological section of the SA node. The SA node (*blue area within three arrows*) has a feeding artery at its center. Each *arrow* also indicates atrionodal connections; *left arrow* indicates connection with the SVC myocardial sleeve, *under arrow* with the CT, and *upper arrow* with pectinate muscles. Bar = 5 mm Azan-Mallory stain.

(**c**) Endocardial aspect of the RA by RAO view. *Crescent dotted line* indicates location of the SA node, and *bifurcate-shape dotted line* shows the AV node. *Double circles* indicate the septum spurium. *Arrows* show the ER/EV-TV isthmus or CSO-TV isthmus. *Triangle* of Koch is demarked by the tricuspid valve annulus, Eustachian ridge, and coronary sinus opening. The development of the Eustachian valve or prevalence the Thebesian valve which covers the os of coronary sinus is highly divers in each individual. Bar = 1 cm. *Ao* aorta, *CSO* coronary sinus opening, *ER/EV* Eustachian ridge/valve, *FO* foramen ovale, *IVC* inferior vena cava, *PM* pectinate muscle, *RA* right atrium, *RAA* right atrial appendage, *RIPV* right inferior pulmonary vein, *RSPV* right superior pulmonary vein, *SVC* superior vena cava, *TC* terminal crest, *TVA* tricuspid valve annulus, *VS* venous sinus

1.1.4 The SVC and IVC Musculature

Above the venous sinus or right atrial appendage, the muscular sleeve of the SVC appears with considerable length. The data of the anatomical length has not yet available, but electrophysiological study by Higuchi et al. revealed the sleeve length of 30 mm or more [10]. In contrast to the SVC, the IVC has no musculature or very short sleeve length within 5 mm (Fig. 1.1a).

1.2 Interatrial Myocardial Connection

1.2.1 Bachmann's Bundle

The Bachmann's bundle is an important musculature that is, along with the coronary sinus musculature, involved in interatrial conduction during sinus rhythm or other arrhythmia [11].

In authors' experience, mean thickness of Bachmann's bundle was 3.7 mm and mean width was 21 mm (Fig. 1.2a). Bachmann's bundle was divided into several parts, the main trunk which bridges the right and left atrial appendages and peripheral extensions which project into the area around the SVC and left pulmonary veins (PV) or both AV annuli [8] (Fig. 1.2b). Bachmann's bundle receives almost half of the myocardium from the septal attachment of the TC. The residual half myocardium of the TC aims to the apex of Koch's triangle and the AV node, through the upper margin of the fossa ovalis.

1.2.2 Coronary Sinus and Surrounding Musculature

The coronary sinus (CS) opens in the lower right atrium consisting the lower rim of the Koch's triangle and plays a

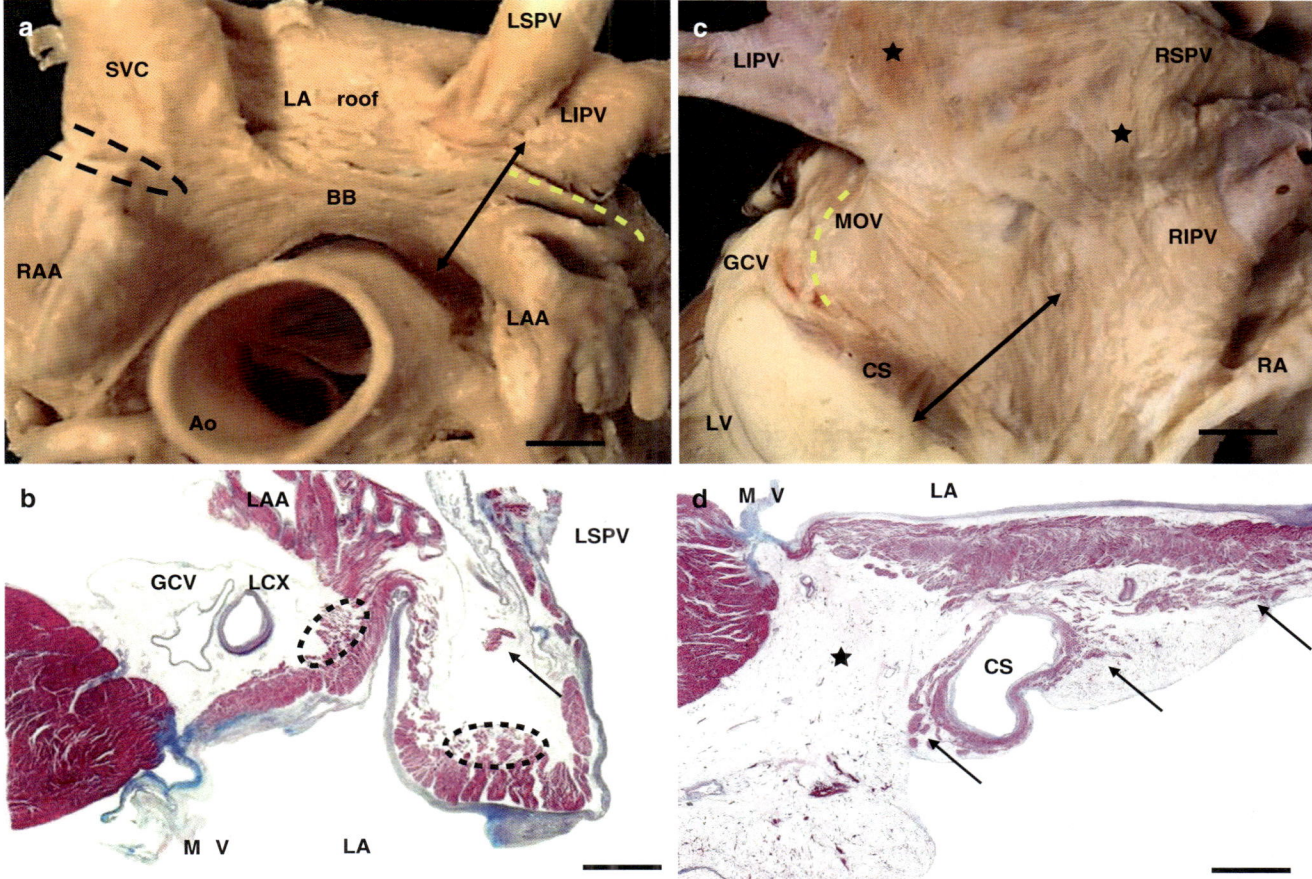

Fig. 1.2 Composite photograph of interatrial connections. (**a**) Short cardiac axis view with Bachmann's bundle. *Dotted area* shows the SA node. Bachmann's bundle is broad musculature sharing anterior part of LA roof. Periphery of the bundle may meet Marshall's bundle (*yellow dotted line*). *Double-headed arrow* shows the area of the histological section shown in (**b**). Bar = 1 cm. (**b**) Bachmann's bundle bifurcates into the anterior and posterior crest shown by *dotted oval* around the opening of the left atrial appendage, with Marshall's bundle (*arrow*) in its periphery. This section also shows LSPV-LAA isthmus. Bar = 5 mm Azan-Mallory stain. (**c**) Overview of the inferior left atrium. *Asterisks* show the disarrangement of the myocardium adjacent to the PV carina. The CS musculature shown by *double-headed arrow* spreads widely, contrary to the limited diameter of the CS. CS musculature ends at Marshall oblique vein (MOV, *yellow dotted line*). Bar = 1 cm. (**d**) Histological section from *arrow* in figure (**c**). Note the distribution of CS musculature shown by *arrows*. Upper margin of CS musculature borders periphery of the right inferior pulmonary vein. *Asterisk* indicates AV groove adipose tissue including nerve fibers. Bar = 5 mm Azan-Mallory stain. *Ao* aorta, *BB* Bachmann's bundle, *CS* coronary sinus, *GCV* great cardiac vein, *LA* left atrium, *LAA* left atrial appendage, *LCX* left circumflex artery, *LIPV* left inferior pulmonary vein, *RSPV* left superior pulmonary vein, *MOV* Marshall's oblique vein, *MV* mitral valve, *RAA* right atrial appendage, *RIPV* right inferior pulmonary vein, *RSPV* right superior pulmonary vein, *RA* right atrium, *RAA* right atrial appendage, *SVC* superior vena cava

secondary significant role in interatrial conduction [12]. The CS is remnant of the fetal right venous sinus (right sinus horn) wearing myocardial sleeve. This sleeve has considerable width which sometimes exceeds 3 times of CS diameter (Fig. 1.2c) [13]. In the right atrial aspect, CS sleeve forms the anteroinferior rim of the fossa ovalis and endocardium of Koch's triangle. The CS musculature ends at the border with the great cardiac vein (GCV) and Marshall's oblique vein (MOV) which is remnant of the left SVC and changes its name to Marshall's bundle. Loose myocardial connection of the CS sleeve in the periphery of the right pulmonary veins may influence the interatrial propagation (Fig. 1.2d).

1.2.3 Marshall Oblique Vein and Its Bundle

Marshall's myocardial bundle (MB) merged with the CS musculature almost 30 mm from the CS opening, at the bifurcation of the GCV [13]. None of the GCV ran along the venous musculature. The diameter of Marshall's oblique vein (MOV) at the CS juncture was almost 1.0 mm. The MB gradually decreased in density toward the distal venous branch and disappeared or joined into the LA myocardium at the anterior left PV-LA junctions (Fig. 1.2b). At closer observation, three distinct myocardial connections between MB and LA were observed in the CS juncture, the left PV-LA junctions (Fig. 1.3d). The lengths of

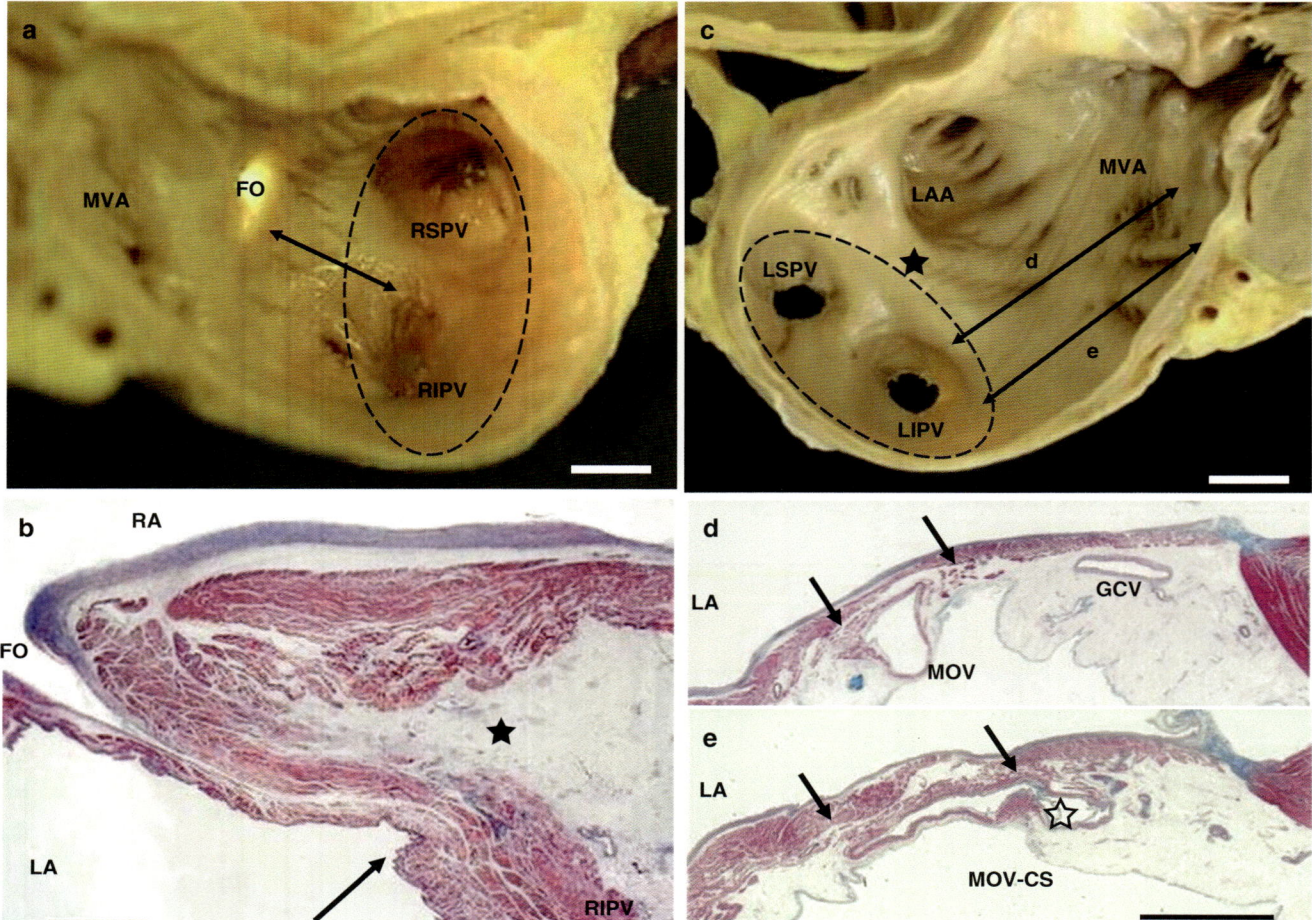

Fig. 1.3 Composite photograph of the left PV openings and isthmus. (**a**) Macroscopic view of the right pulmonary vein ostia with atrial septum. *Dotted oval line* indicates extensive pulmonary vein isolation line. Foramen ovale is emphasized with transillumination. Tissue section (**b**) was excised at *double-headed arrow*. Bar = 1 cm. (**b**) Histological section through FO-RIPV isthmus. The ablation line crosses the hinge of the muscular flap of foramen ovale (*arrow*). *Closed asterisk* shows interatrial adipose tissue with nerve fiber and ganglia. Bar = 5 mm Azan-Mallory stain. (**c**) LA free wall with openings of left PVs and left atrial appendage. *Dotted oval line* indicates extensive left PV isolation ablation line. *Closed asterisk* indicates left anterior ridge constituting LSPV-LAA isthmus and histological section shown in Fig. 1.2b. Tissue sections of the upper (**d**) and lower (**e**) mitral isthmus (LIPV-MVA) shown by *double-headed arrows* were prepared. Bar = 1 cm. (**d, e**) Mitral isthmus attaches Marshall's bundle (*arrows*). Lower mitral isthmus may encounter confluent of GCV and MOV merges into the CS. Vieussens valve shown by *open asterisk* may interfere catheter manipulation. Bar = 1 cm Azan-Mallory stain. *CS* coronary sinus, *FO* foramen ovale, *GCV* great cardiac vein, *LA* left atrium, *LAA* left atrial appendage, *LIPV* left inferior pulmonary vein, *LSPV* left superior pulmonary vein, *MOV* Marshall's oblique vein, *MVA* mitral valve annulus, *RIPV* right inferior pulmonary vein, *RSPV* right superior pulmonary vein, *RA* right atrium

the MB varied widely from 5 to 69 mm and reached the left inferior pulmonary vein (LIPV)-LA junction in some cases. The nerve fibers around MB, most of which were sympathetic fibers, distributed along the entire length of the MB, particularly in the PV-LA junctions. On the other hand, the parasympathetic ganglions scattered around the CS juncture.

1.3 Left Atrium

1.3.1 Pulmonary Vein Myocardial Sleeve and LA Musculature

Because approximately 90% of atrial ectopic beats that triggered atrial fibrillation (AF) derived from myocardial sleeves of pulmonary vein (PV) openings, PV isolation using radio-frequency energy has been widely introduced to treat AF [14].

The origin of ectopic activity attributed to the myocardial sleeve of PV as shown by Nathan and Eliakim [15] and Saito et al. [16]. Despite of the advance in PV isolation procedure, recurrence of AF still remains room for improvement. One postulated mechanism of the AF recurrence may be the reconnection of ablated atrial musculature, presumably derived from incomplete tissue necrosis. Another mechanism may be tissue heterogeneity under the ablation line. Although thickness of the left atrial free wall may be thin, disarrangement of the myocardium or obstacles such as blood vessels may appear under the ablation line. For accomplishing the reliable ablation line in the extended PV isolation procedure, it is crucial to understand the detailed myocardial anatomy around the PV openings.

1.3.2 Left Atrial Isthmus

In particular, the left inferior pulmonary vein opening—mitral valve annulus (LIPV-MVA)—isthmus is known as an additional ablation line (posterior line) in the extensive PV isolation procedure. Despite the prevalence of this application, however, mitral isthmus is wide, and myocardial architecture is thick or laminated with individual diversity. In addition, macroscopic examination revealed an irregular pectinate muscle structure named crevices (Fig. 1.3c) [17]. Crevices make endocardial tissue complexed and may interfere ablation procedure. In addition, an important factor influencing the ablation line may be blood vessels such as the CS or VOM in this isthmus, because of their cooling effect on radio-frequency energy (Fig. 1.3d, e). Under these circumstances, interruption of the CS musculature and Marshall's bundle should be prepared.

The left superior pulmonary vein opening—left atrial appendage (LSPV-LAA) isthmus—is a crucial area because the ablation line for the extensive PV isolation line passes through here (Figs. 1.2 a, b and 1.3c). The LSPV-LAA isthmus is also known as the anterior ridge or fold of the left atrium. Although the LSPV-LAA isthmus is the narrowest (8.4 mm), there are considerable individual differences not only in its width but also in thickness [17]. In addition to macroscopic variation, the myocardial architecture including blood vessels, nerve fibers, and Marshall's bundle enhances tissue nonuniformity.

Concerning about isthmus between the right PV openings and FO, muscularized flap valves and the left and right atrial myocardium form complex architecture (Fig. 1.3a, b). Nerve fibers with ganglionated plexi distribute within interatrial groove fat pad.

1.4 The Septal Part of AV Junction

The septal part of AV junction consists of the offset formed by the tricuspid and mitral valve annuli. In the right atrial aspect, Koch's triangle is the landmark for ablation procedure especially in atrioventricular nodal reentrant tachycardia (AVNRT).

1.4.1 Compact Node and Inferior Extensions

Since slow pathways are considered as inferior extension from the compact part of the AV node, optimal ablation target must be drawn from the orientation of both annuli (Fig. 1.4a) [18, 19]. From the anatomical point of view, dual AV response and slow conduction property attributed to the slow conducting AV nodal tissue with various length, and fast pathway corresponds to the compact part of the node adjacent to His bundle. Extended nodal tissue was considered as the remnant of embryonal AV ring tissue, and tissue preparation could reveal the nodal structure (Fig 1.4c).

1.4.2 Superior Nodal Extension and Retroaortic Node

Recently, Dr. Kaneko and his colleagues reported atypical AVNRT cases who underwent catheter ablation near the His bundle and advocated superior slow pathway [20]. In definition of nodal tissue on AV annulus, spatial myocardial arrangement might be helpful in addition to nodal cell morphology [21]. Concerning about the superior slow pathway, serial sections of the right fibrous trigone revealed that left and right nodal extensions bifurcate from the left inferior extension and not from the compact part of the AV node. These two superior extensions migrate onto the tricuspid and mitral valve annulus behind the noncoronary sinus of Valsalva. Since these ectopic nodal structures distribute on the border of right fibrous trigone, they may meet with the retroaortic node shown in Fig 1.5a, b. Because of the proximity of the His bundle adjacent to the right fibrous trigone, precise measurement of spatial dimensions may help establish the location of the superior slow pathway [22].

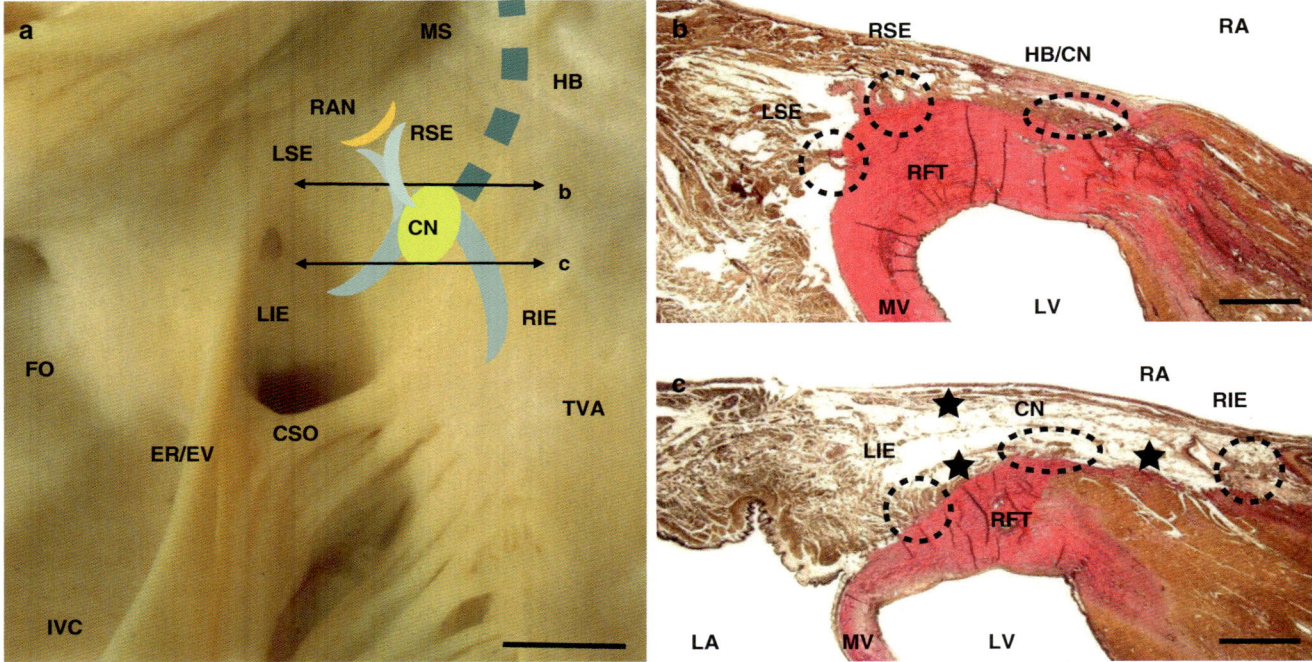

Fig. 1.4 Detailed anatomy of the septal part of AV junction. (**a**) RAO view image of the septal AV junction. The compact node (*yellow*) locates anterosuperior margin of the CS opening, and His bundle (*dark blue*) distributes at the anterior margin of the membranous septum. Right or left inferior extensions (*blue*) may appear along the tricuspid or mitral valve annulus. Recently proposed superior nodal extensions (*light blue*) and retroaortic node (*orange*) are positioned, respectively. Histological section was prepared at the superior or inferior border of the compact node (**b**, **c**) shown by *arrows*. Bar = 1 cm. (**b**) At this level, left inferior nodal extension bifurcates into left and right superior extensions (*dotted circles*) on the right fibrous trigone (*red color*). Both of superior extensions immigrate into the mitral and tricuspid annuli in upper sections. The border of His bundle/compact node is shown by *dotted oval*. Note the difference of the arrangement of the nodal tissues from (**c**). Bar = 1 mm Elastica van Gieson stain. (**c**) At the lower margin of the compact node (*dotted oval*), we could see the left and right inferior nodal extensions (*dotted circles*). *Closed asterisks* show transitional fibers. Bar = 1 mm Elastica van Gieson stain. *CN* compact node, *CSO* coronary sinus opening, *FO* foramen ovale, *HB* His bundle, *LA* left atrium, *LIE* left inferior extension, *LSE* left superior extension, *MS* membranous septum, *MV* mitral valve, *RA* right atrium, *RAN* retroaortic node, *RFT* right fibrous trigone, *RIE* right inferior extension, *RSE* right superior extension, *TVA* tricuspid valve annulus

1.5 The Atrioventricular Junction in Free Wall

1.5.1 Retroaortic Node Adjacent to AV Annuli

At the vicinity of the apex of Koch's triangle or noncoronary sinus of Valsalva, focal AT occasionally underwent catheter ablation [6]. In this area, the retroaortic node appears behind the attachment of the noncoronary leaflet [23]. The central fibrous body, remnant of the embryonal cushion tissue, is composed of the membranous septum (MS) and right fibrous trigone. The His bundle distributes anterior to the MS in RAO view image and locates in proximity in the retroaortic node. Since the retroaortic node may be covered by the vestibule of mitral or tricuspid valve annulus, catheter ablation should be performed from the sinus of Valsalva (Fig. 1.5a, b).

1.5.2 WPW Syndrome

In fetal development of the heart, incomplete formation of the AV ring tissue tends to arrow ectopic AV muscular connection and to establish accessory pathway. For elucidating histological pathway, complete serial sections must be prepared in an estimated area [24]. We experienced accessory pathway in IVC-TVA isthmus in type B WPW syndrome. Figure 1.5c shows myocardium bridging of the right atrial and ventricular musculature. Since accessory pathway distributes behind the attachment of the AV valve leaflet,

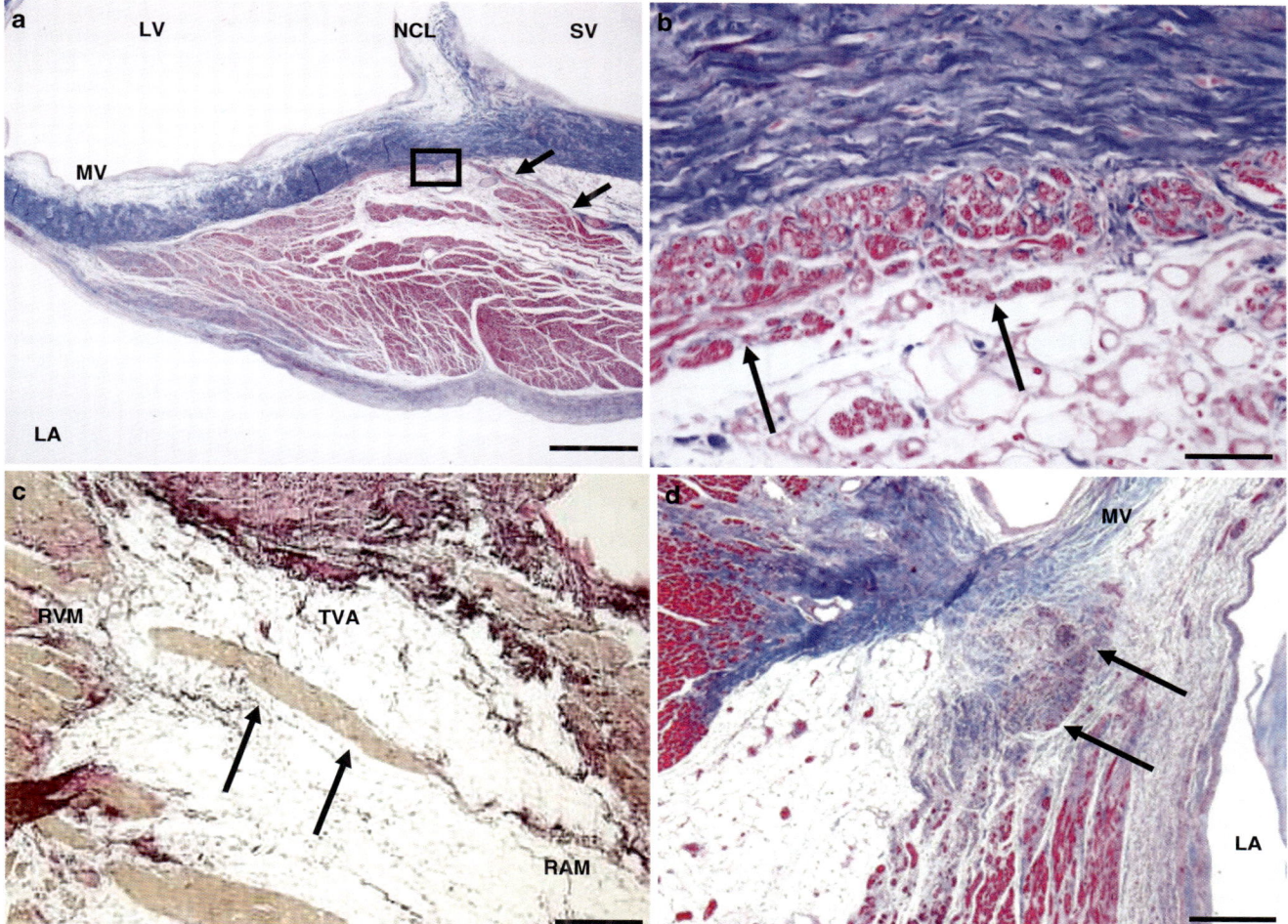

Fig. 1.5 Composite photomicrograph of the atrioventricular ring tissue. (**a**): The retroaortic node observed beneath the attachment of the noncoronary leaflet (NCL). The AV nodal tissue (within *rectangular area*) has atrionodal connection (*arrows*). Bar = 1 mm Azan-Mallory stain. (**b**) High-power photomicrograph of rectangular area in (**a**). Small myocytes (*arrows*) show nodal cell morphology. Bar = 100 μm Azan-Mallory stain. (**c**) Photomicrograph of accessory pathway from autopsied heart of type B WPW syndrome. Full serial section excised from IVC-TVA isthmus revealed myocardial bundle connecting the right atrium and ventricle, beneath the tricuspid valve annulus. Bar = 100 μm Elastica van Gieson stain. (**d**) Photomicrograph of mitral valve ring tissue from the heart underwent catheter ablation for AT from inferolateral mitral annulus. Serial sections reveal the AV nodal tissue (*arrows*) adjacent to ablation scar. Bar = 1 mm Azan-Mallory stain. *LA* left atrium, *LV* left ventricle, *NCL* noncoronary leaflet, *RAM* right atrial myocardium, *RVM* right ventricular myocardium, *MV* mitral valve, *SV* sinus of Valsalva, *TVA* tricuspid valve annulus

ablation energy from the endocardium tends to ablate the surrounding musculature rather than the accessory pathway itself.

1.5.3 Atrial Tachycardia from AV Annulus

Most of AT source from AV ring theorized to ectopic nodal tissue, possibly the remnant of embryonic AV ring tissue. We experienced AT from lower mitral annulus after successful ablation procedure [25]. From the autopsied heart, we made serial sections of the ablation scar tissue with surrounding musculature and found nodal structure adjacent to the ablative lesion (Fig. 1.5d).

References

1. Keith A, Flack M. The form and nature of the muscular connections between the primary divisions of the vertebrate heart. J Anat Physiol. 1907;41:172–87.
2. Anderson KR, Ho SY, Anderson RH. Location and vascular supply of sinus node in human heart. Br Heart J. 1979;41:28–32.

3. Inoue S, Shinohara F, Niitani H, Gotoh K. A new method for the histological study of aging changes in the sinoatrial node. Jpn Heart J. 1986;27:653–60.
4. Matsuyama TA, Inoue S, Kobayashi Y, et al. Anatomical diversity and age-related histological changes in the human right atrial posterolateral wall. Europace. 2004;6:307–15.
5. Boineau JP, Canavan TE, Schuessler RB, et al. Demonstration of a widely distributed atrial pacemaker complex in the human heart. Circulation. 1988;77:1221–37.
6. Kistler PM, Roberts-Thomson KC, Haqqani HM, et al. P-wave morphology in focal atrial tachycardia: development of an algorithm to predict the anatomic site of origin. J Am Coll Cardiol. 2006;48:1010–7.
7. Olgin JE, Kalman JM, Fitzpatrick AP, Lesh MD. Role of right atrial endocardial structures as barriers to conduction during human type I atrial flutter. Activation and entrainment mapping guided by intracardiac echocardiography. Circulation. 1995;92:1839–48.
8. Papez JW. Heart musculature of the atria. Am J Anat. 1920;27:255–85.
9. Ho SY, Anderson RH, Sanchez-Quintana D. Atrial structure and fibres: morphologic bases of atrial conduction. Cardiovasc Res. 2002;54:325–36.
10. Higuchi K, Yamauchi Y, Hirao K, et al. Superior vena cava as initiator of atrial fibrillation: factors related to its arrhythmogenicity. Heart Rhythm. 2010;(7):1186–91. https://doi.org/10.1016/j.hrthm.2010.05.017.
11. Bachmann G. The inter-auricular time interval. Am J Phys. 1916;41:309–20.
12. Markides V, Schilling RJ, Ho SY, et al. Characterization of left atrial activation in the intact human heart. Circulation. 2003;107:733–9.
13. Makino M, Inoue S, Matsuyama TA, et al. Diverse myocardial extension and autonomic innervation on ligament of Marshall in humans. J Cardiovasc Electrophysiol. 2006;17:594–9.
14. Haïssaguerre M, Jais P, Shah DC, et al. Spontaneous initiation of atrial fibrillation by ectopic beats originating in the pulmonary veins. N Engl J Med. 1998;339:659–66.
15. Nathan H, Eliakim M. The junction between the left atrium and the pulmonary veins. An anatomic study of human hearts. Circulation. 1966;34:412–22.
16. Saito T, Waki K, Becker AE. Left atrial myocardial extension onto pulmonary veins in humans: anatomic observations relevant for atrial arrhythmias. J Cardiovasc Electrophysiol. 2000;11:888–94.
17. Ogawa G, Inoue S, Matsuyama TA, et al. Histological study of left atrial wall – a consideration of the compound myocardial architecture and potential durability with respect to catheter ablation in pulmonary vein isolation procedure. Showa University Journal of. Med Sci. 2010;22:211–9.
18. Inoue S, Becker AE. Posterior extensions of the human compact atrioventricular node: a neglected anatomic feature of potential clinical significance. Circulation. 1998;97:188–93. Erratum in: Circulation 1998;97:1216
19. Inoue S, Becker AE, Riccardi R, Gaita F. Interruption of the inferior extension of the compact atrioventricular node underlies successful radio frequency ablation of atrioventricular nodal reentrant tachycardia. J Interv Card Electrophysiol. 1999;3:273–7.
20. Kaneko Y, Naito S, Okishige K, et al. Atypical fast-slow atrioventricular nodal reentrant tachycardia incorporating a "superior" slow pathway: a distinct supraventricular tachyarrhythmia. Circulation. 2016;133:114–23. https://doi.org/10.1161/ciculationaha.115.018443.
21. McGuire MA, de Bakker JM, et al. Atrioventricular junctional tissue. Discrepancy between histological and electrophysiological characteristics. Circulation. 1996;94:571–7.
22. Inoue S, Becker AE. Koch's triangle sized up: anatomical landmarks in perspective of catheter ablation procedures. Pacing Clin Electrophysiol. 1998;21(8):1553.
23. Anderson RH, Boyett MR, Dobrzynski H, Moorman AFM. The anatomy of the conduction system: implications for the clinical cardiologist. J Cardiovasc Trans Res. 2013;6:187–96. https://doi.org/10.1007/s12265-012-9433-0.
24. Fitzpatrick AP, Gonzales RP, Lesh MD, et al. New algorithm for the localization of accessory atrioventricular connections using a baseline electrocardiogram. J Am Coll Cardiol. 1994;23:107–16.
25. Matsuyama TA, Inoue S, Tanno K, et al. Ectopic nodal structures in a patient with atrial tachycardia originating from the mitral valve annulus. Europace. 2006;8:977–9.

Anatomy of Aorta, Pulmonary Artery, and Ventricles

Osamu Igawa

Keywords
Catheter ablation · Anatomy · Aorta · Pulmonary artery · Aortomitral fibrous continuity · Ventricles · Interventricular septum · Papillary muscles

2.1 Introduction

With the development of technology for electrophysiological procedures, the importance of understanding the cardiac anatomy has increased not only for interpreting the information obtained from electroanatomical mapping of the heart but also for analyzing the mechanisms of arrhythmias [1, 2]. It goes without saying that a great deal of anatomical knowledge concerning the cardiac anatomy has already been accumulated in various kinds of textbooks. These textbooks have naturally provided us with very important information regarding imaging the cardiac structures [3]. However, this anatomical knowledge does not seem sufficient for cardiologists, particularly, electrophysiologists, as it fails to provide a complete image of the cardiac structures. Electrophysiologists require not the name of these anatomical structures but practical images of the structures for use in various clinical situations.

During catheter ablation (CA) therapy, operators always reconstruct three-dimensional cardiac structures in their heads based on their knowledge and experiences. They manipulate the catheters based on the reconstructed cardiac image in order to avoid any complications associated with the procedure. When trying to obtain some clues to solve various electrophysiological problems, they have to be aware of potential anatomical pitfalls.

In this chapter, I describe practical cardiac anatomy in an effort to help resolve some of the structure-related clinical problems encountered in various situations. I hope to provide particularly useful anatomical information related to CA to electrophysiologists in order to help them envision an appropriate three-dimensional image of the cardiac structures when manipulating catheters. In addition, I will present new anatomical information and propose a new way of thinking about cardiac structures.

2.2 Anatomy of the Aorta, Pulmonary Trunk, and Ventricles

2.2.1 Anatomy of the Aorta, Pulmonary Trunk, and Ventricular Outflow Tracts

2.2.1.1 The Structure of the Aortic Root and Its Surroundings

The aspect of the aortic root (AoR) as viewed from right upper side of the heart is shown in Fig. 2.1. The ascending aorta (AAo) and pulmonary trunk (PT) are removed from the heart by cutting transversely just above their sinotubular junction (STJ). The left, right, and noncoronary cusps (L/R/NCC) of the aortic valve (AoV) can easily be seen in the AoR. Furthermore, we can roughly make out the structures surrounding the AoR from this picture, which shows both atria and the right ventricle (RV). As demonstrated in Fig. 2.1, the left and right atria are located just behind the AAo. The noncoronary aortic sinus (NAS) faces the anterior wall of the atria, specifically the interatrial septum (IAS). In this specimen, the left atrial appendage (LAA) is slightly elevated and has been pulled posteriorly to facilitate viewing

O. Igawa
Department of Internal Medicine and Cardiology, Nippon Medical School, Tama-Nagayama Hospital,
1-7-1 Nagayama Tama City, Tokyo 206-8512, Japan
e-mail: oigawa@nms.ac.jp

© Springer Nature Singapore Pte Ltd. 2018
K. Hirao (ed.), *Catheter Ablation*, https://doi.org/10.1007/978-981-10-4463-2_2

the area between the LAA and PT. The main trunk of the left coronary artery (LMT) is located in this area. However, the LMT and right coronary artery (RCA) cannot be observed in this figure because they are covered by a large amount of cardiac adipose tissue.

Of note, the LMT descends surrounding the root of the PT and is extremely close to the septal side of the PT: this results in a risk of LMT damage when performing CA just around the septal cusp of the pulmonary valve (SPC). The AAo, which has already been removed from this specimen, is connected to the PT alongside the tough ligament. They form an AAo-PT complex. There is a narrow space between the AAo-PT complex and the atria known as the "pericardial transverse sinus (PTS)," which is a part of the pericardial cavity (PC). The bottom of the PTS (in other words, the pericardial reflection on its lower side) is located at the level of sinotubular junction (STJ) of the aortic valve (AoV). These great cardiac vessels appear to closely follow the posterior side by the left and right atrial appendages (L/RAA).

Of further note, the conduction system (branching portion of the His bundle [bHB]) is located just beneath the commissure between the RCC and NCC. In addition, as described above, the IAS is located just behind the middle point of the NAS.

The terminal groove (TG), which is the border between the RAA and sinus venarum (SV), can clearly be seen at the surface of the right atrium of this specimen.

2.2.1.2 Relationship Between the AoR and Fibrous Cardiac Skeleton

Figure 2.2a, b shows the human heart and the schematic illustration of its fibrous cardiac construction, as viewed from the right upper side. The AoR (balls of three aortic sinuses) and atrioventricular fibrous ring (mitral and tricuspid valve annuli (M/TVA)) are clearly exposed by removing the RA, LA, and IAS muscles and other tissues from the heart. The external aspect of the AoR can be observed in detail.

All spaces between the M/TVA and AoR are filled with fibrous tissue. This fibrous structure plays an important role not only as a framework of the heart but also as a partition, enabling electrical isolation between the atria and ventricles. This structure is called the "fibrous cardiac skeleton (FCS)."

The FCS consists of four valvular annuli (two rings and two coronets) and other fibrous tissues. The two rings are mitral and tricuspid valve annuli (M/TVA), and the two coronets are aortic and pulmonary valve annuli (A/PVA). The other fibrous tissues are trigones and the membranous sep-

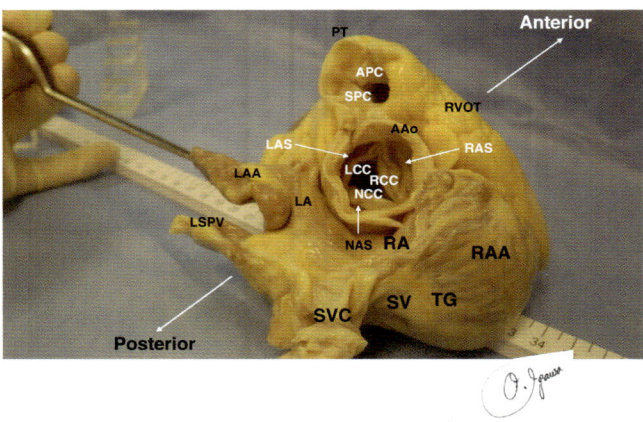

Fig. 2.1 The aspect of the aortic root (AR) viewed from the right upper side. The ascending aorta (AAo) and pulmonary trunk (PT) are removed from the heart by cutting transversely just above their sinotubular junction (STJ)

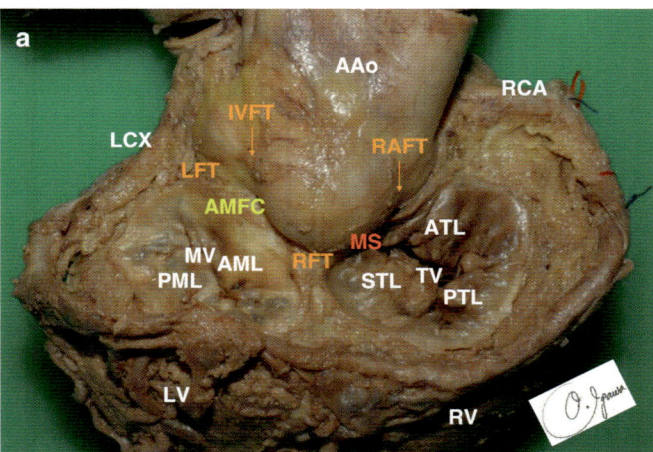
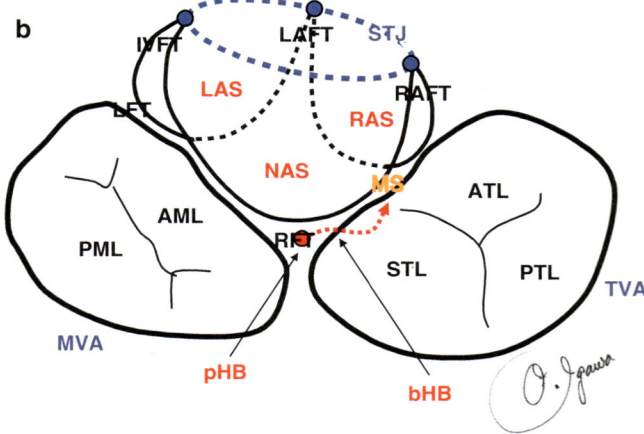

Fig. 2.2 (**a**) The aspect of the fibrous ring or atrioventricular annuli. The atrial muscle was removed from the heart completely to expose atrioventricular annuli. The specimen was observed from the right upper side of the heart. (**b**) Schematic illustration of the fibrous cardiac skeleton and normal conduction system. The HB penetrating the CFB on the side of the atrium and that spreading several branches on the side of the left ventricle are known as the penetrating and branching portions of the HB (pHB and bHB), respectively

tum (MS). The trigones refer to the right and left fibrous trigones (R/LFT), the right anterior and left posterior fibrous trigones (RA/LPFT), and the interventricular trigone (IVT). The contents of the FCS are shown in Fig. 2.2b.

2.2.1.3 Membranous Septum

The MS is a tough fibrous membrane located just beneath the commissure between the RCC and NCC and is a part of central fibrous body (CFB). The area size of this structure I investigated is 11.5 mm × 8.6 mm. When observed from the right side of the heart (Fig. 2.3b), the MS is divided into two parts, an atrial part and a ventricular part, by the septal tricuspid leaflet (STL). As shown in the schematic illustration in Fig. 2.3c, the atrial part of the MS forms a border between the LV and RA and the ventricular part forms a border between the LV and RV. The atrial part is called the "membranous part of the atrioventricular septum (mAVS)", and the ventricular part is called the "membranous part of the interventricular septum (mIVS)." Of note, when observed from the left side of the heart, there are no partitions on this membrane, as shown in Fig. 2.3b. In both figures, the MS can be seen as a translucent area, because it is being illuminated from behind by a flashlight.

2.2.1.4 Relationship Between the AoR and the His Bundle

The CFB (RFT+MS) is a part of the FCS. As described above, the CFB enables electrical isolation between the atria and ventricles. However, electrical excitation originating from the sinus node is able to pass the CFB via a conduction pathway known as the His bundle (HB). The HB is an electrically isolated muscle that penetrates the CFB. After passing through the RFT and crossing the TVA of the STL, the HB advances just beneath the MS (in other words, mAVS). This is just above the muscular part of the IVS. The HB spreads its branches into the left endocardial surface of the IVS. The HB on the side of atrium is known as the "penetrating portion of the HB" (pHB) while that on the side of the ventricle is known as the "branching portion of the HB (bHB)." Of note, the pHB is located beneath the NAS and bHB just below the commissure between the NCC and RCC as described above (Fig. 2.1). This conduction system can be seen in Fig. 2.3d.

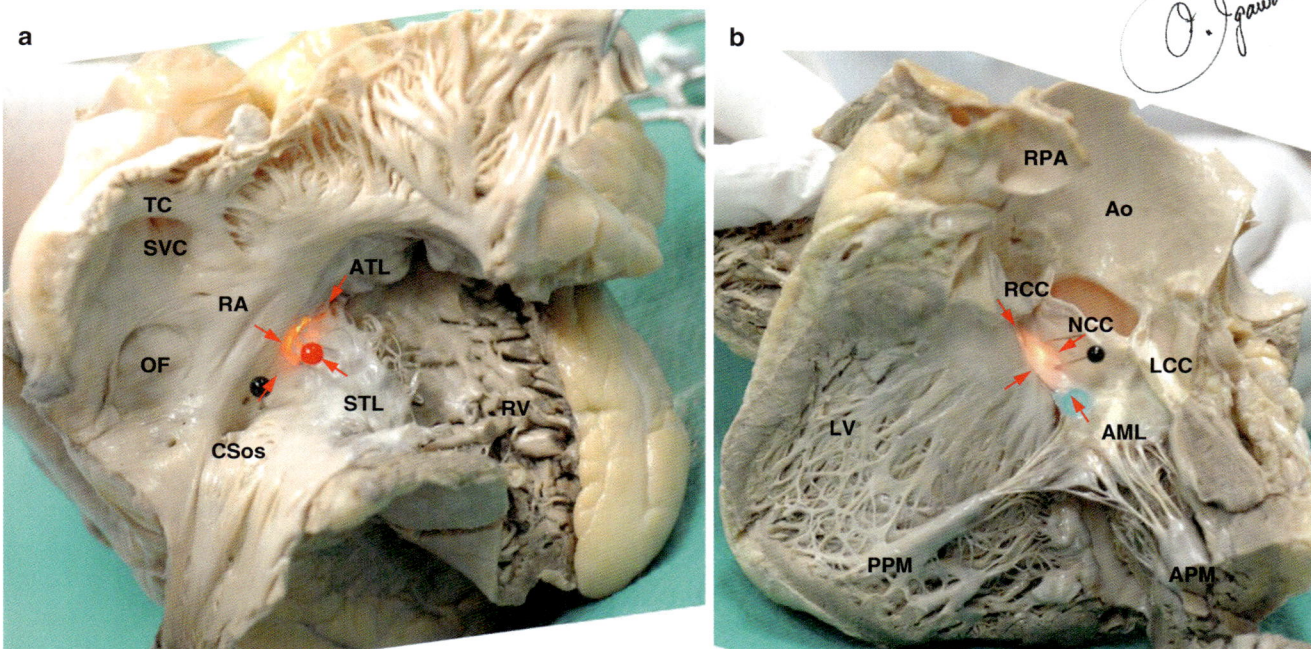

Fig. 2.3 (**a**, **b**) Image of membranous septum (MS). Shown as the internal aspect of the right heart when shining a flashlight from behind (LV side) the specimen. The translucent area (TA) indicated by *red arrows* is noticeable. The MS is divided into two parts by the septal tricuspid leaflet (STL). When looking at the backside (LV side) of the MS, the TA is confirmed just beneath the RCC-NCC commissure. (**c**) Schematic illustration of the MS. The MS consists of the membranous part of the atrioventricular septum (mAVS) and the membranous part of the interventricular septum (mIVS). (**d**) Schematic illustration of the relationship between the ME and HB. The HB is located in the CFB on the atrial side and just beneath the mIVS (just above the muscular portion of the IVS (muIVS)). In the muIVS, the HB spreads its branches into the endocardial surface of the IVS on the left side

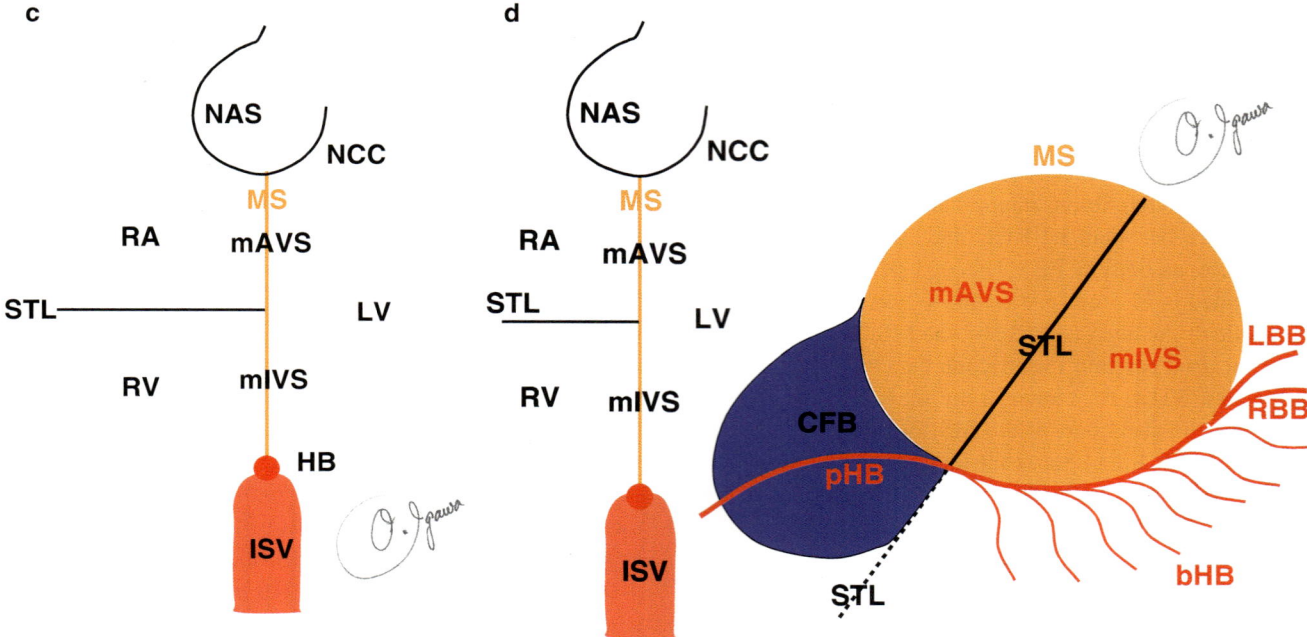

Fig. 2.3 (continued)

2.2.1.5 Structure of Junction Between the PT and the Right Ventricular Outflow Tract

Figure 2.4a is a schematic illustration of the junction between the PT and right ventricular outflow tract (RVOT). This illustration shows the relationship between the PT root and RVOT muscle.

In the real heart, the area around the PT-RVOT junction is covered with a large amount of cardiac adipose tissue, which hampers any external observation. However, this junction can clearly be recognized as a horizontal borderline in the present specimen, as the fat tissue was removed completely before treatment of the PT-RVOT junction (Fig. 2.4b). This horizontal borderline is known as the ventriculoarterial junction (VAJ).

As shown in Fig. 2.4a, the attachment of the pulmonary valve (PV) cusps (also known as the PVA) forms a coronet-shaped structure like annulus of the AoV (AoVA), which is described below. The attachment lines extend into the RVOT muscle crossing the VAJ. This coronet has three apexes. If we draw a line along the inner wall of the PT through these apical points, we create a ring, as shown in Fig. 2.4a. This ring is the STJ, and it sits at a much higher level than VAJ.

We can also imagine three basal points in this coronet. If we draw a line along the inner wall of the RVOT through these basal points, we create another ring known as the "basal ring (BR)." To identify the root of the great vessel, we should always note these three rings, the BR, VAJ, and STJ (Fig. 2.4a).

As demonstrated in Fig 2.4a, b of the PT-RVOT junction, the muscular areas in the pulmonary sinuses and the muscle-free areas in the RVOT can easily be seen. These muscle-free areas, which are a part of the vessel wall, are called the "interleaflet triangle (ILT)." CA carries some risk of perforation at these sites, because the structure of the ILT is very weak to local pressure, such as catheter pushing (Fig. 2.4a).

As described above, the LAA is extremely close to the root of the PT, especially anterior pulmonary sinus (APS). The electrogram of LAA muscle could be documented in APS.

Understanding the detailed structure of the PT-RVOT junction can be extremely helpful when trying to identify the junction between the AoR and left ventricular outflow tract (LVOT), as described below.

2.2.1.6 Structure of Junction Between the AoR and LVOT (AoR-LVOT Junction)

Figure 2.5a is a schematic illustration of the AoR-LVOT junction. In the real heart, this aspect of the AoR-LVOT junction cannot be viewed via external observation because it is surrounded by the RVOT and both atria.

Like the PVA, the attachment of the AoV cusps (also known as the AoVA) also forms a coronet-shaped structure with three apexes and three bases. Furthermore, in the AoR-LVOT junction, the three rings of STJ, VAJ, and BR can also be observed. The STJ is located above the VAJ.

The PT-RVOT connection is relatively simple, as described above. Briefly, three PV annuli connect to the PT wall and the RVOT muscle tightly and in the same manner. However, the Ao-LVOT connection differs substantially from that of the PT-RVOT. Briefly, a portion of

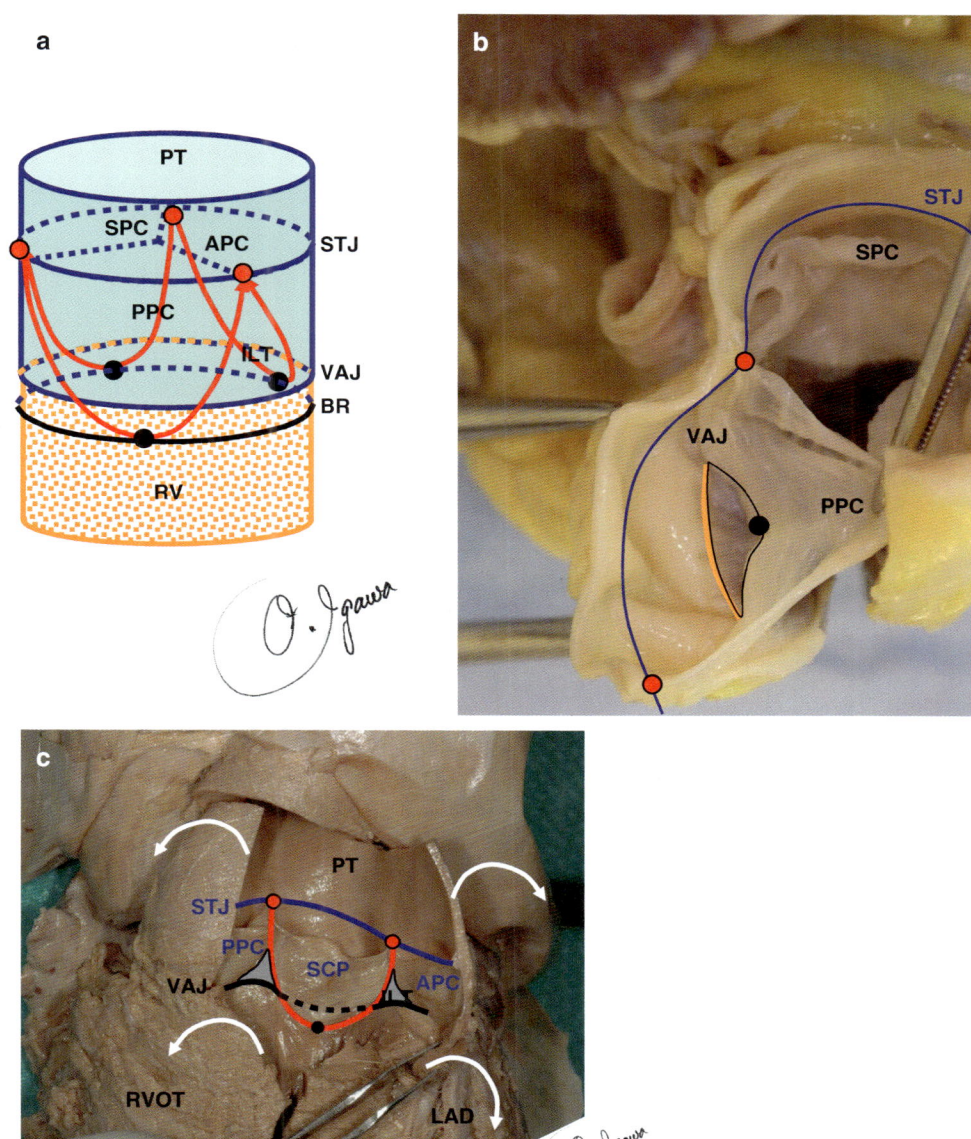

Fig. 2.4 (**a**, **b**) Schematic illustration of the relationship between the RVOT and PT. The PV annulus (attachment of the PV cusps) shows a coronet-shaped structure with three specific rings: the sinotubular junction (STJ), the ventriculoarterial junction (VAJ), and the basal ring (BR). (**c**) The internal aspect of the PV and lower part of the PT. The PT was cut along its short-axis plane at a level 1.5 cm above the STJ, and its anterior wall was then cut along its long axis plane and opened widely. Before cutting, the cardiac adipose tissue surrounding the PT was removed

the AoV annulus connects to the Ao wall and muscular tissue, while another portion connects to the Ao wall and fibrous tissue.

Figure 2.5b presents the characteristics of the subvalvular area of the AoV from its internal aspect. This subvalvular area is an internal aspect of the AoR-LVOT junction.

As shown in Fig. 2.5b, the anterior part of the RCC attaches mainly to muscular tissue (IVS), but the posterior portion partly attaches to fibrous tissue (the MS). The anterior part of the LCC attaches to muscular tissue (left ventricle (LV)), but the posterior portion attaches to fibrous tissue (aortomitral fibrous continuity (AMFC)). The NCC entirely connects to fibrous tissue (MS and AMFC). There are also three ILTs just beneath the three commissures of the AoV. Based on the manner of AoV attachment to the LVOT, the AoR is divided into two parts: a muscular portion and a fibrous one (Fig. 2.5c).

When viewing each AS of Valsalva (AS-V) from the upper side, we can see an IVS muscle in the right aortic sinus of Valsalva (RAS-V) and an LV muscle in the anterior left aortic sinus (LAS-V), with no myocardium in the NAS of Valsalva or posterior LAS-V.

2.2.1.7 Aortomitral Fibrous Continuity

As shown in Fig. 2.5b, the anterior part of anterior mitral leaflet (AML) leads to the posterior part of the LAS and NAS. Strictly speaking, the anterior part of the AMV annulus is connected to the posterior parts of the LAS and NAS

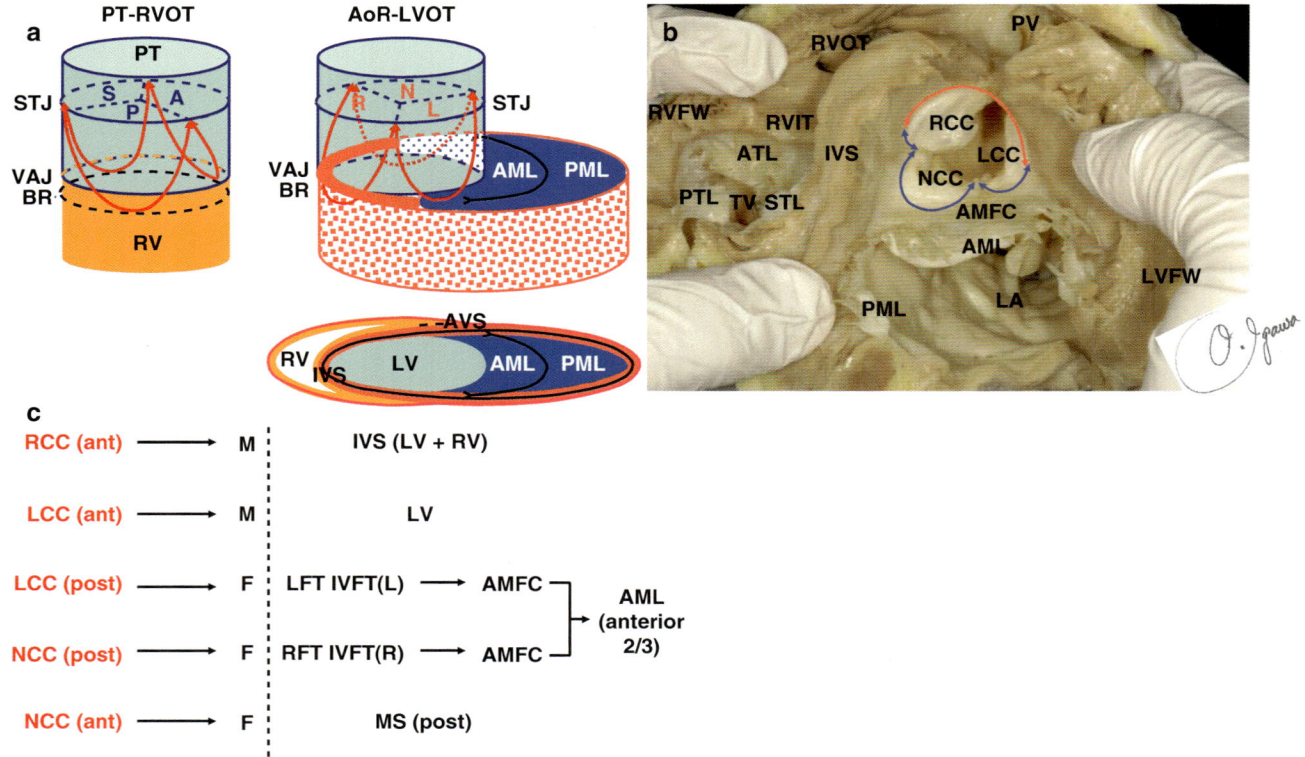

Fig. 2.5 (**a**) Schematic illustration (*right upper*) of the relationship between the AoR and the LVOT. The *right lower* figure shows the schematic illustration of the cross section of the heart cut at the level of just below the basal ring. (**b**) The aspect of the subvalvular area of the AoV. The attachment of AoV cusps and continuation from the AoV to AML (AMFC) can clearly be observed. The anterior and posterior parts of the RCC attach to the muscular (IVS) and fibrous (MS) tissue, respectively. The anterior and posterior parts of the LCC attach to the muscular (LV) and fibrous (AMFC) tissue, respectively. The anterior and posterior parts of NCC attach to the MS and AMFC, respectively. The NCC attaches wholly to fibrous tissue. The attachment sites (muscular and fibrous tissues) are indicated by *red* and *blue lines*, respectively. (**c**) A summary of the AoV attachment. The AoR is divided into two parts: a muscular portion and a fibrous portion, based on the tissue connecting to the AoVA

with specific fibrous tissue. This fibrous connection between the annulus of the AML and that of the aortic valve cusps is the AMFC. Ventricular arrhythmias originating from this fibrous area have been reported. However, to my knowledge, no ventricular cardiac muscle has yet been found in this fibrous area.

2.2.2 Anatomy of the Right and Left Ventricles

2.2.2.1 Anatomy of the Right Ventricle

Structure of the Right Ventricle

The right ventricle (RV) chamber is defined as the space from the tricuspid valve annulus to the PVA. This chamber is a crescent-shaped space when examined in a short-axis view (Fig. 2.6a). The morphology of the RV septum (S) and RV free wall (FW) are convex and concave, respectively.

Several approaches to divide this space have been proposed. The RV chamber can clearly be divided into two parts by specific muscle bundles, as described below: the RV inflow tract (RVIT) and the RVOT.

In the RV, there are two prominent muscle bundles: the septomarginal trabecula (SMT) on the RVS wall and supraventricular crest (SVCr) on the RVFW. These two projected muscle bundles form a ring in the inner wall of the RV. I have proposed calling this ring the "RV ring." The RV chamber is separated by the RV ring into two parts: the RVIT and RVOT (Fig. 2.6b). Accordingly, the RV wall is divided into four parts: RVIT septum and free wall (RVIT-S, RVIT-FW) and the RVOT septum and free wall (RVOT-S, RVOT-FW). The RV apex is included in the RVIT.

As shown in Figure, there is a muscle bundle floating in the RV cavity, known as a moderator band (MB). The MB is a part of the SMT as well as a continuation of it. The MB bridges the RVS and the anterior papillary muscle (APM) of the RV anterior free wall (RVAW). Notably, the right bundle

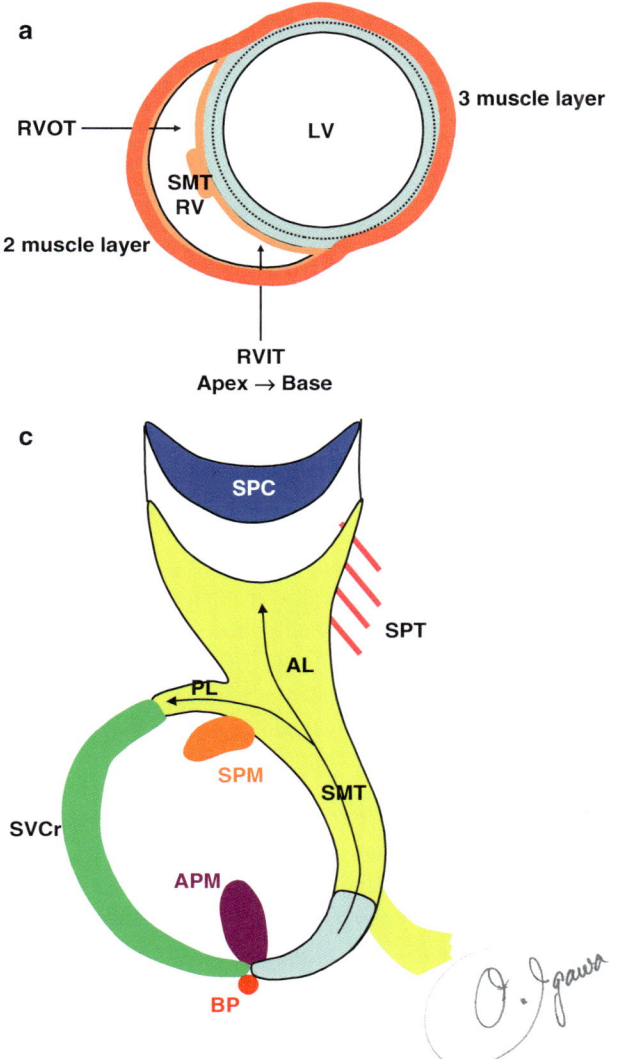
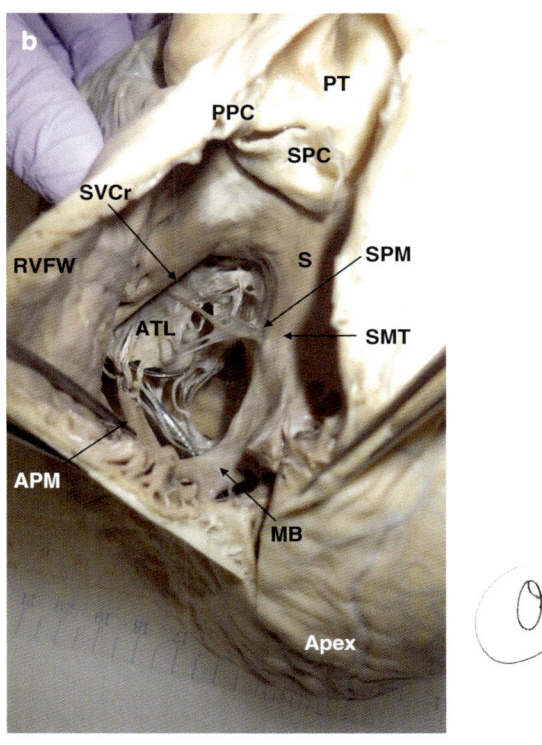

Fig. 2.6 (**a**) Schematic illustration of a ventricular cross section when viewed from apex to base in the short-axis view. The morphology of the RV and LV chamber shows a crescent- shaped and round structure, respectively. The structure of the RV and LV wall are two- and three-muscle layered, respectively. The IVS has three muscle layers: one from the RV (*red*) and two from the LV (*blue*). (**b**) The structure of the RV. There are two prominent muscle bundles: the septomarginal trabecula (SMT)-moderator band (MB) and the supraventricular crest (SVCr). These muscle bundles forms a prominent ring on the inner wall of the RV. I have proposed calling this ring as the "RV ring." The RV chamber is divided into two parts by the RV ring: the RVIT (from the TVA to the RV ring) and the RVOT (from the RV ring to the PVA). (**c**) Schematic illustration of the RV structure. There are two prominent muscle bundles in the RV: the SMT-MB and the SVCr. The SMT-MB on the RV septum consists of an anterior limb (AL) going toward the RVOT septum and a posterior limb (PL) going toward the RVIT septum. The AL-SMT switches over to the infundibular septum. The RV ring, which consists of the SMT-MB and SVr, can be seen on the inner wall of the RV

branch (RBB), which is electrically insulated by fibrous tissue, is in the SMT and MB. Electrical excitation through the AV junction travels down into the RBB and breaks through the APM in the RV. The SVCr connects to the APM as well. Using this anatomical information, we can identify a ring in the inner wall of the RV.

The internal surface of the RV wall, except for that of the RVOT-S wall, is not smooth but rough because of trabeculae. The trabeculae in RVOT-FW just beneath the APC are lined up in good order and known as the septoparietal trabecula (SPT) (Fig. 2.6b,c).

RV Ring and Its Related Structures

As described above, the circular muscle structure known as the RV ring is projected into the RV chamber. Figure 2.6c is a schematic illustration of this structure. RV ring consists of two main muscle bundles, the SMT-MB of the RVS and the SVCr of the RVFW. The septal papillary muscle (SPM) originates at the base of the SMT. The MB connects with the base of the APM. If this ring protrudes enough to divide the RV chamber into two spaces, a condition known as "double-chambered right ventricle (DRV)" develops.

Anterior and Posterior RV Hinge

Based on the structural characteristics of the RV, we can define the inner border between the anterior RVFW and IVS as the "anterior RV hinge." However, another inner border between the posterior RVFW and IVS can be defined as the "posterior RV hinge." The anterior RV hinge line is adjacent to the left anterior descending coronary artery (LAD). The LAD is in cardiac adipose tissue of the anterior interventricular groove (AIVG). Similarly, the "posterior RV hinge" line is close to the right posterior descending coronary artery (RPD). CA performed around the RV hinge therefore carries some risk of coronary artery damage as well as RV wall perforation when manipulating a catheter around the RV hinge. The RV hinge line is structurally weak to catheter pressure.

RV Recess

Interestingly, there is a recess in the RVOT. This structure is located in the area of the posterior free wall of the RVOT just beneath the annulus of the posterior pulmonary cusp (PPA). Strictly speaking, the recess is in the area between the PPA and SVCr (Fig. 2.7). The number, size, and morphology of this recess vary by individual. Some have only one recess, while others have more. Its typical morphology is round, but some have a cleft-shaped morphology.

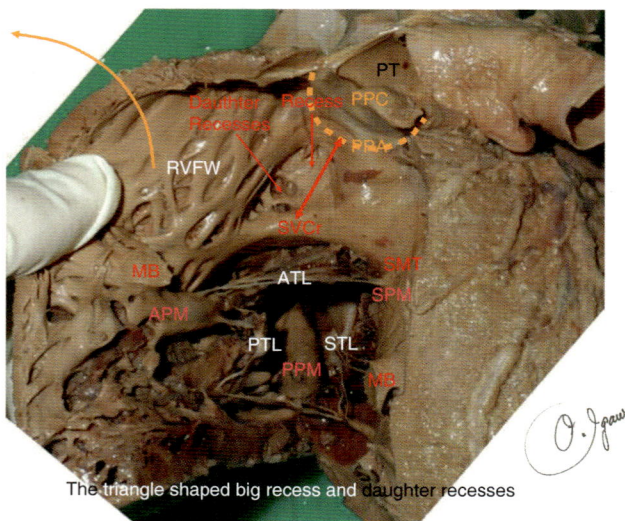

Fig. 2.7 The internal aspect of the RV recess. The RV recess is located in the area between the annulus of the posterior pulmonary cusp (PPA) and the SVCr. In this case, a large, triangle-shaped recess can be seen. Notably, several daughter recesses are located in the bottom of the big recess, as indicated by *red arrows*

Histologically, the muscle structure of this recess wall is normal. The wall thickness of this area is extremely thin compared to that of other areas of the RVOT. There is a large amount of cardiac adipose tissue outside of this recess (on the side of the epicardium).

2.2.2.2 Anatomy of the Tricuspid Valve

Atrioventricular Valves and Atrioventricular Conduction System

The atrioventricular valve consists of the (1) valvular annulus, (2) valvular leaflets, (3) tendinous cords, and (4) papillary muscles (PMs) of the heart. Therefore, the "mitral valve" and "tricuspid valve (TV)" are merely the name of the valvular system and not the leaflets.

Of note, the atrioventricular conduction system dwells in electrically isolated fibrous tissue. This means that the electrical excitation from the sinus node travels down to the ventricles through the electrically insulated atrioventricular conduction system, atrioventricular node (AVN), the HB, the RBB, and the left bundle branch (LBB), breaking through via the Purkinje fibers around the PMs. The muscle structures containing the atrioventricular conduction system, such as the septomarginal trabecula (SMT), connects to the PMs (Fig. 2.8a).

The PMs are the earliest activation and contraction sites in the ventricles. Excitation propagates through the ventricles entirely via the Purkinje network following activation of the PMs. Other ventricular contraction follows this PM-based contraction. The PMs ensure that the atrioventricular valve leaflets do not turn over prior to ventricular muscle contraction (Fig. 2.8b).

Tricuspid Valve (TV)

The TV leaflets are anterior, septal, and posterior ones (A/S/PTLs). The PMs in the RV are anterior, septal, and posterior papillary muscles (A/S/PPMs). The APM supports the anterior part of ATL and PTL, the SPM supports the anterior part of the STL and posterior part of the ATL, and the PPM supports the posterior part of the STL and PTL. There are no second chordae in the subvalvular space of the A/PTL. However, many second chordae can be observed in the space under the STL. The area of the TV leaflets is ATL>STL>PTL.

2.2.2.3 Anatomy of the LV and PMs

Structure of the LV

Figure 2.6a shows a schematic illustration of the short-axis view of the heart at the level of the ventricles. While the RVFW has a two-muscle-layered structure, the LVFW has a three-muscle-layered structure. As shown in Fig. 2.6a, the IVS shows three muscle layers: one from the RV and two from the LV.

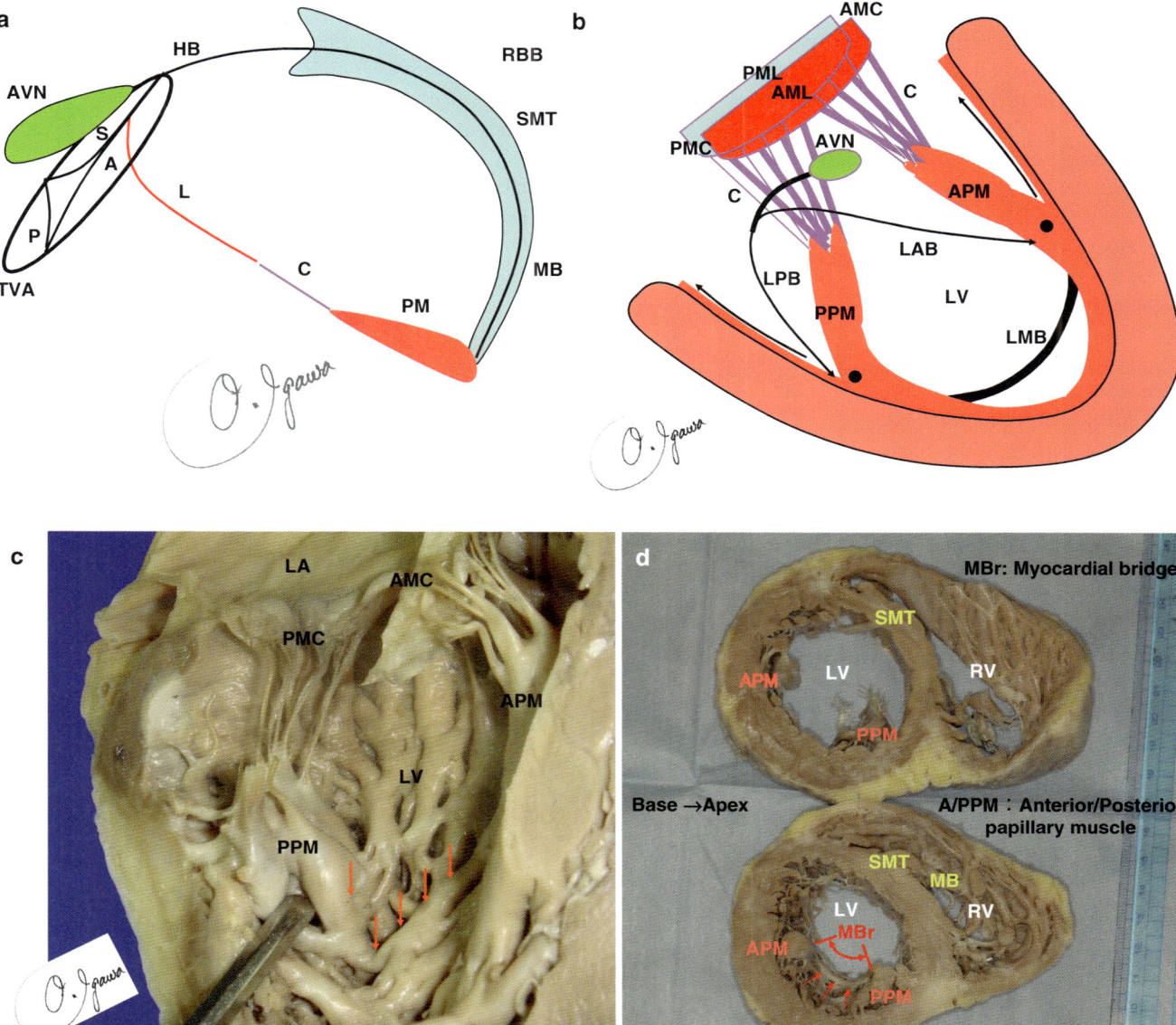

Fig. 2.8 (**a**) Schematic illustration of the relationship between the AV conduction system and AV valvular system in the RV. Normal electrical excitation from the sinus node travels down through the AVN, HB, and RBB and breaks through via the Purkinje fibers around the PM (APM) on the *right side*. The MB containing the RBB connects to the APM structurally. It travels down through the anterior and posterior branches of the LBB and breaks through via the Purkinje fibers around the anterior and posterior PMs on the left side (next figure). (**b**) Schematic illustration of the relationship between normal intraventricular conduction system and the PMs in the LV. Normal electrical excitation from the AV node travels down through the LAB and RAB and breaks through via the Purkinje fibers around the PMs (APM and PPM) in the LV. Both excitations propagate along the endocardial surface of the LV wall via the Purkinje network. A muscle bundle (LMB) linking both PMs can be seen. (**c**) Muscle bundle linking both PMs in the LV (shown by *red arrows*). (**d**) Muscle bundle linking both PMs in LV (shown by *red arrows*)

Definition of the Left Ventricular Inflow Tract and LVOT

The LV chamber is the space from the mitral valve annulus to the aortic valve annulus. This chamber is round when viewed in a short-axis view (Fig. 2.6). The morphology of the LVS and LVFW is concave in both instances.

The LV chamber is divided into two parts (the left ventricular inflow tract (LVIT) and the LVOT) for the purpose of convenience. However, from an anatomical viewpoint, there are no specific structures separating the LV chamber. With respect to the function of the LV chamber, we can imagine a border dividing the LV chamber into two parts. One structure comprises the APM-anterior tendinous cords of the AML-AML-posterior tendinous cords of the AML-PML: in other words, the AML and its subvalvular supporting structures. In addition, as shown in Fig. 2.8b, we can make out the gate to this structure. I have proposed that this border and gate be called the "mitral border" and "mitral window," respectively. Functionally, blood flows into the LVIT from the LA in the diastolic phase and then into the LVOT through the mitral window in systole, subsequently passing through the aortic valve flowing into the AAo. The mitral border then flexibly moves in the LV, anteriorly in the diastolic phase, and posteriorly in the systolic phase. The LVOT and LVIT are defined as the spaces anterior and posterior to the border, respectively. LV apex is in the LVOT. When planning to position a catheter inserted through the AoV retrogradely in the LVIT, we always ensure that it passes through the mitral window.

Mitral Valve and Conduction System in the LV

The APM and PPM are located at the anterolateral and posterolateral LVFW, respectively. These muscle bundles are linked just above the apex (Fig. 2.8b, c).

When considering the pathway of the normal interventricular conduction system, excitation passing through the HB travels down through the RBB on the right side and the left anterior and posterior limb of left bundle branch (LAB, LPB) on the left side, which are electrically insulated from their surroundings. These excitations go down toward the right APM, left APM and left PPM, and the excitations in each branch, breaking through via the Purkinje fibers around the PMs. They then propagate entirely along the endocardial surface of the LV wall through the Purkinje network.

Tendinae from the APM support the anterior part of the AML and PML, including the anterior mitral commissure (AMC). In contrast, tendinae from the PPM support the posterior part of the AML and PML, including the posterior mitral commissure (PMC).

Structural and Electrical Linkage Between the APM and PPM in the LV

Of note, there is another muscle linking both PMs besides those described above. In my studies, I have found that this linking muscle contains Purkinje fibers, suggesting that it may play an important role in connecting both PMs not only structurally but also electrically. There may be fast conduction along Purkinje fibers in this linking muscle between both PMs (Fig. 2.8b).

References

1. Macedo PG, Kapa S, Mears JA, et al. Correlative anatomy for the electrophysiologist: ablation for atrial fibrillation. Part I: pulmonary vein ostia, superior vena cava, vein of Marshall. J Cardiovasc Electrophysiol. 2010;21:721–30.
2. Macedo PG, Kapa S, Mears JA, et al. Correlative anatomy for the electrophysiologist: ablation for atrial fibrillation. Part II: regional anatomy of the atria and relevance to damage of adjacent structures during AF ablation. J Cardiovasc Electrophysiol. 2010;21:829–36.
3. Ho SY, Sánchez-Quintana D. The importance of atrial structure and fibers. Clin Anat. 2009;22:52–63.

Part II

Techniques and Interpretation to Diagnose the Mechanism of Supraventricular Tachycardias

Entrainment Pacing: A Diagnostic Tool for Reentrant Tachycardia and Its Application for Catheter Ablation

Ken Okumura and Hideharu Okamatsu

Keywords

Entrainment • Reentry • Catheter ablation • Slow conduction zone • Critical isthmus

3.1 Introduction

Entrainment is defined as a phenomenon of continuous resetting of tachycardia with pacing at rates faster than the tachycardia rate. It is used as a tool for diagnosing reentry as a mechanism of tachycardias [1–4], localizing and characterizing the reentry circuit including slow conduction zone (SCZ) [5], evaluating the electrophysiologic properties of SCZ [6–12], and identifying a target site suitable for catheter ablation [13–15]. There are two types of entrainment, manifest entrainment and concealed entrainment, according to the pacing site relative to the reentry circuit and SCZ [5]. Entrainment is one of the most important fundamentals of electrophysiologic testing, and its application is quite useful and important in ablating various forms of tachycardias.

3.2 Definition of Entrainment

Every tachycardia can be continuously reset with pacing at rates faster than the tachycardia rate when the tachycardia has an excitable gap, and the pacing impulse can enter to the origin site of the tachycardia [1–3]. During continuous resetting of automatic tachycardias including triggered activity-mediated tachycardia, the excitation rate of the automatic cell is passively increased to the pacing rate, and the intrinsic change in the automaticity rate caused by the enhanced phase 4 depolarization does not occur. On the contrary, in the case of reentrant tachycardias, the pacing impulses do enter the reentrant circuit and continue the tachycardia while activating the circuit at the pacing rate. Thus, entrainment in a narrow sense is defined as a phenomenon of continuous resetting of reentrant tachycardia.

In the clinical point of view, two types of entrainment including manifest entrainment and concealed entrainment should be understood precisely [1–5, 13, 14]. Manifest entrainment is used for diagnosing reentry as a mechanism of tachycardia [1–5] and for exploring and ablating the SCZ which is concealed under routine electrophysiology [15, 16]. Concealed entrainment is useful in identifying the critical isthmus in the reentry circuit for ablation.

3.3 Pacing Method for Entrainment

To demonstrate entrainment, rapid pacing at rate 5–10 beats/min (bpm) faster than the tachycardia rate is initiated, continued for several seconds, and interrupted abruptly [1–5]. The duration of pacing depends on the pacing site relative to the tachycardia site, and it is usually sufficient to pace for 3–5 s when the pacing is done in the same chamber as the tachycardia is. After interruption of pacing, it should be confirmed that not only the ECG but all of the intracardiac electrograms are activated stably at the pacing CL during pacing.

When the tachycardia resumes just after interruption of pacing, rapid pacing is repeated with a rate being further increased by 5–10 bpm. This pacing maneuver with increased pacing rate is repeated until the tachycardia is terminated. In the case that entrainment is used for identifying the target ablation site, one pacing maneuver which obviously captures the tachycardia at the pacing rate, i.e., entrains the tachycardia, is sufficient since pacing at more rapid rate may result in termination of the tachycardia.

K. Okumura, M.D. (✉) • H. Okamatsu, M.D.
Division of Cardiology, Saiseikai Kumamoto Hospital Cardiovascular Center, Chikami 5-3-1, Minami-ku, Kumamoto 861-4193, Japan
e-mail: okumura@hirosaki-u.ac.jp

3.4 Influential Factors in Demonstrating Entrainment

There are several factors that influence demonstrating entrainment. When tachycardia entrainment is attempted and interpreted, all of these factors need to be taken into consideration.

3.4.1 Excitable Gap

Entrainment of tachycardia is impossible even in the reentrant tachycardia if excitable gap is not present in the circuit. This is because the pacing impulse cannot enter the reentry circuit. Also, if the circuit is protected by the surrounding tissue and the pacing impulse cannot reach the circuit, entrainment cannot be observed (concealed perpetuation).

3.4.2 Pacing Site Relative to the Reentry Circuit

For demonstrating entrainment, the pacing site especially in relation to the SCZ within the circuit is critical [5]. As discussed below, pacing from a site proximal to the SCZ usually results in manifest entrainment which indicates entrainment with fusion. On the other hand, pacing from a site distal to or within the SCZ results in concealed entrainment, which indicates entrainment with concealed fusion. In identifying and ablating tachycardias, concealed entrainment with pacing from a site within the SCZ is important [13, 14].

3.4.3 Pacing Rate

Pacing at a rate much faster than the tachycardia rate, for example, at rates >20 bpm faster than the tachycardia rate, may terminate the tachycardia by inducing conduction block in the SCZ. On the other hand, pacing at rates close to the tachycardia rate may not entrain the tachycardia because of a failure to enter the circuit. Thus, as described above, pacing at a rate 5–10 bpm faster than the tachycardia rate is recommended to be performed initially, and it should be confirmed that all of the electrograms are activated stably at the pacing CL.

3.4.4 Pacing Duration

When the duration of pacing is short, the impulse may not be able to enter the reentry circuit completely, especially when the pacing rate is just above the tachycardia rate. Again, it should be confirmed that all of the electrograms are activated stably at the pacing CL.

3.4.5 Stability of Tachycardia

During entrainment, the wavefront from the pacing impulse successively enters the reentry circuit and activates the circuit at the pacing rate. Therefore, in the case of unstable tachycardia whose circuit or rate is unstable or unsustained tachycardia, entrainment is not feasible. For unsustained tachycardias, isoproterenol infusion may be useful in making the tachycardia sustained and stable and therefore entrained.

3.5 Manifest Entrainment and Its Mechanism

Professor Albert L. Waldo has dedicated to exploring the electrophysiologic mechanisms and aspects of entrainment using various forms of reentrant tachycardias including atrial flutter, atrial tachycardia, paroxysmal supraventricular tachycardia, and ventricular tachycardia [1–6]. He then proposed four criteria for demonstrating entrainment (Table 3.1) [1–4]: When at least one of the criteria is fulfilled, entrainment of tachycardia is manifested, and the mechanism of the tachycardia can be best explained by reentry (*manifest entrainment*). Among the criteria supporting reentry as the mechanism of tachycardia, this manifest entrainment is simple and most reliable.

An example of manifest entrainment of ventricular tachycardia (VT) associated with healed anterior myocardial infarction is shown in Fig 3.1 [6]. VT rate is 194 beats/min (cycle length (CL), 309 ms), and VT morphology is right bundle branch block pattern, suggesting the location of VT origin in the left ventricle. Electrode mapping during VT revealed the early action site (EAS) in the LV anterior wall with the local activation time of −10 ms relative to the QRS complex. When rapid pacing at a rate of 200 bpm (CL, 300 ms) is done from the right ventricular apex (RVA) (Fig 3.1 left panel), constant fusion, indicated by black dots, is observed in the ECG during pacing except for the last entrained beat, and with the cessation of the pacing, VT resumes (*criterion 1*). It should be noted that the LV early activation site is captured with a long conduction interval (360 ms) via the SCZ. Thus, in one paced beat, there are two wavefronts activating the ventricles, one from the current

Table 3.1 Criteria for demonstration of entrainment

1. Constant fusion except for the last captured beat
2. Different degrees of constant fusion at different pacing rates (progressive fusion)
3. Localized conduction block associated with interruption of tachycardia
4. Changes in conduction time and electrogram morphology by increasing the pacing rate (electrogram criterion equivalent of progressive fusion)

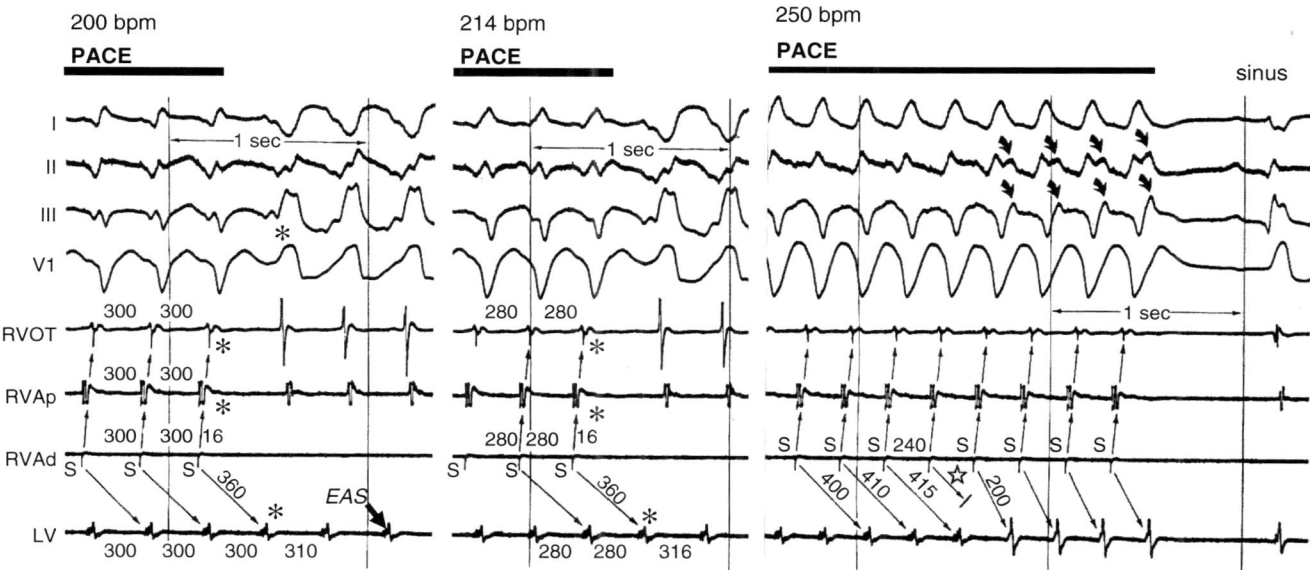

Fig 3.1 Manifest entrainment of ventricular tachycardia associated with healed anterior myocardial infarction [6]. See text for discussion. *RVOT* right ventricular outflow tract, *RVA* right ventricular apex, *LV* left ventricle, *EAS* early activation site

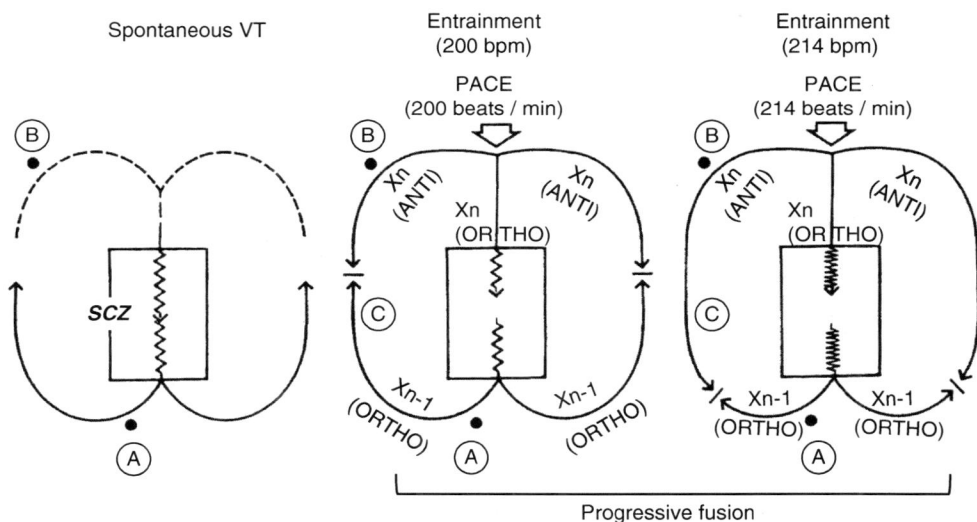

Fig 3.2 Mechanism of manifest entrainment shown in Fig 3.1 [6], *left* and *center panels*. See text for discussion. *VT* ventricular tachycardia, *SCZ* slow conduction zone

pacing impulse and the other from the previous pacing impulse coming via a long conduction interval.

When pacing is done with the rate increased to 214 bpm (CL, 280 ms) (Fig 3.1 center panel), constant fusion is again observed during pacing, while the degree of fusion changed (progressive fusion, *criterion 2*). It is noted that the conduction interval from the pacing impulse to the LV site is further increased to 380 ms. When pacing is done with the rate further increased to 250 bpm (CL, 240 ms) (Fig 3.1 right panel), it results in further prolongation of the conduction interval (400, 410, and 415 ms) to and localized conduction block to the LV site (indicated by ☆), being associated with an abrupt change in the QRS complex (indicated by curved arrows), and VT is terminated with the cession of the pacing (*criterion 3*). Note that the LV site is captured with a relatively short conduction interval (200 ms) after the localized conduction block.

The mechanism of entrainment in Fig 3.1 is schematically shown in Fig 3.2 and Fig 3.3 using the figure of eight type reentry with a SCZ within the circuit (Fig 3.2, left panel) [6]. During pacing from a site proximal to the SCZ done during VT (Fig 3.2, center panel), the orthodromic wavefront (ORTHO) from the pacing impulse Xn enters the reentry circuit and then SCZ, resulting in continuation of reentry at the pacing rate (200 bpm). The antidromic wavefront (ANTI) from Xn activates the ventricular tissue from a different direction from VT and collides with the orthodromic

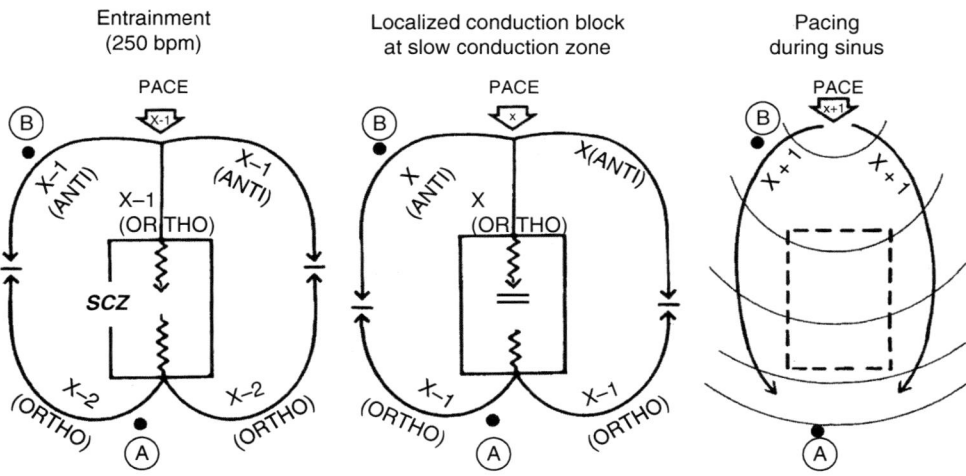

Fig 3.3 Mechanism of tachycardia interruption during manifest entrainment shown in Fig 3.1, right panel. See text for discussion

wavefront from the previous pacing impulse Xn-1. Note that the present ORTHO Xn is still within the SCZ. Since the pacing rate is constant, collision of antidromic wavefront Xn with orthodromic wavefront Xn-1 occurs at the same site constantly during pacing, resulting in constant fusion in the ECG (*criterion 1*). When the pacing is interrupted, the last orthodromic wavefront entering the SCZ no longer collides with antidromic wavefront, thus no fusion beat being created, and results in resumption of the initial tachycardia.

When the pacing rate is increased (Fig 3.2, right panel), the antidromic wavefront activates more area outside the SCZ, which results in a change in the degree of fusion (progressive fusion, *criterion 2*). The site C which is previously activated by the orthodromic wavefront is activated by the antidromic wavefront, being associated with the shortening of the activation time from the pacing to site C and with the change in the electrogram morphology because of the change in the direction of activation (*criterion 4*). When the pacing rate is further increased, entrainment is initially observed (Fig 3.3, left panel), but the orthodromic wavefront is blocked in the SCZ, being associated with termination of the tachycardia (Fig 3.3, center panel). The following pacing impulses activate the ventricles in the same way as pacing is done during sinus rhythm, and therefore the QRS morphology suddenly changes (Fig 3.3, right panel) (*criterion 3*).

3.6 Concealed Entrainment and Its Mechanism

Entrainment of reentrant tachycardia is always associated with collision of the antidromic wavefront with the previous orthodromic one, which is recognized as fusion beats in manifest entrainment [5]. When the pacing is done from a site within the SCZ or distal the to the SCZ (site A in Fig 3.2), however, collision occurs in the SCZ and therefore is hardly recognized (concealed fusion) [5].

Using these entrainment phenomena with manifest and concealed fusion, Stevenson et al. proposed entrainment mapping for localizing the pacing site relative the VT reentry circuit (Fig 3.4) [17]. When entrainment is associated with QRS fusion, the pacing site is mostly in the outer loop, i.e., outside the SCZ. When entrainment is associated with concealed fusion, the pacing site is mostly in the central pathway, i.e., within the SCZ. In this case, if post-pacing interval (PPI) is equal to or within 30 ms of the tachycardia CL (TCL) or stimulus-to-QRS interval (S-QRS) is equal to or within 20 ms of the electrograms at the pacing site-to-QRS interval (EG-QRS), then the pacing site is on the central SCZ (concealed entrainment). Further, when the ratio of S-QRS to TCL (S-QRS/TSL) is <30%, the pacing site is at the exit of the SCZ; when it is 31–50%, the pacing site is at the center of the SCZ; when it is 51–70%, the pacing site is at the proximal SCZ. Thus, with this diagnostic algorithm, the pacing site relative to the reentry circuit, especially to the SCZ, can be identified. Above all, the pacing site with S-QRS/TCL 31–50% strongly suggests a successful ablation site for the cure of VT. It should be reminded that in concealed entrainment, PPI is equal or close to TCL in many cases, but it may be longer by >30 ms than TCL when the reentry circuit contains the SCZ with a decremental conduction property such as the atrioventricular (AV) node [18]. Similar criteria for concealed entrainment (entrainment mapping) were reported by El-Shalakany subsequently [19].

An example of concealed entrainment of VT associated with nonischemic cardiomyopathy is shown in Fig 3.5 (left panel). VT rate is 129 beats/min (cycle length (CL), 465 ms), and VT morphology is right bundle branch block pattern, suggesting the location of VT origin in the left ventricle. CARTO mapping during VT revealed reentry around the mitral and aortic complex with abnormal low voltage (≤0.5 mV) area in the lateral LV close to the mitral annulus (Fig 3.5, center and right panels). When rapid pacing at

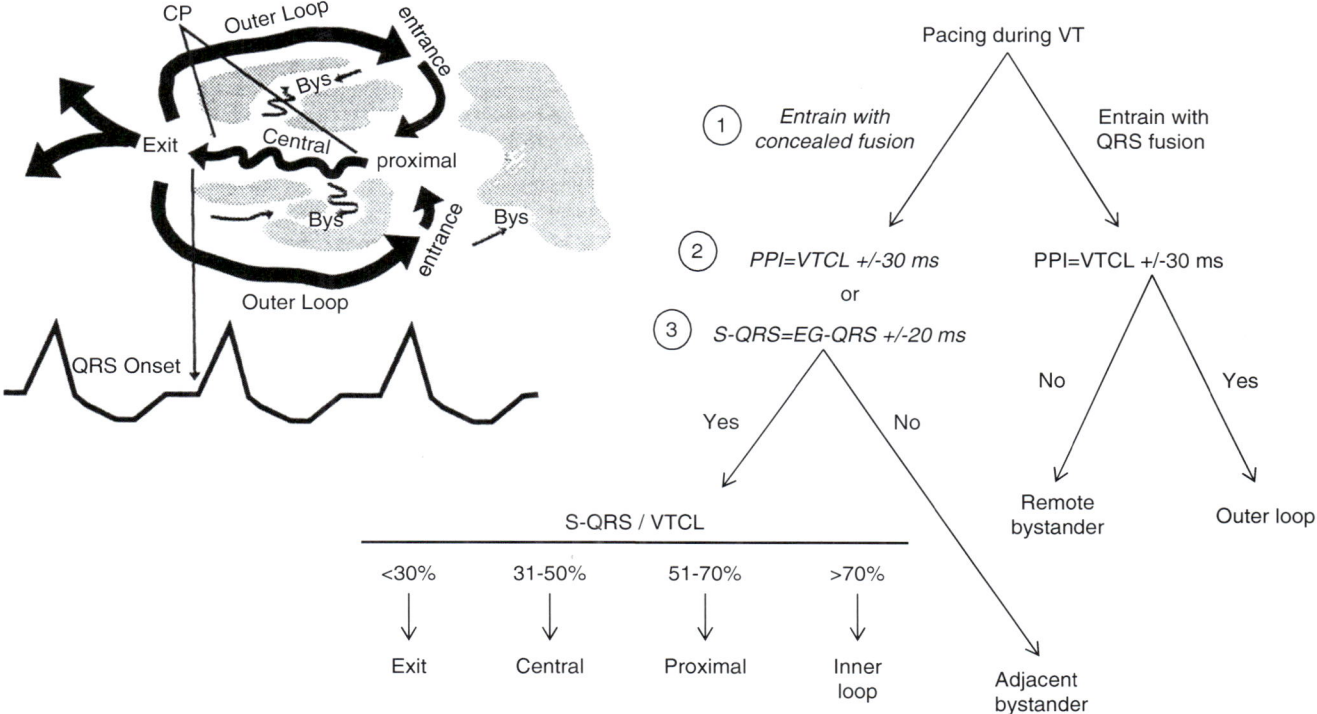

Fig 3.4 Entrainment mapping for localizing the pacing site relative the reentry circuit of ventricular tachycardia [17]. See text for discussion

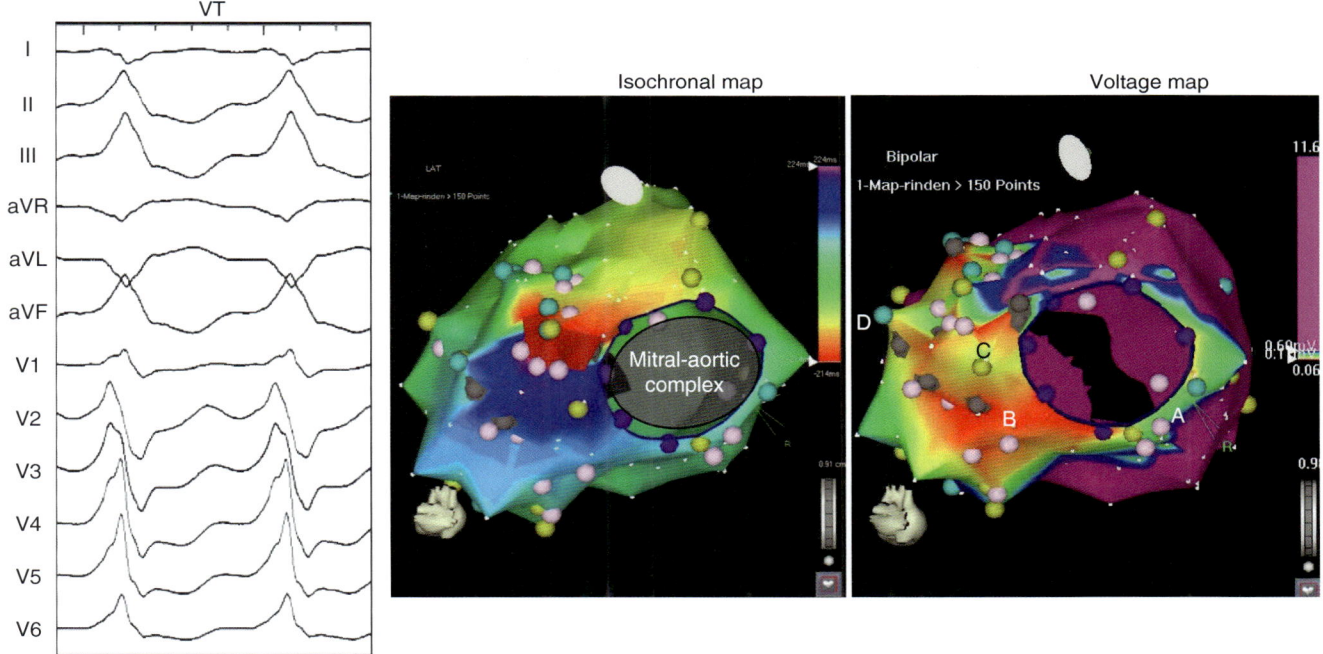

Fig 3.5 Ventricular tachycardia associated with nonischemic cardiomyopathy. *Left panel*, 12 leads ECG during tachycardia; *center* and *right panels*, CARTO activation and voltage maps, respectively, during tachycardia (posterior view of the left ventricle with right anterior oblique projection)

140 bpm (CL, 430 ms) is done from site A (Fig 3.5 right panel), concealed entrainment indicated by exactly the same QRS complexes during pacing as those during VT is observed (Fig 3.6a). It is also noted that the morphology and relative activation sequence of the electrogram recorded at the right ventricular outflow tract (RVOT) during pacing remain consistent to those during VT, indicating that RVOT is captured orthodromically. Following the Stevenson's algorithm, PPI is 465 ms, which is equal to TCL, and S-QRS 340 ms, which is to EG-QRS. Further, S-QRS/TCL is 73%, suggesting the pacing site is just at the entrance to the SCZ or inner loop. When rapid pacing is done from site B, concealed entrainment is again observed with PPI 465 ms equal to TCL and S-QRS 210 ms equal to EG-QRS (Fig 3.6b). Since S-QRS/TCL is 45%, the pacing site is suggested at the center of the SCZ. When rapid pacing is done from site D, the QRS morphology during pacing is slightly but definitely different from that during VT, and thus entrainment with fusion (manifest entrainment) is observed, indicating site D outside the SCZ (Fig 3.6c).

3.6.1 Electrogram Characteristics Equivalent to Concealed and Manifest Entrainment

It should be reminded that in the case of supraventricular tachycardias, P wave or flutter wave is not clearly recognized during tachycardia and rapid pacing. Therefore, the presence or absence of fusion needs to be judged by the characteristics of the electrograms recorded at multiple sites: In one paced beat, when some of them are activated in the same way as during the tachycardia, indicating orthodromic capture, and others in different ways, indicating antidromic capture, then the presence of fusion is strongly suggested, and the pacing site is considered to be proximal to the SCZ. On the other hand, when all of the electrograms are activated orthodromically, then the pacing site may be on the SCZ or critical narrow isthmus (concealed entrainment). When all are activated antidromically, then the pacing site may be distal to the SCZ or critical isthmus and far from the circuit (another form of concealed entrainment).

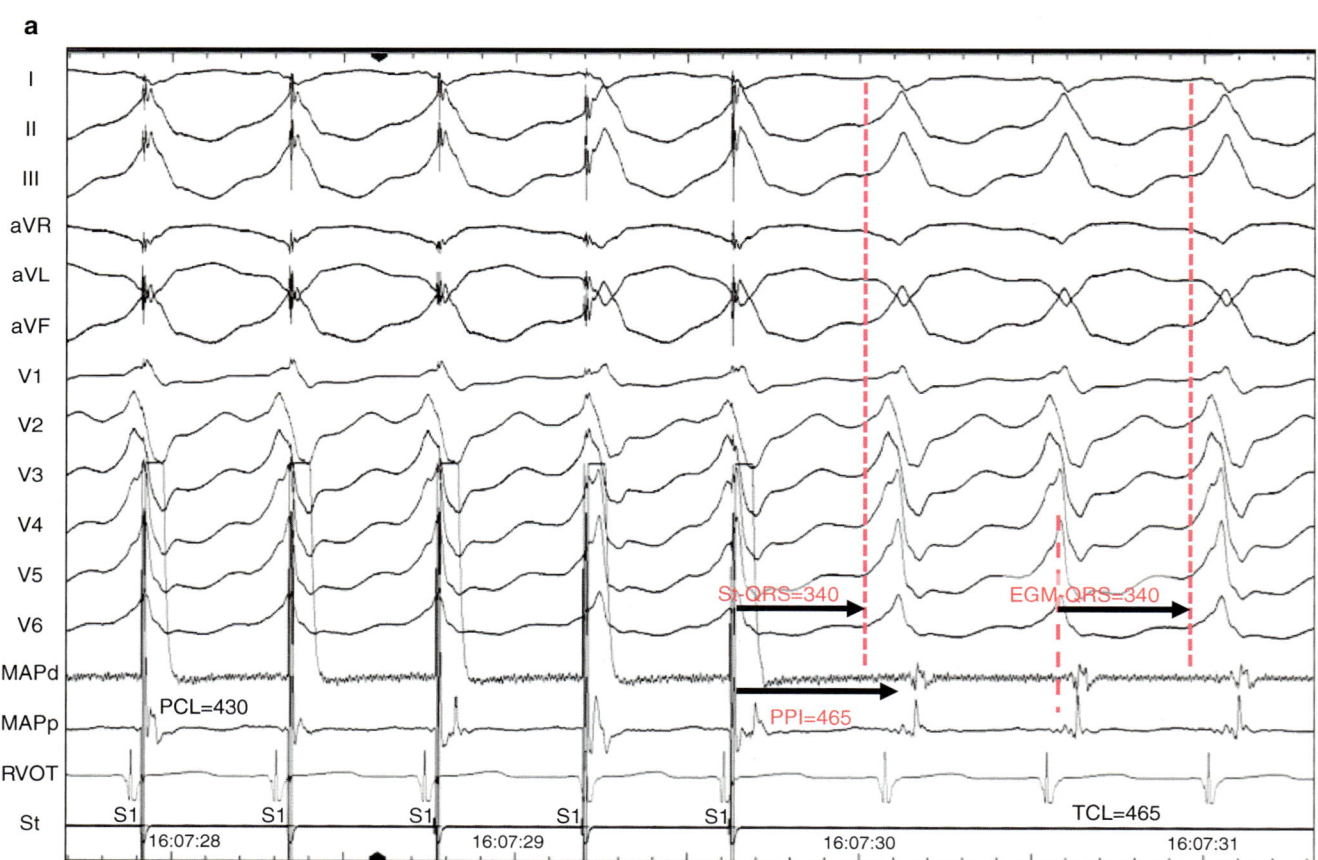

Fig 3.6 Concealed entrainment of ventricular tachycardia shown in Fig 3.5. Panel (**a**), rapid pacing (CL, 430 ms) done from site A shown in the *right panel* of Fig 3.5; panel (**b**), rapid pacing from site B; panel (**c**), rapid pacing from site D. See text for discussion. *MAPd and MAPp* electrograms recorded from the distal and proximal pairs of electrode, respectively, placed at the left ventricular site, *RVOT* right ventricular outflow tract

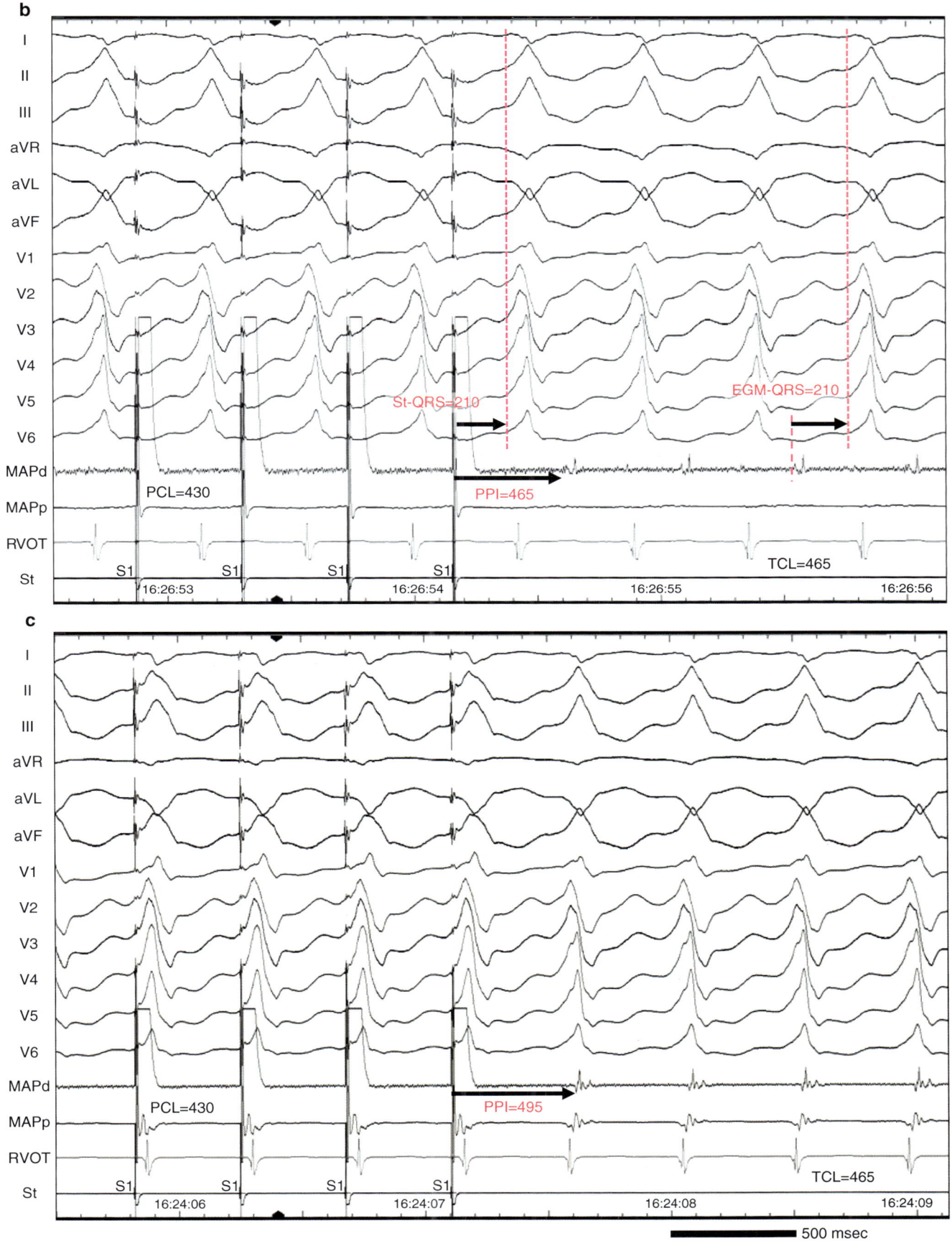

Fig 3.6 (continued)

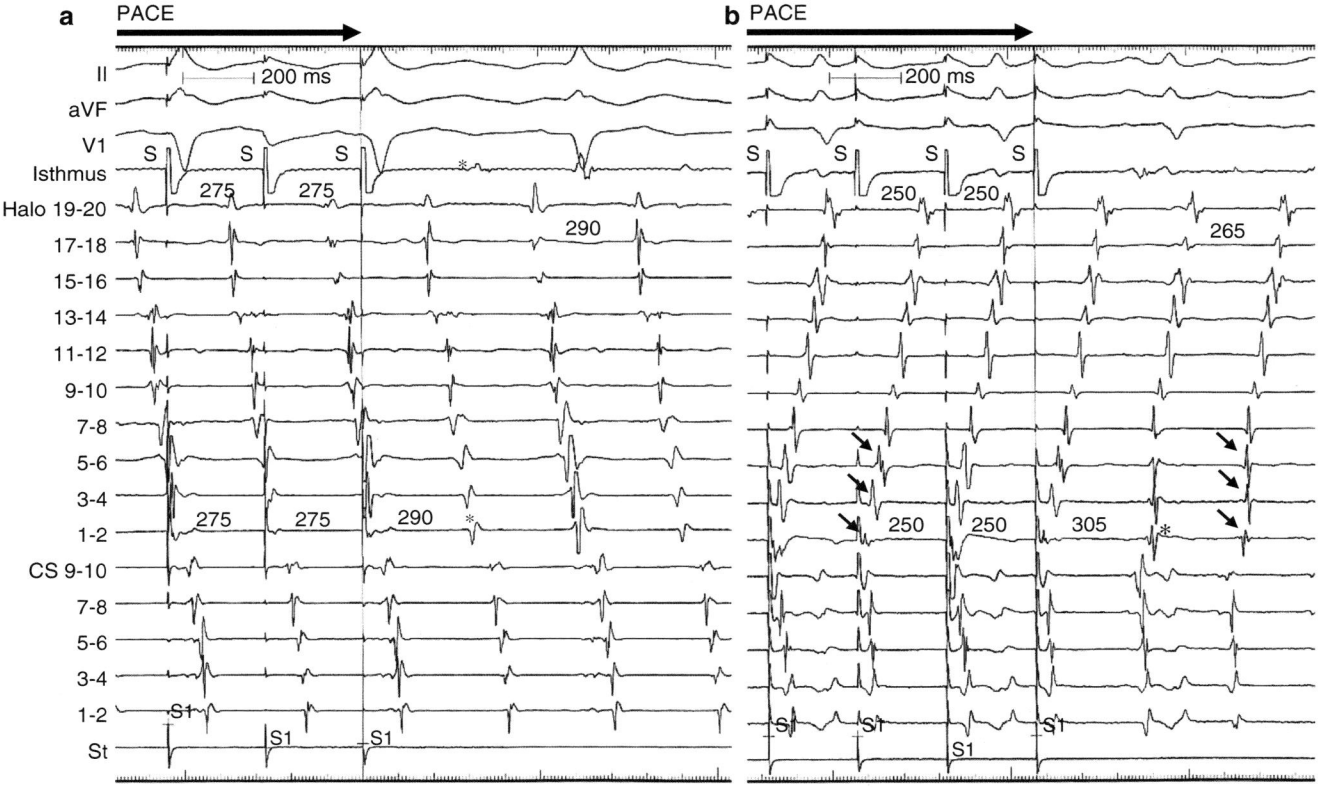

Fig 3.7 Concealed (panel **a**) and manifest entrainment (panel **b**) of typical and atypical atrial flutter, respectively. See text for discussion

An example of concealed entrainment of typical atrial flutter (AFL) is shown in Fig 3.7a. Rapid pacing at 218 bpm (CL, 275 ms) was performed from the cavotricuspid isthmus (CTI) during AFL with a rate of 207 bpm (TCL, 290 ms). It is noted that the morphologies and activation sequences of all electrograms recorded in the right atrium (RA), from Halo 1–2 to Halo 19–20, and on the left atrium (LA), from CS 1–2 to CS 9–10, remain consistent with those during AFL, suggesting concealed entrainment. PPI measured from the last pacing impulse to the first post-pacing electrogram at the pacing site (*) is 290 ms and equal to TCL. It is difficult to measure precisely the stimulus-to-F wave interval or electrogram-to-F wave interval. Thus, the pacing site CTI is on the reentry circuit although it is not clear if the CTI is the SCZ or not. Since the CTI is a narrow conduction pathway sandwiched by the two anatomical barriers, it can serve as a critical pathway for reentry circuit just as the SCZ for VT.

An example of manifest entrainment of atypical AFL is shown in Fig 3.7b. Rapid pacing at 240 bpm (CL, 250 ms) was done from the CTI during AFL with a rate of 226 bpm (TCL, 265 ms). During pacing, the morphologies and activation sequences of all electrograms recorded in the RA and LA look as if they are consistent with those during AFL, but careful observation of the electrograms at Halo 1–2 to 5–6 (arrows) reveals that these electrogram morphologies and activation sequence are different from those during AFL, indicating antidromic capture. Further, the timing of activation of CS 9–10 relative to Halo 1–2 is different between pacing and AFL. Thus, these electrogram characteristics during pacing indicate manifest entrainment by the presence of both antidromic (indicated by arrows) and orthodromic capture by the previous pacing impulse (the other Halo electrograms). PPI from the last pacing impulse to the first post-pacing electrogram at the pacing site (*) is 305 ms and longer than TCL. Thus, the pacing site CTI is not included in the reentry circuit of this AFL.

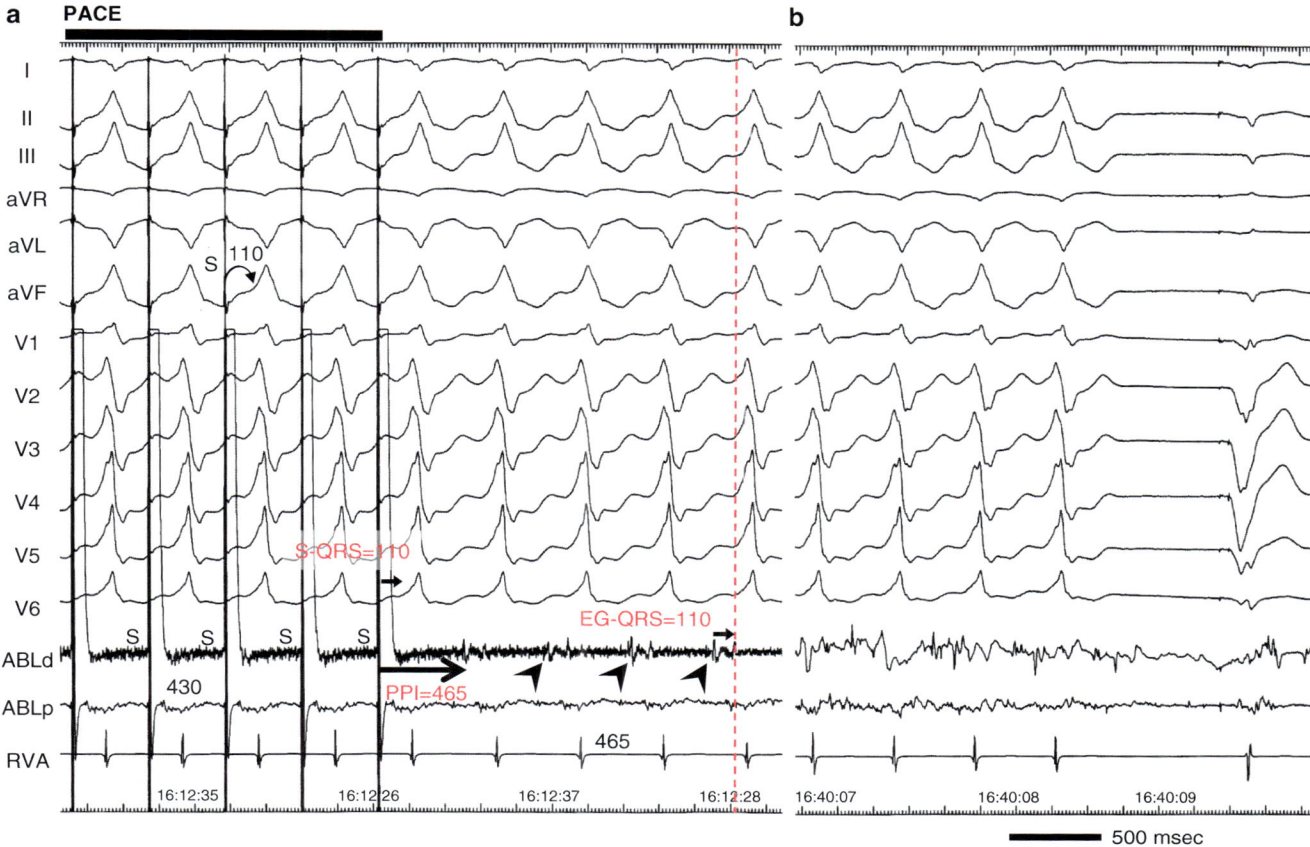

Fig 3.8 Concealed entrainment and ablation of ventricular tachycardia at site C shown in the *right panel* of Fig 3.5. Panel **a**, concealed entrainment with S-QRS/TCL 24%; panel **b**, termination of the tachycardia by application of radio-frequency energy. See text for discussion

3.7 Application of Entrainment to Identifying Ablation Target

3.7.1 Concealed Entrainment

It should be reminded that a concept of concealed entrainment is applied to reentrant tachycardia and not to focal (automatic) tachycardia. Therefore, when discussing concealed entrainment, reentry as a mechanism of the tachycardia needs to be proven in advance. For this purpose, the presence of manifest entrainment should be first confirmed as described above, and then concealed entrainment is tested. In clinical practice, however, when an electroanatomical map such as CARTO map during tachycardia suggests reentry as a mechanism, then the proof of manifest entrainment may not be necessary.

In reentrant tachycardias, concealed entrainment with PPI equal or close to TCL strongly suggests the pacing site being on the critical conduction pathway or SCZ within the circuit [13, 14, 17, 19], and this pacing site can be a target for catheter ablation. Fig 3.8 shows an example of VT ablation done at the site where concealed entrainment is demonstrated (Site C in Fig 3.5 right panel). According to Stevenson's algorithm (Fig 3.4) [17], the pacing site is close to the exit of the SCZ since S-QRS/TCL is 24% (Fig 3.8a). It is noted that a mid-diastolic potential indicated by arrowheads is recorded at this site. Application of radio-frequency energy abruptly terminated VT (Fig 3.8b).

In clinical practice, mapping and detecting the mid-diastolic potential during the tachycardia are important, and when such a potential is detected, then it should be examined whether concealed entrainment with rapid pacing can be fulfilled or not.

3.7.2 Manifest Entrainment

As compared with concealed entrainment, the role of manifest entrainment in identifying the target ablation site is limited. So far, manifest entrainment was reported to be useful in ablating ATP-sensitive atrial tachycardia (ATP-AT) originating from the AV node vicinity [15, 16].

An example of entrainment and ablation of ATP-AT is shown in Fig 3.9 [16]. TCL is 420 ms and CARTO mapping during the tachycardia revealed focal activation in the RA with the EAS being 8 mm above the His recording site. Entrainment pacing is done from the anterior RA at a cycle length of 400 ms (Fig 3.9a). The asterisks indicate the last electrograms captured by the last pacing stimulus, occurring at the cycle length of 400 ms. It is noted that some of the RA sites are activated antidromically (indicated by black asterisks), while the others including the His bundle recording site and coronary sinus are orthodromically with long conduction intervals (indicated by red asterisks). Thus, in one paced beat, two wavefronts, antidromic and orthodromic, are present, and fusion is likely to be present, indicating manifest entrainment. This suggests the presence of the SCZ between the pacing site and the His bundle recording site and EAS (Fig 3.9b). Radio frequency energy was applied to the SCZ, which resulted in termination of the tachycardia. The fluoroscopy image showed the ablation site remote from the His bundle recording site.

Disclosure Both authors have nothing to disclose in relation to this article.

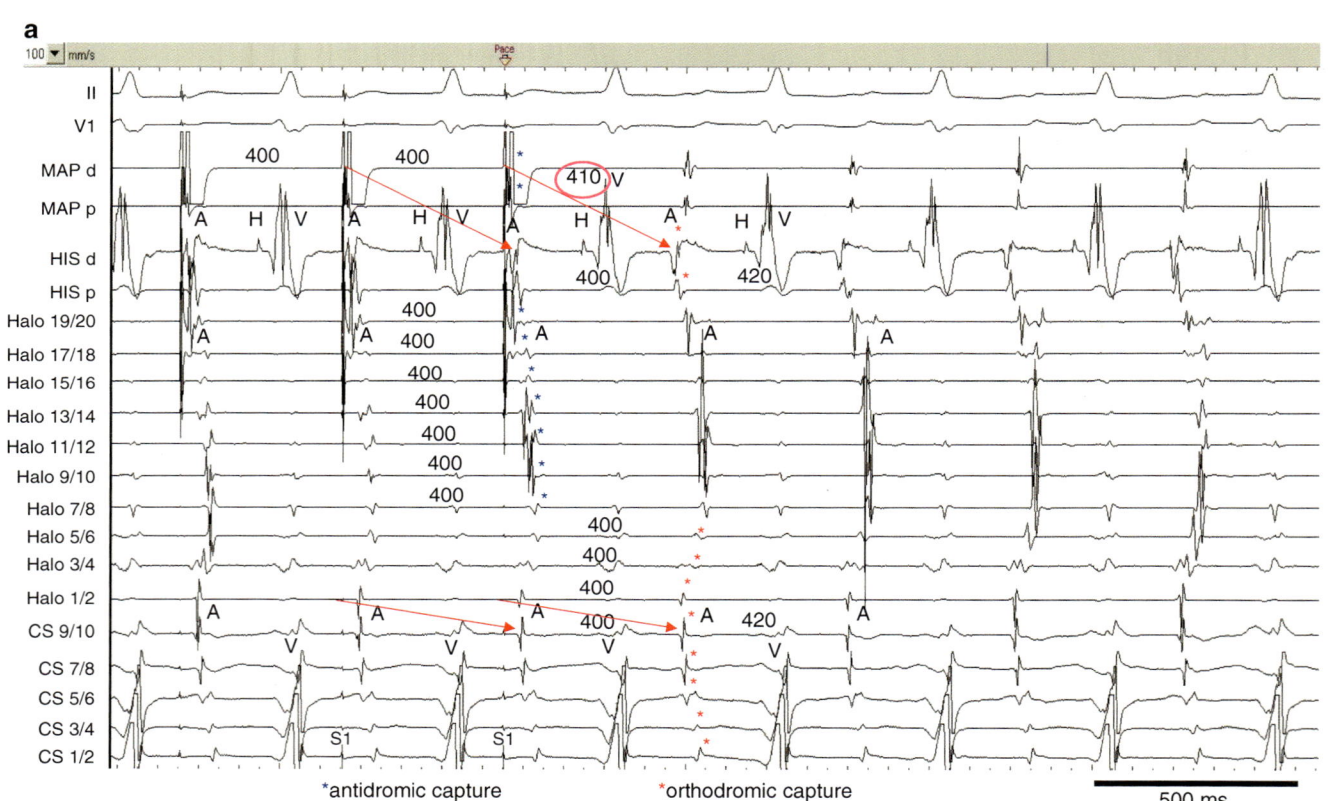

Fig 3.9 Entrainment and ablation of ATP-sensitive atrial tachycardia (ATP-AT) originating from the atrioventricular node vicinity [16]. Panel **a**, manifest entrainment with pacing done at the right anterior right atrium (RA). Halo catheter was placed around the tricuspid annulus. See text for discussion. *MAPd* and *MAPp* electrograms recorded from the distal and proximal pairs of the electrode placed at the right anterior RA. *CS* coronary sinus. Panel **b**, application of radio frequency energy (RF) to a site between the right anterior RA (manifest entrainment site) and earliest activation site (EAS) close to the His bundle recording site where slow conduction zone (SCZ) was suggested to be present. Tachycardia was terminated 8 s after RF application. Fluoroscopic images in the *right* (RAO) and left anterior oblique projections (LAO) show the position of ablation catheter (ABL) relative to the His bundle electrogram recording catheter (His)

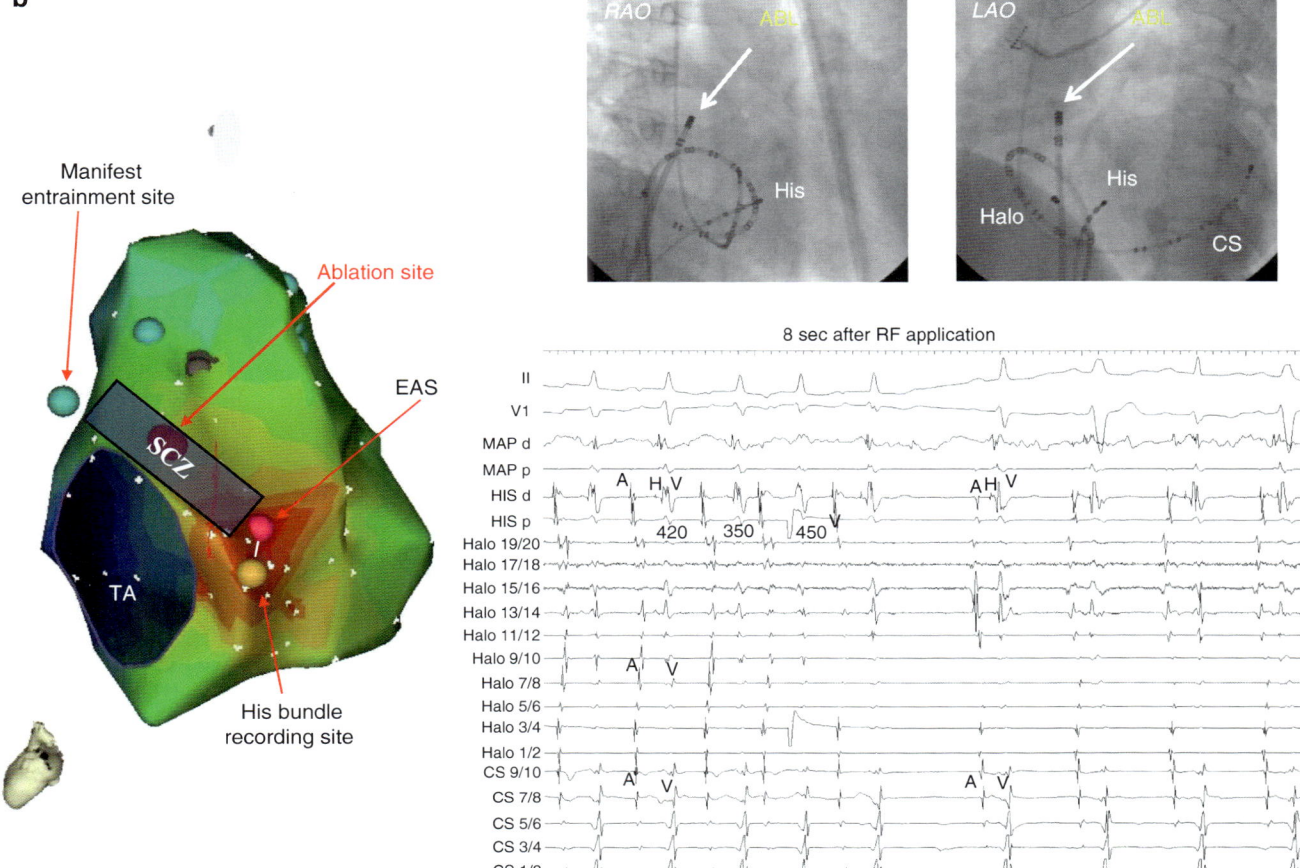

Fig 3.9 (continued)

References

1. Waldo AL, MacLean WA, Karp RB, et al. Entrainment and interruption of atrial flutter with atrial pacing: studies in man following open heart surgery. Circulation. 1977;56:737–45.
2. Waldo AL, Plumb VJ, Arciniegas JG, et al. Transient entrainment and interruption of the atrioventricular bypass type of paroxysmal atrial tachycardia. A model for understanding and identifying reentrant arrhythmias. Circulation. 1983;67:73–83.
3. Waldo AL, Henthorn RW, Plumb VJ, MacLean WA. Demonstration of the mechanism of transient entrainment and interruption of ventricular tachycardia with rapid atrial pacing. J Am Coll Cardiol. 1984;3:422–30.
4. Henthorn RW, Okumura K, Olshansky B, et al. A fourth criterion for transient entrainment. The electrogram equivalent of progressive fusion. Circulation. 1988;77:1003–12.
5. Okumura K, Henthorn RW, Epstein AE, et al. Further observations on transient entrainment. Importance of pacing site and properties of the components of the reentry circuit. Circulation. 1985;72:1293–307.
6. Okumura K, Olshansky B, Henthorn RW, et al. Demonstration of the presence of slow conduction during sustained ventricular tachycardia in man. Use of transient entrainment of the tachycardia. Circulation. 1987;75:369–78.
7. Okumura K, Matsuyama K, Miyagi H, et al. Entrainment of idiopathic ventricular tachycardia of left ventricular origin with evidence for reentry with an area of slow conduction and effect of verapamil. Am J Cardiol. 1988;62:727–32.
8. Olshansky B, Okumura K, Hess PG, et al. Use of procainamide with rapid atrial pacing for successful conversion of atrial flutter to sinus rhythm. J Am Coll Cardiol. 1988;11:359–64.
9. Okumura K, Honda T, Nishigami K, Hayasaki K. Facilitation of localized conduction block with procainamide during entrainment of sustained ventricular tachycardia. Am Heart J. 1989;118:630–2.
10. Olshansky B, Okumura K, Hess PG, Waldo AL. Demonstration of an area of slow conduction in human atrial flutter. J Am Coll Cardiol. 1990;16:1639–48.
11. Okumura K, Yamabe H, Tsuchiya T, et al. Characteristics of slow conduction zone demonstrated during entrainment of idiopathic ventricular tachycardia of left ventricular origin. Am J Cardiol. 1996;77:379–83.

12. Tsuchiya T, Okumura K, Honda T, et al. Effects of verapamil and lidocaine on two components of the re-entry circuit of verapamil-sensitive idiopathic left ventricular tachycardia. J Am Coll Cardiol. 2001;37:1415–21.
13. Stevenson WG, Khan H, Sager P, et al. Identification of reentry circuit sites during mapping and radiofrequency ablation of ventricular tachycardia late after myocardial infarction. Circulation. 1993;88:1647–70.
14. Bogun F, Bahu M, Knight BP, et al. Comparison of effective and ineffective target sites that demonstrate concealed entrainment in patients with coronary artery disease undergoing radiofrequency ablation of ventricular tachycardia. Circulation. 1997;95:183–90.
15. Yamabe H, Okumura K, Morihisa K, et al. Demonstration of anatomical reentrant tachycardia circuit in verapamil-sensitive atrial tachycardia originating from the vicinity of the atrioventricular node. Heart Rhythm. 2012;9:1475–83.
16. Okumura K, Sasaki S, Kimura M, et al. Usefulness of combined CARTO electroanatomical mapping and manifest entrainment in ablating adenosine triphosphate-sensitive atrial tachycardia originating from the atrioventricular node vicinity. J Arrhythm. 2016;32:133–40.
17. Stevenson WG, Friedman PL, Sager PT, et al. Exploring postinfarction reentrant ventricular tachycardia with entrainment mapping. J Am Coll Cardiol. 1997;29:1180–9.
18. Kinjo T, Sasaki S, Kimura M, et al. Long postpacing interval after entrainment of tachycardia including a slow conduction zone within the circuit. J Cardiovasc Electrophysiol. 2016;27:923–9.
19. El-Shalakany A, Hadjis T, Papageorgiou P, et al. Entrainment/mapping criteria for the prediction of termination of ventricular tachycardia by single radiofrequency lesion in patients with coronary artery disease. Circulation 1999;99:2283-2289.

Para-Hisian Pacing

Kenzo Hirao

Keywords

Supraventricular tachycardia · Para-Hisian pacing · Atrioventricular accessory pathway · Atrioventricular node

4.1 Introduction

The accurate diagnosis of supraventricular tachycardias (SVTs) is crucial for the successful catheter ablation. To differentiate these SVTs, several pacing maneuvers are useful in the invasive electrophysiological (EP) study.

The para-Hisian (PH) pacing technique is employed to identify the route of retrograde electrical conduction from the ventricle to the atrium. It has been considered as one of the reliable tools to establish whether a paraseptal atrioventricular (AV) accessory pathway (AP) is present or absent. Proper interpretation of the PH pacing, however, requires a systemic approach and an understanding of the potential pitfalls.

4.2 Concept of Para-Hisian Pacing

There are three factors affecting the ventricular-atrial (V-A) conduction in patients with Wolff-Parkinson-White (WPW) syndrome, which include the pacing site in the ventricle, pacing cycle length, and pacing stimulus strength.

As shown in Fig. 4.1, in a case with only retrograde conduction over the AV node, a high output pacing stimulus captures both the right ventricle (RV) and His bundle; hence, a low output pacing stimulus captures only the RV, which changes the stimulus-atrial (S-A) interval dramatically.

K. Hirao, M.D.
Cardiovascular Medicine, Tokyo Medical and Dental University, Tokyo, Japan
e-mail: 0160.cvm@tmd.ac.jp

On the other hand, in a WPW syndrome case, either a high output or low output pacing stimulus causes a short S-A interval because the activation propagates similarly to the ventricular end of the AP as in Fig. 4.1b.

4.3 Techniques for Para-Hisian Pacing

This maneuver is not possible in cases with an absence of retrograde conduction, and in whom an isoproterenol administration should be considered to enhance the retrograde conduction over a concealed AV accessory pathway or the AV node.

4.3.1 Pacing Technique

For PH pacing, a deflectable quadripolar catheter is positioned at the anterobasal right ventricular septum 1–2 cm anterior and apical to the His bundle best recording site, where a tiny His bundle potential can be recorded from the distal bipolar electrodes.

The pacing is performed at a cycle length just shorter than the native rhythm, and the pacing output is started from a high value (20–40 mA), which may produce a narrower QRS complex indicating that the high output pacing has captured both the His bundle and local RV myocardium, HB/RV capture.

Once having successfully achieved producing a narrower QRS complex, the pacing strength is decreased gradually until the QRS complex becomes wider, which indicates that the pacing is capturing only the RV septum (=only RV capture).

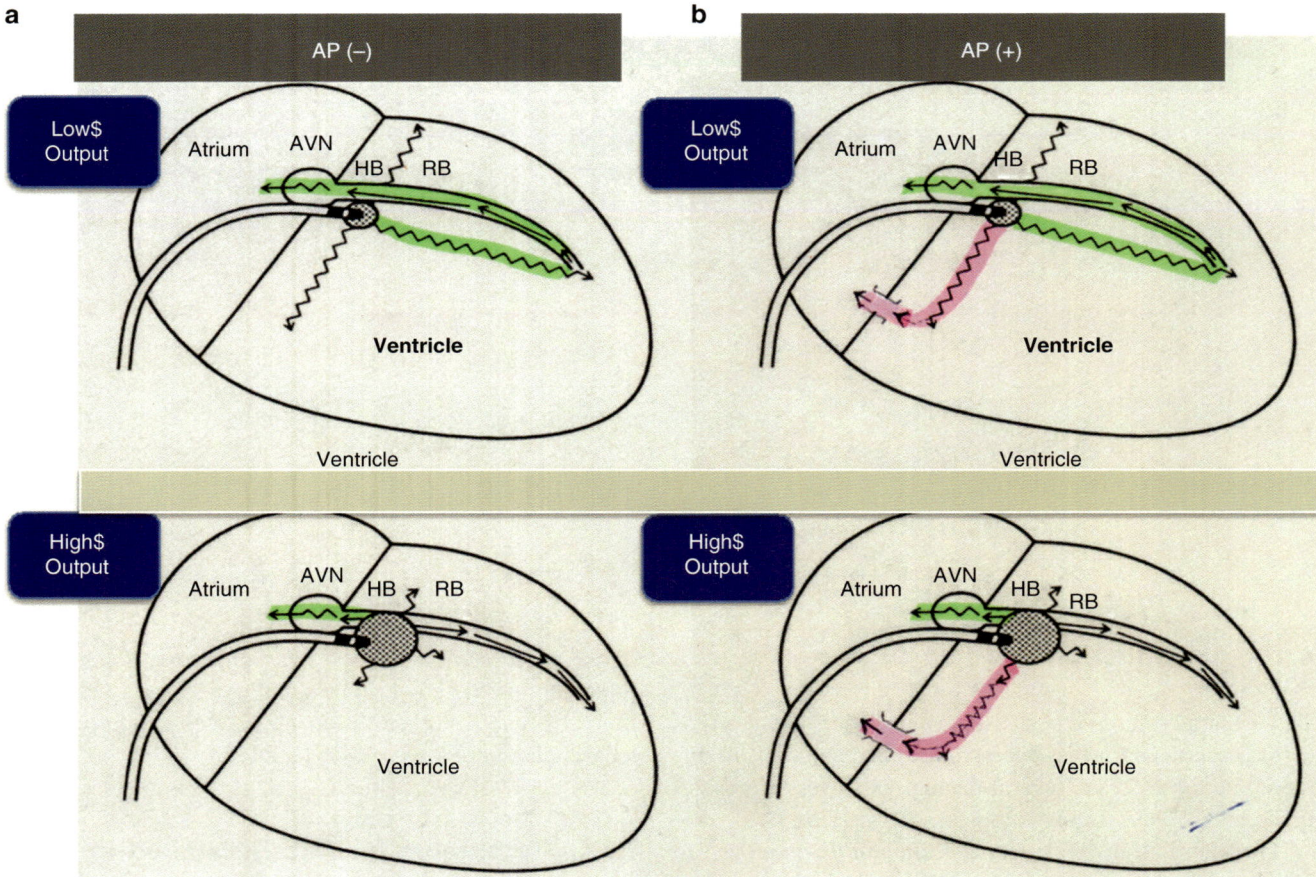

Fig. 4.1 Schema of the intracardiac propagation during (**a**, **b**) high and low pacing output at the para-Hisian site

4.3.2 Recording Technique

As in the standard EP study, at least three multielectrode catheters are positioned in the right atrial appendage, His bundle region, and coronary sinus to map the retrograde atrial activation in both the right and left atrium.

4.4 Interpretation of Para-Hisian Pacing

The response to PH pacing is determined by the change in the following variables between HB/RV capture and only RV capture: (1) the atrial activation sequence, (2) the S-A interval, and (3) the local V-A interval recorded at the earliest atrial activation site. If the His bundle-atrial (H-A) interval can be recorded, the H-A interval is also measured for a more detailed interpretation. The schema for the interpretation is depicted in Fig. 4.2. Five patterns of response to PH pacing are recognized using two of the variables mentioned above, and by adding the H-A interval, the variable responses are classified in more detail into the seven patterns.

4.4.1 Case Presentation

4.4.1.1 Case 1: 68-Year-Old Female – Concealed WPW Syndrome

During RV pacing, the earliest atrial activation is recorded in the HB region, and the V-A conduction demonstrates no decremental properties as in Fig. 4.3b, c. PH pacing is interpreted as retrograde conduction over a septal AV accessory pathway as in Fig. 4.4.

4.4.1.2 Case 2: 50-Year-Old Male – Permanent Form of Junctional Reentrant Tachycardia (PJRT)

SVT is induced by RV pacing and the atrial activation sequence during the SVT is identical to that during RV pacing as shown in Fig. 4.5. Before the catheter ablation, PH pacing demonstrates the presence of the retrograde VA conduction over a slow Kent bundle because the retrograde atrial sequence is identical, and the SA intervals are identical between the narrow and wide QRS complexed as shown in Fig. 4.6a. After ablation, the PH pacing demonstrates VA

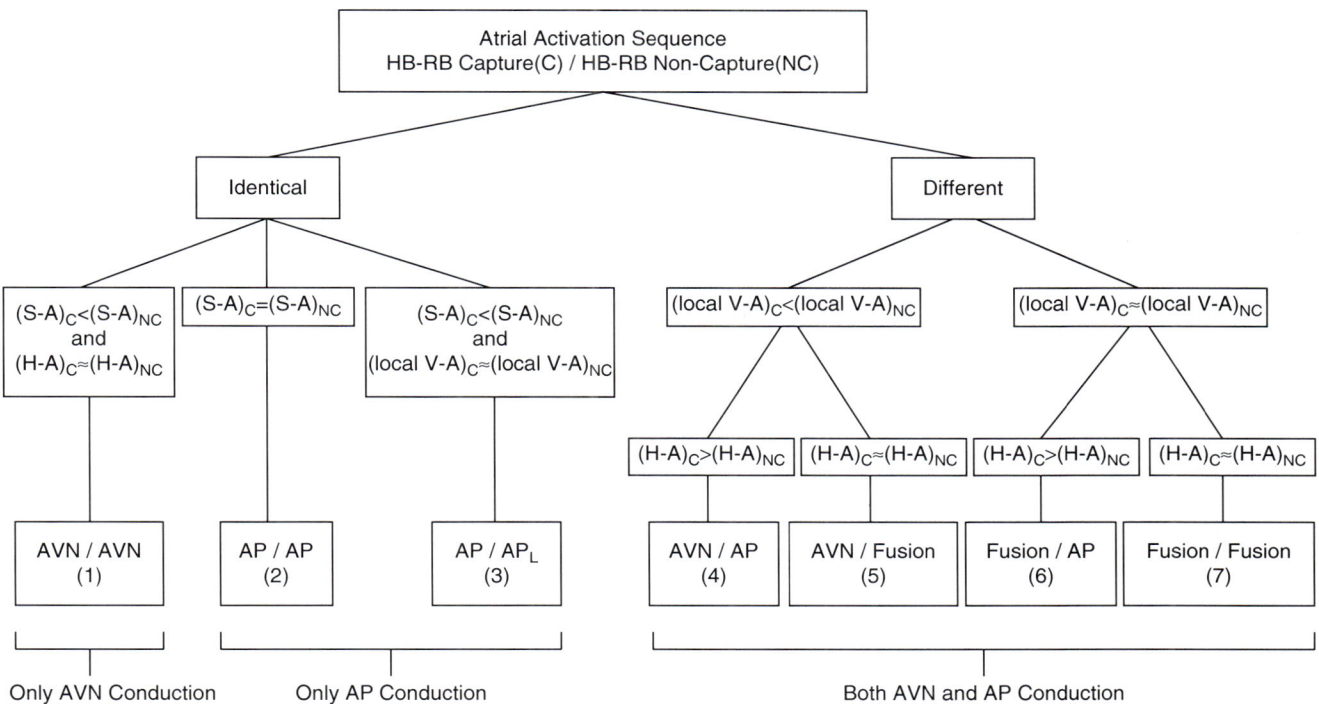

Fig. 4.2 Diagram of the interpretation of para-Hisian pacing [1]

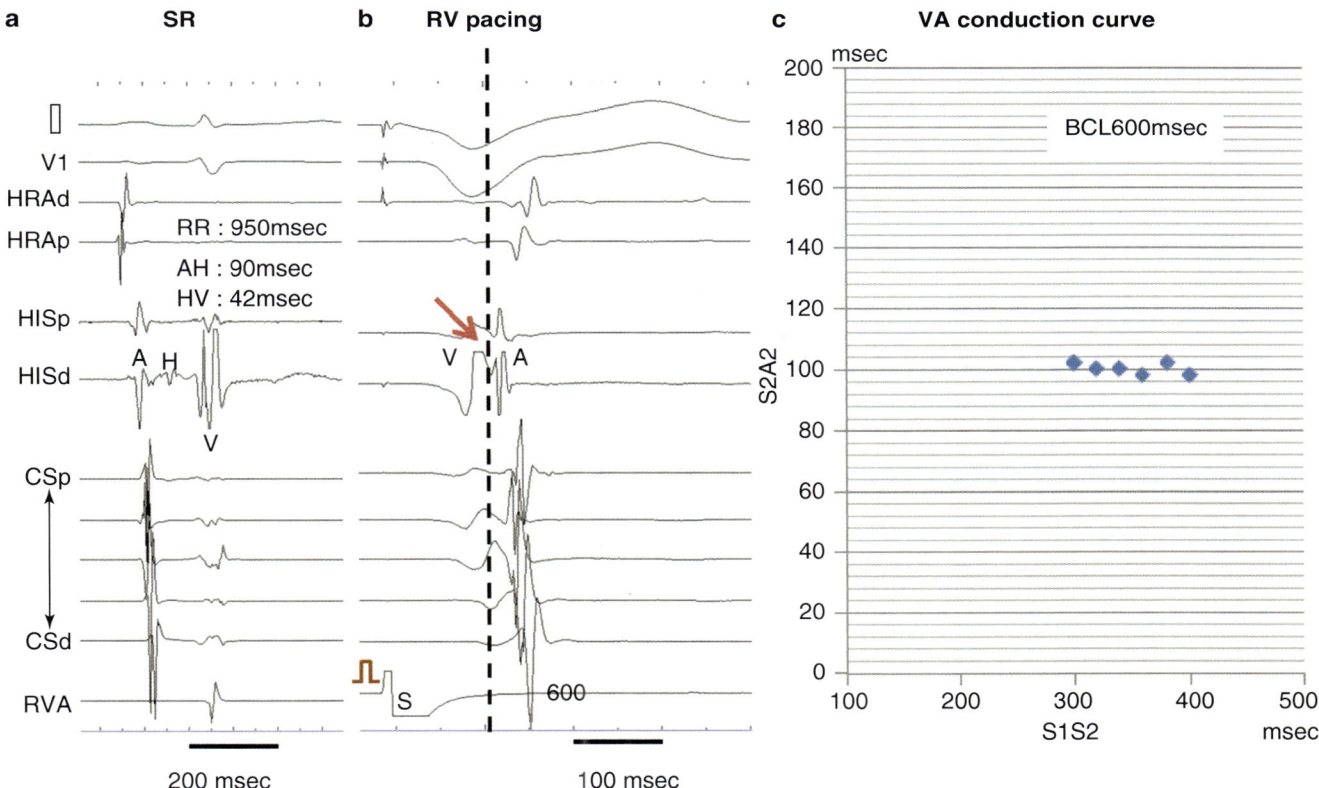

Fig. 4.3 Intracardiac recordings and the V-A conduction curve

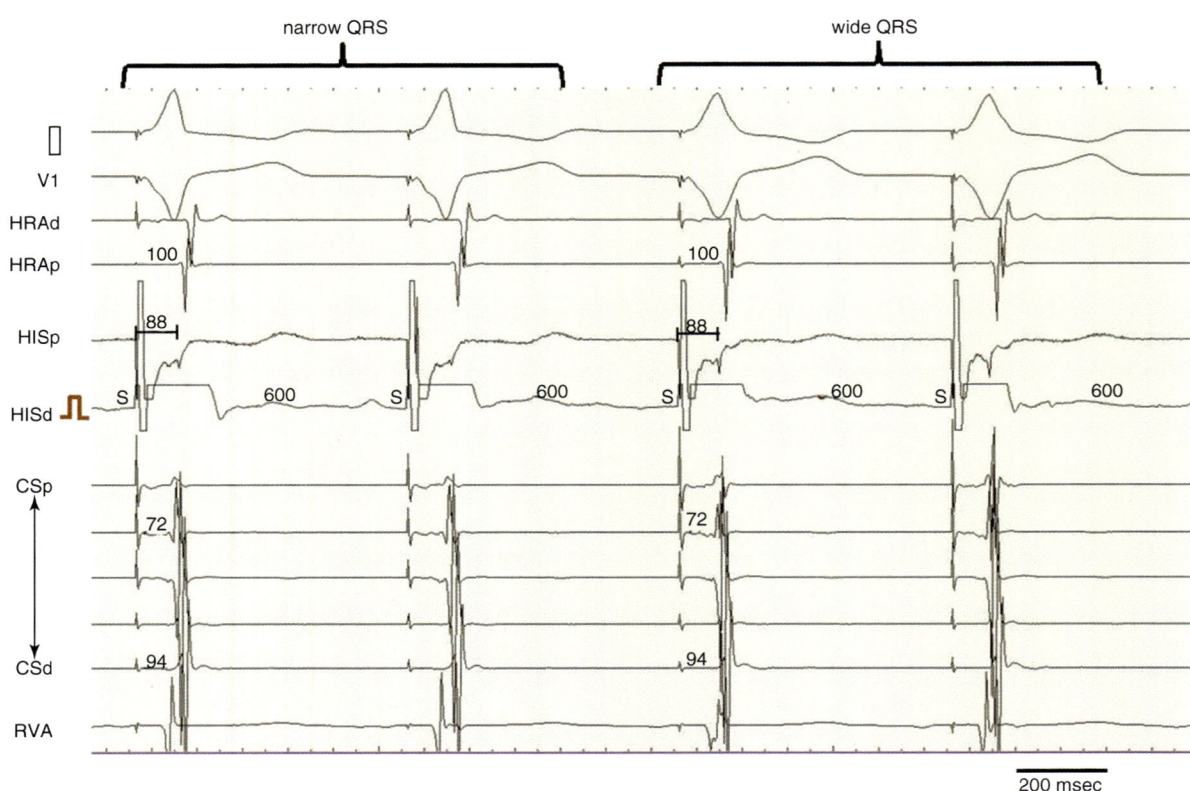

Fig. 4.4 Para-Hisian pacing in concealed septal AP case

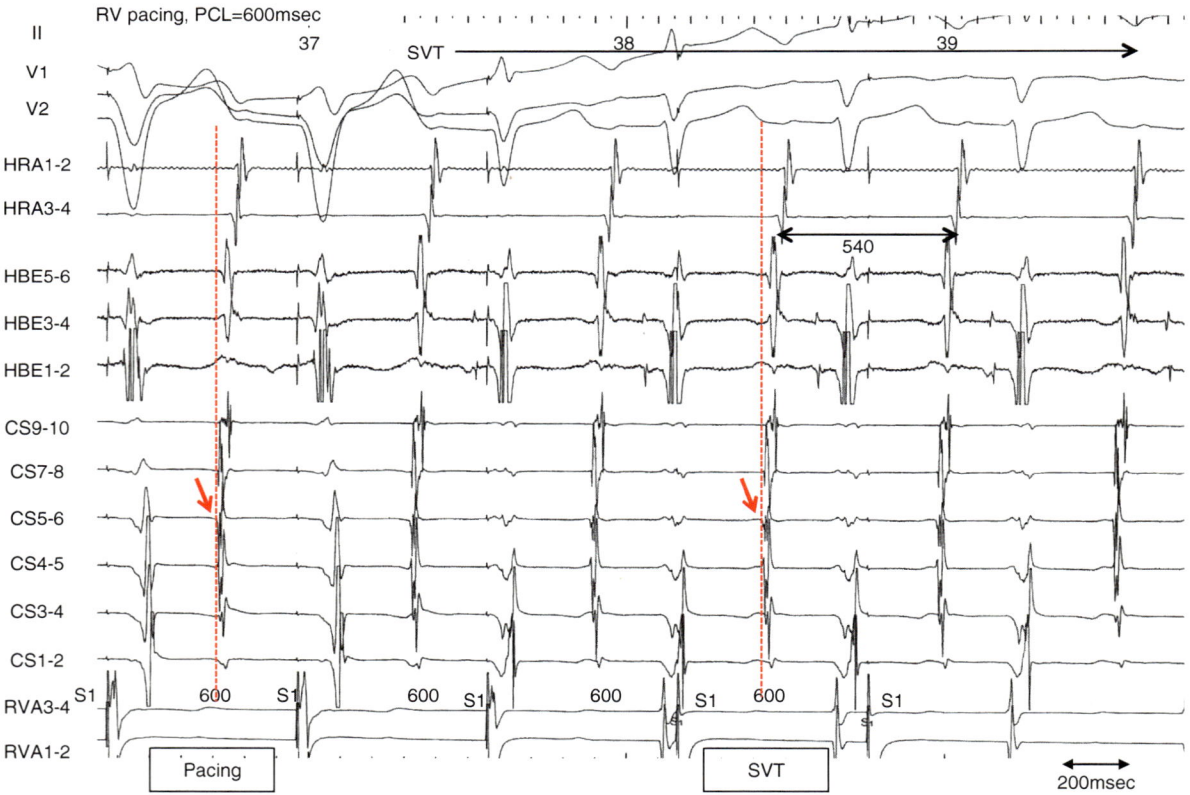

Fig. 4.5 Induction of PJRT during ventricular burst pacing

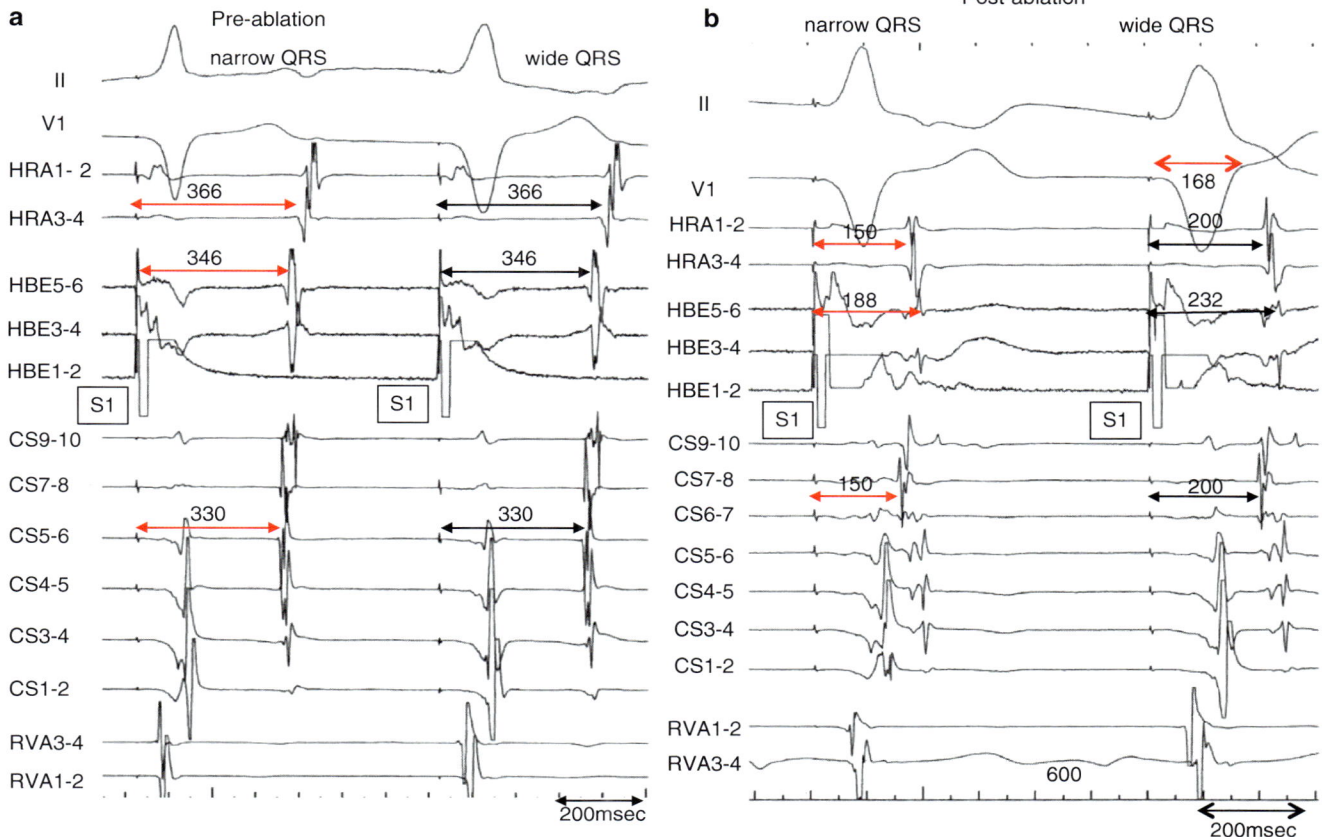

Fig. 4.6 (**a**, **b**) PHP after ablation

conduction over the fast AV nodal pathway only during an isoproterenol infusion (Fig. 4.6b).

4.4.1.3 Case 3: 37-Year-Old Female – Slow-/Fast-Type and Slow-/Slow-Type AVNRT

In an ECG recorded during palpitations, a SVT transforms to another form of SVT. A SVT is induced when at jump-up of the AH interval occurs during atrial extrastimulus pacing. A slow-/fast-type AV nodal reentrant tachycardia transforms to a slow-/slow-type AVNRT as in Fig. 4.7. During PH pacing with 500 msec pacing cycle length, the atrial activation sequence is identical and the S-A interval prolongs during a wide QRS complex, and the earliest atrial activation site is in the HB region, which is interpreted as V-A conduction occurs over the fast AV nodal pathway as in Fig. 4.8a. Of note, PH pacing at 20 ms shorter pacing cycle length demonstrates the presence of retrograde slow AV nodal pathway conduction as in Fig. 4.8b.

4.5 Limitations

4.5.1 RBBB

In a patient with right bundle branch block (RBBB), high output PH pacing does not produce a narrow QRS complex. However, the V-A interval will behave similarly as in those without RBBB [2].

4.5.2 Left Lateral AP

In patients with the AV accessory pathway located far from the septum, such as a left free wall AP, the local ventricle near the ventricular end of the AP may not be affected by high or low output PH pacing. In such a case, the S-A interval does not become shortened even by high output PH pacing, resulting in an AV nodal pattern.

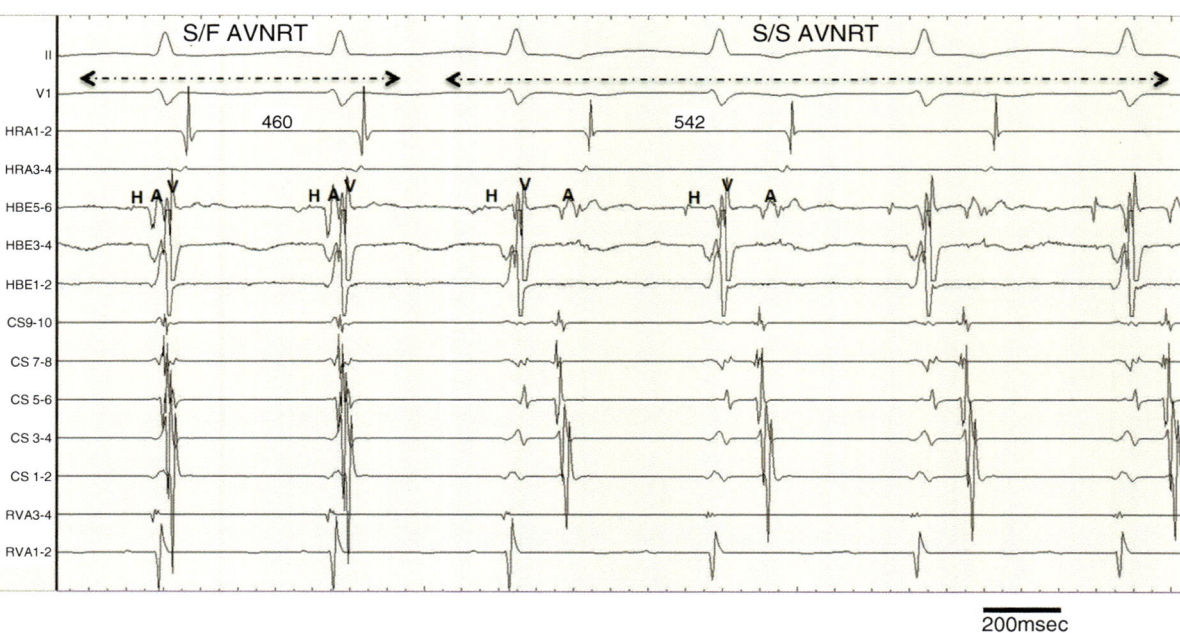

Fig. 4.7 Transformation of the S-/F-type AVNRT to an S-/S-type AVNRT

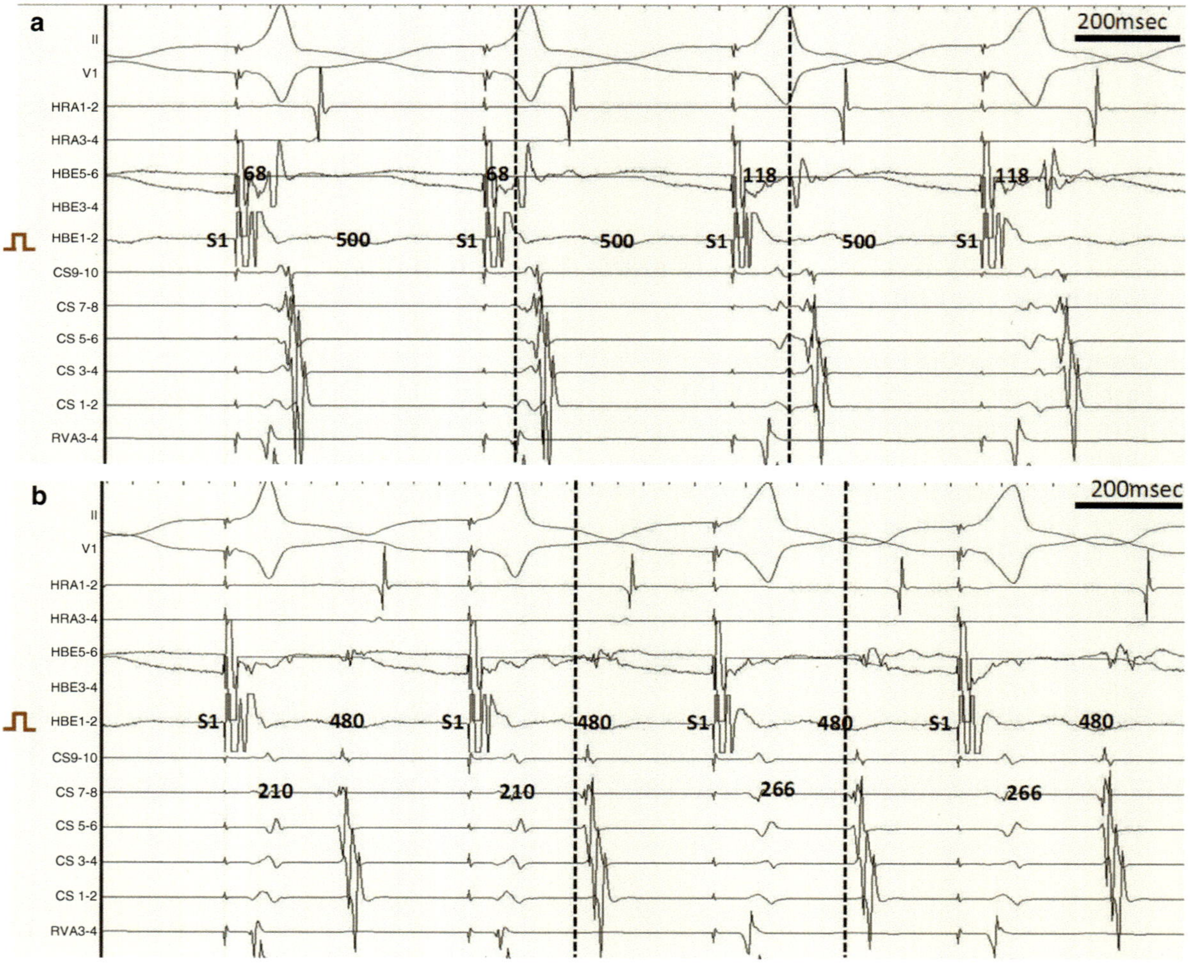

Fig. 4.8 (**a**, **b**) Para-Hisian pacing under different pacing cycle lengths

4.5.3 PJRT

In patients with PJRT, in one thirds, the presence of an AP cannot be diagnosed because of the long conduction time over the slow conducting AP. If the V-A conduction over the AV node is absent or its refractory period is longer than the AP and the PH pacing period is shorter than that, PH pacing effectively demonstrates the presence of an AP.

4.6 Summary

PH pacing, which is a valuable diagnostic pacing method for demonstration of the presence and absence of an AV accessory pathway, needs proper pacing skill and techniques as well as an accurate knowledge about its interpretation.

References

1. Hirao K, Otomo K, wang X, et al. Para-Hisian pacing: a new method for differentiating retrograde conduction over an accessory AV pathway from conduction over the AV node. Circulation. 1996;94:1027–35.
2. Sheldon SH, Asirvatham SJ, McLeod CJ. Parahisian pacing: technique, utility, and pitfalls. J Interv Card Electrophysiol. 2014;40:105–16.

5. Entrainment Pacing for Differential Diagnosis of Supraventricular Tachycardias

Mitsunori Maruyama

Keywords
Supraventricular tachycardia • Differential diagnosis • Entrainment • pacing

5.1 Introduction

Supraventricular tachycardia (SVT) is a common cardiac tachyarrhythmia with the estimated prevalence and incidence of 2.25/1000 persons and 35/100,000 person-years, respectively [1]. Various cardiac arrhythmias underlie regular narrow QRS complex SVT, including physiological sinus tachycardia, inappropriate sinus tachycardia, sinoatrial nodal reentrant tachycardia, atrial tachycardia (AT), orthodromic reciprocating tachycardia (ORT) using an accessory pathway (AP), atrioventricular nodal reentrant tachycardia (AVNRT), and junctional tachycardia. Clinical characteristics and surface electrocardiogram are useful for differential diagnosis of SVT, but an invasive electrophysiologic study is usually required for a definite diagnosis of the three most common SVT, namely, AT, ORT, and AVNRT. A correct diagnosis is of particular importance because catheter ablation now offers a definitive cure in these SVT. This chapter addresses how to distinguish among AT, ORT, and AVNRT in the electrophysiologic laboratory.

Knight et al. [2] prospectively evaluated diagnostic values of tachycardia features and pacing maneuvers for SVT. They demonstrated that those findings rarely provide a final diagnosis when used individually. In practice, false-positive and false-negative findings from conventional diagnostic techniques cause conflicting results that occasionally mislead us in the differential diagnosis. However, several more specific techniques have recently been reported. Incorporating the newer pacing techniques will allow us to make the differential diagnosis more rapid and conclusive. Here, a comprehensive stepwise approach using entrainment pacing maneuvers is proposed for differentiating AT, ORT, and AVNRT.

5.2 Difficulties with Diagnosis of Atypical SVT

In typical SVT, differential diagnosis is generally straightforward. However, this is not necessarily the case for diagnosis of SVT with atypical electrophysiologic features. For instance, a poor retrograde conduction at baseline suggests AT, but it does not always exclude AVNRT and ORT [2]. If the atrial activation sequences during both ventricular pacing and SVT are eccentric, ORT is the most likely diagnosis. However, AVNRT can also display an eccentric atrial activation during ventricular pacing and SVT [3]. If the atrial activation sequence is eccentric during SVT but concentric during ventricular pacing, one may consider AT. However, an eccentric retrograde activation via AP can be concealed during ventricular pacing in ORT patients with a concomitant retrograde conduction via the AV node. A short septal VA interval (<70 ms) during SVT indicates typical AVNRT [2], but it can also occur in AT with a prolonged AV conduction and in ORT with a left-sided AP [4]. In fact, the presence of a dual AV nodal physiology and AP offers no guarantee of AVNRT and ORT, respectively. Diagnostic pacing maneuvers help correctly diagnose SVT with such atypical electrophysiologic findings.

M. Maruyama, M.D., Ph.D., F.H.R.S.
Department of Cardiovascular Medicine, Nippon Medical School Chiba Hokusoh Hospital, 1715 Kamakari, Inzai, Chiba 270-1694, Japan
e-mail: maru@nms.ac.jp

5.3 Diagnostic Algorithm for SVT with 1:1 AV Relationship (Fig. 5.1)

In this section, diagnostic approaches to SVT with a 1:1 AV relationship are discussed. The differential diagnoses of SVT with AV block or VA block are separately described later in this chapter. Figure 5.1 shows a diagnostic algorithm that is composed of three steps. First, AT is distinguished from ORT and AVNRT (Step I). Next, ORT is differentiated from AVNRT (Step II). In case of ORT using a septal AP, an additional step is necessary to determine whether the AP is atrioventricular (ORT-AV) or node-ventricular/node-fascicular (ORT-NV/NF) (Step III).

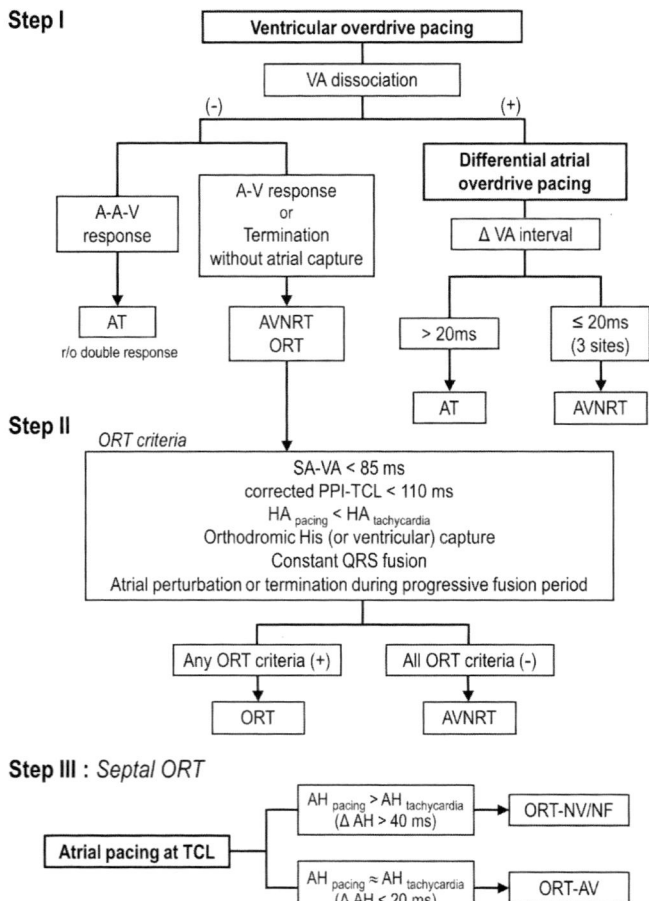

Fig. 5.1 Stepwise approach for differential diagnosis of narrow QRS complex supraventricular tachycardias with a 1:1 AV relationship. Pacing maneuvers necessary to perform are shown in *bold*. *AT* atrial tachycardia, *AH* atrial-His interval, *AV* atrioventricular, *AVNRT* atrioventricular nodal reentrant tachycardia, *HA* His-atrial interval, *NV/NF* node-ventricular/node-fascicular, *ORT* orthodromic reciprocating tachycardia, *PPI* post-pacing interval, *SA* stimulus-atrial interval, *TCL* tachycardia cycle length, *VA* ventriculoatrial. See text for details

5.3.1 Step I: AT Versus ORT/AVNRT

The principal maneuver for the SVT diagnosis is ventricular overdrive pacing (VOP) from the right ventricular apex (RVA) during SVT that is typically performed at the pacing cycle length (PCL) of 10–40 ms below the tachycardia cycle length (TCL). The VOP results in three patterns of response: (1) successful entrainment of the SVT with 1:1 VA conduction, (2) termination of the SVT, and (3) inability to affect the SVT with VA dissociation.

If SVT is successfully entrained (all the atrial electrograms are required to be accelerated to the PCL), the electrogram sequence after cessation of VOP is useful to distinguish AT from ORT and AVNRT. Knight et al. reported that an atrial-atrial-ventricular (A-A-V) sequence after VOP was specific for AT [2, 5]. However, we should be aware that this criterion demands special attention. A pseudo A-A-V response can occur when a decremental conduction property in the retrograde limb of ORT or AVNRT is prominent although it is distinguishable by careful analysis of the last captured atrial electrograms (the interval between the first and second atrial electrograms after VOP coincides with the PCL, and the activation sequences of the first and second atrial electrograms are identical). However, a true A-A-V response can also occur even in AVNRT and ORT by the phenomenon called "double atrial response," especially when they are presented as a long-RP tachycardia [6–8]. Therefore, an additional diagnostic work-up is needed if the double atrial response is suspected.

An atrial-ventricular (A-V) sequence after successful entrainment of SVT by VOP excludes AT. Also, if the SVT is terminated during VOP without any perturbation of the atrial cycle length, AT is excluded. In either case, we can proceed to the next step to differentiate ORT and AVNRT (see Step II).

If VOP does not affect SVT (i.e., VA dissociation), implying that the ventricle is not a part of the SVT circuit, ORT is excluded. To distinguish AT from AVNRT in this situation, examining whether the atrial activation is linked to the ventricular activation (i.e., VA linking) is helpful. VA linking can be assessed by atrial overdrive pacing (AOP) that is independent of the presence or absence of VA conduction. Obviously, ORT and AVNRT have VA linking, while AT does not. In the conventional method to evaluate VA linking, AOP is performed until SVT is entrained (the ventricular cycle length must be synchronized to the PCL with 1:1 AV conduction). If the post-pacing VA interval (the interval from the last entrained ventricular electrogram to the first atrial electrogram after cessation of AOP) is fixed when compared to the VA interval during the tachycardia, the presence of VA linking is suggested. However, this conventional method has limited sensitivity and specificity [2] because it cannot exclude a coincidental match of those VA intervals in the absence of VA linking, or a longer post-pacing VA interval due to a retrograde decremental conduction even in the presence of VA linking. To overcome such limitations, differential AOP method is useful for the assessment of VA linking (Fig. 5.2), where the post-pacing VA interval is measured from two different atrial sites (typically, the right atrial appendage and proximal coronary sinus) at the same PCL. Then, the difference in the post-pacing VA intervals between the different pacing sites is calculated (delta-VA interval). If the delta-VA interval is >20 ms, AT is diagnosed with 100% specificity [9]. Because the delta-VA interval can also coincidentally display a small value in AT patients, another pacing site should be added (typically, the distal coronary sinus) when the delta-VA interval from the two atrial sites is ≤20 ms. If the delta-VA interval remains ≤20 ms, AVNRT is diagnosed in cases with VA dissociation during VOP. If the delta-VA interval from the three atrial sites becomes >20 ms, a diagnosis of AT is made. The differential AOP is also useful for diagnosis of AT when the double atrial response is suspected as the cause of an A-A-V response after VOP.

5.3.2 Step II: ORT Versus AVNRT

After exclusion of AT in Step I, the next step is differentiation between ORT and AVNRT. Several criteria for VOP from the RVA have been reported for that purpose. One of the most validated criteria is the difference between the post-pacing interval (PPI) and TCL (PPI − TCL). As a rule, the PPI − TCL reflects the proximity of the pacing site to the reentrant circuit. Since the RVA is closer to the reentrant circuit for ORT than AVNRT, the PPI − TCL should be a smaller value in ORT. For the same reason, the stimulus-atrial (SA) interval during VOP from the RVA is expected to more closely approximate the VA interval during tachycardia in ORT, while the SA interval minus tachycardia VA interval (SA − VA) should be larger in AVNRT because the VA interval during tachycardia is a pseudo-interval (simultaneous conduction from the lower turnaround site of the AVNRT circuit toward the atrium and ventricle) but the SA interval during VOP is a true interval (sequential conduction from the ventricle to the atrium) in AVNRT. Michaud et al. [10] first reported the usefulness of the PPI − TCL and SA − VA for differentiation of AVNRT from ORT. They showed that all AVNRT and none of ORT using a septal AP had the SA − VA > 85 ms and PPI − TCL > 115 ms (Fig. 5.3).

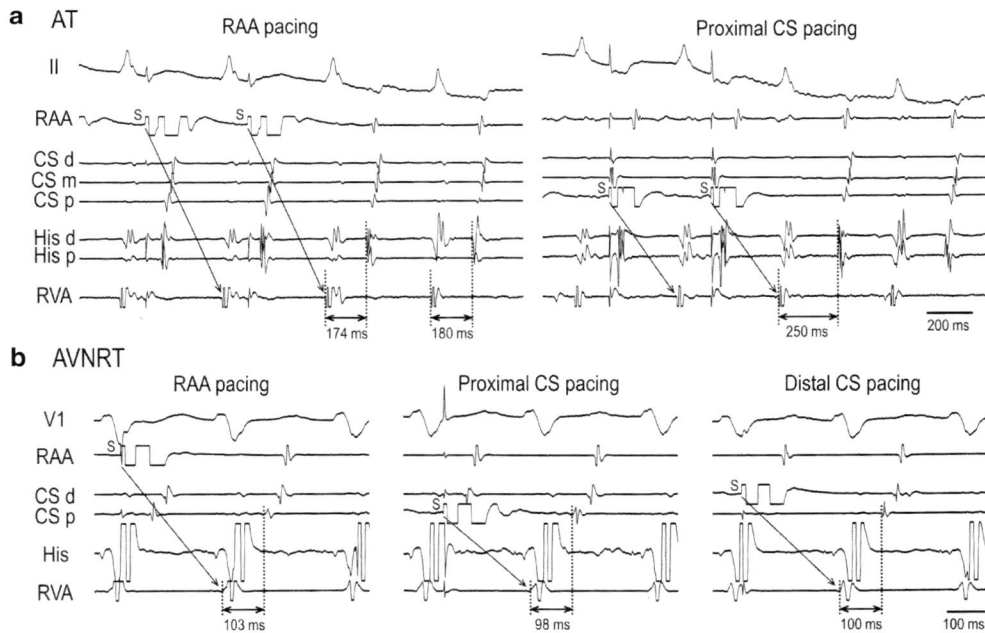

Fig. 5.2 Differential atrial overdrive pacing in a patient with AT (**a**) and AVNRT (**b**). In the AT patient, the post-pacing VA interval was 174 and 250 ms after pacing from the right atrial appendage (RAA) and proximal coronary sinus (CS), respectively. Thus, the delta-VA interval was 76 ms in this case. Note that the post-pacing VA interval from the RAA pacing was coincidentally similar to the VA interval of the AT. In the AVNRT patient, the differences in the post-pacing VA interval among triple sites (i.e., the RAA, proximal and distal CS) were small, and the delta-VA interval was 5 ms. *RVA* right ventricular apex (Modified from Maruyama et al. [9], with permission)

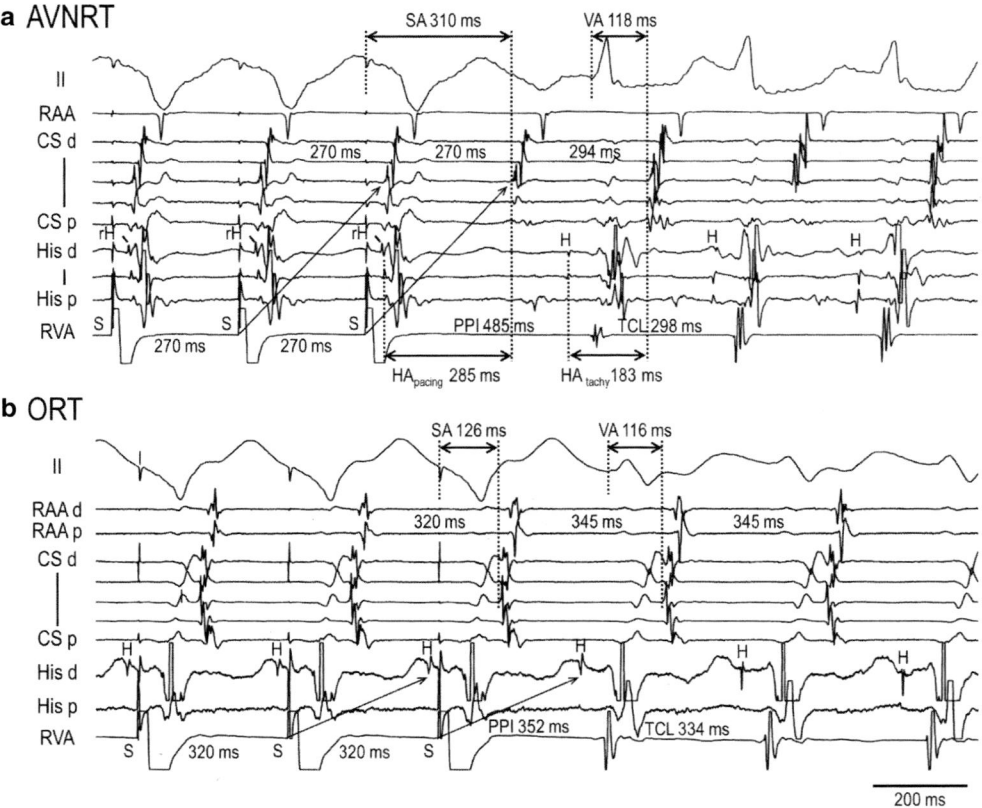

Fig. 5.3 Various diagnostic criteria after ventricular overdrive pacing. (**a**) Fast-slow type AVNRT. The electrogram sequence after pacing was an A-A-V, but the last captured atrial electrogram was the second one due to decremental conduction in the retrograde slow pathway. Therefore, this pattern was considered as an A-V response, which excludes AT (i.e., a pseudo A-A-V response). The difference between the stimulus-atrial and ventriculoatrial intervals (SA − VA) was 192 ms, and the difference between the post-pacing interval and tachycardia cycle length (PPI − TCL) was 187 ms, both of which are consistent with AVNRT. The His bundle electrograms were retrogradely captured (rH), and the His-atrial interval was longer during pacing than during tachycardia ($HA_{pacing} > HA_{tachy}$). (**b**) ORT. The activation sequence after pacing was an A-V. The SA − VA and PPI − TCL were 10 and 18 ms, respectively. Note that the His bundle electrograms were orthodromically captured during pacing

Although ORT with a left free-wall AP (i.e., with an eccentric atrial activation), whose reentrant circuit is relatively remote from the RVA, can have the SA − VA > 85 ms and PPI − TCL > 115 ms, these criteria are helpful in diagnosing SVT with a concentric atrial activation in which the differential diagnosis is most important. Gonzalez-Torrecilla et al. [11] reported that some ORT using a septal AP had the PPI − TCL > 115 ms due to a delay in AV nodal conduction during VOP. They demonstrated that if the PPI − TCL was corrected by subtracting the AV nodal delay (the difference between the post-pacing atrial-His [AH] interval and AH interval during tachycardia) from the measured PPI − TCL, all septal ORT had the corrected PPI − TCL < 110 ms. However, these studies did not include ORT using a slowly conducting AP which may also cause a prolongation of the PPI − TCL. Bennett et al. [12] studied 12 patients with a long-RP ORT using a slowly conducting septal AP and found that half of the studied patients had the SA − VA > 85 ms and PPI − TCL > 115 ms due to a conduction delay in the AP. Taken together, if the SA − VA is ≤85 ms or the corrected PPI − TCL is ≤110 ms, ORT is diagnosed, but neither the SA − VA > 85 ms nor corrected PPI − TCL > 110 ms exclude ORT using a slowly conducting AP. Thus, further criteria are needed to cover the limitation of the SA − VA and PPI − TCL.

Another criterion is a comparison between His-atrial (HA) intervals during tachycardia and VOP. This is available if retrograde His bundle electrograms is recorded during VOP. In AVNRT, the His bundle and atrium are activated sequentially during VOP but simultaneously during tachycardia ($HA_{pacing} > HA_{tachycardia}$, Fig. 5.3a). In ORT, however, the His bundle and atrium are activated in parallel during VOP but sequentially during tachycardia ($HA_{pacing} < HA_{tachycardia}$). Therefore, the value of $HA_{pacing} − HA_{tachycardia}$ is positive for AVNRT and negative for ORT [13]. The diagnosis of ORT using this criterion is also affected by a slowly conducting AP which can cause the positive $HA_{pacing} − HA_{tachycardia}$ by a prolongation of the

HA_{pacing} [14]. Thus, the negative $HA_{pacing} - HA_{tachycardia}$ is diagnostic for ORT but the positive $HA_{pacing} - HA_{tachycardia}$ does not completely exclude ORT as is the case in the SA − VA and PPI − TCL criteria.

The His bundle electrogram is orthodromically captured during entrainment of ORT from the RVA, provided that collision of antidromic and orthodromic wavefronts occurs below the site where the His bundle electrogram is recorded (Fig. 5.3b). In contrast, AVNRT can never be entrained unless the His bundle is antidromically activated. Therefore, the orthodromic capture of the His bundle electrogram during VOP is diagnostic for ORT [15]. In theory, a conduction delay in AP does not prevent the His bundle from being orthodromically captured, but the efficacy of this criterion remains to be sufficiently validated in ORT using a slowly conducting AP. One limitation is that the His bundle electrograms need to be recorded during VOP, as with the $HA_{pacing} - HA_{tachycardia}$ criterion.

If the antidromic wavefront collides with the orthodromic wavefront at a ventricular level during VOP, constant QRS fusion occurs during entrainment in ORT (i.e., manifest entrainment). On the other hand, manifest entrainment is never observed in AVNRT, which always shows a fully paced QRS morphology during VOP. Therefore, the constant QRS fusion criterion is specific for ORT without the need for the His bundle recording during VOP although this criterion is less sensitive especially when pacing from the RVA [16].

Traditionally, ventricular extrastimuli during SVT have been used as a standard maneuver to distinguish ORT from AVNRT. Resetting SVT by ventricular extrastimulus delivered at the timing when the His bundle is refractory is a specific finding for ORT. However, failure to reset the SVT does not exclude the presence of AP when the location of the AP is relatively far from the pacing site such as the RVA because the paced wavefront may not just be able to enter the reentrant circuit of ORT. One advantage of entrainment over a single extrastimulus is better capability for the paced wavefront to enter the reentrant circuit particularly when pacing from the remote site. AlMahameed et al. [17] reported that perturbation of atrial timing or tachycardia termination during the transition zone of progressive QRS fusion at the beginning of VOP was diagnostic for ORT. The strength of this criterion is that it is also available when ORT is terminated during VOP. The significance of the QRS fusion during VOP is similar to ventricular extrastimulus delivered when the His bundle is refractory, but this entrainment criterion seems to have a higher sensitivity for ORT. The 100% sensitivity and specificity for distinguishing ORT from AVNRT were reported in another study using an analogous criterion [18]. In AlMahameed's report, the "transition zone" during VOP included fused QRS complexes and the first paced complex with a stable QRS morphology. However, determining the timing when the QRS morphology becomes stable is subjective, and false-positive cases were shown in a subsequent study using this criterion [19]. In our experience with 225 SVT, exclusion of the first stable QRS complex from the "transition zone" makes this criterion 100% specific for ORT although the sensitivity is diminished. Hence, atrial perturbation or tachycardia termination during a progressive fusion period (not including the first stable QRS complex) is used as a criterion for ORT in this algorithm.

In this proposed algorithm, entrainment criteria from the right ventricular base in comparison with those from the RVA (i.e., differential entrainment [20, 21]) are not included because it obviates the need for manipulation of the ventricular catheter, and more importantly, they can be misleading in the presence of retrograde right bundle branch block [22], node-fascicular AP, or long insulated atrioventricular AP [23].

In summary of Step II, every ORT criterion for VOP (SA − VA < 85 ms, corrected PPI − TCL < 110 ms, $HA_{pacing} < HA_{tachycardia}$, orthodromic His bundle electrogram capture, constant QRS fusion, atrial perturbation, or tachycardia termination during a progressive fusion period) is specific with an incomplete sensitivity. If any of these ORT criteria is positive, ORT is diagnosed. Application of multiple criteria overcomes their limited sensitivities. Thus, AVNRT is diagnosed if none of the ORT criteria is observed.

5.3.3 Step III: Septal ORT (ORT-AV Versus ORT-NV/NF)

If Step I and II determine that ORT is responsible for SVT with a concentric atrial activation pattern (septal ORT), ORT using an atrioventricular AP of the septal location is not the only possibility. In case the AP connects the ventricle/fascicle with the AV node, but not with the atrium (i.e., ORT-NV/NF), responses to diagnostic pacing maneuvers also meet the ORT criteria. Since the His bundle and atrium are simultaneously activated from the upper turnaround of the ORT-NV/NF circuit (i.e., the AP insertion site into the AV node), the AH interval during ORT-NV/NF becomes paradoxically short. Ho et al. [7] described that the AH interval during tachycardia ($AH_{tachycardia}$) was >40 ms shorter than the AH interval during atrial pacing at the TCL (AH_{pacing}) in ORT-NV/NF, whereas they were comparable in ORT-AV (the difference between $AH_{tachycardia}$ and AH_{pacing} was <20 ms). This AH behavior of ORT-NV/NF is analogous to that of AVNRT. In AVNRT, the $AH_{pacing} - AH_{tachycardia}$ difference becomes large probably because the presence of an upper common pathway would cause simultaneous activation of the atrium and His bundle from the upper turnaround of the AVNRT circuit in a similar way to ORT-NV/NF [24].

5.4 Diagnostic Algorithm for SVT with VA Block (Fig. 5.4)

Although uncommon, VA block may occur during SVT. In such cases, AT and ORT-AV are excluded, and the differential diagnosis includes AVNRT with an upper common pathway and ORT-NV/NF. The diagnostic algorithm for SVT with VA block is shown in Fig. 5.4. The ORT criteria such as the PPI − TCL < 115 ms, orthodromic His bundle electrogram capture, and constant QRS fusion indicate ORT-NV/NF, although the SA − VA, HA_{pacing} − $HA_{tachycardia}$, and correction of the PPI − TCL with an AV nodal delay are not available because of the presence of VA block [25]. Likewise, tachycardia termination during a progressive fusion period is diagnostic for ORT-NV/NF although perturbation of atrial timing cannot be assessed in SVT with VA block.

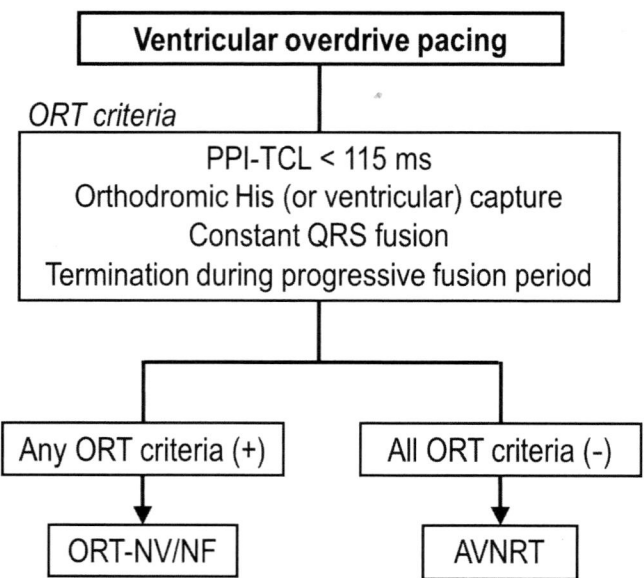

Fig. 5.4 Diagnostic algorithm for supraventricular tachycardias (SVT) with VA block. In this special situation, a possible diagnosis is confined to AVNRT or ORT-NV/NF. See text for details. Abbreviations as in Fig. 5.1

5.5 Diagnostic Algorithm for SVT with AV Block

Because AV block never occurs during ORT, either AT or AVNRT is responsible for SVT with AV block. In the presence of AV block, an eccentric atrial activation usually indicates AT, while it may be challenging to distinguish AT from AVNRT if the atrial activation pattern is concentric. In this situation, there are limitations to the utility of entrainment pacing in the differential diagnosis between AT and AVNRT. If VOP terminates SVT with AV block before the atrium is captured, AVNRT is diagnosed. There is no reliable diagnostic pacing maneuver if VA dissociation occurs during VOP. Enhancing the AV nodal conduction with isoproterenol may restore 1:1 AV conduction, or change the response of the SVT to VOP. Careful observations of the SVT features and/or examining pharmacologic responses (e.g., adenosine bolus) may be required for diagnosis of the SVT with AV block that is inconclusive with pacing maneuvers.

5.6 Limitations of the Proposed Algorithm

In principle, the diagnostic algorithm using entrainment pacing cannot be used for non-sustained SVT. Isoproterenol infusion may help sustain SVT. If sustained SVT are not inducible, baseline observations and tachycardia features would provide important clues to a diagnosis. In addition, pacing maneuvers such as para-Hisian pacing are useful for differential diagnosis (see Chap. 4).

5.6.1 Prediction of PPI − TCL for SVT Terminated with Entrainment Pacing

Even when SVT is sustained, the tachycardia is occasionally terminated during entrainment pacing. If the SVT termination reproducibly occurs during a progressive fusion period after initiation of VOP, ORT can be diagnosed as mentioned above. However, other ORT criteria are not available when VOP terminates SVT. We previously reported that the number of pacing stimuli needed to entrain (NNE) highly correlated with the PPI − TCL [26]. If SVT is terminated during VOP after resetting the tachycardia, the PPI − TCL can be predicted from the NNE using the following formula [27]:

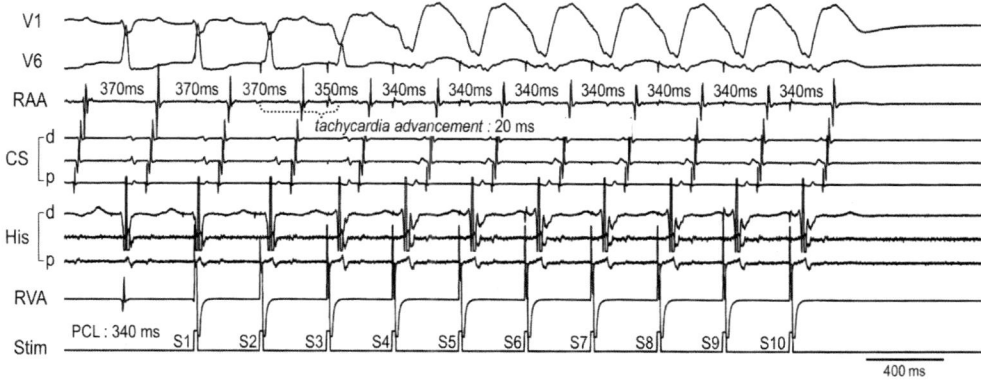

$$\text{Predicted PPI} - \text{TCL} = (\text{NNE} - 1) \times (\text{TCL} - \text{PCL}) - \text{tachycardia advancement}$$
$$= (4 - 1) \times (370\ ms - 340\ ms) - 20\ ms$$
$$= 70\ ms$$

Fig. 5.5 Prediction of the difference between post-pacing interval and tachycardia cycle length (PPI – TCL) from the number of pacing stimuli needed to entrain (NNE) during ventricular overdrive pacing in a patient with ORT. In this example, the atrium was reset first with the third stimulus (S3) and entrained from the fourth stimulus (S4). The amount of tachycardia advancement on the first reset was 20 ms. Therefore, the predicted PPI – TCL was calculated as 70 ms (<115 ms). Note that the atrial resetting occurred during a progressive fusion period at the beginning of the ventricular overdrive pacing, which is consistent with ORT

$$\text{PPI} - \text{TCL} = (\text{NNE} - 1) \times (\text{TCL} - \text{PCL}) - \text{tachycardia advancement}.$$

Figure 5.5 shows an example of calculation of the predicted PPI – TCL. Since the predicted PPI – TCL is well correlated to the observed PPI – TCL [27], the predicted PPI – TCL < 115 ms seems diagnostic for ORT although it should be confirmed in future studies.

Conclusions

Entrainment pacing is an indispensable technique for differential diagnosis of SVT. The proposed stepwise approach will provide a definite diagnosis in an efficient way. We should be aware that atypical SVT can exhibit confusing electrophysiologic findings. Appropriate pacing maneuvers are necessary for a correct diagnosis and successful catheter ablation.

References

1. Orejarena LA, Vidaillet H Jr, DeStefano F, Nordstrom DL, Vierkant RA, Smith PN, et al. Paroxysmal supraventricular tachycardia in the general population. J Am Coll Cardiol. 1998;31(1):150–7.
2. Knight BP, Ebinger M, Oral H, Kim MH, Sticherling C, Pelosi F, et al. Diagnostic value of tachycardia features and pacing maneuvers during paroxysmal supraventricular tachycardia. J Am Coll Cardiol. 2000;36(2):574–82.
3. Otomo K, Okamura H, Noda T, Satomi K, Shimizu W, Suyama K, et al. "Left-variant" atypical atrioventricular nodal reentrant tachycardia: electrophysiological characteristics and effect of slow pathway ablation within coronary sinus. J Cardiovasc Electrophysiol. 2006;17(11):1177–83.
4. Nagashima K, Watanabe I, Okumura Y, Kaneko Y, Sonoda K, Kogawa R, et al. Ventriculoatrial intervals ≤70 ms in orthodromic atrioventricular reciprocating tachycardia. Pacing Clin Electrophysiol. 2016;39(10):1108–15.
5. Knight BP, Zivin A, Souza J, Flemming M, Pelosi F, Goyal R, et al. A technique for the rapid diagnosis of atrial tachycardia in the electrophysiology laboratory. J Am Coll Cardiol. 1999;33(3):775–81.
6. Yamabe H, Okumura K, Tabuchi T, Tsuchiya T, Yasue H. Double atrial responses to a single ventricular impulse in long RP' tachycardia. Pacing Clin Electrophysiol. 1996;19(4 Pt 1):403–10.
7. Ho RT, Frisch DR, Pavri BB, Levi SA, Greenspon AJ. Electrophysiological features differentiating the atypical atrioventricular node-dependent long RP supraventricular tachycardias. Circ Arrhythm Electrophysiol. 2013;6(3):597–605.
8. Kaneko Y, Naito S, Okishige K, Morishima I, Tobiume T, Nakajima T, et al. Atypical fast-slow atrioventricular nodal reentrant tachycardia incorporating a "superior" slow pathway: a distinct supraventricular tachyarrhythmia. Circulation. 2016;133(2):114–23.
9. Maruyama M, Kobayashi Y, Miyauchi Y, Ino T, Atarashi H, Katoh T, et al. The VA relationship after differential atrial overdrive pacing: a novel tool for the diagnosis of atrial tachycardia in the electrophysiologic laboratory. J Cardiovasc Electrophysiol. 2007;18(11):1127–33.

10. Michaud GF, Tada H, Chough S, Baker R, Wasmer K, Sticherling C, et al. Differentiation of atypical atrioventricular node re-entrant tachycardia from orthodromic reciprocating tachycardia using a septal accessory pathway by the response to ventricular pacing. J Am Coll Cardiol. 2001;38(4):1163–7.
11. Gonzalez-Torrecilla E, Arenal A, Atienza F, Osca J, Garcia-Fernandez J, Puchol A, et al. First postpacing interval after tachycardia entrainment with correction for atrioventricular node delay: a simple maneuver for differential diagnosis of atrioventricular nodal reentrant tachycardias versus orthodromic reciprocating tachycardias. Heart Rhythm. 2006;3(6):674–9.
12. Bennett MT, Leong-Sit P, Gula LJ, Skanes AC, Yee R, Krahn AD, et al. Entrainment for distinguishing atypical atrioventricular node reentrant tachycardia from atrioventricular reentrant tachycardia over septal accessory pathways with long-RP tachycardia. Circ Arrhythm Electrophysiol. 2011;4(4):506–9.
13. Ho RT, Mark GE, Rhim ES, Pavri BB, Greenspon AJ. Differentiating atrioventricular nodal reentrant tachycardia from atrioventricular reentrant tachycardia by ΔHA values during entrainment from the ventricle. Heart Rhythm. 2008;5(1):83–8.
14. Ho RT, Patel U, Weitz HH. Entrainment and resetting of a long RP tachycardia: which trumps which for diagnosis? Heart Rhythm. 2010;7(5):714–5.
15. Nagashima K, Kumar S, Stevenson WG, Epstein LM, John RM, Tedrow UB, et al. Anterograde conduction to the His bundle during right ventricular overdrive pacing distinguishes septal pathway atrioventricular reentry from atypical atrioventricular nodal reentrant tachycardia. Heart Rhythm. 2015;12(4):735–43.
16. Veenhuyzen GD, Coverett K, Quinn FR, Sapp JL, Gillis AM, Sheldon R, et al. Single diagnostic pacing maneuver for supraventricular tachycardia. Heart Rhythm. 2008;5(8):1152–8.
17. AlMahameed ST, Buxton AE, Michaud GF. New criteria during right ventricular pacing to determine the mechanism of supraventricular tachycardia. Circ Arrhythm Electrophysiol. 2010;3(6):578–84.
18. Dandamudi G, Mokabberi R, Assal C, Das MK, Oren J, Storm R, et al. A novel approach to differentiating orthodromic reciprocating tachycardia from atrioventricular nodal reentrant tachycardia. Heart Rhythm. 2010;7(9):1326–9.
19. Rosman JZ, John RM, Stevenson WG, Epstein LM, Tedrow UB, Koplan BA, et al. Resetting criteria during ventricular overdrive pacing successfully differentiate orthodromic reentrant tachycardia from atrioventricular nodal reentrant tachycardia despite interobserver disagreement concerning QRS fusion. Heart Rhythm. 2011;8(1):2–7.
20. Segal OR, Gula LJ, Skanes AC, Krahn AD, Yee R, Klein GJ. Differential ventricular entrainment: a maneuver to differentiate AV node reentrant tachycardia from orthodromic reciprocating tachycardia. Heart Rhythm. 2009;6(4):493–500.
21. Khan AH, Khadem A, Basta MN, Gardner MJ, Parkash R, Gula LJ, et al. Differential entrainment distinguishes atrioventricular nodal reentry tachycardia from atrioventricular reentrant tachycardia. Pacing Clin Electrophysiol. 2010;33(11):1335–41.
22. Platonov M, Schroeder K, Veenhuyzen GD. Differential entrainment: beware from where you pace. Heart Rhythm. 2007;4(8):1097–9.
23. Ho RT, Yin A. Spontaneous conversion of a long RP to short RP tachycardia: what is the mechanism? Heart Rhythm. 2014;11(3):522–5.
24. Man KC, Niebauer M, Daoud E, Strickberger SA, Kou W, Williamson BD, et al. Comparison of atrial-His intervals during tachycardia and atrial pacing in patients with long RP tachycardia. J Cardiovasc Electrophysiol. 1995;6(9):700–10.
25. Quinn FR, Mitchell LB, Mardell AP, Dal Disler RN, Veenhuyzen GD. Entrainment mapping of a concealed nodoventricular accessory pathway in a man with complete heart block and tachycardia-induced cardiomyopathy. J Cardiovasc Electrophysiol. 2008;19(1):90–4.
26. Maruyama M, Yamamoto T, Abe J, Yodogawa K, Seino Y, Atarashi H, et al. Number needed to entrain: a new criterion for entrainment mapping in patients with intra-atrial reentrant tachycardia. Circ Arrhythm Electrophysiol. 2014;7(3):490–6.
27. Kaiser DW, Hsia HH, Dubin AM, Liem LB, Viswanathan MN, Zei PC, et al. The precise timing of tachycardia entrainment is determined by the postpacing interval, the tachycardia cycle length, and the pacing rate: theoretical insights and practical applications. Heart Rhythm. 2016;13(3):695–703.

Part III

Special Sites for Ablation

Aortic Sinus Cusps for Catheter Ablation of Supraventricular and Ventricular Arrhythmias

Takumi Yamada

Keywords

Aortic sinus cusp · Supraventricular arrhythmia · Ventricular arrhythmia · Catheter ablation

6.1 Introduction

For the past decade, the aortic sinus cusps (ASCs) have been increasingly recognized as sites of catheter ablation of ventricular arrhythmias (VAs) [1–7], ventricular tachycardias (VTs), or premature ventricular contractions (PVCs), as well as supraventricular tachycardias (only atrial tachycardias [ATs] [8–12] are described in this chapter although a para-Hisian accessory pathway and "superior" slow pathway can be ablated within the ASCs). There is no myocardium within the ASCs, and catheter ablation from the ASCs ablates an arrhythmogenic substrate in the adjacent myocardium [13]. VAs and ATs arising from this specific anatomical location exhibit specific electrocardiographic and electrophysiological characteristics [1–14]. Catheter ablation of these VAs and ATs is highly successful and safe [1–13]. However, since important structures such as the coronary arteries and atrioventricular conduction system are located around the ASCs, there is a potential risk of collateral damage to those structures in catheter ablation from the ASCs [1–13]. In this chapter, the anatomical background, electrocardiographic and electrophysiological characteristics, and catheter ablation of VAs and ATs that can be ablated within the ASCs are described.

T. Yamada, M.D., Ph.D.
Division of Cardiovascular Disease, University of Alabama at Birmingham, FOT 930E, 510 20th Street South, Birmingham, AL 35294-0019, USA
e-mail: takumi-y@fb4.so-net.ne.jp

6.2 Anatomy Relevant to Catheter Ablation

The left ventricular outflow tract (LVOT) is the second most common site of idiopathic VA origins only to the right ventricular outflow tract (RVOT) [14, 15]. The most common site of idiopathic VA origins in the LVOT is the aortic root followed by the sites underneath the ASCs [13–15]. Anatomically, the aortic and mitral valves are in direct apposition and attach to the elliptical opening at the base of the left ventricle (LV) known as the LV ostium [13, 14] (Fig. 6.1a). Because there is no myocardium between the aortic and mitral valves (fibrous trigone), most idiopathic LV VAs can originate from along the LV ostium. The LV myocardium comes in direct contact with the aorta at the base of the ASCs (Fig. 6.1a). When idiopathic VAs arise from the most superior portion of the LV ostium (the aortic sinus of Valsalva), they can be ablated within the base of the ASCs. It has been reported that some idiopathic VAs can be ablated from the junction (commissure) between the left and right coronary cusps (L-RCC) [4]. In these VAs, catheter ablation from underneath the ASCs is often required for their elimination. Anatomically, the superior edge of the LV myocardium makes a semicircular attachment to the aortic root at the bottom of the right and left coronary cusps. However, because of the semilunar nature of the attachments of the aortic valvular cusps, the superior edge of the LV myocardium is located underneath the aortic valves at the L-RCC (Fig. 6.1a). Therefore, idiopathic VAs that can be ablated at the L-RCC should be classified into the same group as the VAs that can be ablated within the ASCs. In this setting, these idiopathic VAs may be defined as idiopathic VAs arising from the aortic root [6]. It has been reported that

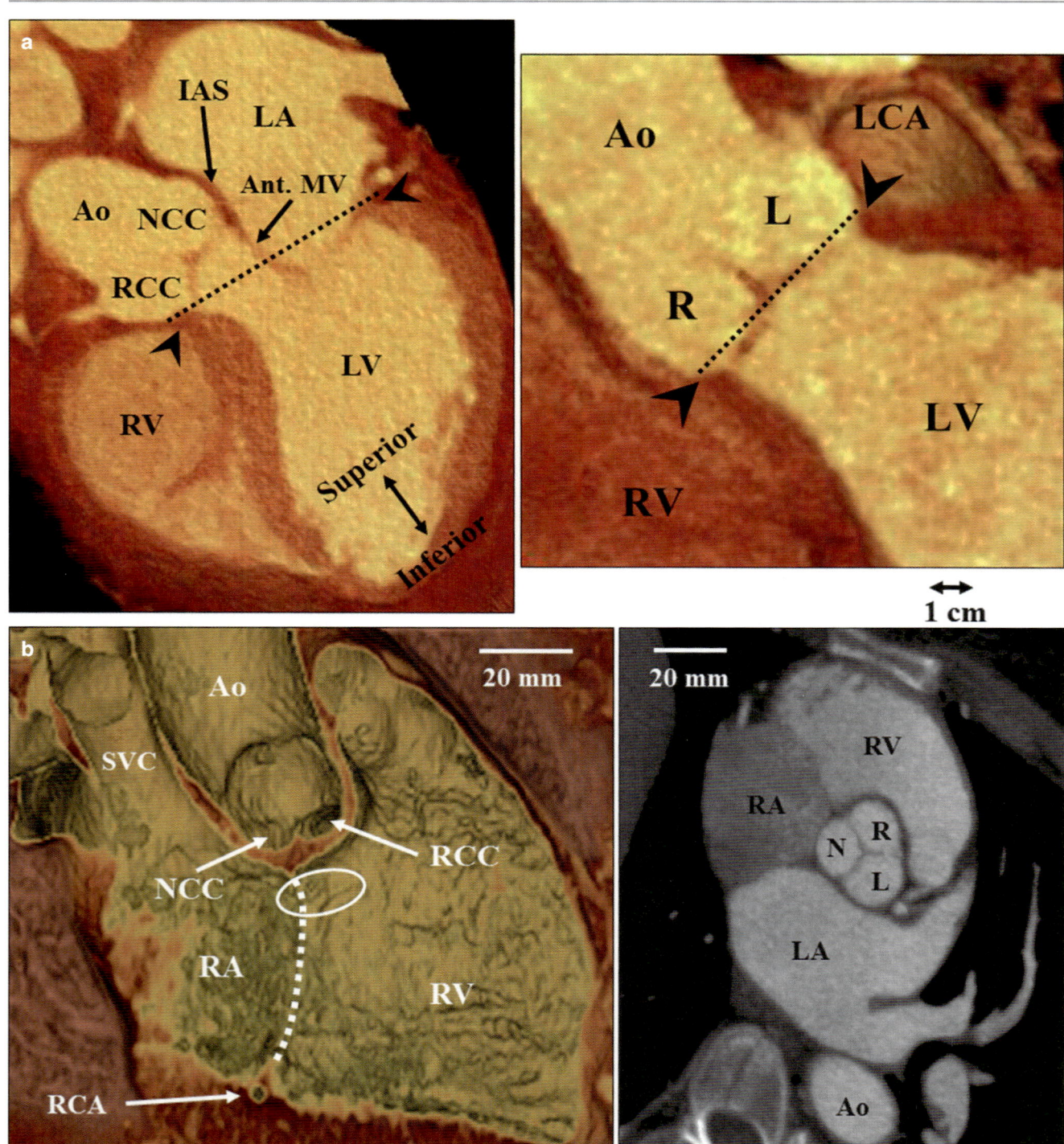

Fig. 6.1 Computed tomography images exhibiting the anatomy around the aorta. (**a**) Two-dimensional computed tomography (CT) images showing the relationships between the ventricular myocardium and aortic sinus cusps. The *arrowheads* indicate the superior edge of the ventricular myocardium connecting with the left coronary cusp and right coronary cusp (RCC) and the dotted line the ventriculo-arterial junction (the ostium of the left ventricle). *Ant.* anterior, *Ao* aorta, *IAS* interatrial septum, *L* left coronary cusp, *LA* left atrium, *LCA* left coronary artery, *LV* left ventricle, *MV* mitral valve, *NCC* noncoronary cusp, *R* right coronary cusp, *RV* right ventricle. This figure was cited from ref. [6] with permission. (**b**) Two-dimensional (*right panel*) and three-dimensional (*left panel*) CT images. The *dotted line* indicates the tricuspid annulus and *solid circle* the right ventricular His bundle (HB) region. *N* noncoronary cusp, *RA* right atrium, *RCA* right coronary artery, *SVC* superior vena cava. The other abbreviations are as in the previous figure. This figure was cited from ref. [5] with permission

idiopathic VAs can rarely be ablated from within the noncoronary cusp of the aorta (NCC) [6, 7, 14]. Spatially, the aortic root occupies a central location within the heart, with the NCC anterior and superior to the paraseptal region of the left and right atria close to the superior atrioventricular junctions (Fig. 6.1b) [13]. In normal human hearts, the NCC is adjacent to the atrial myocardium on the epicardial aspect, and the NCC does not directly come in contact with the ventricular myocardium (Fig. 6.1b). Indeed, ATs that can be ablated from within the NCC are far more common than VAs [1–12]. However, the clinical observation that a noncoronary sinus of Valsalva aneurysm can rupture into the right ventricle (RV) as well as the right atrium supports the assumption that the NCC may be attached to the ventricular myocardium where idiopathic VAs can arise from [16]. Idiopathic VAs can arise from the pulmonary artery with a ventricular myocardial extension from the RVOT [17]. However, it should be noted that ventricular myocardial extensions never occur in the aorta [13].

Anatomically, the NCC overrides the roof of the interatrial septum. Therefore, ATs originating from that region can be ablated only from the NCC [13]. It has been reported that ATs can be ablated within the RCC or LCC presumably because of anatomical variations [11, 12]. The successful ablation site of ATs within the LCC is located posterior to the left main coronary artery and that within the RCC is located at the junction with the NCC [11, 12]. Among ATs that can be ablated within three ASCs, NCC ATs are most prevalent, and LCC and RCC ATs are relatively and very rare, respectively [9, 11, 12].

The posterior part of the RCC is adjacent to the central fibrous body, which carries within it the penetrating portion of the His bundle (HB) [13]. Anteriorly, the RCC is related to the bifurcating atrioventricular bundle and the origin of the left bundle branch. The NCC lies superior to the central fibrous body. The HB penetrates through the central fibrous body and continues as the atrioventricular conduction bundle that then passes to the crest of the muscular ventricular septum, immediately beneath the membranous septum. Therefore, there is a potential risk of damage to atrioventricular conduction system in catheter ablation within the RCC and NCC [13].

6.3 Electrocardiographic Characteristics

6.3.1 Ventricular Arrhythmias

Electrocardiographic characteristics are helpful for predicting the site of origin of idiopathic VAs originating from the aortic root [1–7, 14, 18]. The electrocardiograms (ECGs) of these idiopathic VAs are characterized by positive R waves in all inferior leads and deep S waves in both leads aVR and aVL (almost QS pattern) (Fig. 6.2). The most important diagnosis to make by an ECG may be whether the VAs originate from the right or left side. It is often challenging because anatomically the RVOT and LVOT are located next to each other [1, 3, 19]. The bundle branch block pattern, precordial transition zone, and some ECG algorithms may be helpful for localizing the site of origin. A right bundle branch block (RBBB) QRS morphology clearly suggests a VA origin on the left side. When a left bundle branch block (LBBB) QRS morphology is observed, it is often difficult to predict whether the VA originates from the right or left side. Because the LVOT is anatomically located posterior to the RVOT, LVOT VAs exhibit a taller and wider R wave in the right precordial leads than RVOT VAs [3, 19]. Therefore, the precordial transition zone is helpful for predicting whether a VA originates from the RVOT or LVOT. A precordial transition of ≥ lead V4 most likely predicts an RVOT VA origin, while a precordial transition of ≤ lead V2 predicts an LVOT VA origin. When there is a precordial transition in lead V3, it is most difficult to predict RVOT or LVOT VA origins [19]. Several ECG algorithms to predict RVOT or LVOT VA origins have been proposed, and the author would like to recommend two ECG algorithms: the R/S amplitude index and R wave duration index [3] and the V2S/V3R ratio [19] because they are simple and accurate and also can make a diagnosis by looking at the ECG of the VA alone. The R-/S-wave amplitude ratio in leads V1 and V2 is calculated as the amplitude of the QRS complex peak or nadir to the isoelectric line. The R-/S-wave amplitude index, calculated from the percentage of the R/S-wave amplitude ratio in lead V1 or V2 (whichever is greater), is considered more useful than the R-/S-wave amplitude ratio alone in lead V1 or V2. The R wave duration index is calculated by dividing the longer R wave duration in lead V1 or V2 by the QRS complex duration. A precordial transition later than lead V4 or R/S amplitude index of <0.3 and R wave duration index of <0.5 may strongly suggest a VA origin on the right side. Otherwise, a VA origin on the left side may be suggested. A V2S/V3R ratio is calculated by dividing an S-wave amplitude in lead V2 by an R wave amplitude in lead V3. Ratios of the V2S/V3R of >1.5 and ≤1.5 predict RVOT and LVOT VA origins, respectively. This ECG algorithm has proven to be useful in VAs with a precordial transition in lead V3 and may be the most accurate among the previously proposed ECG algorithms. The presence of S waves in lead I may also be helpful for differentiating the VA origins in the aortic root or RVOT [1]. The presence of S waves in lead V6 may suggest a VA origin in the endocardial LV which indicates the area below the aortic valve [1].

Although the three ASCs are anatomically located next to each other, it may be possible to differentiate VAs that can be ablated within each ASC (Fig. 6.2) [6]. An RBBB pattern is very rarely observed during VAs that can be ablated within

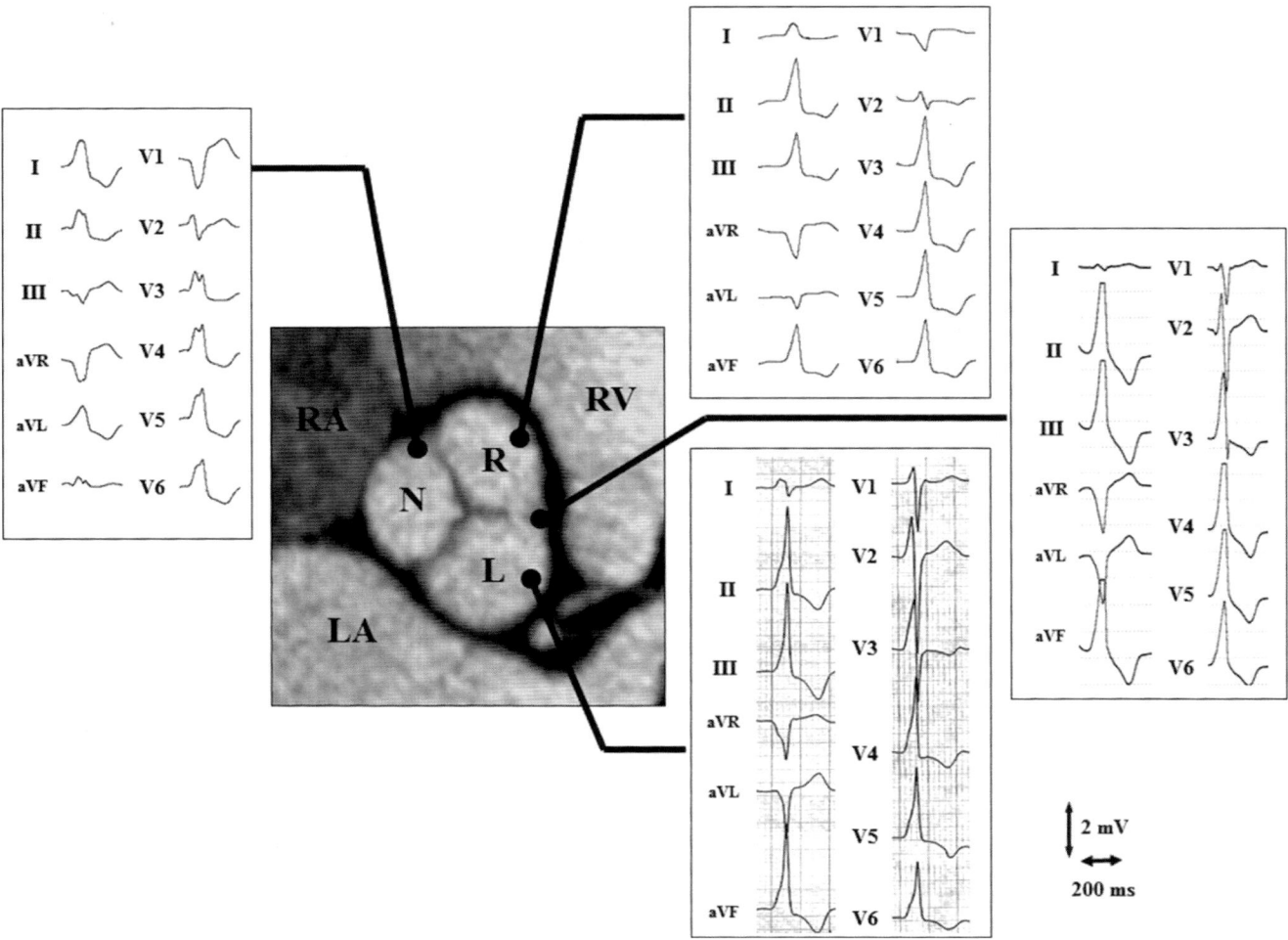

Fig. 6.2 Two-dimensional CT images and representative 12-lead electrocardiograms of ventricular arrhythmias originating from the aortic root. *L* left coronary cusp, *N* noncoronary cusp, *R* right coronary cusp. The other abbreviations are as in the previous figures. This figure was cited from ref. [6] with permission

the right coronary cusp (RCC), and only an LBBB is observed during VAs that can be ablated within the NCC. Therefore, when an RBBB pattern is observed, the VAs are likely to be ablated within the left coronary cusp (LCC). The ratio of the R wave amplitude in leads III to II (III/II) may be helpful for differentiating between LCC VAs and RCC VAs. When the III/II ratio is >0.9, the VAs are more likely to be ablated within the LCC [6]. A qrS pattern in the right precordial leads may be highly specific for a VA origin at the L-RCC [4]. The ECG characteristics of NCC VAs are similar to those of RCC VAs. However, S waves are often observed in lead III during NCC VAs although they are not during RCC VAs. When the III/II ratio is <0.65, the VAs are more likely to be ablated within the NCC [7].

The electrocardiographic features as to whether VAs can be successfully ablated from the endocardial or epicardial side are also important to recognize. The maximum deflection index (MDI) which is calculated by dividing the shortest time to the maximum deflection in any precordial lead by the QRS duration [20] and the ratio of the Q wave amplitude in leads aVL to aVR (aVL/aVR ratio) [1] may be helpful for making such a diagnosis. An MDI of >0.55 and aVL/aVR ratio of >1.4 suggest that VAs may be ablated epicardially, although these algorithms are reliable for VAs arising from the LVOT underneath the ASCs and less reliable for those arising from the aortic root [21].

Because of their anatomical close proximity, VAs originating from the RVOT, LVOT underneath the ASCs, and aortic root may exhibit similar electrocardiographic features. In addition, the complex anatomy of these regions may limit the reliability of these ECG algorithms. In the pre-procedural planning, these limitations should be kept in mind and all possibilities should be considered.

6.3.2 Atrial Tachycardia

ATs that can be ablated within the ASCs exhibit distinctive P wave characteristics [9–12]. The common P wave characteristics among these ATs are a shorter P wave duration than a sinus P wave and a negative/positive P wave in lead V1 because of the anteromedial location of the AT origins. P waves in leads I and aVL are likely to be positive during NCC ATs, while they are likely to be negative/positive or isoelectric during LCC ATs because of the more leftward position of the LCC as compared with the NCC. The P wave polarity in the inferior leads can be negative/positive, positive, or negative during NCC ATs and is always positive during LCC ATs.

6.4 Mapping and Catheter Ablation

6.4.1 Ventricular Arrhythmias

For mapping and pacing, a quadripolar catheter is positioned at the HB region and a deflectable decapolar catheter in the coronary sinus (CS) via the right femoral vein [18, 22]. The CS catheter is advanced into the great cardiac vein (GCV) as far as possible, even into the anterior interventricular vein until the proximal electrode pair records an earlier ventricular activation than the most distal electrode pair during the VAs. Anatomically, the RVOT and LVOT are located next to each other, and it is often difficult to predict idiopathic VA origins from the RVOT or LVOT by the ECGs prior to the procedure. Therefore, mapping in the RV should be first performed in all patients with idiopathic VAs exhibiting an LBBB QRS morphology [18]. Idiopathic VAs originating from the aortic root occur with a focal mechanism. Therefore, activation mapping seeking the earliest bipolar activity and/or a local unipolar QS pattern during VAs is most reliable for identifying a site of a VA origin [18]. Pace mapping is especially helpful for idiopathic RVOT VAs, but is less helpful for idiopathic aortic root VAs because pacing within the ASCs may not exactly reproduce the QRS morphology of the VAs due to preferential conduction across the ventricular septum [23] or the inability to obtain myocardial capture despite the use of a high pacing current. A comparison of the pace maps from the right and left side may be helpful to predict whether a VA origin can be ablated from the RV or LV. When an earlier precordial transition during VAs cannot be reproduced by pace mapping from the RV, a VA origin may be considered to be located in the LV. A comparison of the pace maps from the ASCs, endocardial LVOT, and GCV may be helpful to predict whether a VA origin can be ablated from the endocardial or epicardial side. In this comparison, the MDI as well as the pace map score should be evaluated. When the MDI during VAs is closer to that during pace mapping from the GCV than that during pace mapping from the ASCs and LVOT, a VA origin may be considered to be located on the epicardial surface.

When the earliest ventricular activation in the RV precedes the QRS onset by more than 20 ms and is earlier than that recorded in the GCV, radiofrequency catheter ablation (RFCA) may be performed at that site when there is confirmation of an excellent pace map match to the QRS complex of the clinical VAs. When there are no suitable sites for ablation in the RV or when RV catheter ablation is unsuccessful, mapping in the ASCs and LVOT should follow. When the QRS morphology of the VAs changes after the unsuccessful ablation in the RV, the presence of a preferential conduction from the VA origin in the aortic root to the breakout in the RV is suggested [23]. Because the posterior portion of the RVOT is in close apposition to the LV near the aortic root, when catheter ablation has not been successful in the LVOT, the RV should be carefully remapped before determining that an epicardial approach is required.

Mapping and catheter ablation within the ASCs are performed through a retrograde transaortic approach. Before mapping and catheter ablation within the ASCs, selective angiography of the coronary artery and aorta should be performed to delineate the ASCs and coronary artery (Fig. 6.3) [13]. The three ASCs can be readily identified during biplane aortography or coronary angiography. The LCC is most easily identified in the left anterior oblique (LAO) projection where this cusp is on the far lateral aspect of the aortic root, leftward and superior to the HB catheter (Fig. 6.3a). The RCC usually requires coronary angiography in both the right anterior oblique (RAO) and LAO projections for an accurate identification of the cusp relative to the right coronary artery (RCA) ostium (Fig. 6.3b). In the RAO projection, the ablation catheter is typically located anterior and inferior to the RCA ostium. In the LAO projection, the typical ablation site is more leftward in the RCC than the RCA ostium. The NCC is readily identified as the most inferior of the three cusps and by its close relation to the HB catheter (Fig. 6.3c). In the RAO projection, a catheter in the NCC is posterior and inferior to the RCA ostium, just above the HB catheter. In the LAO projection, the NCC is just superior to the HB catheter, well posterior to the RCA ostium. Intracardiac echocardiography may also be useful for identifying the site of the ablation catheter (Fig. 6.4a). Because the NCC overlies the interatrial septum, the amplitude of an atrial electrogram is usually larger than that of the ventricular electrogram within the NCC.

The NCC and L-RCC may be confounded in the fluoroscopic identification because both the NCC and L-RCC are

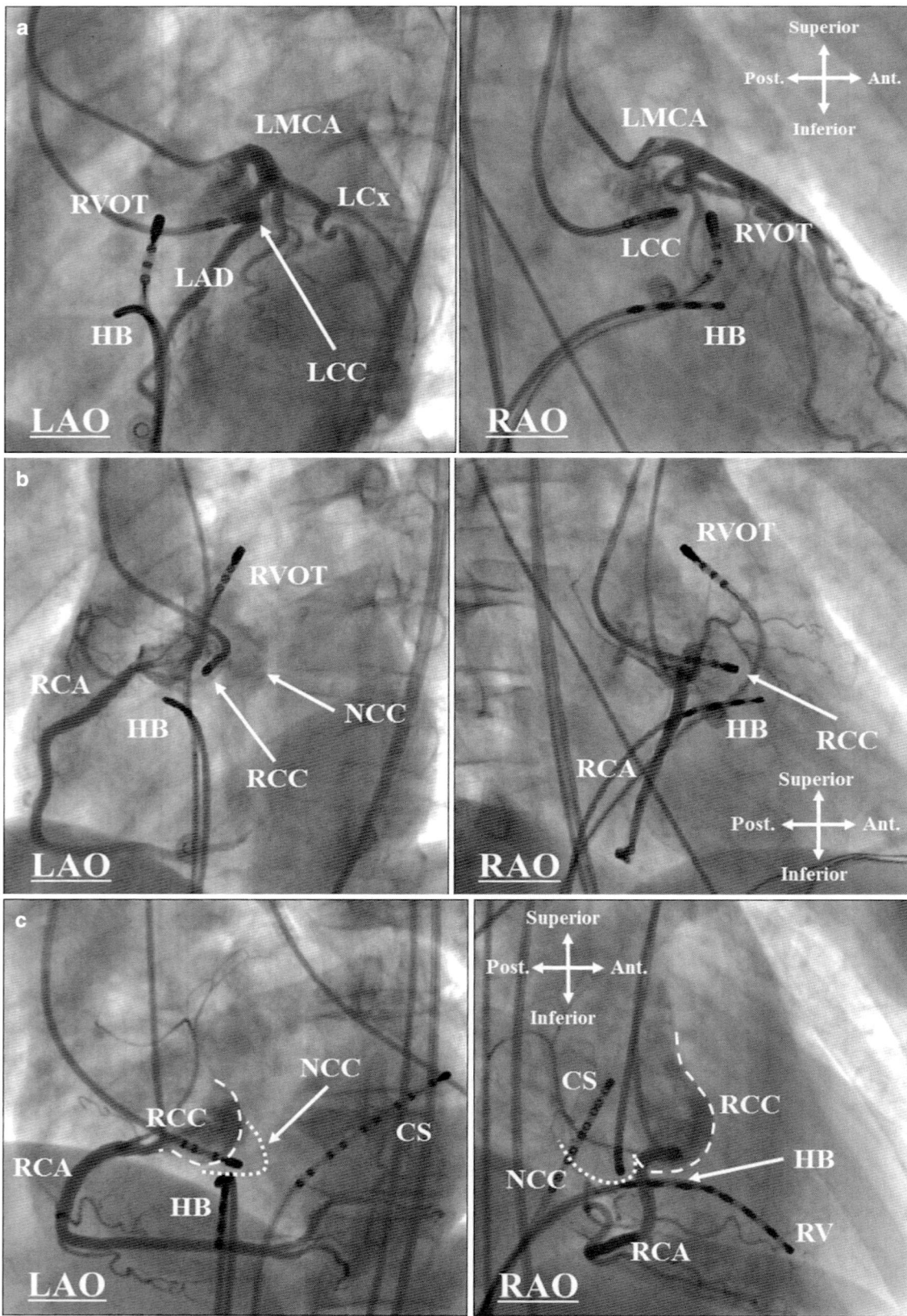

Fig. 6.3 Coronary angiograms and the catheter positions. (**a**) The left main coronary angiogram. (**b**) The right coronary angiograms. (**c**) The right coronary angiograms with the ablation catheter within the NCC. Note that the typical site of the successful catheter ablation within the left coronary cusp (LCC) and RCC is at the nadir of those cusps. *CS* coronary sinus, *LAD* left anterior descending coronary artery, *LAO* left anterior oblique projection, *LCC* left coronary cusp, *LCx* left circumflex coronary artery, *LMCA* left main coronary artery, *RAO* right anterior oblique projection, *RVOT* right ventricular outflow tract. The other abbreviations are as in the previous figures. This figure was cited from ref. [13] with permission

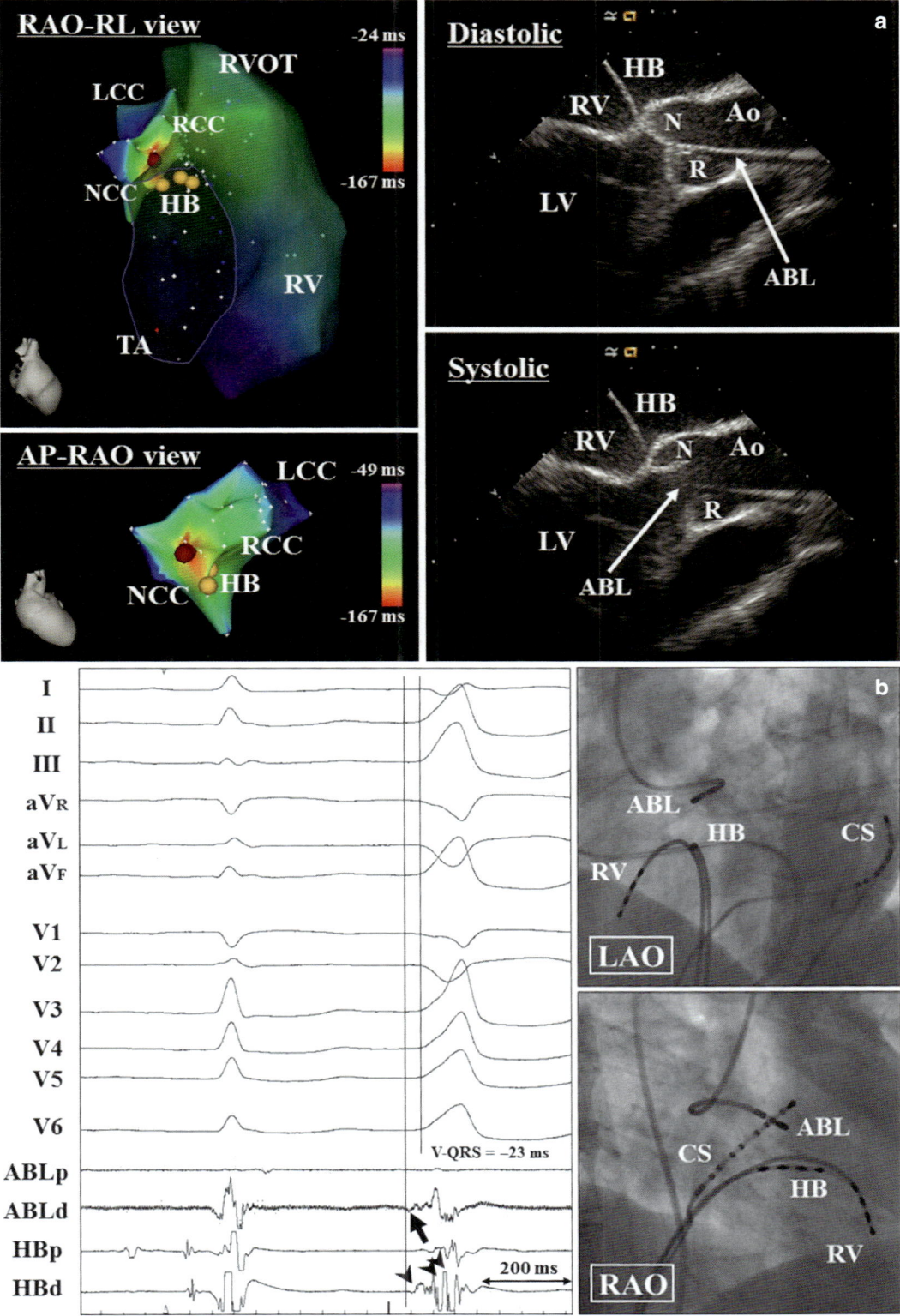

Fig. 6.4 Successful ablation sites of idiopathic ventricular arrhythmias within the noncoronary cusp (**a**) and right coronary cusp (**b**). (**a**) Activation maps (*left panels*) and intracardiac echocardiograms (*right panels*) exhibiting the successful ablation site within the noncoronary cusp at the junction with the right coronary cusp. The *red* and *yellow* tags indicate the successful ablation site and the sites where His bundle electrograms were recorded. *Ao* aorta, *AP* anteroposterior, *RL* right lateral. The other abbreviations are as in the previous figures. This figure was cited from ref. [7] with permission. (**b**) Intracardiac tracings (*left panel*) and fluoroscopic images (*right panels*) exhibiting the successful ablation site within the right coronary cusp. The first beat is a sinus beat and the second one is a premature ventricular contraction (PVC). During the PVC, a far-field electrogram (*single arrowhead*) preceding the QRS onset by 18 ms and the following near-field electrogram (*double arrowheads*) were recorded in the right ventricular HB region. The local ventricular electrogram at the successful ablation site (*arrow*) preceded the QRS onset by 23 ms. Note that the ablation catheter was located close to the HB catheter. *V-QRS* the local ventricular activation relative to the QRS onset, *Xd(p)* the distal (proximal) electrode pairs of the relevant catheter. The other abbreviations are as in the previous figures. This figure was cited from ref. [5] with permission

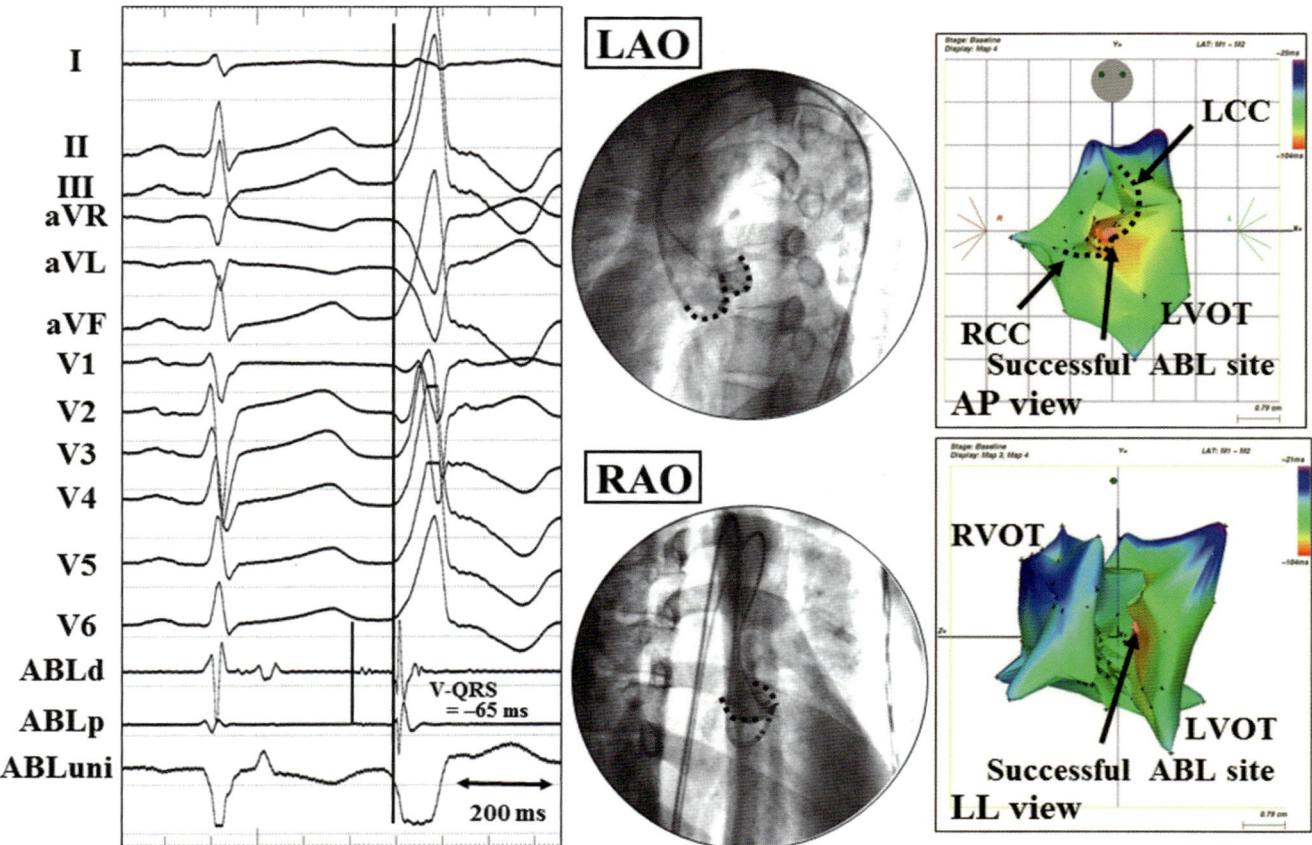

Fig. 6.5 Successful ablation site of the premature ventricular contractions (PVCs) originating from the junction of the left and right aortic sinus cusps (L-RCC). The first beat is a sinus beat and the second one is a PVC. At the successful ablation site, two ventricular activation components were recorded during sinus rhythm. The sequence of the two components was reversed during the PVC. The first of the two components preceded the QRS onset by 65 ms. The aortogram showed that the ablation catheter was located in the L-RCC (*mid panels*). Note that the tip of the ablation catheter was positioned at the L-RCC by deflecting the loop of the ablation catheter in the left ventricular cavity. The activation map during the PVCs revealed the earliest activation at the L-RCC (*right panel*). *ABL uni* the distal unipolar electrode of the ablation catheter, *LL* left lateral, *LVOT* left ventricular outflow tract. This figure was cited from ref. [4] with permission

located in the middle between the LCC and RCC in the LAO projection (Fig. 6.5) [4]. Therefore, it should be noted that the NCC is located just above the HB catheter, while the L-RCC is located far above the HB catheter. It is easy to identify the NCC and L-RCC in the RAO projection because the L-RCC is located most anteriorly in the aortic root while the NCC is located most posteriorly.

When VAs exhibit an R wave in lead I and a local ventricular activation recorded from the HB catheter precedes the QRS onset, mapping in the RCC, NCC, and sites underneath those cusps should be added to accurately identify the site of the VA origin (Fig. 6.4b) [5]. In this setting, two components are often observed in the local ventricular electrogram recorded in the HB region. They consist of a far-field electrogram reflecting the activity of the left-sided VA origin followed by a near-field electrogram reflecting the activity of the RV myocardium (Fig. 6.4b) [5]. Otherwise, mapping in the LCC and aorto-mitral continuity should be first performed because VAs are more likely to arise from these sites. A ventricular prepotential preceding the QRS onset is often recorded at the aortic root during idiopathic VAs, and it may predict a successful ablation site (Fig. 6.5) [4, 6, 13]. Pacing within the ASCs often exhibits a long stimulus to QRS interval (more likely in the LCC than the RCC), whereas pacing below the aortic valves gives no latency between the pacing stimulus and QRS onset [13]. When the earliest ventricular activation in the ASCs precedes the QRS onset by more than 20 ms, RFCA may be performed at this site. An HB electrogram is sometimes recorded within the RCC and NCC, and RFCA should be avoided at those sites.

In RFCA within the ASCs, both irrigation and non-irrigation ablation catheters can be used because the blood flow through the aorta is great enough to provide a sufficient cooling effect [18]. Nonirrigated radiofrequency (RF) current is delivered in the temperature-control mode with a target temperature of 55–60 °C and maximum power output of

50 W. Irrigated RF current is delivered in the power-control mode starting at 30 W with irrigation flow rates of 30 ml/min. The RF power is titrated up to 40 W. The goal of RF applications is to achieve a decrease in the impedance of 8–10 Ω and with care taken to limit the temperature to <41 °C. When an acceleration or reduction in the frequency of the VT or PVCs is observed during the first 10 seconds of the application, the RF delivery is continued for 30–60 s. Otherwise, the RF delivery is terminated, and the catheter is repositioned.

When an RF application is delivered close to the coronary arteries, the coronary arteries will be susceptible to heat damage, which may result in spasms, stenosis, and an occlusion [24, 25] of the coronary arteries and thrombus formation. The damage to the coronary artery can occur acutely [25] or chronically [24]. In order to prevent this complication during catheter ablation within the ASCs, selective angiography of the coronary artery and/or aorta should be performed prior to the ablation to assess the anatomical relationships between the coronary arteries and the location of the ablation catheter. Calcifications of the coronary arteries in older patients may also facilitate delineation of the ostium of the coronary arteries. RF ablation should be applied under continuous fluoroscopic observation with an angiographic catheter positioned within the ostium of the coronary artery. The outline of the ASCs and flow in the coronary artery are observed by hand injections of contrast every 15 s during RF applications. An RF application should be avoided within 5 mm of the coronary artery [18]. A rare complication of a transient vasovagal reflex during RFCA within the RCC has been reported [26]. There is also a potential risk of aortic insufficiency associated with the RFCA within the ASCs.

6.4.2 Atrial Tachycardia

All ATs that can be ablated within the ASCs will be first mapped from the right atrium (RA) with the earliest atrial activation recorded adjacent to the HB region because these ATs activate the RA through the interatrial septum near the HB region (Fig. 6.6) [8–12]. In this setting, mapping within the ASCs should be added to accurately identify the site of

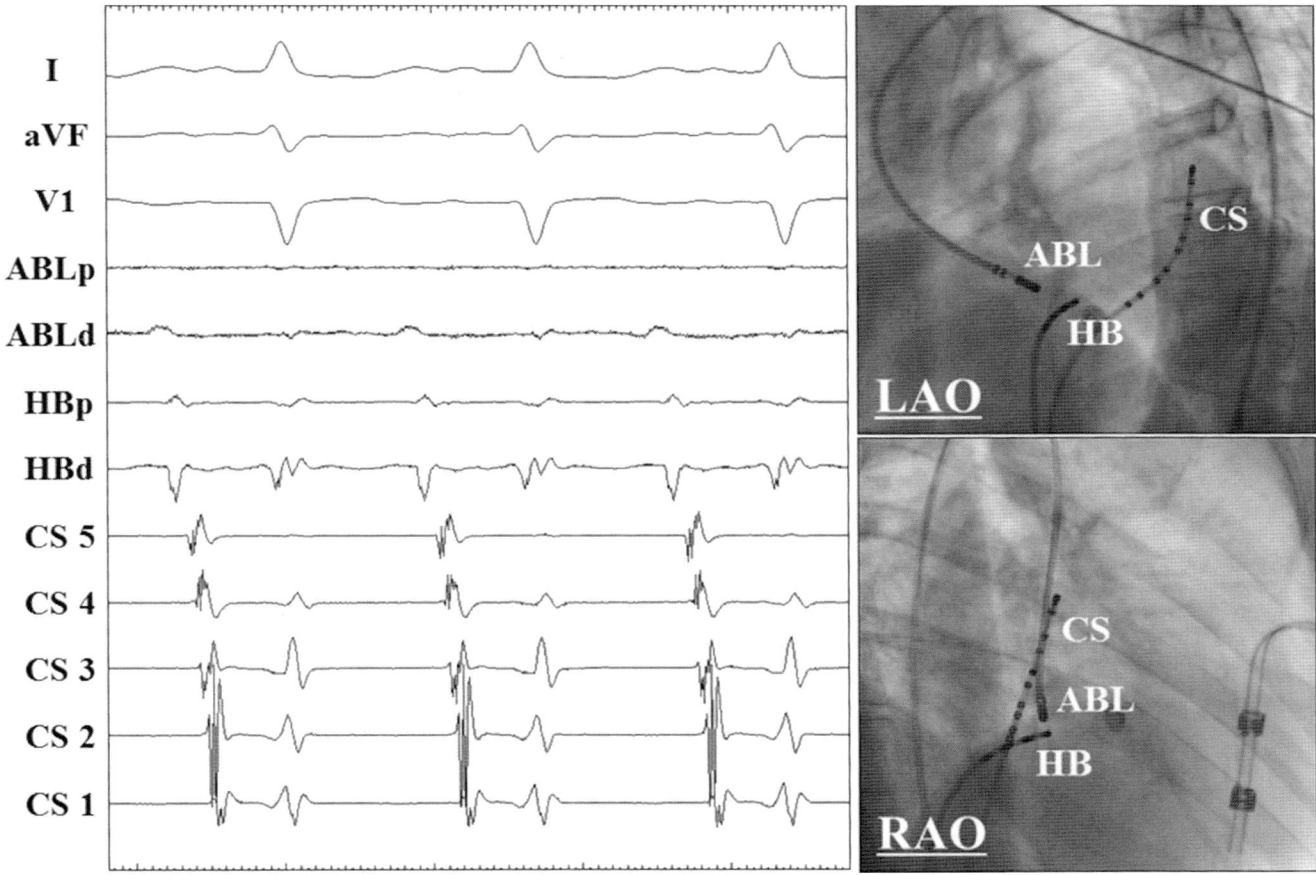

Fig. 6.6 Intracardiac tracings (*left panel*) and fluoroscopic images (*right panels*) exhibiting the successful ablation site of the atrial tachycardia within the noncoronary cusp. Note that the amplitude of the atrial electrogram was larger than that of the ventricular electrogram at the successful ablation site. Also, note that the ablation catheter was located close to the HB catheter. The abbreviations are as in the previous figures

AT origin. Basically, mapping and catheter ablation of ATs within the ASCs can be performed in the same way as those of VAs. When ATs are mapped seeking the earliest atrial activation within the ASCs, the amplitude ratio of the local atrial and ventricular electrogram (A/V ratio) is helpful for identifying which ASC is mapped [8–13]. The A/V ratio should be >1 within the NCC adjacent to the interatrial septum (Fig. 6.6), but it gets smaller toward the junction with the RCC and LCC. It should be <1 within the RCC and LCC because of the relatively thicker ventricular myocardium underneath the RCC and LCC. When the earliest atrial activation is recorded within the ASCs during the ATs, RFCA may be applied at that site [8–12]. When the earliest atrial activation recorded within the ASCs is as early as or even later than that in the RA adjacent to the HB region, RFCA may be applied at that site because it can be successful and safer than that in the RA [12].

Conclusion

The ASCs are one of the major sites of catheter ablation of idiopathic VAs, and catheter ablation of VAs within the ASCs is highly successful and safe. ATs originating from the interatrial septum can be ablated within the ASCs. Catheter ablation in this region may cause critical damage to important anatomical structures such as the coronary arteries and AV conduction system because of their close proximity. Accurate recognition of the anatomy of this region is essential for a successful catheter ablation and the prevention of complications associated with catheter ablation.

References

1. Ito S, Tada H, Naito S, Kurosaki K, Ueda M, Hoshizaki H, Miyamori I, Oshima S, Taniguchi K, Nogami A. Development and validation of an ECG algorithm for identifying the optimal ablation site for idiopathic ventricular outflow tract tachycardia. J Cardiovasc Electrophysiol. 2003;14:1280–6.
2. Kanagaratnam L, Tomassoni G, Schweikert R, Pavia S, Bash D, Beheiry S, Neibauer M, Saliba W, Chung M, Tchou P, Natale A. Ventricular tachycardias arising from the aortic sinus of valsalva: an under-recognized variant of left outflow tract ventricular tachycardia. J Am Coll Cardiol. 2001;37:1408–14.
3. Ouyang F, Fotuhi P, Ho SY, Hebe J, Volkmer M, Goya M, Burns M, Antz M, Ernst S, Cappato R, Kuck KH. Repetitive monomorphic ventricular tachycardia originating from the aortic sinus cusp: electrocardiographic characterization for guiding catheter ablation. J Am Coll Cardiol. 2002;39:500–8.
4. Yamada T, Yoshida N, Murakami Y, Okada T, Muto M, Murohara T, McElderry HT, Kay GN. Electrocardiographic characteristics of ventricular arrhythmias originating from the junction of the left and right coronary sinuses of Valsalva in the aorta: the activation pattern as a rationale for the electrocardiographic characteristics. Heart Rhythm. 2008;5:184–92.
5. Yamada T, McElderry HT, Doppalapudi H, Kay GN. Catheter ablation of ventricular arrhythmias originating from the vicinity of the his bundle: significance of mapping of the aortic sinus cusp. Heart Rhythm. 2008;5:37–42.
6. Yamada T, McElderry HT, Doppalapudi H, Murakami Y, Yoshida Y, Yoshida N, Okada T, Tsuboi N, Inden Y, Murohara T, Epstein AE, Plumb VJ, Singh SP, Kay GN. Idiopathic ventricular arrhythmias originating from the aortic root: prevalence, electrocardiographic and electrophysiological characteristics, and results of the radiofrequency catheter ablation. J Am Coll Cardiol. 2008;52:139–47.
7. Yamada T, Lau YR, Litovsky SH, Thomas McElderry H, Doppalapudi H, Osorio J, Plumb VJ, Kay GN. Prevalence and clinical, electrocardiographic, and electrophysiologic characteristics of ventricular arrhythmias originating from the noncoronary sinus of Valsalva. Heart Rhythm. 2013;10:1605–12.
8. Tada H, Naito S, Miyazaki A, Oshima S, Nogami A, Taniguchi K. Successful catheter ablation of atrial tachycardia originating near the atrioventricular node from the noncoronary sinus of Valsalva. Pacing Clin Electrophysiol. 2004;27:1440–3.
9. Ouyang F, Ma J, Ho SY, Bänsch D, Schmidt B, Ernst S, Kuck KH, Liu S, Huang H, Chen M, Chun J, Xia Y, Satomi K, Chu H, Zhang S, Antz M. Focal atrial tachycardia originating from the noncoronary aortic sinus: electrophysiological characteristics and catheter ablation. J Am Coll Cardiol. 2006;48:122–31.
10. Yamada T, Huizar JF, McElderry HT, Kay GN. Atrial tachycardia originating from the noncoronary aortic cusp and musculature connection with the atria: relevance for catheter ablation. Heart Rhythm. 2006;3:1494–6.
11. Gami AS, Venkatachalam KL, Friedman PA, Asirvatham SJ. Successful ablation of atrial tachycardia in the right coronary cusp of the aortic valve in a patient with atrial fibrillation: what is the substrate? J Cardiovasc Electrophysiol. 2008;19:982–6.
12. Wang Z, Liu T, Shehata M, Liang Y, Jin Z, Liang M, Han Y, Amorn A, Liu X, Liu E, Chugh SS, Wang X. Electrophysiological characteristics of focal atrial tachycardia surrounding the aortic coronary cusps. Circ Arrhythm Electrophysiol. 2011;4:902–8.
13. Yamada T, Litovsky SH, Kay GN. The left ventricular ostium: an anatomic concept relevant to idiopathic ventricular arrhythmias. Circ Arrhythm Electrophysiol. 2008;1:396–404.
14. Yamada T. Idiopathic ventricular arrhythmias: relevance to the anatomy, diagnosis and treatment. J Cardiol. 2016;68:463–71.
15. Stevenson WG, Soejima K. Catheter ablation for ventricular tachycardia. Circulation. 2007;115:2750–60.
16. Hoevelborn T, Doering J, Lindemann S, Haas CS. Images in cardiovascular medicine. Newly discovered heart murmur: noncoronary sinus of valsalva aneurysm with rupture into the right atrium and right ventricle. Circulation. 2009;119:e15–6.
17. Sekiguchi Y, Aonuma K, Takahashi A, Yamauchi Y, Hachiya H, Yokoyama Y, Iesaka Y, Isobe M. Electrocardiographic and electrophysiologic characteristics of ventricular tachycardia originating within the pulmonary artery. J Am Coll Cardiol. 2005;45:887–95.
18. Yamada T, Kay GN. Optimal ablation strategies for different types of ventricular tachycardias. Nat Rev Cardiol. 2012;9:512–25.
19. Yoshida N, Yamada T, McElderry HT, Inden Y, Shimano M, Murohara T, Kumar V, Doppalapudi H, Plumb VJ, Kay GN. A novel electrocardiographic criterion for differentiating a left from right ventricular outflow tract tachycardia origin: the V2S/V3R index. J Cardiovasc Electrophysiol. 2014;25:747–53.
20. Daniels DV, Lu YY, Morton JB, Santucci PA, Akar JG, Green A, Wilber DJ. Idiopathic epicardial left ventricular tachycardia originating remote from the sinus of Valsalva: electrophysiological characteristics, catheter ablation, and identification from the 12-lead electrocardiogram. Circulation. 2006;113:1659–66.
21. Yamada T, McElderry HT, Okada T, Murakami Y, Doppalapudi H, Yoshida N, Yoshida Y, Inden Y, Murohara T, Epstein AE, Plumb VJ, Kay GN. Idiopathic left ventricular arrhythmias originating adjacent to the left aortic sinus of valsalva: electrophysiological rationale for the surface electrocardiogram. J Cardiovasc Electrophysiol. 2010;21:170–6.

22. Yamada T, Kay GN. How to diagnose and ablate ventricular tachycardia from the outflow tract and aortic cusps. In: Al-Ahmad A, Callans D, Hsia HH, Natale A, Oseroff O, Wang PJ, editors. Hands-on ablation: the experts' approach. Mineapolis, MN: Cardiotext; 2013. p. 292–301.
23. Yamada T, Murakami Y, Yoshida N, Okada T, Shimizu T, Toyama J, Yoshida Y, Tsuboi N, Muto M, Inden Y, Hirai M, Murohara T, McElderry HT, Epstein AE, Plumb VJ, Kay GN. Preferential conduction across the ventricular outflow septum in ventricular arrhythmias originating from the aortic sinus cusp. J Am Coll Cardiol. 2007;50:884–91.
24. Pons M, Beck L, Leclercq F, Ferriere M, Albat B, Davy JM. Chronic left main coronary artery occlusion: a complication of radiofrequency ablation of idiopathic left ventricular tachycardia. Pacing Clin Electrophysiol. 1997;20:1874–6.
25. Waciński P, Głowniak A, Czekajska-Chehab E, Dąbrowski W, Wójcik J, Wysokiński A. Acute left main coronary artery occlusion following inadvertent delivery of radiofrequency energy during ventricular tachycardia ablation successfully treated by rescue angioplasty with stenting: a two-year follow-up. Cardiol J. 2013;20:100–2.
26. Yamada T, Yoshida Y, Inden Y, Murohara T, Kay GN. Vagal reflex provoked by radiofrequency catheter ablation in the right aortic sinus cusp: a Bezold-Jarisch-like phenomenon. J Interv Card Electrophysiol. 2008;23:199–204.

7. Coronary Sinus for Ablation of Ventricular Tachyarrhythmia and Supraventricular

Seiichiro Matsuo

Keywords
Coronary sinus • Epicardial ablation and mitral isthmus

7.1 Catheter Ablation Inside Coronary Sinus (CS)

7.1.1 Venography for Evaluation of the CS Anatomy

The coronary sinus (CS) is in the epicardium between the left atrium and ventricle around mitral valve. The epicardial ablation could be performed from the CS without epicardial puncture. The CS ablation is effective for patients with Wolf-Parkinson-White (WPW) syndrome, atrial fibrillation (AF), and ventricular arrhythmia. The CS, however, has limited space and its ablation may cause unique complications. The venography of CS would be useful to recognize the anatomy of CS because the size (diameter) and anatomy of CS vary among the patients (Fig 7.1a, b). In addition, the ability to recognize CS anomalies may help to interpret the anatomical cause for arrhythmogenic substrates and provides valuable information to guide catheter manipulation in the search for the target site of RF current application [1, 2]. The venography of CS can be simply performed with use of catheter with the lumen (Inquiry™ Luma-Cath™, St. Jude Medical). Although the CS catheter is sometime challenging to reach the distal CS legion, a guidewire is also accessed via the central lumen and the catheter could be placed at the distal CS in most patients.

7.1.2 Ablation Setting of CS

To avoid complications, radiofrequency energy should be delivered with maximum power of 25 W. Jais et al. reported that the incidence of cardiac tamponade was high in AF patients with radiofrequency application inside the CS with maximum power output of 30 W to complete mitral isthmus line [3]. The open-irrigated ablation catheter would be favorable to ablate the CS because the value of resistance could be higher compare to the normal endocardial lesions inside the CS. Where the impedance of ablation catheter is higher than normal value (the value of normal impedance is different according to the kind of ablation catheter), the maximum of power output should be limited to 20 W at the first application. Especially at the distal the CS (up to 3 or 4 o'clock), the impedance of ablation catheter is commonly high. In addition, radiofrequency energy should also be limited to 20 W in patients with narrow CS presenting the high impedance all along the CS. Recently, the ablation catheters can measure the contact force to tissue would be more favorable to perform CS ablation (SmartTouch, Biosense Webster, Inc. and TactiCath™ Quartz Contact Force Ablation Catheter, St. Jude Medical). These ablation catheters with contact force sensor can evaluate not only the value of contact force but also the force direction. Although the ablation where the ablation catheter is oriented to cardiac muscle (endocardial direction) is safe (Fig. 7.1a), the ablation for epicardial direction may be needed for completing procedure (Fig. 7.2b). In case of ablation with epicardial direction, the lower power output of radiofrequency energy (<20 W) and the lower value of contact force of ablation catheter (<10 g) would be feasible.

S. Matsuo
The Department of Cardiology, The Jikei University School of Medicine, 3-25-8, Nishi-shinbashi, Minato-ku, Tokyo 105-8471, Japan
e-mail: mattsuu@tc4.so-net.ne.jp

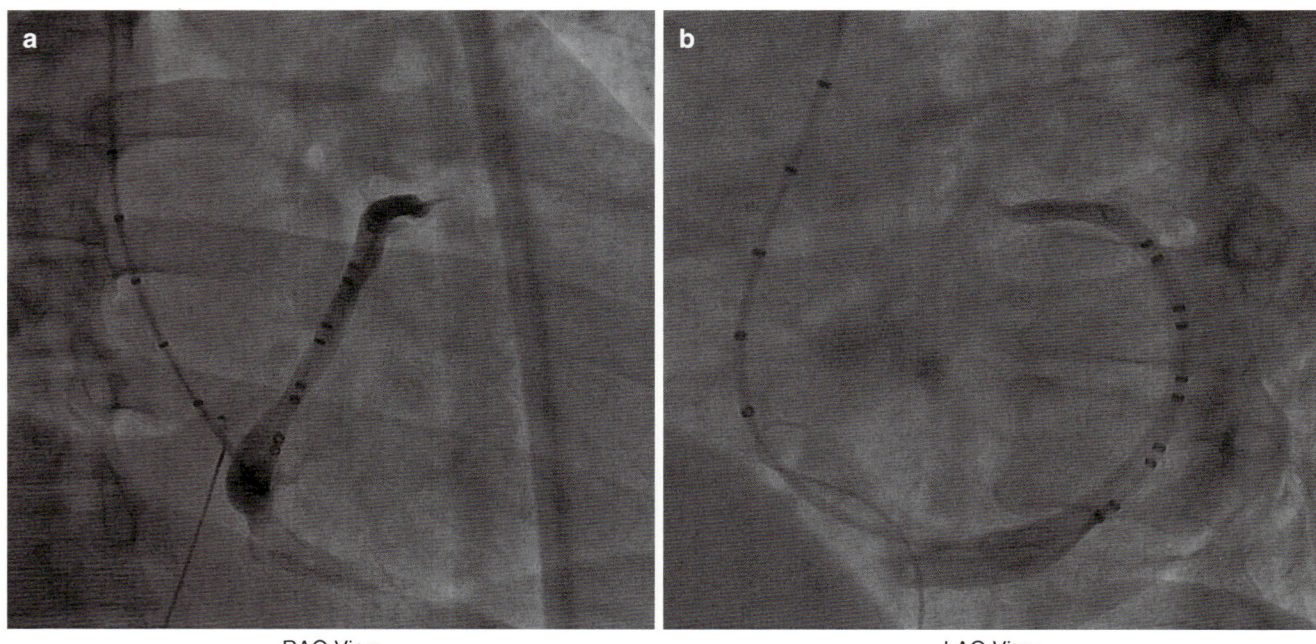

Fig. 7.1 The venography of coronary sinus with the use of electrode catheter with a lumen (Right anterior oblique (**a**) and left anterior oblique view (**b**))

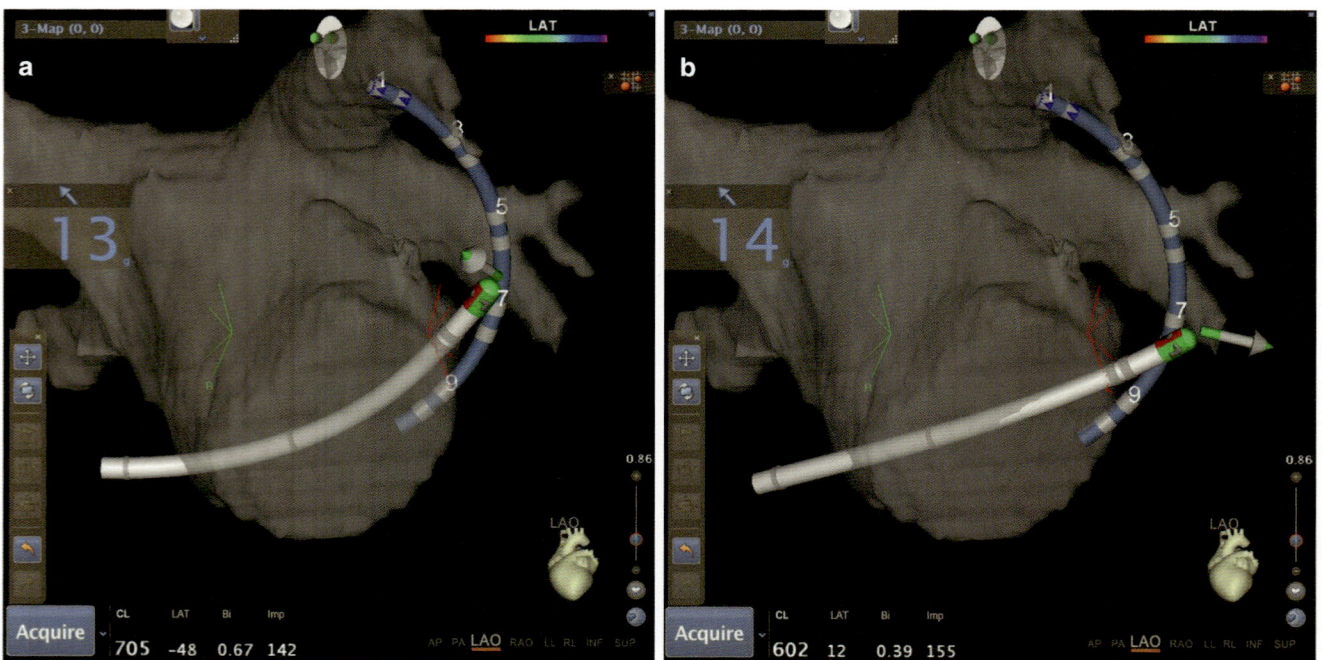

Fig. 7.2 (**a**) Fluoroscopic image of ablation catheter inside coronary sinus which is oriented to the direction of cardiac muscle. Three-dimensional mapping system presents the direction of ablation catheter with the value of contact force. (**b**) Ablation catheter is oriented against the direction cardiac muscle

7.2 Catheter Ablation of Wolf-Parkinson-White (WPW) Syndrome

Accessory pathways in patients with Wolff-Parkinson-White (WPW) syndrome usually have endocardial ventricular and atrial insertions located close to the atrioventricular valve rings, making endocardial standard ablation relatively easy and yielding a high success rate. The elimination of accessory pathway by endocardial radiofrequency ablation can be challenging in some patients with WPW syndrome because the accessory pathway can be at the epicardial lesion or its insertion of atrium or ventricle may be located far from the atrioventricular groove. Sacher F, et al. summarized the challenging cases with WPW syndrome [4]. In their study, catheter ablation for WPW syndrome failed in 7.6% (89/1171) of patients. Of 89 patients who were resistant to standard catheter ablation, radiofrequency application from the CS successfully eliminated the accessory pathway in 19 (21.3%) patients.

The posteroseptal and left posterior accessory pathways are sometimes located in the epicardial region and associated with ablation failure due to the complex anatomic arrangement [5]. This kind of epicardial accessory pathway results from a connection between an extension of CS myocardial coat along the middle cardiac vein, the posterior coronary sinus vein, or the neck of a CS diverticulum and the left ventricular epicardium [6]. A surface electrocardiogram is useful to predict the epicardial accessory pathway in WPW syndrome. The finding of steep negative delta wave in lead II is known to be predictive of epicardial accessory pathways. It has been reported that the sensitivity of negative delta wave in lead II in identifying a CS accessory pathway >70% [7]. A 46 years old man presenting narrow QRS tachycardia was referred to catheter ablation. Narrow QRS tachycardia was diagnosed as atrioventricular reciprocate tachycardia via left posterolateral accessory pathway by electrophysiological study. Endocardial RF application at this site resulted slight prolongation of the ventriculoatrial interval of the CS 5–6 but failed to eliminate the accessory pathway. Detailed mapping in the CS revealed the continuous VA electrogram was recorded within the posterolateral branch of the CS (Figs. 7.3 and 7.4a). However, application of RF energy in the CS branch could not be delivered by a non-irrigated ablation catheter due to the rise of the temperature. The ablation catheter was then replaced to an open-irrigated ablation catheter (Navistar Thermo-cool EZ DD, Biosense Webster) to be able to deliver enough energy within the CS branch. Epicardial ablation within the posterolateral branch of the CS under temperature control with maximum pre-set energy of 25 W achieved successful elimination of ventriculoatrial conduction via an accessory pathway (Fig. 7.4b). Even in the epicardial region within the CS, radiofrequency application should be delivered in the lesion demonstrating continuous activity or accessory pathway potential between atrial and ventricular potentials.

There are several strategies of catheter ablation for accessory pathway in patients with WPW syndrome. Although the epicardial ablation inside the CS is one of those approaches

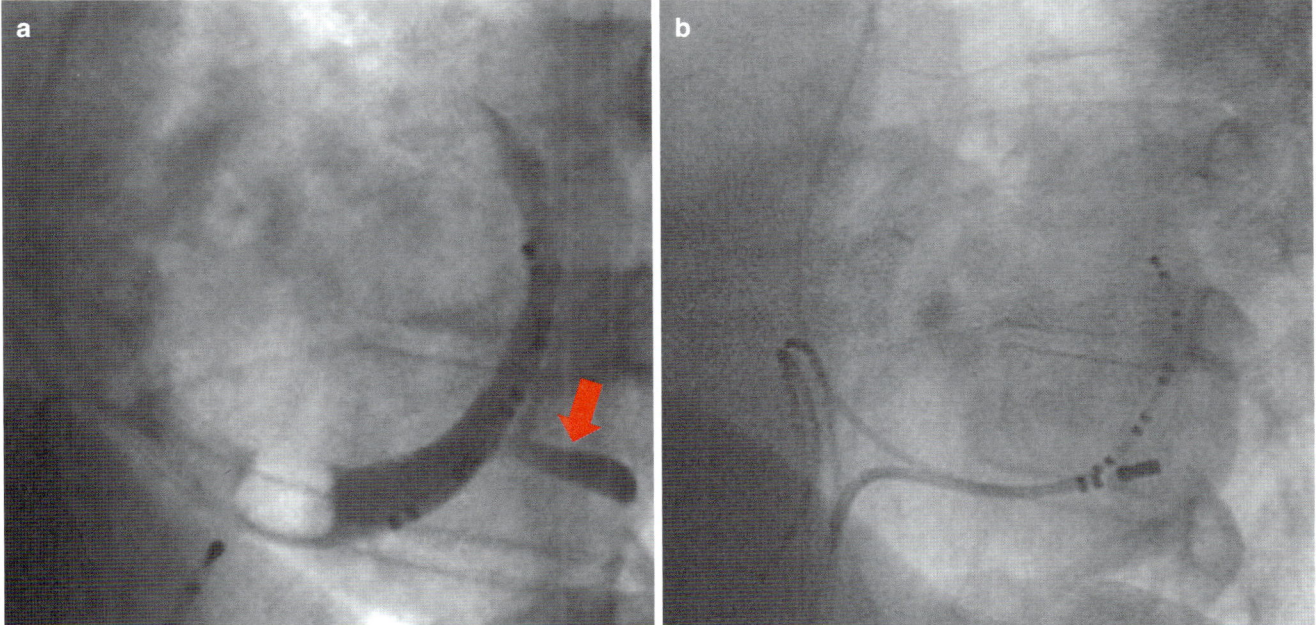

Fig. 7.3 (**a**) Venography of the CS was performed before mapping and ablation of coronary sinus. *Red arrow* indicates posterolateral branch of the CS. (**b**) The open-irrigated ablation catheter was positioned into the posterolateral branch of coronary sinus

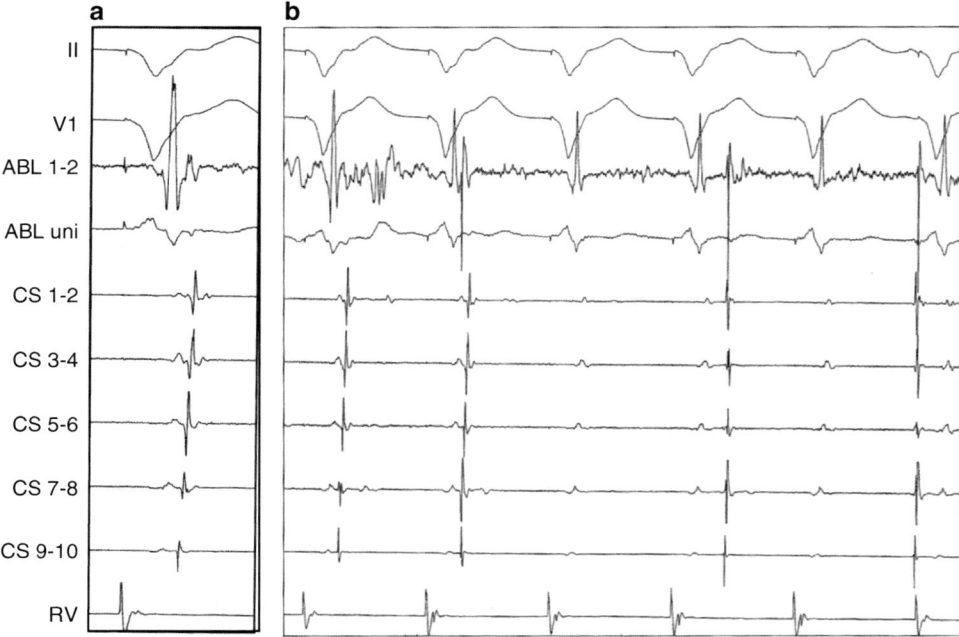

Fig. 7.4 (**a**) The intracardiac recordings demonstrated the continuous activity between atrial and ventricular potentials. (**b**) Electrical conduction between atrium and ventricle via accessory pathway was disappeared 3 s after radiofrequency application from coronary sinus

to ablate an accessory pathway, it should be performed after attempting several standard endocardial ablation methods. Ablation catheter could be advanced by either retrograde transaortic or trans-septal approaches for ablating the accessory pathway in the left side. In addition, radiofrequency energy can be delivered in not only the atrium but also ventricle. The epicardial ablation from the CS may cause complications including cardiac tamponade and coronary artery injury. The epicardial ablation from the CS should be considered after all endocardial ablation strategies were attempted and failed to eliminate an accessory pathway.

In patients with posteroseptal accessory pathway, the diverticulum of the CS was observed [8]. The diverticula of the CS were frequently observed in patients with manifest posteroseptal accessory pathways who have a previous failed ablation, documented AF, or typical electrocardiographic signs demonstrating a negative delta wave in lead II on the surface electrocardiogram. A clear accessory pathway potential is commonly seen at the successful site, but the local ventricular electrogram is not as early as in other accessory pathways.

7.3 Catheter Ablation of Atrial Fibrillation

7.3.1 Trigger of Atrial Fibrillation in the Coronary Sinus

Catheter ablation is a common treatment for patients with AF. The pulmonary veins are the major source of AF initiation, and thus its isolation from the left atrium resulted in the maintenance of sinus rhythm in AF patients. The trigger of AF originated from CS had been reported [9]. In that report, 3% of patients who underwent AF ablation demonstrated arrhythmogenicity inside the CS with the evidence of repetitive activities within the vein. The ablation of CS targeting focal origin initiating AF was basically performed by focal ablation strategy. The isolation of CS is usually challenging because the CS is a complex structure comprising a mesh of circumferential muscular fibers with oblique connections to both right and left atria. Thus, AF foci inside the CS will be focally ablated following detailed mapping of the vein.

7.3.2 Substrate of Atrial Fibrillation

In patients with non-paroxysmal AF, atrial ablation to modify the AF substrate in addition to PV isolation is performed. Haissaguerre et al. reported the impact of catheter ablation of the CS region in patients with AF [10]. In their study, CS ablation was commenced endocardially with use of dragging technique along the inferior peri-mitral legion in left atrium. Following endocardial CS ablation, it was continued from within the vessel (epicardial) if CS electrograms had cycle lengths shorter than that of the left atrial appendage. Radiofrequency energy was delivered with maximum power output of 35 W endocardially and 25 W epicardially. Although the primary objective of CS ablation in patients with AF is the modification and elimination of electrical interaction between the CS and atria through the CS musculature, the complete electrical isolation of CS is usually challenging. The endpoint of CS ablation is the organization of CS activity during AF and the decrease of atrial potential voltage of CS catheter. Another possible mechanism of modification of AF substrate by CS ablation is the effect for ganglionated plexi which is located at inferior and lateral left atrium. There are three ganglionated plexi around CS which are right inferior, left inferior, and Marshall ganglionated plexi. In the previous report by Haissaguerre [8], the cycle length of CS was significantly prolonged by 17 ms and its activation sequence was organized by endocardial CS ablation. In addition, further epicardial ablation in the CS increased the local cycle length by 32 ms. AF cycle length in the left atrial appendage at a lesion distant from CS was also prolonged significantly both during endocardial and epicardial CS ablation by 15 ms ($P < 0.03$). Finally, CS ablation terminated AF in 35% of AF patients (paroxysmal AF: 46% and persistent AF: 30%). Stepwise ablation is involved of pulmonary vein isolation, electrogram-based ablation targeting complex atrial fractionated potentials, linear ablation (roof line and mitral isthmus line), and CS ablation. During stepwise ablation, the CS ablation terminated AF directory to sinus rhythm in some patients. Based on their results, the CS is perpetuating AF as well as initiating AF in some patients.

7.3.3 Coronary Sinus Ablation for Mitral Isthmus Ablation

The linear ablation technique is performed in addition to PV isolation in persistent AF patients and enhances the efficacy of persistent AF ablation [11, 12]. Among linear ablation lesion sets, the mitral isthmus linear ablation is performed by connecting the left inferior PV to the mitral annulus. Although the mitral isthmus linear ablation commonly undergoes to modify the AF substrate in patients with non-paroxysmal AF, it will also be required to terminate the macro-reentrant tachycardia circulating around the mitral annulus. Unfortunately, the mitral reentrant atrial tachycardia is frequently observed in persistent AF patients who underwent catheter ablation [13]. It is widely recognized that completion of the mitral isthmus line block is challenging, requiring extensive ablation with irrigation catheters, the use of high ablation power, and epicardial ablation within the CS. Although the use of steerable sheath (The Agilis™ NxT steerable introducer, St. Jude Medical) is effective to establish the mitral isthmus block without the epicardial ablation from the CS [14], some patients still required the CS ablation for completing the mitral isthmus ablation ranging from 60% to 97% of patients [15–17]. Wong et al. reported that larger diameter of the CS was significantly associated with a need for CS ablation during the mitral isthmus ablation [18]. They also evaluated the correlation between the circumflex coronary artery diameter and need of epicardial ablation for the mitral isthmus ablation. In their results, the circumflex coronary artery diameter did not correlate with total mitral ablation time and CS ablation time. Although the blood flow in both the CS and circumflex coronary artery may act as a heat sink and reduce the efficacy of radiofrequency ablation of the mitral isthmus lesion, the CS but not the circumflex coronary artery acts as a heat sink phenomenon based on their results. The venography of CS and the cardiac multi-detector computed tomography which is performed prior to the procedure are helpful not only to recognize the anatomy of CS but also to evaluate whether the epicardial ablation from the CS will be needed for completion of the mitral isthmus line block or not. The epicardial ablation is commonly performed following the significant reduction of the atrial electrogram on the mitral isthmus or the long duration of endocardial radiofrequency application. Although the distinct indication of the epicardial ablation for the completion of the mitral isthmus block remains unclear, the CS ablation should be considered when the separated double potentials of the atrial electrograms with the opposite activation sequence were recorded by the CS catheter.

7.4 Catheter Ablation of Ventricular Arrhythmia

Ventricular arrhythmia could be originated from the epicardial regions [19–21]. Among those, ventricular arrhythmia originating from the CS is not uncommon accounting for about 9% of idiopathic ventricular arrhythmia cases. Although the epicardial ventricular arrhythmia usually required the direct epicardial access through the epicardial puncture, some arrhythmia may occur and be ablated in the regions close to the CS. The epicardial mapping and ablation through the CS is effective and safe and increasingly favored. The most common ventricular arrhythmia which can be treated into the CS is originated from the left ventricular summit [22]. The left ventricular summit was anatomically defined as the region on the epicardial left ventricular surface near the bifurcation of the left main coronary artery that is bounded by an arc from the left anterior descending artery superior to the first septal perforating branch anterior to the left circumflex laterally [22]. Among the ventricular arrhythmias in the left ventricular summit, the prevalence of left ventricular summit arrhythmia origins was much higher within the CS (the great cardiac vein and the anterior interventricular cardiac vein) than on the epicardial surface of either side of these veins. In detail, radiofrequency ablation in the distal CS eliminated the left ventricular summit arrhythmia 13 of 27 patients (nine in the great cardiac vein and four in the anterior interventricular cardiac vein) [22]. Catheter ablation or mapping of the left ventricular summit arrhythmias could be challenging because of the difficulty to position the ablation catheter within the distal part of the CS. The 2 Fr mapping catheter with eight electrodes (EP star Fix; Japan Lifeline Co. Ltd., Tokyo, Japan) is convenient to map the distal CS. To access the distal CS and map the left ventricular summit arrhythmias, the 2 Fr EP star catheter can be advanced through the lumen of CS mapping catheter (Inquiry™ Luma-Cath™, St. Jude Medical., Tokyo, Japan) (Fig. 7.5a, b). The pace mapping is also able to perform with use of this catheter. With this fine mapping catheter (2 Fr size), ablation catheter can smoothly advance into the deep CS lesion and radiofrequency energy is more easily delivered compared to it with a normal size CS catheter (8 Fr size). (Fig. 7.6a, b).

Coronary angiography should be performed to identify the anatomy of coronary artery because the ablation catheter within either the great cardiac vein or the anterior interven-

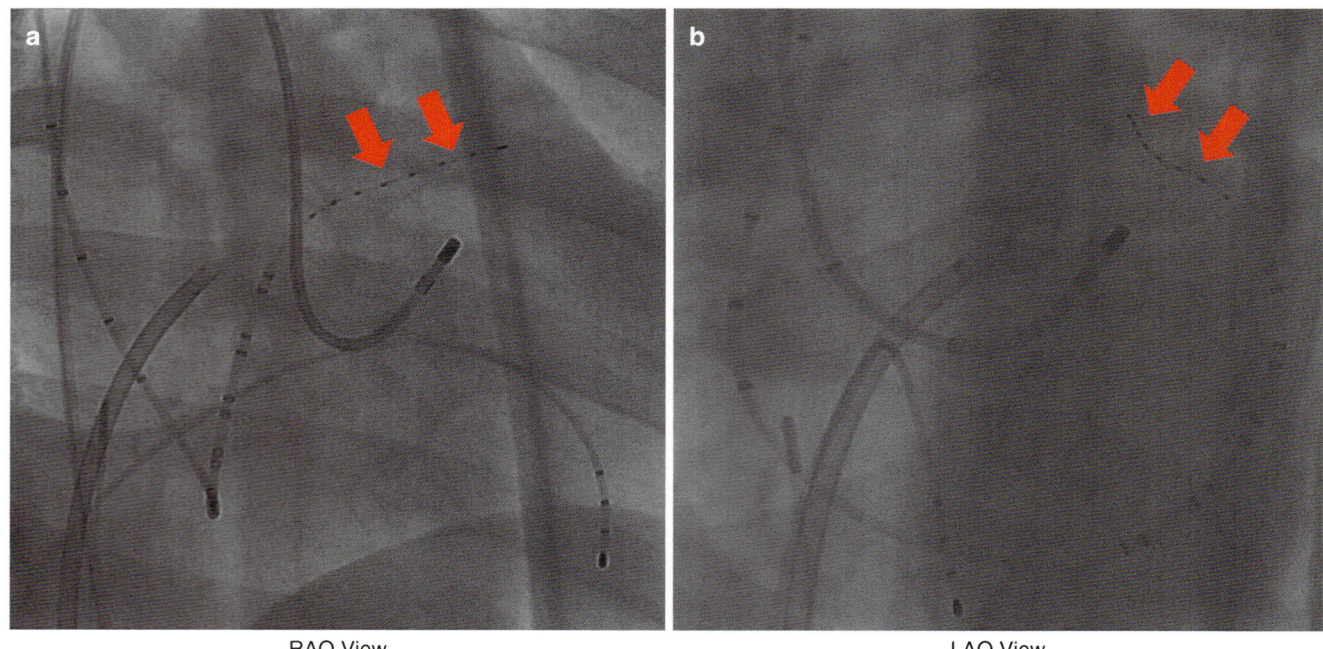

Fig. 7.5 The 2 Fr mapping catheter (*red arrows*) is introduced to the distal lesion of the coronary sinus (CS) via the central lumen of the CS catheter (Right anterior oblique (**a**) and left anterior oblique view (**b**))

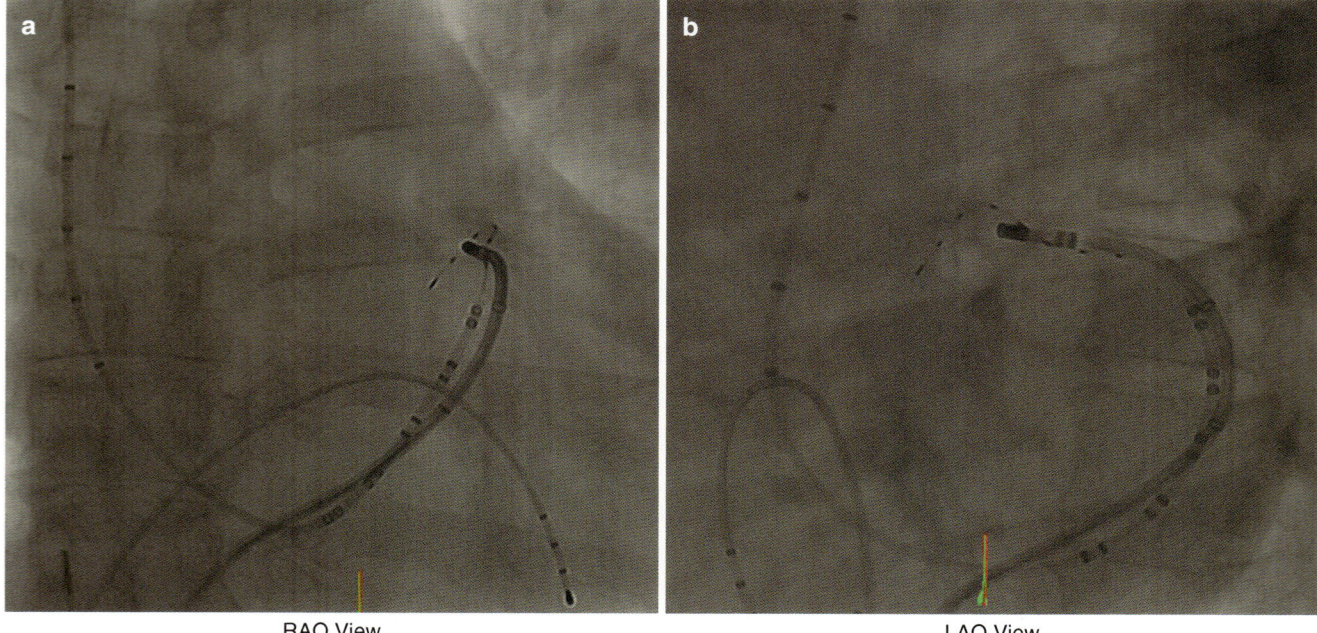

Fig. 7.6 Ablation catheter is advanced into the distal lesion of CS with the 2 Fr mapping catheter (Right anterior oblique (**a**) and left anterior oblique view (**b**))

tricular cardiac vein can be in close proximity to the left coronary arteries. The biplane fluoroscopic images and left coronary angiography are recommended to identify whether the site of origin is within the accessible or inaccessible regions of the left ventricular summit. Radiofrequency application should be abandon in the patients with the ablation sites close to the artery to protect the coronary arteries from inadvertent damage by radiofrequency ablation. An irrigated radiofrequency current was delivered in the power-control mode starting at 20 W in the CS (both the great cardiac vein and the anterior interventricular cardiac vein) with an irrigation flow rate of 30 mL/min (maximum flow). Radiofrequency energy is limited up to 30 W in the CS with the goal being to achieve a decrease in the impedance of 8–10 Ω and with care taken to limit the temperature to <40 °C. Although the non-irrigated ablation catheter was used for ablation of the left ventricular summit arrhythmias from the CS in the previous report [20], an open-irrigated ablation catheter would be favorable to use for this technique because the impedance of ablation catheter tip could be high and its temperature easily raises. In case in whom the high impedance of the ablation catheter was observed (>300 Ω), the abort of radiofrequency ablation is highly recommended.

7.5 Complication of Coronary Sinus Ablation

Although the CS is useful to deliver the radiofrequency energy from the epicardial lesion, some severe complications might occur. The CS ablation could injure coronary artery. CS is running parallel to the left circumflex artery. Stavrakis et al. reported that the stenosis of the left circumflex artery was observed in 15.4% (12/78) of patients who underwent CS ablation and the risk of a coronary artery injury with radiofrequency ablation delivered within the CS is inversely related to the distance of the coronary artery from the ablation site, with high (50%) risk of coronary artery injury for radiofrequency ablation within 2 mm of the artery [23]. The mechanism of injury of the coronary artery remains unclear. The direct thermal injury or coronary artery spasm might be considered as possible mechanism of coronary injury by radiofrequency energy. In order to avoid the coronary injury by radiofrequency application, the maximum power output should be limited to 30 W. The high-power output, however, will be required to complete ablation especially in patients with ventricular arrhythmia. In patients who require the high-power output (>30 W) ablation to eliminate arrhythmia, the coronary angiography would be better to perform before the ablation. The leads I, II, III, aVL, and aVF of surface 12 leads electrogram should be carefully monitored both during and after catheter ablation inside the CS to aware the ischemic change especially in patients with deep sedation. The coronary angiography should be performed as soon as possible in patients with ST-T change to avoid the myocardial infarction. In case with coronary artery stenosis and occlusion, nitro vasodilator is administered because the coronary artery spasm may be responsible. The percutaneous of coronary intervention will be conducted without improvement of the stenosis by nitro vasodilator. Finally, the ablation of CS ostium could be risk of injury of atrioventricular node. The interval between atrial and ventricular potential should be monitored during the CS ostium ablation. Additionally, the position of ablation catheter would be favorable to continuously observed by either fluoroscopy imaging or three-dimensional mapping system.

References

1. Chiang CE, Chen SA, Yang CR, Cheng CC, Wu TR, Chiang BN, et al. Radiofrequency ablation of posteroseptal accessory pathways in patients with abnormal coronary sinus. Am Heart J. 1993;126:1213–6.
2. Haissaguerre M, Gaita F, Fischer B, Egloff P, Lemetayer P, Warin JF. Radiofrequency catheter ablation of left lateral accessory pathways via the coronary sinus. Circulation. 1992;86:1464–8.
3. Jaïs P, Hocini M, Hsu LF, Sanders P, Scavee C, Weerasooriya R, et al. Technique and results of linear ablation at the mitral isthmus. Circulation. 2004;110:2996–3002. https://doi.org/10.1161/01.CIR.0000146917.75041.58.
4. Sacher F, Wright M, Tedrow UB, O'Neill MD, Jais P, Hocini M, et al. Wolff-Parkinson-White ablation after a prior failure: a 7-year multicentre experience. Europace. 2010;12:835–41. https://doi.org/10.1093/europace/euq050.
5. Wen MS, Yeh SJ, Wang CC, King A, Lin FC, Wu D. Radiofrequency ablation therapy of the posteroseptal accessory pathway. Am Heart J. 1996;132:612–20.
6. Sun Y, Arruda M, Otomo K, Beckman K, Nakagawa H, Calame J, et al. Coronary sinus-ventricular accessory connections producing posteroseptal and left posterior accessory pathways: incidence and electrophysiological identification. Circulation. 2002;106:1362–7.
7. Arruda MS, JH MC, Wang X, Beckman KJ, Widman LE, Gonzalez MD, et al. Development and validation of an ECG algorithm for identifying accessory pathway ablation site in Wolff-Parkinson-White syndrome. J Cardiovasc Electrophysiol. 1998;9:2–12.
8. Selvaraj RJ, Sarin K, Singh VR, Satheesh S, Pillai AA, Kumar M, et al. Radiofrequency ablation of posteroseptal accessory pathways associated with coronary sinus diverticula. J Interv Card Electrophysiol. 2016;47:253–9. https://doi.org/10.1007/s10840-016-0113-x.
9. Knecht S, O'Neill MD, Matsuo S, Lim KT, Arantes L, Derval N, et al. Focal arrhythmia confined within the coronary sinus and maintaining atrial fibrillation. J Cardiovasc Electrophysiol. 2007;18:1140–6. https://doi.org/10.1111/j.1540-8167.2007.00927.x.
10. Haïssaguerre M, Hocini M, Takahashi Y, O'Neill MD, Pernat A, Sanders P, et al. Impact of catheter ablation of the coronary sinus on paroxysmal or persistent atrial fibrillation. J Cardiovasc Electrophysiol. 2007;18:378–86. https://doi.org/10.1111/j.1540-8167.2007.00764.x.
11. Fassini G, Riva S, Chiodelli R, Trevisi N, Berti M, Carbucicchio C, et al. Left mitral isthmus ablation associated with PV Isolation: long-term results of a prospective randomized study. J Cardiovasc Electrophysiol. 2005;16:1150–6. https://doi.org/10.1111/j.1540-8167.2005.50192.x.
12. Willems S, Klemm H, Rostock T, Brandstrup B, Ventura R, Steven D, Risius T, et al. Substrate modification combined with pulmonary vein

isolation improves outcome of catheter ablation in patients with persistent atrial fibrillation: a prospective randomized comparison. Eur Heart J. 2006;27:2871–8. https://doi.org/10.1093/eurheartj/ehl093.
13. Matsuo S, Wright M, Knecht S, Nault I, Lellouche N, Lim KT, et al. Peri-mitral atrial flutter in patients with atrial fibrillation ablation. Heart Rhythm. 2010;7:2–8. https://doi.org/10.1016/j.hrthm.2009.09.067.
14. Matsuo S, Yamane T, Date T, Hioki M, Narui R, Ito K, et al. Completion of mitral isthmus ablation using a steerable sheath: prospective randomized comparison with a nonsteerable sheath. J Cardiovasc Electrophysiol. 2011;22:1331–8. https://doi.org/10.1111/j.1540-8167.2011.02112.x.
15. Matsuo S, Yamane T, Date T, Tokutake K, Hioki M, Narui R, et al. Substrate modification by pulmonary vein isolation and left atrial linear ablation in patients with persistent atrial fibrillation: its impact on complex-fractionated atrial electrograms. J Cardiovasc Electrophysiol. 2012;23:962–70. https://doi.org/10.1111/j.1540-8167.2012.02322.x.
16. Sawhney N, Anousheh R, Chen W, Feld GK. Circumferential pulmonary vein ablation with additional linear ablation results in an increased incidence of left atrial flutter compared with segmental pulmonary vein isolation as an initial approach to ablation of paroxysmal atrial fibrillation. Circ Arrhythm Electrophysiol. 2010;3:243–8. https://doi.org/10.1161/CIRCEP.109.924878.
17. Fassini G, Riva S, Chiodelli R, Trevisi N, Berti M, Carbucicchio C, et al. Left mitral isthmus ablation associated with PV Isolation: long-term results of a prospective randomized study. J Cardiovasc Electrophysiol. 2005;16:1150–6. https://doi.org/10.1111/j.1540-8167.2005.50192.x.
18. G Wong KC, Jones M, Sadarmin PP, De Bono J, Qureshi N, Rajappan K, et al. Larger coronary sinus diameter predicts the need for epicardial delivery during mitral isthmus ablation. Europace. 2011;13:555–61. https://doi.org/10.1093/europace/eur019.
19. Daniels DV, Lu YY, Morton JB, Santucci PA, Akar JG, Green A, et al. Idiopathic epicardial left ventricular tachycardia originating remote from the sinus of Valsalva: electrophysiological characteristics, catheter ablation, and identification from the 12-lead electrocardiogram. Circulation. 2006;113:1659–66. https://doi.org/10.1161/circulationaha.105.611640.
20. Soejima K, Stevenson WG, Sapp JL, Selwyn AP, Couper G, Epstein LM. Endocardial and epicardial radiofrequency ablation of ventricular tachycardia associated with dilated cardiomyopathy: the importance of low-voltage scars. J Am Coll Cardiol. 2004;43:1834–42. https://doi.org/10.1016/j.jacc.2004.01.029.
21. Della Bella P, Brugada J, Zeppenfeld K, Merino J, Neuzil P, Maury P, et al. Epicardial ablation for ventricular tachycardia: a European multicenter study. Circ Arrhythm Electrophysiol. 2011;4:653–9. https://doi.org/10.1161/CIRCEP.111.962217.
22. Yamada T, McElderry HT, Doppalapudi H, Okada T, Murakami Y, Yoshida Y, et al. Idiopathic ventricular arrhythmias originating from the left ventricular summit: anatomic concepts relevant to ablation. Circ Arrhythm Electrophysiol. 2010;3:616–23. https://doi.org/10.1161/CIRCEP.110.939744.
23. Stavrakis S, Jackman WM, Nakagawa H, Sun Y, Xu Q, Beckman KJ, et al. Risk of coronary artery injury with radiofrequency ablation and cryoablation of epicardial posteroseptal accessory pathways within the coronary venous system. Circ Arrhythm Electrophysiol. 2014;7:113–9. https://doi.org/10.1161/CIRCEP.113.000986.

Vein of Marshall Chemical Ablation of Atrial Tachyarrhythmias

Kaoru Okishige

Keywords
Atrial fibrillation • Chemical ablation • Vein of Marshall

8.1 Introduction Remarks

Chemical ablation therapy has been shown to be an effective modality in the treatment of a variety of arrhythmias. Haines et al. performed an experimental study of intracoronary ethanol ablation in swine hearts [1]. They demonstrated that ethanol infused into a specific coronary artery could provide an ablation bed that was smaller than the perfused bed, and an ethanol reflux was observed in 29% of the lesions resulting in injury beyond the targeted perfusion bed. Wang et al. also experimentally demonstrated that permanent atrioventricular block or modification of the atrioventricular node (AVN) function could be provoked by a selective AVN artery ethanol infusion [2]. Sneddon et al., Kay et al. and Okishige et al. performed successful intracoronary ethanol ablation procedures of the AVN conduction system, and Brugada et al. also demonstrated the transcoronary chemical ablation of ventricular tachycardia [3–6]. Wright et al. experimentally demonstrated the feasibility and effects of a retrograde coronary venous infusion of ethanol to ablate canine ventricular myocardium [7]. They infused ethanol through a branch of the middle cardiac vein and found that low volume infusions resulted in the creation only small epimyocardial lesions, whereas infusion volumes of 3 or 5 cc uniformly created transmural left ventricular necrosis. The coronary arteriograms and left ventriculograms remained unchanged from the pre- to post-ablation studies. However, nonsustained monomorphic ventricular tachycardia (with runs lasting 9–26 s at a maximal rate of 250 beats/min) occurred during and up to 90 s immediately following the infusions of ethanol in eight out of nine dogs. A histological examination confirmed the presence of necrosis in all sections taken from the affected region. In addition, numerous epicardial veins with partial or complete thrombosis were observed in many sections. Often the epicardial coronary artery was located near the vein; however, a coronary arterial thrombosis was never present. Of note, the ischemic regions were sharply demarcated from the surrounding normal myocardium. That experimental study elegantly showed that retrograde coronary venous infusions of ethanol are effective in ablating ventricular myocardium when subselective cannulation with a balloon infusion catheter is used, and chemical ablation does not significantly alter the hemodynamic measurements in the normal dogs.

The Marshall vein is a vestigial fold of the pericardium that contains fibrous bands, small blood vessels, and venous filaments enveloped in fat [8]. It courses obliquely above the left atrial appendage and lateral to the left superior pulmonary veins. Doshi et al. showed that the Marshall vein is a catecholamine-sensitive automatic focus in the canine left atrium, and it may be a source of adrenergic atrial tachyarrhythmias [9]. Hwang et al. demonstrated that the Marshall vein plays an important role in inducing chronic atrial fibrillation by providing a source of rapid activation [10, 11]. Kim et al. also found that the ligament of Marshall in humans consists of Marshall bundles that have multiple insertions into the coronary sinus musculature and the free wall of the left atrium, and the presence of multiple insertions provides a possible anatomical substrate for reentrant activation [12]. Kurotobi et al. also showed that mapping the ends of the Marshall vein branches during an isoproterenol infusion facilitates the identification of localized sites of

K. Okishige
Heart Center, Yokohama-City Bay Red Cross Hospital,
3-12-1 Shinyamashita, Naka-ku, Yokohama, Kanagawa
231-8682, Japan
e-mail: okishige@yo.rim.or.jp

high-frequency activity potentially responsible for the initiation and maintenance of atrial fibrillation (AF) [13]. These reports proposed the important clinical implications of the Marshall vein associated with AF.

Valderrabano et al. performed an experimental and clinical study regarding the feasibility and effects of a retrograde ethanol infusion into the Marshall vein [14]. They infused ethanol into the Marshall vein through a balloon catheter, which was utilized for coronary angioplasty, and constructed a three-dimensional voltage map of the left atrium. Successful cannulation of the Marshall vein with an angioplasty wire could be performed in 11 out of 12 dogs, and the angioplasty balloon was advanced over the wire into the proximal Marshall vein through which ethanol was infused into the Marshall vein. The low-voltage surface areas varied in their extent and distribution, depending on the course, size, and length of the Marshall vein. They also measured the effective refractory period (ERP) of the left atrium with a basket catheter inserted into the left atrium during vagal stimulation performed through a cuff electrode positioned on the vagus nerve exposed by a surgical cervical dissection. In the control status, a decrease in the ERP was demonstrated after the vagal stimulation; however, a significant blunting of the vagally mediated decrease in the ERP was observed after the ethanol infusion in the Marshall vein. This effect was observed only in the neighborhood of the ablated tissue exhibiting the blunting of the vagal effect and was not uniform across the three left atrial sites tested. They elegantly demonstrated that an ethanol infusion in the Marshall vein is able to exert parasympathetic denervation, and that this effect can be expected when this treatment option is applied for AF associated with an increase vagal tone.

8.2 Rationale for an Ethanol Infusion into the Marshall Vein

Several animal experiments have already demonstrated the feasibility, effects, and safety of an ethanol infusion into the Marshall vein, and this technique can be expected to compensate for the clinical efficacy of catheter ablation using radiofrequency (RF) energy current in patients with AF.

An ethanol infusion into the Marshall vein is attractive for the following reasons:

1. In the setting of the ablation of AF, the local toxicity of ethanol would be limited to the tissue in direct contact with it and would spare the neighboring structures such as the esophagus.
2. An ethanol infusion into the Marshall vein would directly address the mechanistic sources of AF located in the Marshall vein such as the autonomic nerves and ectopic foci triggering AF.
3. An ethanol infusion into the Marshall vein could help achieve an adequate ablation of the lateral ridge from the epicardial side.
4. A large area of tissue could be ablated at once with a simple infusion maneuver.
5. This technique is a purely right-sided procedure, obviating the need for a trans-septal puncture and anticoagulation.

The multiple factors described above can contribute to the improvement in the success rate of treating AF by catheter ablation.

8.3 Methods for Performing an Ethanol Infusion into the Marshall Vein

Under general anesthesia, the Marshall vein can be cannulated using a sheath (GCS aim SL, St. Jude. Medical, Inc., St. Paul, Minnesota) designed for a left ventricular pacing lead delivery that is inserted into the coronary sinus via the right jugular vein (Fig 8.1a). A subselector sheath (GCS direct SL II, St. Jude Medical, Inc.,) can be inserted through the outer sheath (GCS aim SL, St Jude. Medical, Inc.) and manipulated so that its tip faces posteriorly and superiorly (Fig. 8.1b). Angiographic contrast medium can be injected slowly and the Marshall vein can be identified as an atrial branch of the coronary sinus that arises from the level of the valve of Vieussens and is directed posteriorly. An angioplasty wire can then be advanced into the Marshall vein, and an angioplasty balloon (8 mm length, 1.5–2.0 mm diameter) can be advanced over the wire as distally as possible without perforating the distal end of the Marshall vein. Depending on the length of the Marshall vein, up to three balloon occlusive injections of 98% ethanol (1.5–2.0 cc over 90 s) can be delivered. Starting in the most distal part of the Marshall vein, the balloon is slightly retracted sequentially after each injection of ethanol, so that the last injection is performed from the most proximal portion of the Marshall vein. In that setting, as a result the distal half of the balloon is positioned inside the Marshall vein, whereas the proximal half of the balloon is located in the coronary sinus.

If the patient is not under the total anesthesia, the patient may experience serious chest pain during the ethanol infusion into the Marshall vein, and always should disappear soon after the end of the ethanol infusion. If the angioplasty wire perforates the most distal part of the Marshall vein, the angioplasty balloon has to be positioned just proximal to the perforated portion, and the balloon has to be inflated in order

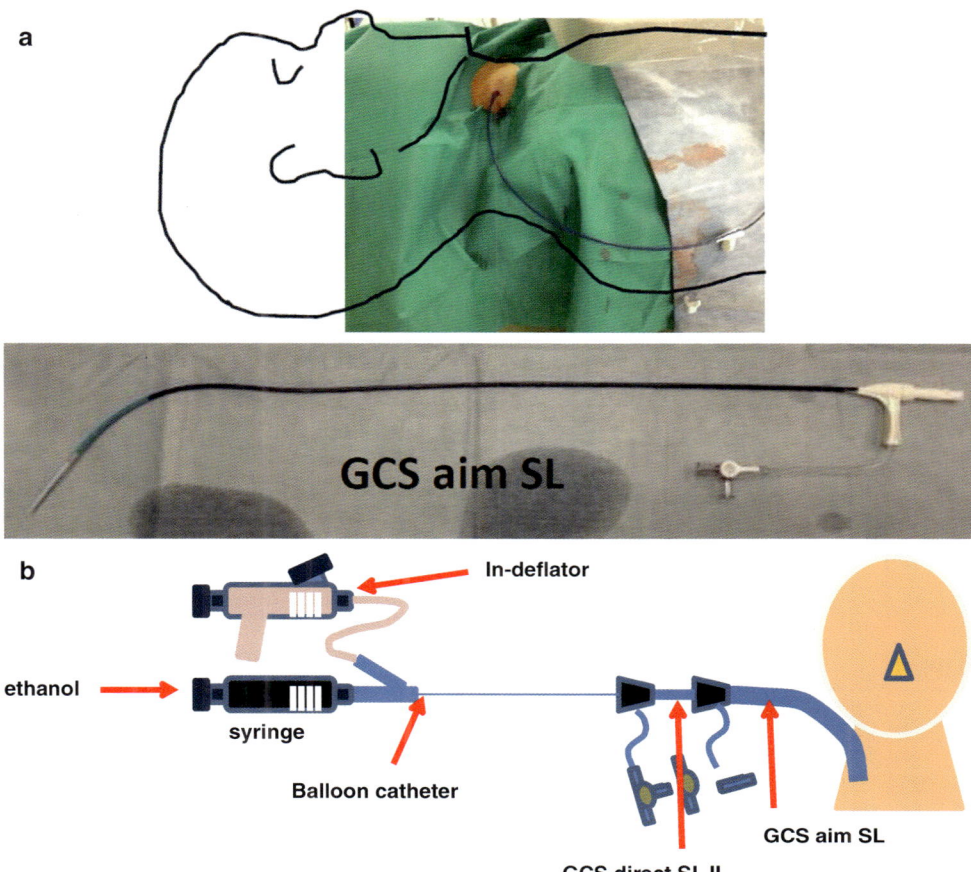

Fig. 8.1 (**a**) The right-sided jugular vein is punctured, and a long guiding sheath (GCS aim SL) is inserted deep into the right atrium through the superior vena cava. (**b**) Device setup for the ethanol infusion into the Marshall vein. A subselector sheath (GCS direct SL II, St. Jude Medical Inc.) is inserted through the outer sheath (GCS aim SL, St. Jude Medical Inc.) and manipulated so that its tip face posteriorly and superiorly for an appropriate cannulation into the Marshall vein. An angioplasty wire is advanced into the Marshall vein, and an angioplasty balloon is advanced over the wire as distally as possible without perforating the distal end of the Marshall vein. After inflating the balloon, ethanol is infused into the Marshall vein using a syringe

to occlude the Marshall vein for at least 1 h. If such a procedure is able to occlude the perforation of the Marshall vein, which has to be ascertained by venography of the coronary sinus, the ethanol infusion into the Marshall vein can be performed. The ethanol infusion into the Marshall vein is expected to acutely occlude the perforation by forming a blood clot in some cases; however, an ethanol infusion should be avoided. There is little chance of provoking a cardiac tamponade due to a perforation of the Marshall vein because a blood pressure inside the Marshall vein is very low and almost the entire perforated pore can be compressed by the epicardium.

8.4 Clinical Effect on the Autonomic Tone

Kim et al. demonstrated that the human ligament of Marshall contains multiple sympathetic nerve fibers and suggested that the ligament of Marshall plays a role in the genesis and maintenance of adrenergic AF [12]. The ligament of Marshall has been regarded as a target to identify the source of AF [15, 16]. Ulphani et al. experimentally demonstrated that the ligament of Marshall contains predominantly parasympathetic nerves and that these nerves originate from the left vagus nerve, travel through the ligament of Marshall, and innervate a number of structures in the posterior left atrium [17]. Valderranabo et al. tested the effects of a retrograde ethanol infusion in the vein of Marshall [18]. First, they experimentally demonstrated that the vagally mediated ERP decrease was eliminated after the ethanol infusion into the vein of Marshall. They also showed that cannulation of the vein of Marshall and an ethanol infusion was feasible and could create new scar involving the infero-posterior left atrial wall extending toward the left pulmonary veins.

We performed a clinical study to investigate the clinical effect on the autonomic tone provoked by an ethanol infusion in the vein of Marshall [19]. AF was induced by high-frequency electrical stimulation in eight patients in the control state; however, an ethanol infusion in the vein of Marshall abolished any AF induction upon repeated high-frequency stimulation (Fig. 8.2). In 32 patients undergoing AF catheter ablation for the first time, burst high-frequency stimulation provoked an asystolic response in 23 out of 32 and a significant R-R prolongation (of 228 ± 70%) in 9 out

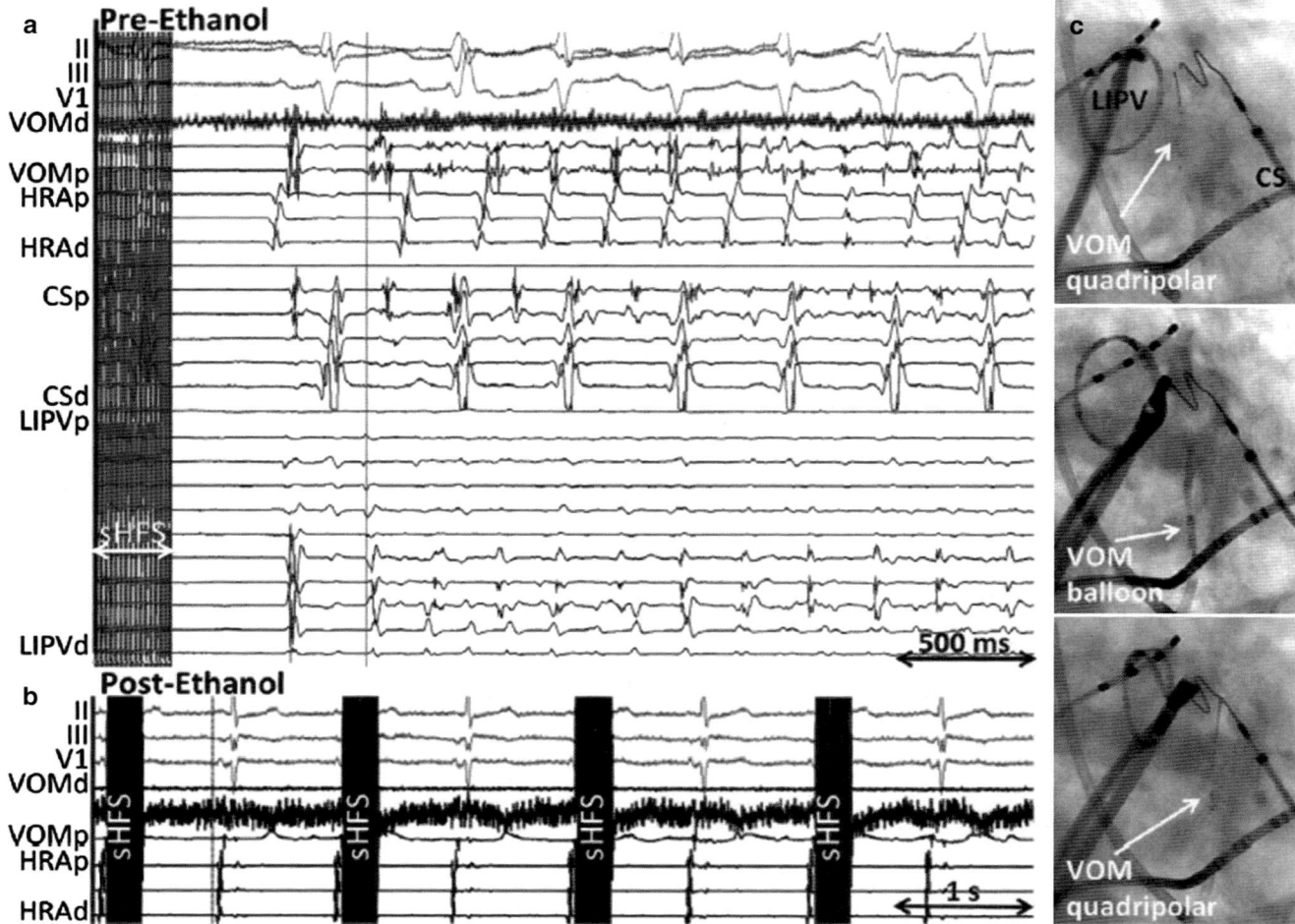

Fig. 8.2 AF was induced by high-frequency electrical stimulation in the control state (**a**); however, an ethanol infusion into the vein of Marshall abolished any further AF induction upon repeated high-frequency stimulation (**b**) (Reprinted from J Am Coll Cardiol. 2014;63(18):1892–901)

of 32 patients as shown in Fig. 8.3. However, such parasympathetic responses were not obtained after an ethanol infusion in the vein of Marshall. We also performed high-frequency electrical stimulation from different electrode sites to observe the parasympathetic response depending on the stimulation sites along the Marshall vein. When we performed stimulation from the most distal and middle electrodes, a significant vagal response was provoked. However, when we stimulated from the most proximal electrode, no significant parasympathetic response could be induced such as a significant slowing of the rate during AF. These findings might mean that the parasympathetic nervous innervation was more prominent in the distal portion of the ligament of Marshall. The significant vagotonic response was totally abolished after the ethanol infusion in the vein of Marshall (Fig. 8.4a–d).

8.5 Clinical Effect of the Chemical Ablation on the Cardiac Tissue

A retrograde ethanol infusion into the vein of Marshall has the capability of provoking ablative effects on left atrial tissue. We previously demonstrated that an ethanol infusion into the vein of Marshall could have therapeutic value in creating conduction block across the mitral isthmus between the inferior pulmonary vein and mitral annulus [20]. Using a NavX (St. Jude Medical Inc.) three-dimensional mapping system, we constructed voltage map after the ethanol infusion into the vein of Marshall. Scar was defined as areas with a bipolar voltage amplitude of <0.1 mV. Pacing from the left atrial appendage (LAA) and coronary sinus was used to assess the peri-mitral conduction. When a gap conduction was recognized after the ethanol infusion, the procedure was

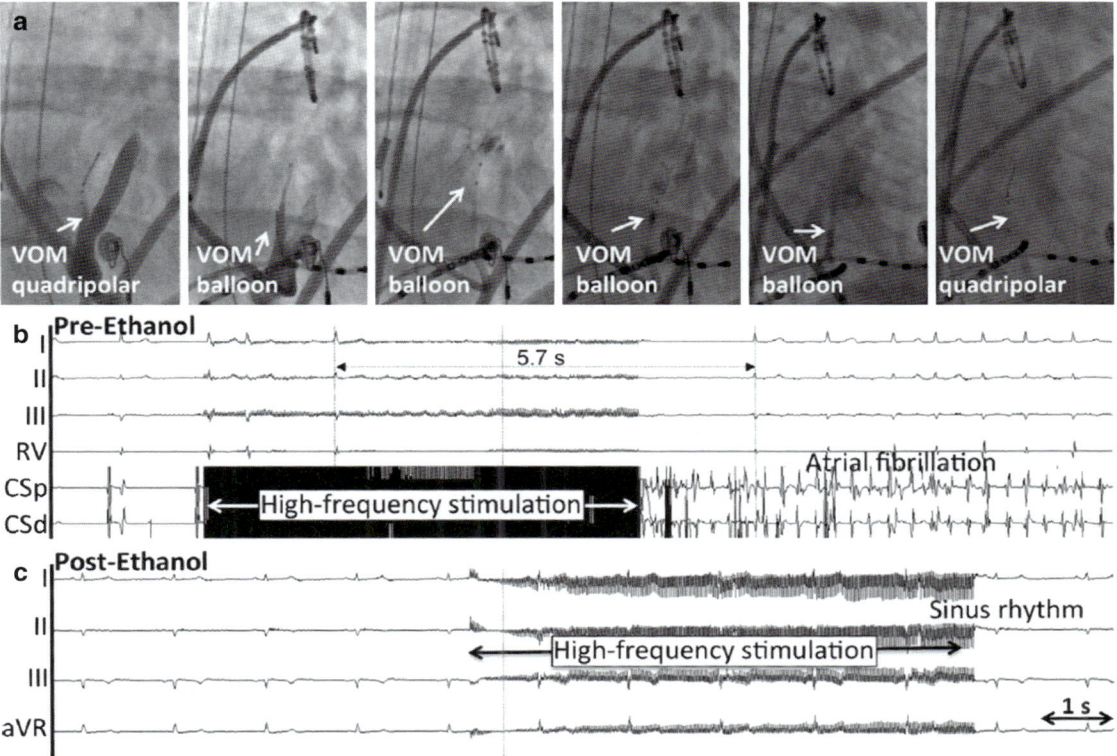

Fig. 8.3 (**a**) High-frequency stimulation provoked an asystolic response that lasted for 5.7 s (**b**); however, such a response was abolished after an ethanol infusion into the Marshall vein (**c**) (Reprinted from J Am Coll Cardiol. 2014;63(18):1892–901)

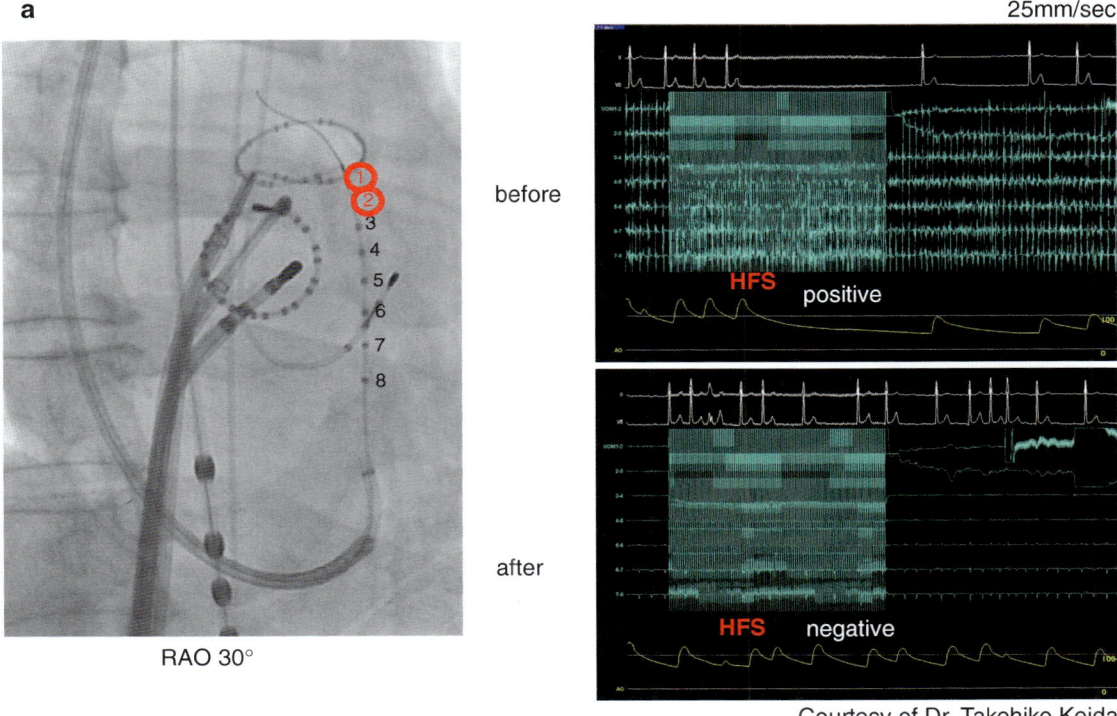

Fig. 8.4 We performed high-frequency electrical stimulation through different electrode sites to observe the parasympathetic response depending on the stimulation site along the Marshall vein (**a**–**c**). When we performed stimulation from the most distal and middle electrodes, a significant vagal response was provoked. The *red* colored portions are high-frequency stimulation sites. However, when we simulated through the most proximal electrode, no significant parasympathetic response could be induced exhibiting any significant slowing of the rate during AF (**d**). That finding might mean that parasympathetic nerve innervation was more prominent in the distal portion of the Marshall vein. A significant vagotonic response was totally abolished after the ethanol infusion into the vein of Marshall. *HFS* high-frequency stimulation (Courtesy of Dr. Takehiko Keida, Cardiology Department, Edogawa Hospital, Japan)

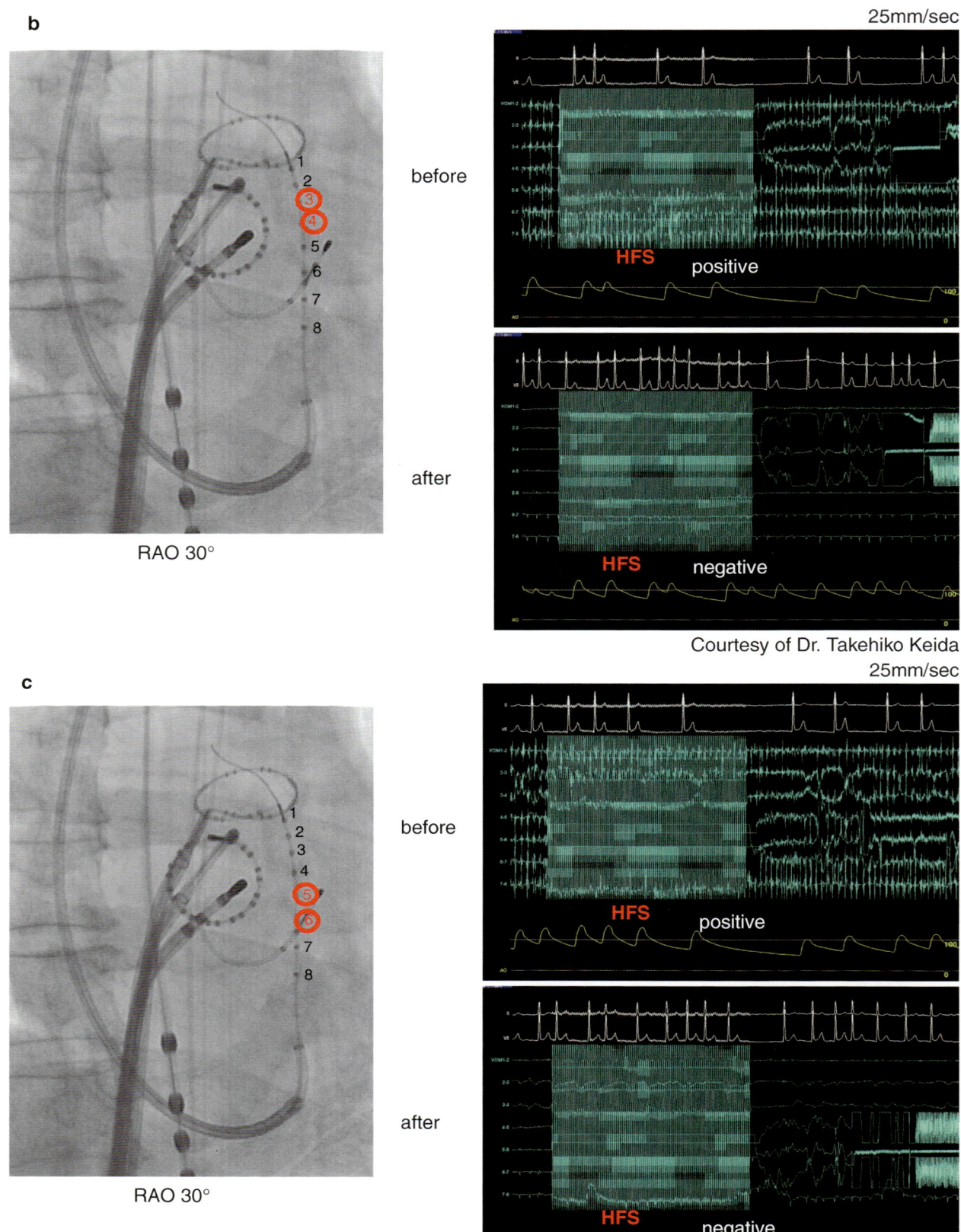

Fig. 8.4 (continued)

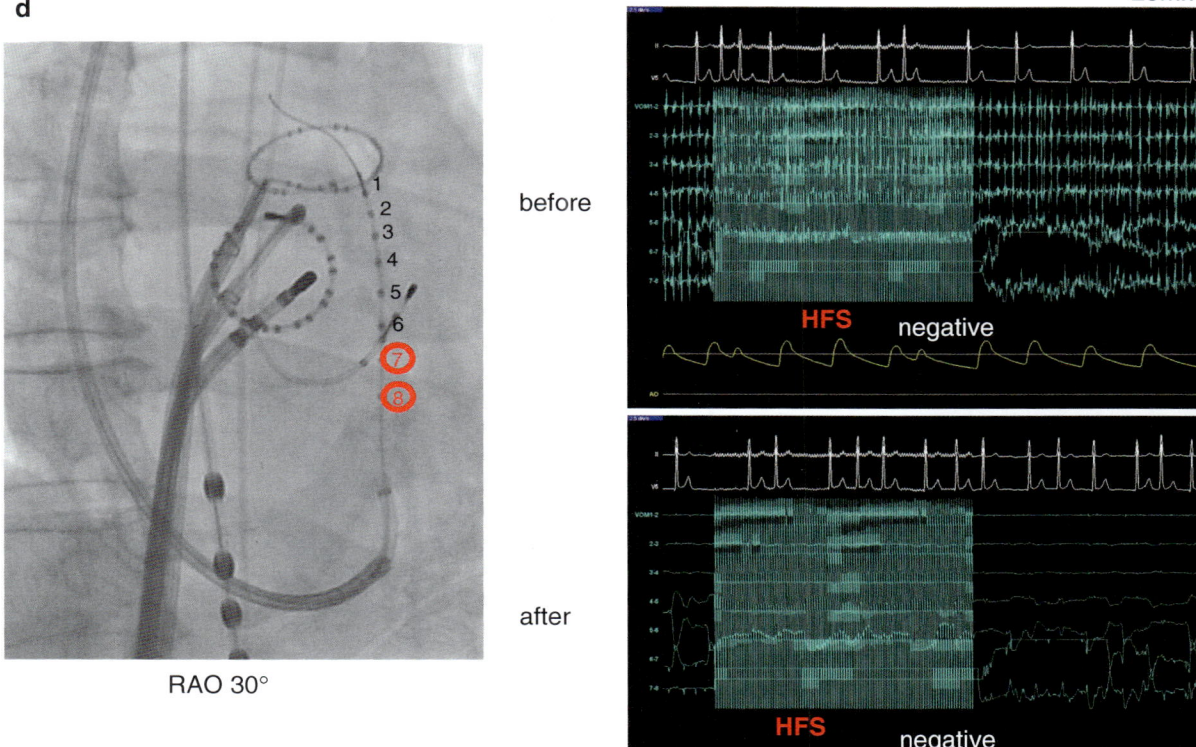

Fig. 8.4 (continued)

continued with radiofrequency (RF) energy using an irrigated catheter. The RF was applied to areas of the endocardial scar where signals were still present, by delivering a power of 25–35 W with a 20 cc/min saline irrigation. Mitral isthmus block was confirmed by differential pacing.

The time course of the lesion expansion created by the ethanol infusion into the Marshall vein was observed as shown in Fig. 8.5. Compared to the lesion at 30 min after the ethanol infusion, the lesion at 90 min demonstrated a significantly larger lesion size using the NavX system.

The anatomical course of the Marshall vein arises from the coronary sinus at its middle portion, and the anatomical location of the coronary sinus is shifted upwards in the left atrium. Therefore, injurious effects of the ethanol infusion into the vein of Marshall would not be expected in the area between the coronary sinus and mitral annulus (Fig. 8.6). We speculated that undiscernible small branches of the Marshall vein take an anatomical course around the area between mitral annulus, and the injurious effects of the ethanol infusion into the vein of Marshall could be provided as a result because conduction block at the mitral isthmus can be achieved solely by an ethanol infusion into the Marshall vein in sporadic cases. As an example, peri-mitral flutter was provoked by atrial stimulation after a pulmonary vein electrical isolation with radiofrequency current as shown in Fig. 8.7a. This atrial tachycardia could be terminated during the ethanol infusion into the Marshall vein (Fig. 8.7b), which meant that conduction block could be created solely by the ethanol infusion into the Marshall vein without any touch-up ablation.

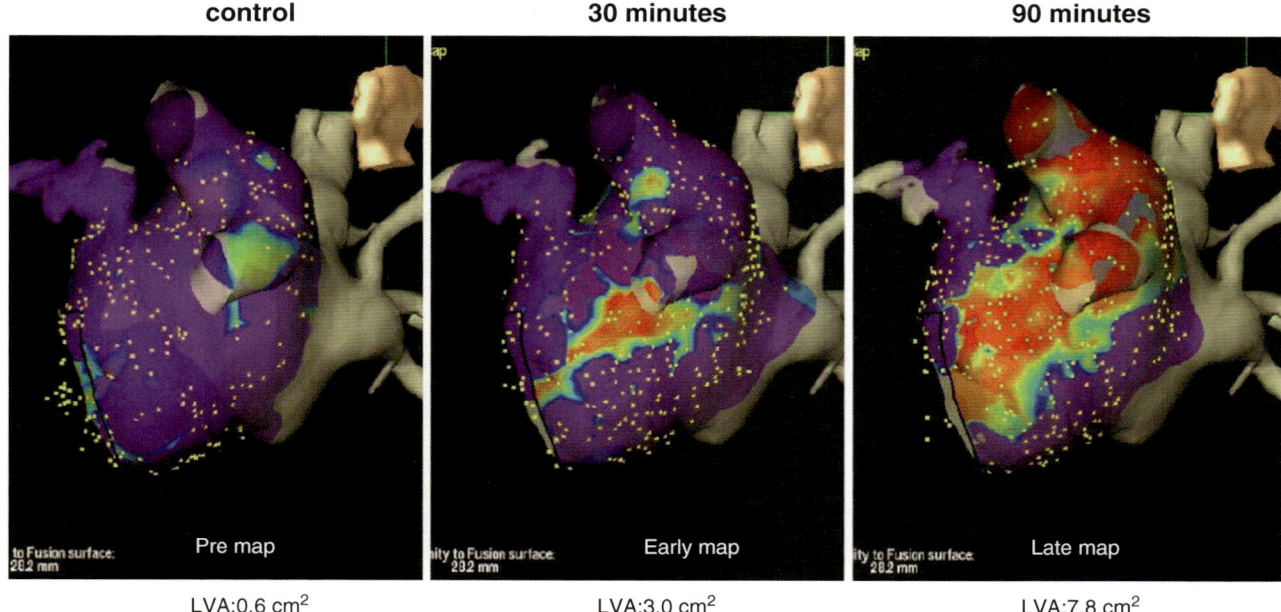

Fig. 8.5 The time course of the lesion expansion created by the ethanol infusion into the Marshall vein. There was a significant difference regarding the lesion size between the lesion at 30 min and that at 90 min after the ethanol infusion using the NavX system

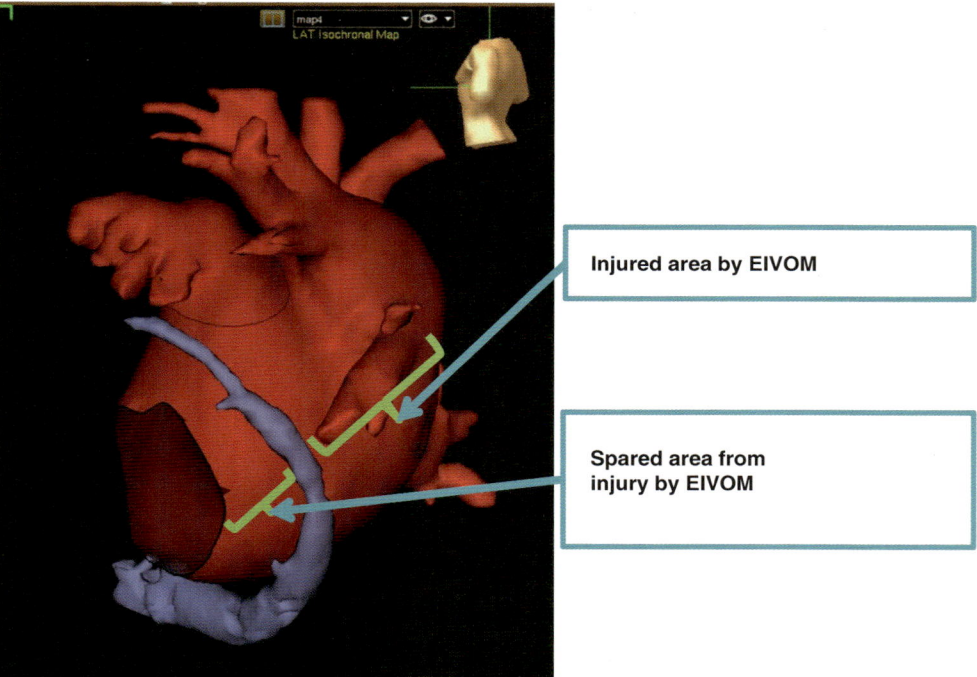

Fig. 8.6 The anatomical course of the Marshall vein arises from the coronary sinus, and the anatomical location of the coronary sinus is shifted upward in the left atrium. Therefore, the area of the left atrium between the coronary sinus and mitral annulus could be spared from injury by the ethanol infusion into the vein of Marshall. *EIVOM* ethanol infusion into the Marshall vein

a Activation map

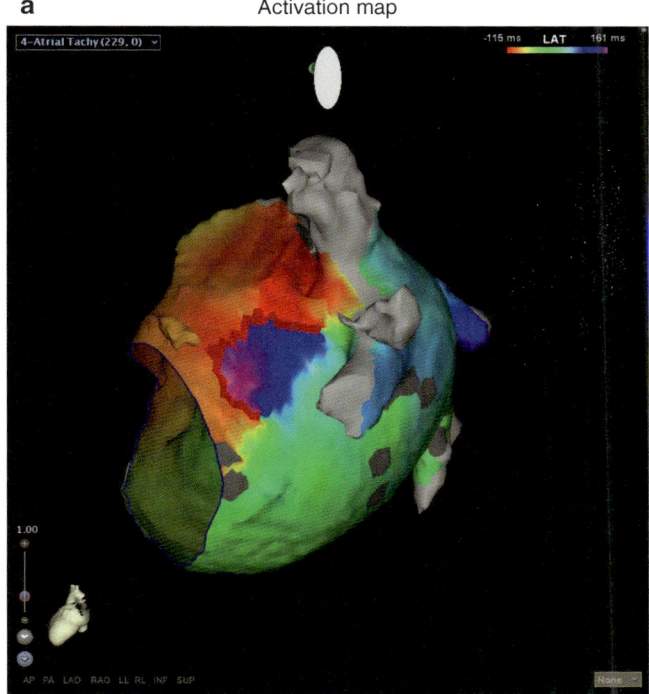

b AT termination during injection of ethanol

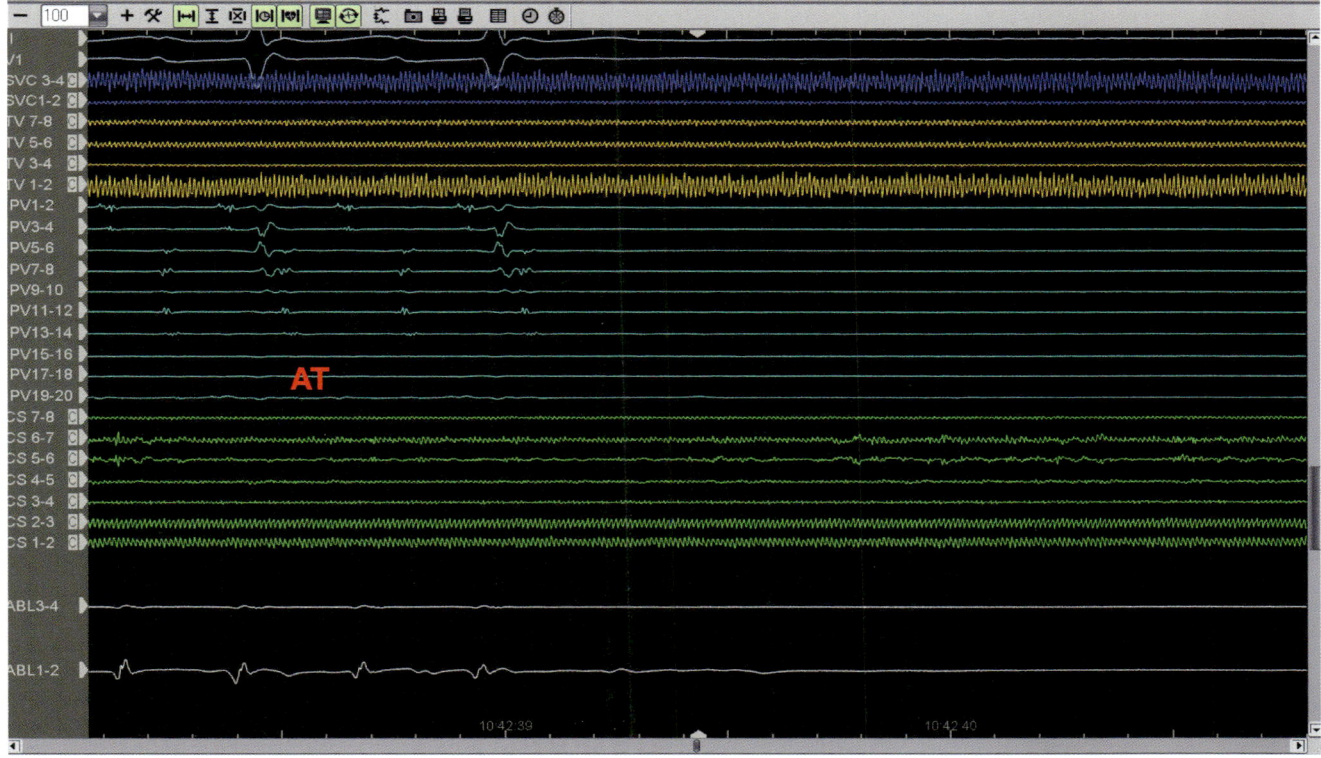

Fig. 8.7 (**a**) An activation map using the CARTO system (Biosense Webster, Diamond Bar CA) showing an example of a peri-mitral flutter provoked by atrial stimulation after pulmonary vein electrical isolation with radiofrequency current. This demonstrates a counterclockwise rotation around the mitral isthmus. (**b**) This atrial tachycardia terminated during the ethanol infusion in the Marshall vein, and a transient sinus pause was observed

8.6 Clinical Effect on the Isolation of the Pulmonary Veins

The Marshall vein takes an anatomical course arising from the middle portion of the coronary sinus and runs toward the ridge between the left atrial appendage and left-sided pulmonary veins. A low-voltage zone created by an infusion of ethanol into the vein of Marshall can be located at the mitral isthmus between the mitral annulus and left inferior pulmonary vein. When the Marshall vein covers the ostium of the left-sided pulmonary veins, injurious effects of the ethanol infusion into the Marshall vein could be expected. In 5 out of 436 patients who underwent chemical ablation of the Marshall vein, bidirectional conduction block at the mitral isthmus could be created solely by the ethanol into the Marshall vein. As shown in Fig. 8.8, we were able to electrically isolate the left-sided pulmonary veins solely by the ethanol infusion into the Marshall vein. In the control state, the vein of Marshall was identified by the venography of the coronary sinus, which could be annotated with the NavX 3-D mapping system (Fig. 8.8a). After the ethanol infusion into the Marshall vein, a low-voltage area could be noted along the Marshall vein. During pacing from the left atrial appendage, conduction block at the mitral isthmus was created in the low-voltage area along the Marshall vein (Fig. 8.8b).

8.7 Clinical Effect on the Epicardial Fat Pad

Several recent reports have demonstrated that the epicardial fat pad plays an important role in the initiation and maintenance of atrial fibrillation [21–23]. Ethanol of a high concentration has been considered to be able to dissolve fat tissue. On a workstation (Zio M900 Quadra; Amin, Tokyo), the total epicardial fat pad could be detected and its volume could be semi-automatically reconstructed. We measured the total volume of the epicardial fat pad during the control state and measured it after the ethanol infusion into the Marshall vein (Fig. 8.9a). As shown in Fig. 8.9b, a reduction in the total volume of the epicardial fat pad was observed, but it did not reach a statistical significance. However, the magnitude of the volume reduction after the ethanol infusion into the Marshall vein showed a significant difference (Fig. 8.9c). In addition, that magnitude of the volume reduction was significantly larger in persistent than paroxysmal AF (Fig. 8.9d).

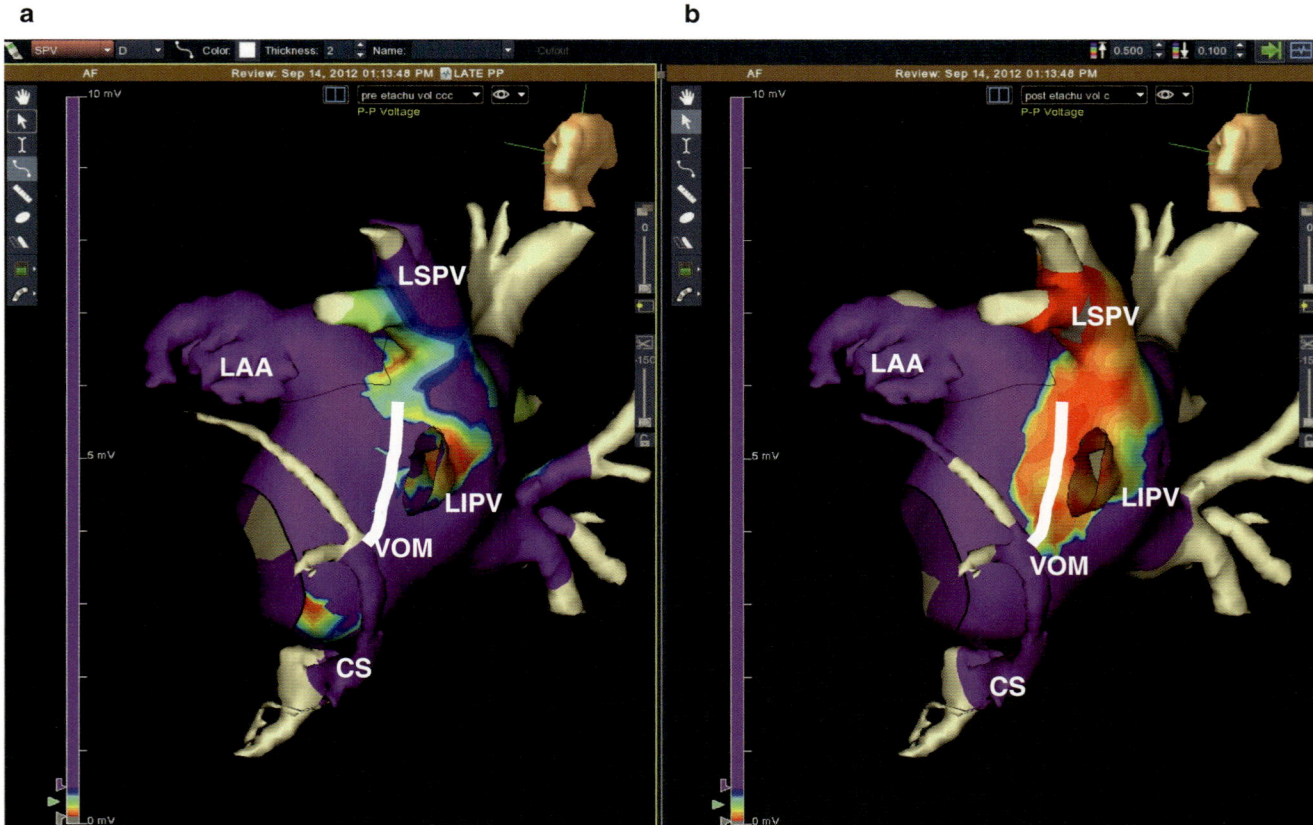

Fig. 8.8 In the control state (**a**), the vein of Marshall was identified by venography of the coronary sinus and is annotated in the 3-D NavX mapping system. After the ethanol infusion into the Marshall vein, a low-voltage area could be observed along the Marshall vein (**b**). *LSPV* left superior pulmonary vein, *LIPV* left inferior PV, *LAA* left atrial appendage, *VOM* vein of Marshall, *CS* coronary sinus

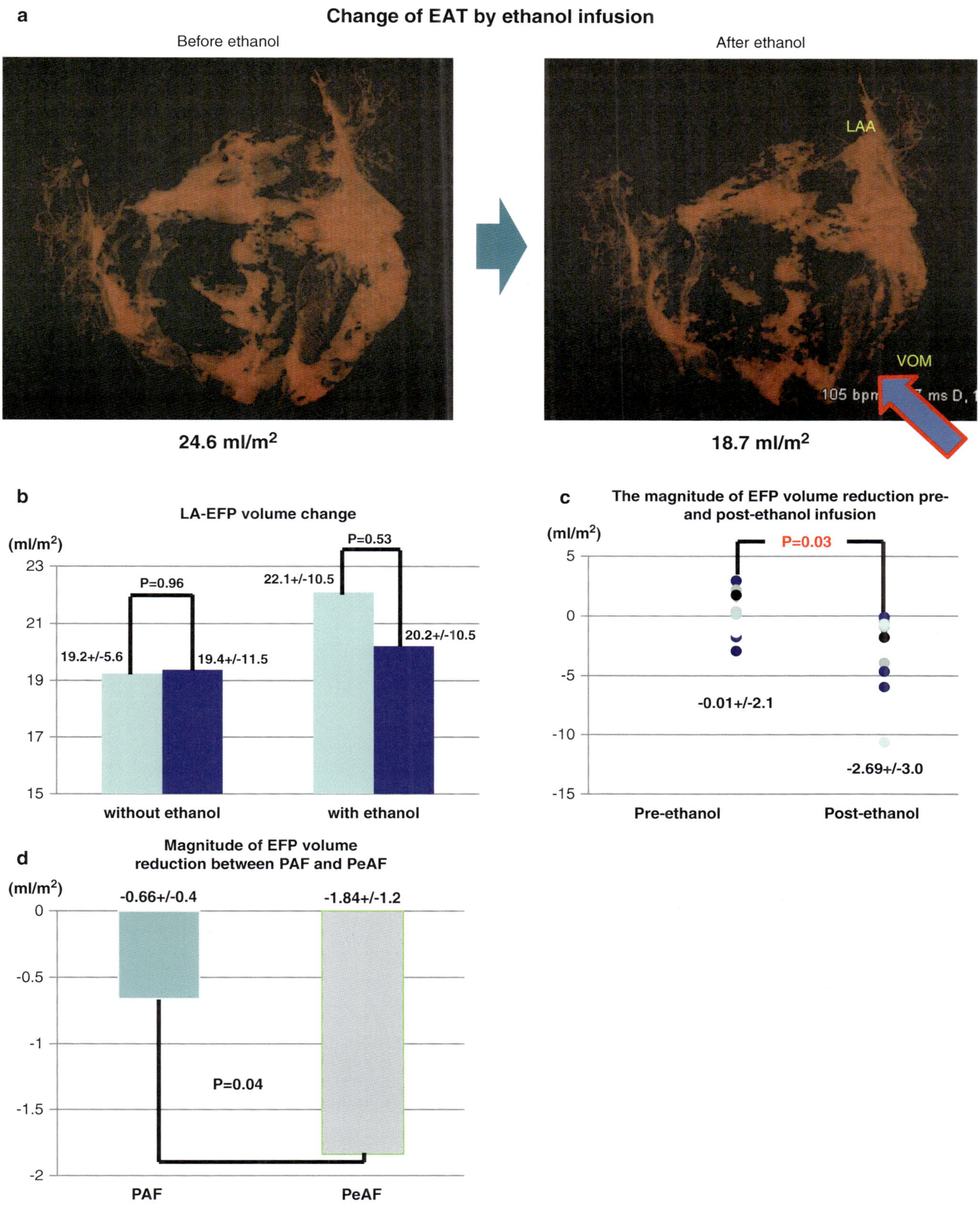

Fig. 8.9 (a) The total epicardial fat pad (EFP) can be detected and their volume semi-automatically reconstructed. We measured the total volume of the epicardial fat pad in the control state, and remeasured that after an ethanol infusion into the Marshall vein. A significant volume reduction of the fat tissue was observed after the ethanol infusion into the Marshall vein. *LAA* left atrial appendage, *VOM* vein of Marshall. (b) In those patients with an ethanol infusion, a reduction in the total volume of the epicardial fat pad was observed compared to that in those without an ethanol infusion, but it did not reach a statistical significance ($p = 0.53$). (c) There was a significant difference in the magnitude of the volume reduction after the ethanol infusion into the Marshall vein. (d) The magnitude of the volume reduction of the EFPs was significantly larger in those with persistent (PeAF) rather than paroxysmal atrial fibrillation (PAF)

8.8 Clinical Effect on the Complexed Fractionated Atrial Electrograms

The elimination of areas that exhibit complexed fractionated atrial electrograms (CFEs) has demonstrated a significant improvement in suppressing the recurrence of AF [24, 25]. We mapped the CFE areas in the control state during sustained AF (Fig. 8.10a upper panel). Such CFE areas could be significantly eliminated after the ethanol infusion into the Marshall vein (Fig. 8.10a lower panel). Of interest, the CFE areas distant from the location of the Marshall vein also disappeared after the ethanol infusion. That suggested there was an interference between the CFE areas. When focusing on the area of the Marshall vein's anatomical course, a significant reduction in the total CFE area was observed (Fig. 8.10b). Although the clinical implication of the elimination of CFEs by an ethanol infusion into the Marshall vein has never been investigated, we might be able to expect a therapeutic effect involving the prevention of any recurrence of AF.

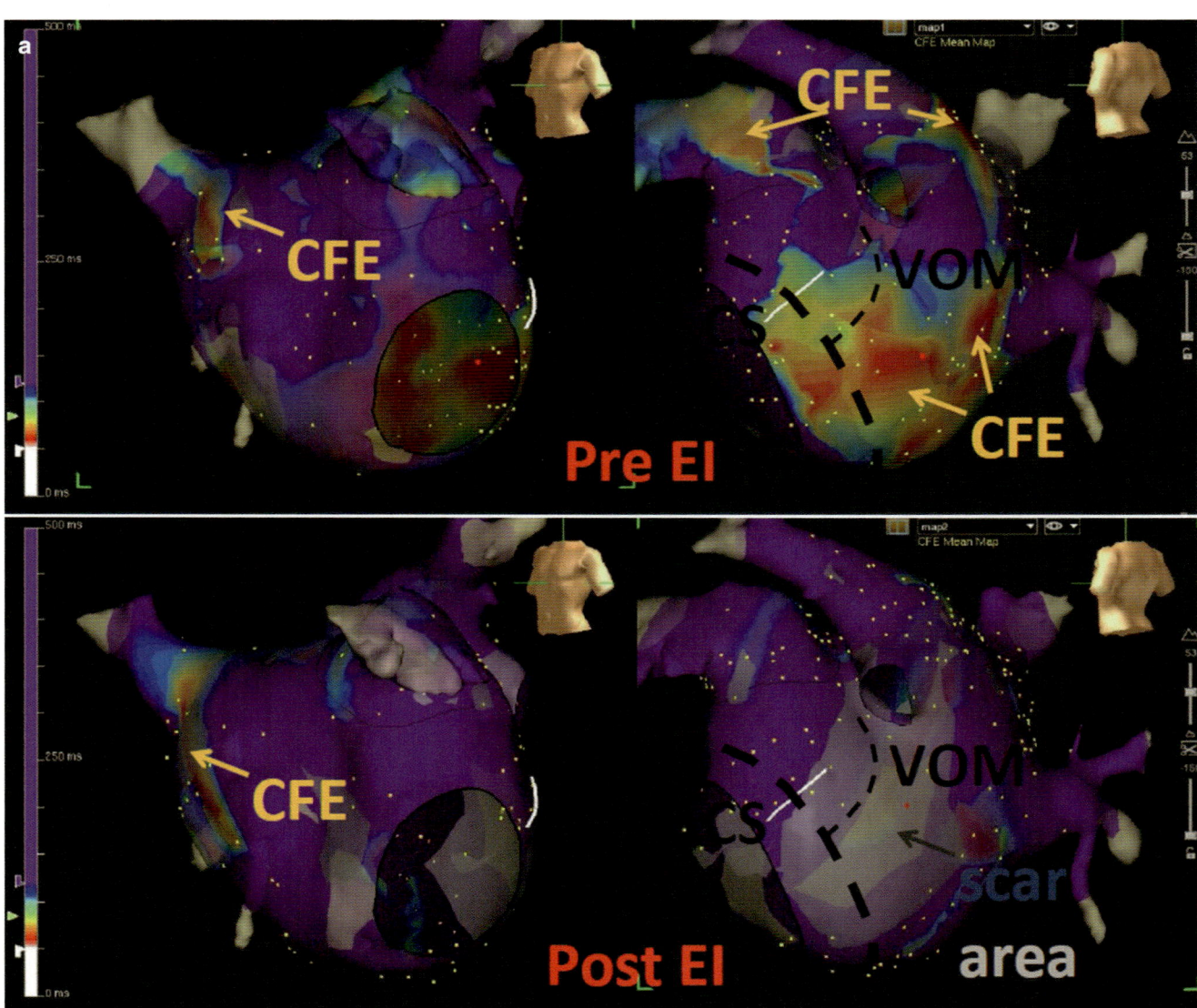

Fig. 8.10 We mapped the complex fractionated atrial electrogram (CFE) areas in the control state (pre-EI) during sustained atrial fibrillation. The CFE area was significantly eliminated after an ethanol infusion into the Marshall vein (post EI), and a scar area was created along the Marshall vein. Of interest, the CFE area distant to the location of the Marshall vein also disappeared after the ethanol infusion (**a**). The total area of the CFEs was calculated by NavX, and it became significantly reduced after the ethanol infusion into the Marshall vein (**b**). *EI* ethanol infusion

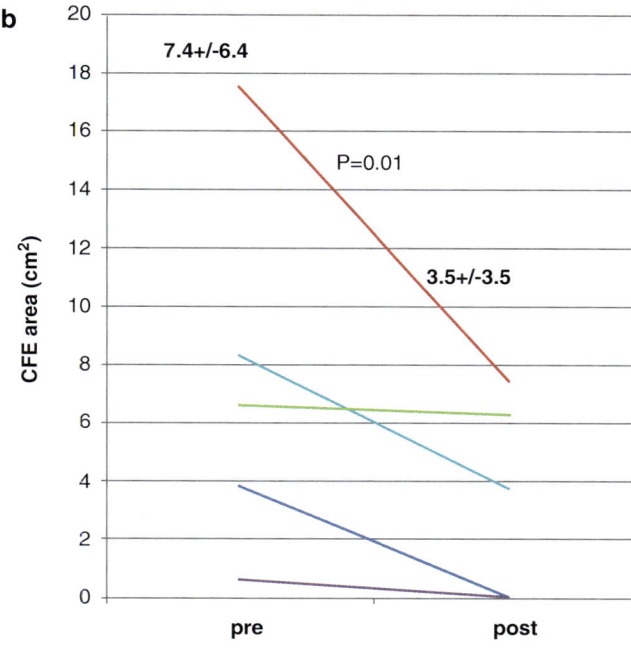

Fig. 8.10 (continued)

8.9 Clinical Effect on Treating Atrial Fibrillation

We reported a case in which ectopic atrial beats (EABs) arising from the Marshall vein appeared in a bigeminal fashion and provoke sustained AF (Fig. 8.11a). This patient complained of palpitations during the EABs and suffered from dizziness during AF. When a micro-electrode catheter was inserted into the Marshall vein, we found that the EAB arose from the Marshall vein. We successfully cannulated the Marshall vein with the micro-infusion catheter and slowly infused a total of 5 cc of ethanol. The EABs could be completely abolished after the ethanol infusion as shown in Fig. 8.11b, and AF also was eliminated after the procedure. We constructed a voltage map after the ethanol infusion into the Marshall vein, and a significant low-voltage area could be created along the Marshall vein as shown in Fig. 8.11c.

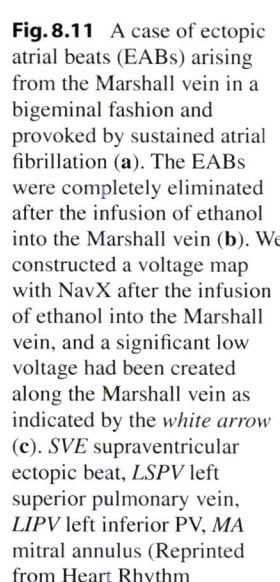

Fig. 8.11 A case of ectopic atrial beats (EABs) arising from the Marshall vein in a bigeminal fashion and provoked by sustained atrial fibrillation (**a**). The EABs were completely eliminated after the infusion of ethanol into the Marshall vein (**b**). We constructed a voltage map with NavX after the infusion of ethanol into the Marshall vein, and a significant low voltage had been created along the Marshall vein as indicated by the *white arrow* (**c**). *SVE* supraventricular ectopic beat, *LSPV* left superior pulmonary vein, *LIPV* left inferior PV, *MA* mitral annulus (Reprinted from Heart Rhythm 2013;10(9):1354–1356)

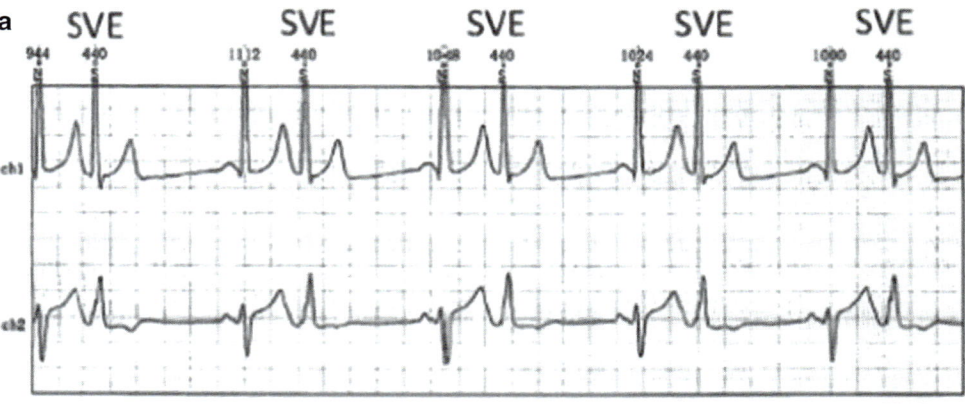

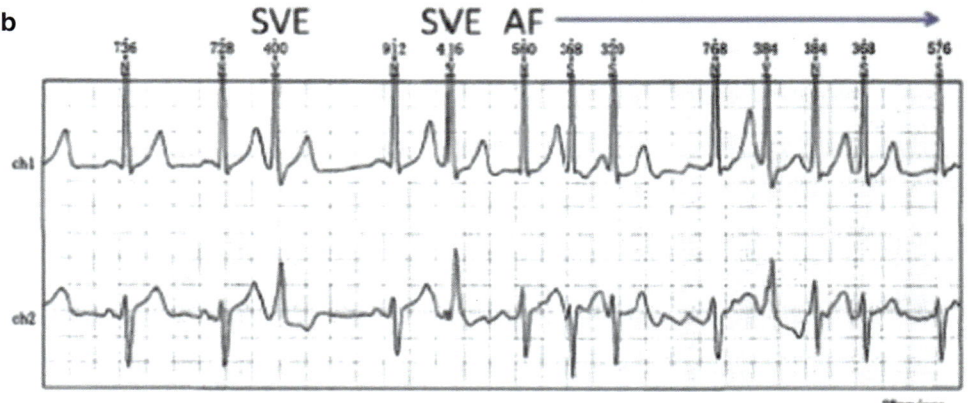

Fig. 8.11 (continued)

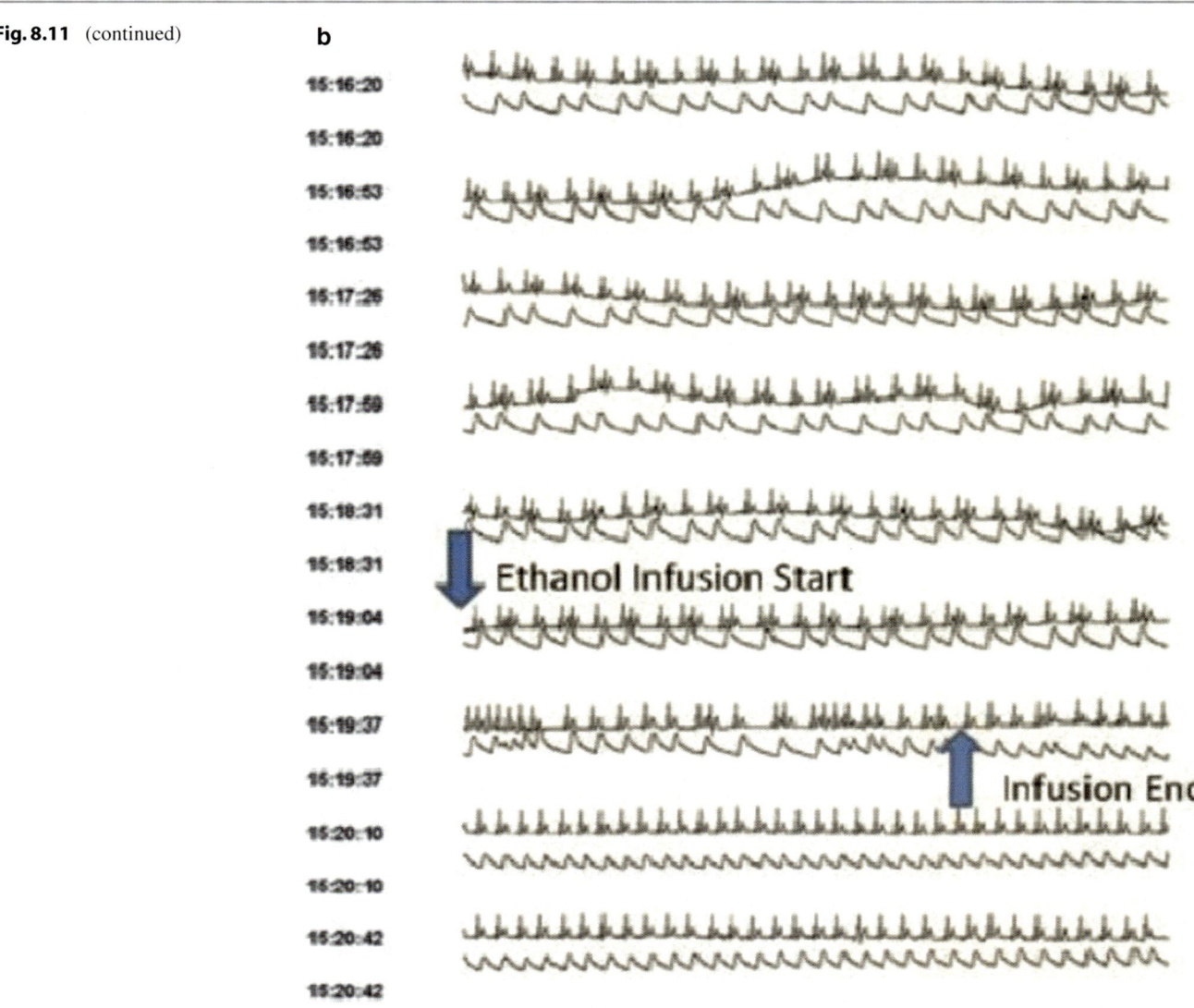

Fig. 8.11 (continued)

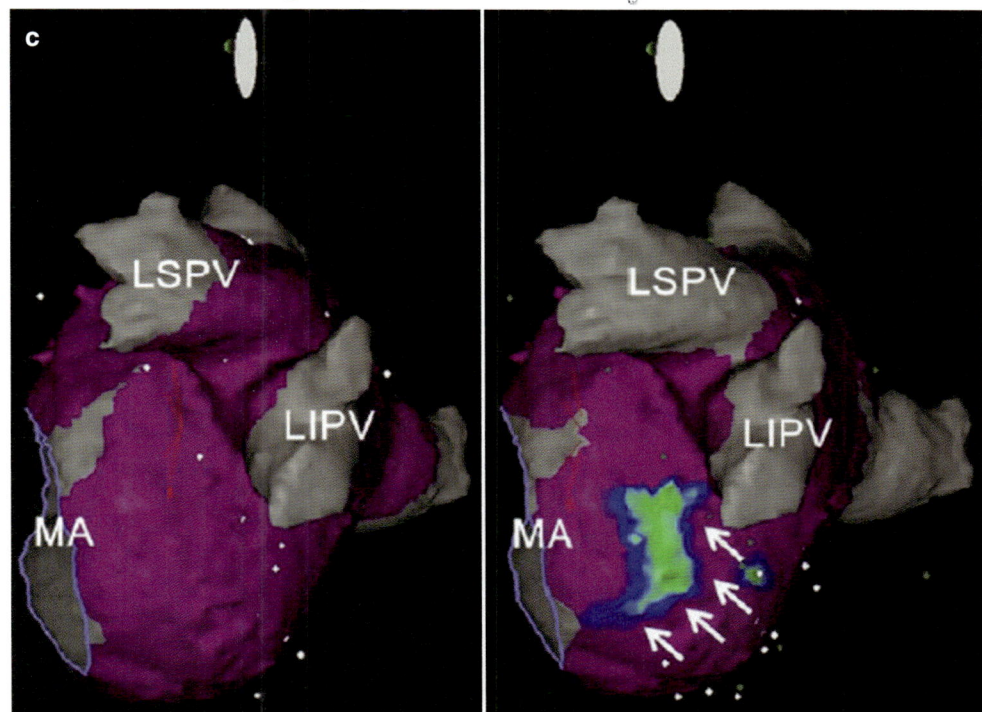

Voltage map after ethanol infusion into VOM

Low voltage zone 0.05–0.5mV

8.10 Adverse Events

For cannulation into the Marshall vein, a long guiding sheath can be utilized. Further, contrast medium can be injected through that guiding sheath in order to evaluate the status of the cannulation into the Marshall vein. If too large a dose of the contrast medium is injected, or if the contrast medium is infused too rapidly, a dissection of the coronary sinus or Marshall vein can be provoked (Fig. 8.12). However, in such a case no bleeding into the pericardial space is observed. A dissection of the coronary sinus was provoked in four patients (0.9%), and the dissection of the Marshall vein was also induced in three patients (0.6%). One patient suffered from a dissection of the coronary sinus after undergoing a re-do ablation session. Venography of the coronary sinus revealed the full recovery of the anatomy of this vessel with patency of the Marshall vein.

When a guidewire is introduced into the Marshall vein and advanced as deep as possible, the guidewire may penetrate the distal end of the Marshall vein. In such a case, a balloon catheter can be advanced in an over-the-wire fashion and inflated just proximal to the perforated portion for a complete occlusion of the Marshall vein. The ablation procedure is undertaken under anticoagulation with intravenous heparin

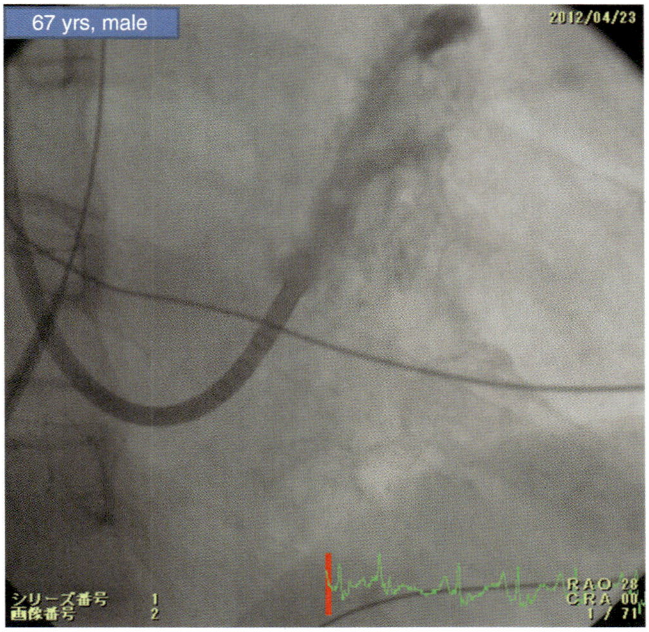

Fig. 8.12 When contrast medium was injected through the outer long guiding sheath inserted into the coronary sinus (CS) for visualization of the Marshall vein, a dissection of the CS was provoked. However, no pericardial effusion was detected by transthoracic echocardiography

to maintain the ACT level at longer than 300 s. The balloon is deflated after the completion of the ablation procedure. No significant bleeding into the pericardial space has never been recognized, and there have been no cases that required pericardiocentesis to restore the hemodynamic status.

In all instances when ethanol was infused into the Marshall vein, according to the patient interviews all patients complained of serious chest pain that was comparable to that of ablation using RF energy on the posterior wall of the left atrium or cavo-tricuspid annulus. That pain disappeared immediately after the infusion of ethanol within 3–5 s.

Two out of 443 patients (0.5%) suffered from pericarditis after undergoing an ethanol infusion into the Marshall vein; however, all symptoms associated with pericarditis, such as chest pain, had resolved within a day. Any slight ST-segment elevation that was observed on the 12-lead ECG had also disappeared within a day without any medications. Two-dimensional echocardiography could not identify any pericardial effusions, and no findings were suggestive of a pathological status associated with pericarditis.

References

1. Haines DE, Verow AF, Sinusas AJ, Whayne JG, DiMarco JP. Intracoronary ethanol ablation in swine: characterization of myocardial injury in target and remote vascular beds. J Cardiovasc Electrophysiol. 1994;5:41–9.
2. Wang PJ, Ursell PC, Sosa-Suarez G, Okishige K, Friedman PL. Permanent AV block or modification of AV nodal function by selective AV nodal artery ethanol infusion. PACE. 1992;15:779–82.
3. Sneddon JF, Ward DE, Simpson IA, Linker NJ, Wainwright RJ, Camm AJ. Alcohol ablation of atrioventricular conduction. Br Heart J. 1991;65:143–7.
4. Kay GN, Bubien RS, Dailey SM, Epstein AE, Plumb VJ. A prospective evaluation of intracoronary ethanol ablation of the atrioventricular conduction system. J Am Coll Cardiol. 1991;17:1634–40.
5. Okishige K, Friedman PL. Alcohol ablation for tachycardia therapy. J Cardiovasc Electrophysiol. 1992;3:354–64.
6. Brugada P, de Swart H, Smeets JLRM, Wellens HJJ. Transcoronary chemical ablation of ventricular tachycardia. Circulation. 1989;79:475–82.
7. Wright KN, Morley T, Bicknell J, Bishop SP, Walcott GP, Kay GN. Retrograde coronary venous infusion of ethanol for ablation of canine ventricular myocardium. J Cardiovasc Electrophysiol. 1998;9:976–84.
8. Marshall J. On the development of the great anterior veins an man and mammalia: including an account of certain remnents of foetal structure found in the adult, a comparative view of these great veins in the different mammalia, and an analysis of their occasional peculiarities in the human subject. Phil Trans R Soc Lond. 1850;140:133–69.
9. Doshi RN, Wu TJ, Robinson MJ. Relation between ligament of marshall and adrenergic atrial tachyarrhythmia. Circulation. 1999;100:876–83.
10. Hwang C, Karagueuzian HS, Chen PS. Idiopathic paroxysmal atrial fibrillation induced by a focal discharge mechanism in the left superior pulmonary vein: possible roles of the ligament of Marshall. J Cardiovasc Electrophysiol. 1999;10:636–48.
11. Hwang C, Wu TJ, Doshi RN, Peter CT, Chen PS. Vein of Marshall cannulation for the analysis of electrical activity in patients with focal atrial fibrillation. Circulation. 2000;101:1503–5.
12. Kim DT, Lai AC, Hwang C, Fan LT, Karagueuzian HS, Chen PS. The ligament of Marshall: a structural analysis in human hearts with implications for atrial arrhythmias. J Am Coll Cardiol. 2000;36:1324–7.
13. Kurotobi T, Ito H, Inoue K, Iwakura K, Kawano S, Okamura A, Date M, Fujii K. Marshall vein as arrhythmogenic source in patients with atrial fibrillation: correlation between its anatomy and electrophysiological findings. J Cardiovasc Electrophysiol. 2006;17:1062–7.
14. Valderrabano M, Chen HR, Sidhu J, Rao L, Ling Y, Khoury DS. Retrograde ethanol infusion in the vein of Marshall. Regional left atrial ablation, vagal denervation, and feasibility in humans. Circ Arrhythm Electrophysiol. 2009;2:50–6.
15. Omichi C, Chou CC, Lee MH, Chang CM, Lai AC, Hayashi H, Zhou S, Miyauchi Y, Okuyama Y, Hamabe A, Hwang C, Fishbein MC, Lin SF, Karagueuzian HS, Chen PS. Demonstration of electrical and anatomic connections between Marshall bundles and left atrium in dogs: Implications on generation of P waves on surface electrogram. J Cardiovasc Electrophysiol. 2002;13:1283–91.
16. Wu TJ, Ong JJC, Chang CM, Doshi RN, Yashima M, Huang HL, Fishbein MC, Ting CT, Karagueuzian HS, Chen PS. Pulmonary veins and ligament of Marshall as source od rapid activations in a canine model of sustained atrial fibrillation. Circulation. 2001;103:1157–63.
17. Ulphani JS, Arora R, Cain JH, Villuendas R, Shen S, Gordon D, Inderyas F, Harvey LA, Morris A, Goldberger JJ, Kadish AH. The ligament of Marshall as a parasympathetic conduit. Am J Phys. 2007;293:1629–35.
18. Valderrabano M, Chen HR, Sidhu J, Rao L, Ling Y, Khoury DS. Retrograde ethanol infusion in the vein of Marshall. Regional left atrial ablation, vagal denervation, and feasibility in humans. Circ Arrhythm Electrophysiol. 2009;2:50–6.
19. Baez-Escudero JL, Keida T, Dave AS, Okishige K, Valderrabano M. Ethanol infusion in the vein of Marshall leads to parasympathetic denervation of the human atrium. J Am Coll Cardiol. 2014;63:1892–901.
20. Baez-Escudero JL, Morales PF, Dave AS, Sasaridis CM, Kim YH, Okishige K, Valderabano M. Ethanol infusion the vein of Marshall facilitates mitral isthmus ablation. Heart Rhythm. 2012;9:1207–15.
21. White CM, Sanders S, Coleman CI, Gallagher R, Takata H, Humphrey C, Henyan N, Gillespie EL, Kluger J. Impact of epicardial anterior fat pad retention on postcardiothoracic surgery atrial fibrillation incidence: the AFIST-III study. J Am Coll Cardiol. 2007;49:298–303.
22. Nagashima K, Okumura Y, Watanabe I, Nakai T, Ohkubo K, Kofune T, Kofune M, Mano H, Sonoda K, Hirayama A. Association between epicardial adipose tissue volumes on 3-dimensional reconstructed CT images and recurrence of atrial fibrillation after catheter ablation. Circ J. 2011;75:2559–65.
23. Wong CX, Abed HS, Molaee P, Nelson AJ, Brooks AG, Sharma G, Leong DP, Lau DH, Middeldorp ME, Roberts-Thomson KC, Wittert GA, Abhayaratna WP, Worthley SG, Sanders P. Pericardial fat is associated with atrial fibrillation severity and ablation outcome. J Am Coll Cardiol. 2011;57:1745–51.
24. Oral H, Chung A, Good E, Wimmer A, Dey S, Gadeela N, Sankaran S, Crawford T, Sarrazin JF, Kuhne M, Chalfoun N, Wells D, Frederick M, Fortino J, Benloucif-Moore S, Jongnarangsin K, Pelosi F Jr, Bogun F, Morady F. Radiofrequency catheter ablation of chronic atrial fibrillation guided by complex electrograms. Circulation. 2007;115:2606–12.
25. Li WJ, Bai YY, Zhang HY, Tang RB, Miao CL, Sang CH, Yin XD, Dong JZ, Ma CS. Additional ablation of complex fractionated atrial electrograms (CFAEs) after pulmonary vein isolation (PVAI) in patients with atrial fibrillation: a meta-analysis. Circ Arrhythm Electrophysiol. 2011;4:143–8.

Part IV

Catheter Ablation of Atrial Tachycardias and Flutter

9. Cavo-tricuspid Isthmus-Dependent Atrial Flutter

Shinsuke Miyazaki

Keywords
Cavo-tricuspid isthmus • Atrial flutter • Catheter ablation

9.1 Introduction

Cavo-tricuspid isthmus (CTI)-dependent atrial flutter (AFL) is the most frequently encountered right atrial (RA) macroreentrant tachycardia. The electrophysiologic substrate underlying AFL has been shown to be a combination of a slow conduction velocity in the CTI between the tricuspid annulus (TA) and inferior vena cava (IVC) [1], and anatomic or functional conduction block along the crista terminalis and Eustachian ridge. These electrophysiologic characteristics enable sustainable macroreentrant tachycardias around the tricuspid valve. The triggers of AFL might be premature atrial contractions and/or atrial fibrillation (AF). Both clockwise (reverse typical or uncommon) and counterclockwise (typical or common) CTI-dependent AFL can occur, and counterclockwise AFL is the most commonly encountered in clinical practice presumably because the majority of triggers come from the left atrium (LA) and pulmonary veins (PVs). AFL is refractory to medical therapy and has now become routinely amenable to curative treatment by catheter ablation [2, 3]. Radiofrequency (RF) catheter ablation of the CTI is considered a first-line therapy for treating CTI-dependent AFL. This chapter focuses on the practical points for catheter ablation of CTI-dependent AFL.

9.2 Mechanisms and Anatomy

Intraoperative and transcatheter activation mapping revealed that CTI-dependent AFL was a macroreentrant circuit rotating in either the counterclockwise or clockwise direction around the tricuspid valve annulus. The predominant slow conduction zone in the circuit has been shown to be in the CTI [1]. Maintenance of reentrant circuits requires not only the presence of slow conduction zones but also functional block produced by natural obstacles or barriers. The crista terminalis forms a boundary and functional or anatomic block perhaps due to anisotropy, which is necessary to sustain AFL and to prevent short-circuiting the reentrant wavefront (Fig. 9.1). Since slow conduction exists in the CTI, counterclockwise AFL is more likely to be induced when pacing is performed from the coronary sinus (CS) ostium, and clockwise AFL when pacing is from the low lateral RA. Lower loop reentry is also a CTI-dependent AFL in which the caudal-to-cranial limb of the wavefront crosses over gaps in the crista terminalis in the inferior to mid-RA. This variant activation sequence may be sustained, or convert to other forms of AFL.

The CTI is anatomically bounded by the IVC and Eustachian ridge posteriorly and by the TA anteriorly (Fig. 9.2). Postmortem studies have shown that, in human hearts, the average size of the CTI region measures about 30 mm in length [4, 5]. Other clinical studies using angiography, computed tomography, and magnetic resonance imaging have reported a 34 mm length from the IVC to TA, and the length is longer in patients with AFL than those without [6]. The central isthmus marks the shortest distance and thinnest portion. The anterior CTI adjacent to the

S. Miyazaki
Cardiovascular Center, Tsuchiura Kyodo Hospital,
4-1-1 Otsuno, Tsuchiura, Ibaraki 300-0028, Japan
e-mail: mshinsuke@k3.dion.ne.jp

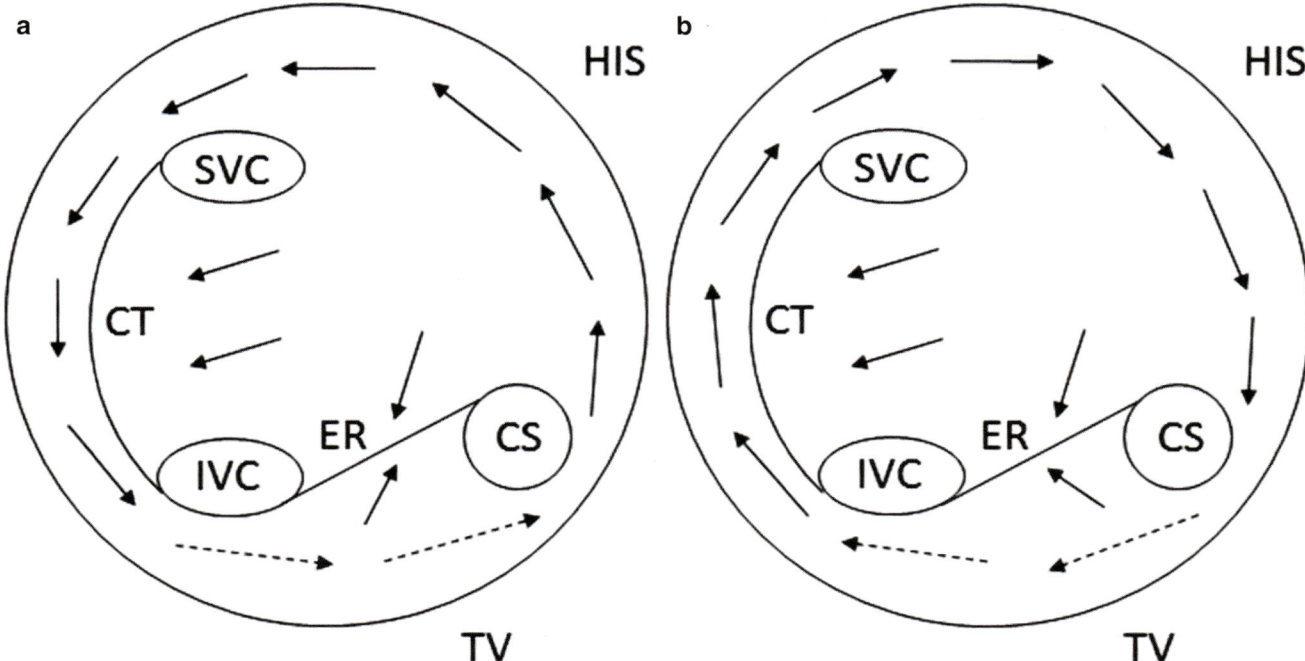

Fig. 9.1 Circuits of typical AFL (**a**) and reverse typical AFL (**b**) are shown. The *dotted arrow* indicates slow conduction. *SVC* superior vena cava, *IVC* inferior vena cava, *CT* crista terminalis, *ER* Eustachian ridge, *TV* tricuspid valve, *HIS* His recording area, *CS* coronary sinus

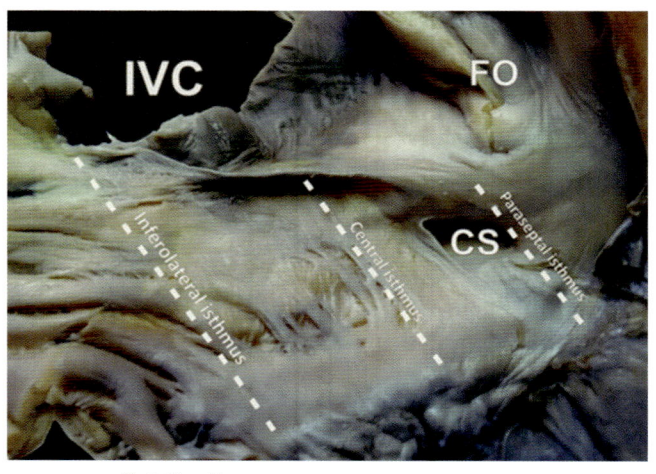

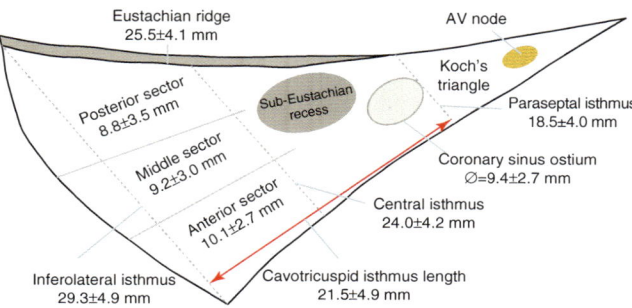

Fig. 9.2 Photograph of a cadaveric heart specimen showing the CTI area and schematic view of the investigated heart region (mean ± standard deviations). *AV* atrioventricular, *CS* coronary sinus ostium, *FO* fossa ovalis, *IVC* inferior vena cava (from Klimek-Piotrowska W, et al. PLoS One. 2016;11:e0163383)

tricuspid valve is entirely muscular, while the posterior CTI closest to the IVC is primarily fibrofatty tissue. The CTI configuration is subdivided into straight, concave, and pouch-like recess configurations [7]. The presence of intertrabecular recesses, trabecular bridges, and sub-Eustachian recesses within the CTI is identified in 25.0%, 12.9%, and 48.6% of patients, respectively [5]. The anatomy of the CTI in individual patients is highly variable and unpredictable prior to the procedure. These specific anatomic features form variations of the CTI and influence the catheter ablation at CTI.

9.3 Diagnosis

The surface 12-lead ECG of typical AFL exhibits an inverted saw-tooth F-wave pattern in the inferior leads, upright F waves in precordial lead V1, and inverted F waves in lead V6 (Fig. 9.3a) [8]. Leads I and aVL characteristically exhibit low-voltage defections. The saw-tooth pattern consists of a downsloping segment, followed by a sharper negative defection, then a sharp positive defection with a positive "overshoot" leading to the next downsloping plateau. In contrast, reverse typical AFL often exhibits a sine wave pattern in the inferior leads (Fig. 9.3b). Wide negative deflections in lead V1 may be a specific diagnostic sign, but the pattern is much less specific than typical AFL. A typical saw-tooth morphology is highly predictive of typical AFL. Of note, CTI-dependent flutter that occurs

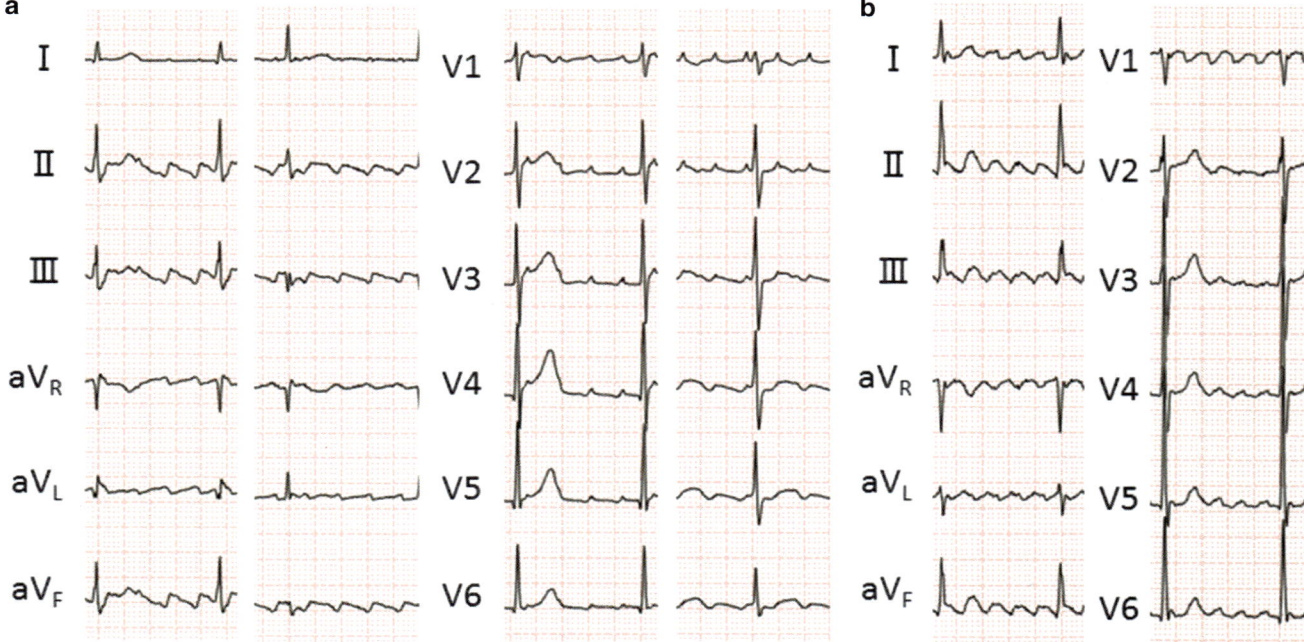

Fig. 9.3 Twelve lead electrograms of typical AFL (**a**) and reverse typical AFL (**b**) are shown

after LA ablation of AF often has atypical ECGs since the determinants of the F-wave pattern on the ECG largely depend on the LA activation pattern [9]. When the F waves are not evaluable due to a rapid ventricular response, an adenosine injection might be useful to evaluate the morphology.

For the precise diagnosis, an electrophysiologic study with mapping and entrainment must be performed. For patients who present in sinus rhythm, it is recommended to induce AFL to confirm its mechanism. In this situation, as abovementioned, the selection of the pacing site is important. Activation mapping during sustained tachycardia is necessary, and 3-D mapping systems and multipolar mapping catheters can facilitate mapping. Entrainment mapping is performed with pacing at a cycle length 10–20 ms shorter than the tachycardia cycle length and ideally at multiple sites. It should be noted that the activation remains the same before and after pacing because the rhythm can change with the maneuver. Reentry could be demonstrated by concealed entrainment during pacing from the CTI including an acceleration of the tachycardia to the pacing cycle length without a change in the F waves or endocardial activation, post-pacing interval nearly equal to the tachycardia cycle length (<20 ms difference) at the CTI, lateral RA, anterior RA, and septal RA wall, and manifest entrainment by pacing at sites outside the CTI (Fig. 9.4). The differential diagnosis of AFL from the other atrial arrhythmias is generally easy by the response to entrainment from the CTI and a radial activation pattern.

9.4 Management of the Peri-Procedural Period

It is not necessary to discontinue antiarrhythmic drugs before the procedure. Concomitant AF is common in patients with AFL. Indeed, patients with class Ic antiarrhythmic agents for AF who organize into AFL are good candidates for CTI ablation. In this situation, AF might be easily induced mechanically or by pacing during the procedure. The endpoint of the procedure cannot be evaluated during AF. Therefore, in patients with a history of concomitant AF, ongoing antiarrhythmic drugs therapy during the peri-procedural period is recommended.

The indication for anticoagulation therapy should be decided based on the stroke risk just as for AF. Generally, the prevalence of vascular complications and cardiac tamponade are low in catheter ablation of the CTI because the vascular access is limited to veins and the procedure is not relatively complex. Therefore, performing ablation with ongoing anticoagulation therapy is reasonable. Restoration of sinus rhythm from sustained AFL can lead to thromboembolic events during the period of atrial stunning. Thus, anticoagulation therapy should be continued during the peri-procedural period and at least until 1 month after the procedure when recovery of atrial function is expected. In patients with persistent AFL under insufficient anticoagulation therapy and with a high risk of thromboembolic events, pre-procedural transesphageal echocardiography is recommended to explore for intracardiac thrombi. Alternatively,

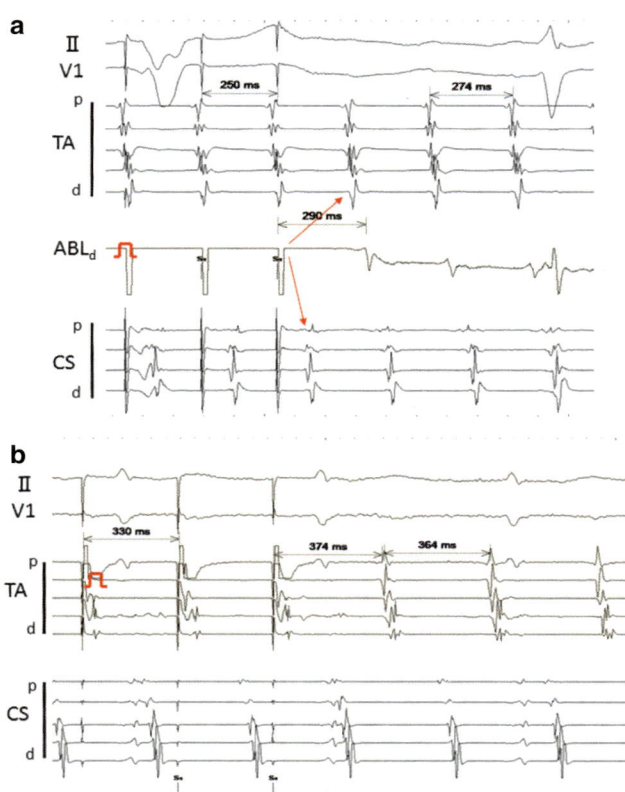

Fig. 9.4 Entrainment pacing during typical AFL is shown. A decapolar catheter is placed along the tricuspid annulus (TA). (**a**) The tachycardia cycle length is 274 ms, and post-pacing interval following pacing from ablation catheter (ABL) positioned on the CTI is 290 ms. (**b**) The tachycardia cycle length is 364 ms, and post-pacing interval following pacing from low lateral RA is 374 ms. *p* proximal, *d* distal

therapeutic anticoagulation for >4 weeks prior to the procedure is reasonable to avoid transesphageal echocardiography. After the procedure, careful monitoring should be performed. Patients will typically lie flat for 3 h. AFL recurrence is rare if the acute endpoint can be achieved; however, AF could be identified in about half of the population if implantable loop recorder are implanted [10]. This information is critical to consider for further treatment and anticoagulation therapy.

9.5 Ablation Protocol

9.5.1 Mapping Catheters

The procedure can be completed by local anesthesia. However, RF applications at the posterior isthmus (IVC edge) are generally painful. If patients complain of pain, opiates should be used for pain control. A urinary catheter is not required due to the short procedure time.

Although catheter configurations vary greatly among institutes, at least one ablation catheter and another pacing catheter (quadripolar catheter) is required to create a blockline along the CTI. The two catheters are introduced into the femoral vein via two sheaths. The pacing catheter is placed in the proximal CS or low lateral RA, then ablation is performed during pacing from the catheter. A multipolar catheter (decapolar or duodecapolar catheter) is placed along the TA to facilitate mapping of the activation anterior to the crista. If three catheters are used, two mapping catheters are placed in the lateral RA and proximal CS, respectively. Bi-directional conduction block (see below) can be more easily evaluated. When a catheter is placed into the CS, the internal jugular vein is an alternative access. After the venous sheaths are in place, an intravenous heparin bolus of 5000 U is given to minimize the risk of venous thromboses.

9.5.2 CTI Ablation

The surface electrocardiogram and bipolar intracardiac electrograms are continuously monitored and stored on a computer-based digital recording system. The system is configured to monitor and provide the mean power, temperature, and impedance during each RF application. The initial ablation line should be at the central isthmus because the distance between the TA and IVC is shortest and the musculature the thinnest. The medial isthmus region has the thickest muscular content along the CTI. In patients with cardiac rotation, it is recommended to place one catheter at the His bundle area or right ventricular (RV) apex once to confirm the degree of cardiac rotation. In the left anterior oblique (LAO) view, the catheter direction should be right in front. The initial ablation line is set at 6 o'clock in the LAO view. The catheter position can be easily recognized on fluoroscopy. In the LAO view, the catheter is located at the central (6 o'clock), lateral (7 o'clock), or medial isthmus (5 o'clock). In the right anterior oblique (RAO) view, the catheter is located between the TA and IVC. During the procedure, low lateral RA pacing is recommended for a medial isthmus ablation line, and proximal CS pacing for a lateral isthmus ablation line for better electrogram recognition to avoid overlapping of the pacing spikes with local signals.

The initial ablation point is decided based on the ratio of the atrial and ventricular electrogram amplitudes recorded by the distal bipolar electrode pair, and 1:3–1:4 is recommended. It should be ensured that the ablation catheter is positioned beneath the mapping catheter if multi-electrode catheters cross the CTI. Ablation is performed using a continuous application or point-by-point application technique from the TA to IVC with a duration of 30–60 s each. Electrogram recordings may be employed in addition to fluo-

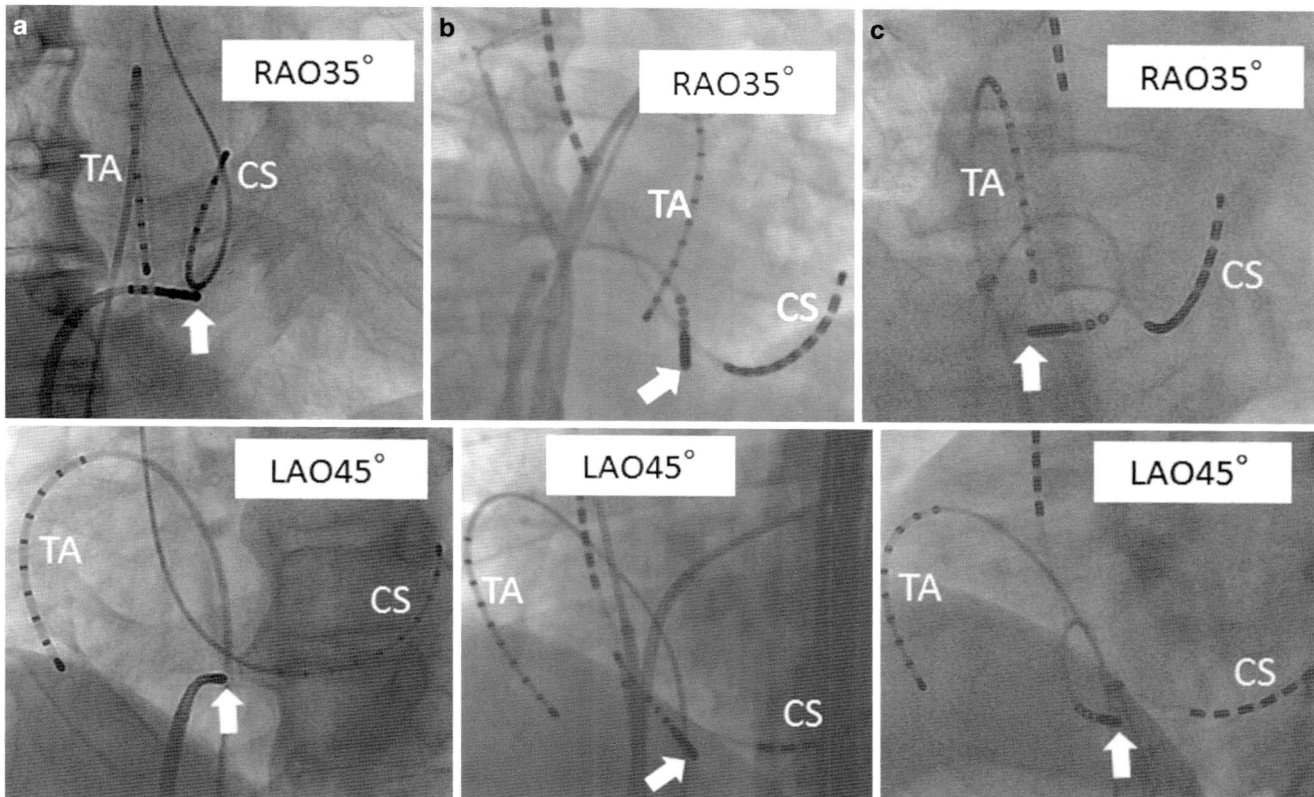

Fig. 9.5 Various catheter positions during the CTI ablation are shown. The CS catheter is placed from the right internal jugular vein with the proximal electrodes placed just inside the CS ostium. The TA catheter is positioned just anterior to the crista terminalis. The ablation catheter is positioned on the CTI. (**a**) The ablation catheter is placed on the CTI in a horizontal fashion. (**b**) The ablation catheter is perpendicularly placed on the CTI (a 180° curvature). (**c**) "Loop technique" to map the CTI pouch. The *white arrows* indicate the tip of the ablation catheter. *RAO* right oblique view, *LAO* left oblique view, *TA* tricuspid annulus, *CS* coronary sinus

roscopy to ensure that the ablation electrode is in contact with viable CTI tissue throughout each energy application. The catheter should be gradually withdrawn until the distal ablation electrode records no atrial electrograms, or the ablation electrode is fluoroscopically noted to abruptly slip off the Eustachian ridge (Fig. 9.5a). RF applications should be immediately interrupted when RF applications venous structures cause significant pain to the patients. Generally, stable placement of the catheter tip at the IVC edge is challenging due to the sharp angle (anatomical specificity), patient respirations, and pain during the application. When complete block cannot be created on the first line, conduction gaps should be explored along the line.

9.5.3 Endpoint of the Procedure

The procedural endpoint is defined as complete bidirectional conduction block along the CTI line. AFL termination by an application in the CTI is no longer considered a suitable endpoint because of both high recurrence rates and a lack of correlation with isthmus block. If ablation is performed during ongoing AFL, atrial pacing should be prepared, for the possible occurrence of a sinus pause when the AFL terminates. The creation of CTI block is accompanied by prolongation of the intervals required for the pacing stimulus on one side of the line to propagate to the opposite side (Fig. 9.6). The achievement of complete block is verified through documentation of a change in the activation of the septal or lateral RA during pacing from the opposite side of the lesion as evidence of an actual detour around the area of block, through sequential multipoint mapping along the ablation line to document double potentials, or both [11]. An interval separating the two components of double potentials of <90 ms is associated with a local gap, whereas a double potential interval of >110 ms is associated with local block [12]. It seems important to pace at relatively slow rates during assessment of block to discriminate functional conduction block.

A consistent change in the P-wave morphology in the inferior leads during low lateral RA pacing after achieving isthmus block is helpful for recognizing CTI block [13, 14].

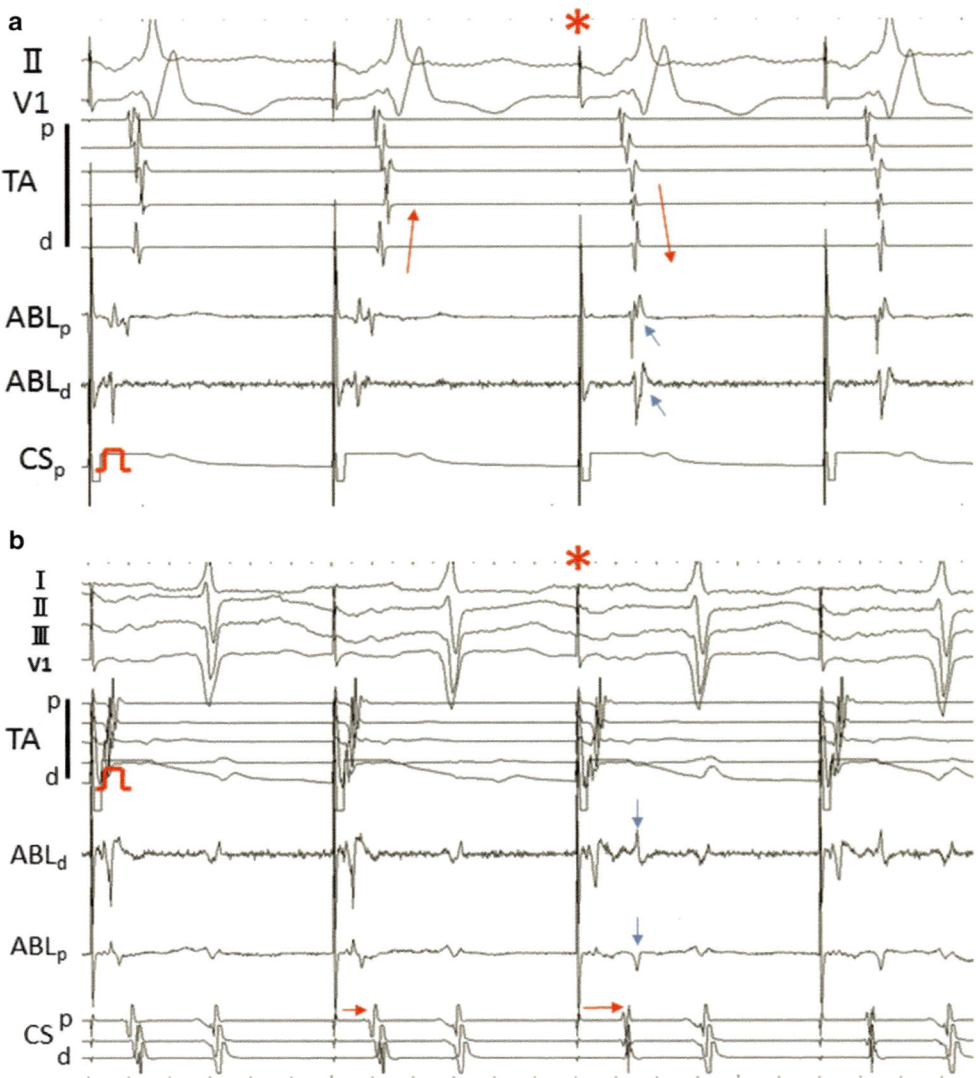

Fig. 9.6 Intracardiac electrograms when CTI block is achieved are shown. (**a**) During pacing from the proximal CS, CTI block was achieved (*asterisk*). Note that the activation sequence along the TA abruptly changed (*red arrows*) together with the splitting of the potentials on the ablation catheter (*blue arrows*). (**b**) During pacing from the low lateral RA, CTI block was achieved (*asterisk*). Note that the interval between the pacing spike and proximal CS abruptly prolonged (*red arrows*) together with the splitting of the potentials on the ablation catheter (*blue arrows*)

During low lateral RA pacing, the septal wall activation changes from caudocephalic to cephalocaudal when block is created and results in a positive change in the terminal portion of the P wave. After confirming bidirectional block, a 30 min waiting time should be taken. Although the temporal kinetics indicate the highest incidence of recovery soon after RF deliveries, conduction recovery does not always indicate recovery of the last delivered lesion. Conduction resumption is not rare during this period regardless of the energy sources, and it is important to create sustainable conduction block and decrease the incidence of AFL recurrence.

9.5.4 Conduction Gaps and the Differential Pacing Technique

When block is not achieved after the initial line, the remaining atrial signals along the line are targeted. The gap can be identified as a single or fractionated potential along the line bounded by split electrograms. Confusing or inconclusive electrograms can be encountered along the ablation line. The differential pacing technique is a simple and sensitive technique to reliably distinguish persisting conduction from complete isthmus block without catheter movement [11]. Pacing from another site farther away from the ablation line would obviously delay the stimulus to initial component timing, but the response of the terminal component would depend on the presence or absence of conduction through the ablation line. The terminal component would be delayed like the initial component if it was activated by the same wavefront penetrating through the ablation line, indicating persistent conduction, but would be advanced if it was activated by the wavefront going around, indicating conduction block, instead of through the line because the length of the detour is shortened by withdrawal of the pacing site. In this technique, it is essential that the initial pacing site be as close as possible to the ablation line and that the more remote pacing site be of limited distance from the first to maintain similar propagation wavefronts.

9.5.5 Selection of the Ablation Catheter

A variety of ablation catheters, with different shapes and curve lengths, as well as RF generators, are available from several commercial manufactures. The use of 8-mm tip or irrigated ablation electrodes reduces procedure durations and improves success rates compared with standard 4-mm RF electrodes [15, 16]. Long fixed curves or deflectable sheaths are useful to improve the catheter reach, stability, and contact. In our experience, dumbbell-shaped 8-mm tip RF ablation catheters are the most useful for CTI ablation, and irrigated tip catheters aid in eliminating residual conduction due to insufficient power deliveries by non-irrigated catheters. In our laboratory, to obtain a similar current density at the tip with different tip sizes during RF applications, a temperature controlled RF delivery is performed with a maximum power output of 70, 50, and 30 W, and temperature limit of 70, 55, and 43 °C, with 10-, 8-, and 3.5- or 4-mm irrigation-tip catheters, respectively. 3-D mapping systems and contact force sensing catheters might potentially be useful for procedures, however generally they are not necessary.

The 10-mm tip ablation catheter further reduces the number of applications and procedure time for achieving block [17, 18]. The disadvantage of the catheter is the difficulty in manipulating the large tip in the complex structures of the CTI and poor signal resolution. Sufficient power cannot be obtained without sufficient blood flow, particularly in a CTI pouch. The impaired near-field electrogram resolution is another limitation. A novel ablation catheter equipped with mini-electrodes has been recently introduced into clinical use to enhance the spatial resolution of the mapping. However, currently the data is limited in humans.

Cryoablation is an alternative choice for CTI ablation [19, 20]. Ablation is performed at a target temperature of −80 °C, and each cryoenergy delivery lasts 180–300 s with an 8-mm tip cryocatheter. Cryoablation has specific advantages over RF catheter ablation, including a greater safety resulting from the catheter stability during ablation due to adherence to the myocardial tissue, lower risk of thrombus formation, and lower risk of myocardial perforations. In addition, cryoablation is relatively painless, which should improve the patient tolerability and reduce the analgesic demand, notably, when ablation of the posterior isthmus is attempted. The limitation is the difficulty in manipulating the large tip in the complex structures of the CTI and the lower durability of conduction block when compared to RF ablation [21].

9.5.6 Ablation Techniques

There are several approaches for CTI ablation, and the selection is best guided by the operator's experience and preference. A prospective study revealed that, when using 8-mm tip RF catheters, a continuous RF delivery approach could shorten the procedure and fluoroscopic times, and required lower RF energies compared to the point-by-point ablation strategy [22]. The mapping duration may contribute to the spread of endocardial edema, leading to difficulty in making transmural myocardial lesions adjacent to ablative lesions. This approach might be recommended in patients with a simple CTI anatomy. On the contrary, the point-by-point approach is superior for evaluating local signals and ensuring catheter contact, and therefore is recommended in patients with complex CTI anatomies.

Jacobsen et al. proposed a practical ablation strategy that selectively targeted high amplitude signals on a line across the isthmus, regardless of their anatomic position on the line [23]. This voltage-guided ablation technique resulted in reducing the ablation time and fewer recurrences. A pathological study demonstrated that the CTI is composed of a series of distinct anatomically defined bundles. The bundle anatomy frees the operator from being confined to a single line since the bundle can theoretically be interrupted at more than one location. Thus, difficulty in positioning at one point is often overcome by moving laterally or medially to a position with better contact to more effectively ablate that "cable."

The presence of sub-Eustachian recesses significantly prolongs ablation times and is associated with a lower rate of success [7]. In these cases, ablation within the pouch is accomplished by forming a 180° curvature on the ablation catheter and withdrawing the catheter to enter the pouch perpendicularly (Fig. 9.6b). The size of the Eustachian valve and ridge may hinder catheter access to regions located anterior to the ridge and valve. In addition, the Eustachian ridge, due to the presence of muscle fibers, is able to conduct electrical impulses and represents the site of conduction gaps that are difficult to ablate. Making an acute flexion of the ablation catheter ("loop technique") can enable better mapping and stability around the Eustachian ridge (Fig. 9.6c). These techniques are particularly useful when block cannot be created by standard catheter manipulation.

9.5.7 Challenging Cases

Occasionally creating CTI block is challenging, and multiple energy applications and prolonged procedure and fluoroscopic times are required owing to highly variable isthmus anatomies [4]. The majority of anatomical obstacles are unfortunately detected only at the time of the CTI ablation, which significantly prolongs the procedure time and reduces the success rate.

If the tachycardia is not terminated after multiple applications, the tachycardia mechanism should be re-evaluated using activation and entrainment mapping. Major causes of difficulty in creating block are (1) difficulty in obtaining stable catheter contact during RF deliveries, (2) insufficient power deliveries because of insufficient blood flow may impede efficient tip cooling, (3) difficulty in mapping conduction gaps located in specific anatomies, and (4) conduction gaps cannot be identified due to tissue edema after multiple energy applications. Isthmus pouches may not be ablated without specific catheter maneuvers to enter as abovementioned. Long formed sheaths enable better catheter contact and stability than short sheaths, and steerable sheaths enhance further stability and more flexible mapping rather than long formed sheaths. Creating a new ablation line medially or laterally is another approach. For prominent pouches, it may be easier to ablate more laterally, and for a prominent pectinate musculature, a more medial approach may be easier. It should be noted that ablation at the medial isthmus is associated with a higher risk of atrioventricular conduction injury. It can be helpful to change the rhythm and pacing site to see the signals differently. In deep recesses where sufficient power cannot be obtained, irrigation tip catheters should be used. In this situation, a lower power setting is recommended to avoid steam pops in the recesses. Scheduling a second procedure after tissue recovery is the final option if extensive ablation cannot achieve block.

9.6 Complications

According to a meta-analysis, the incidence of acute complications during CTI ablation was 2.6% (77/6293), and most common complications were vascular complications, complete heart block, and pericardial effusions [24]. Rarely, spasms of the right coronary artery, manifested by ST elevation in the inferior leads, could occur regardless of a history of angina. This can be observed not only during the procedure but also several hours after the procedure. For progressive ST elevation, intravenous nitroglycerin should be administered, then emergent coronary angiography is considered. A pacing catheter should be placed in right ventricle for back-up pacing. Surface ECG leads need to be carefully monitored during the procedure, and monitoring is continued for at least several hours after the procedure. Cardiac tamponade can rarely occur due to steam pops during RF deliveries, and the risk is especially higher when using irrigation-tip catheters. Excessive impedance drops should be avoided to prevent tissue overheating and steam pops. In cases with pacemakers and defibrillators, care should be taken to avoid dislodgement or damage to the leads.

9.7 Procedure and Clinical Outcomes

The acute success rate has been provided for 153 studies and was 91.1% [24]. There were strong trends toward higher acute success rates when using 8- to 10-mm or irrigated RF electrodes compared to 4- to 6-mm RF electrodes (92.7% vs. 87.9%). The AFL recurrence rate reported for 155 studies with 9942 patients was 10.9% over 13.8 months of follow-up; however, it was lower for the use of 8- to 10-mm or irrigated RF electrodes compared to 4- to 6-mm RF electrodes (6.7% vs. 13.8%). The AFL recurrence rate for cryoablation was 11.2%. Recurrence of AFL was lower for the use of bidirectional block as a procedural endpoint compared with not using isthmus block as the endpoint (9.3% vs. 23.6%). The cryoablation acute success was 88.6%, and the procedure time was longer than that of RF ablation, but the fluoroscopic time and clinical outcomes were similar to RF ablation. On the other hand, the durability of the conduction block is likely lower than that of RF ablation. Kuniss et al. reported the durability was 65.6% 3 months after creating block using an 8-mm tip cryocatheter in contrast to 85% after RF ablation using 8-mm tip catheters [21].

The use of antiarrhythmic medications after ablation was described in 59 studies that comprised 4430 patients. During an average of 13.1 months of follow-up, 31.6% were taking antiarrhythmic medications after ablation almost exclusively for AF. In six studies, including 538 patients that commented specifically on the use of warfarin beyond that time mandated for the ablation procedure, 65.9% remained on coumadin at 10.6 months after ablation. Ninety-nine studies that comprised 7328 patients reported the occurrence of AF after ablation of AFL. The overall incidence of AF was 33.6%, with an average follow-up for those studies of 15.2 months. That suggests that atrial electrical disease may be less advanced in patients with AFL alone, but is still progressive despite prevention of AFL. Thirty-seven studies that comprised 3433 patients reported the mortality after ablation. During an average follow-up of 12.1 months, the total mortality rate was 3.3%. Cardiac mortality was reported in 30 studies with 2616 patients. During an average of 12.1 months of follow-up, the cardiac mortality was 1.8% [24].

Conclusions

CTI-dependent AFL is a commonly encountered atrial arrhythmia in clinical practice. RF catheter ablation is highly effective and safe and is considered as a first-line therapy for the treatment of CTI-dependent AFL. The precise diagnosis, creating bidirectional block, and implementing a waiting time are required for a successful procedure.

References

1. Olshansky B, Okumura K, Hess PG, Waldo AL. Demonstration of an area of slow conduction in human atrial flutter. J Am Coll Cardiol. 1990;16:1639–48.
2. Feld GK, Fleck P, Chen PS, Boyce K, Bahnson TD, Stein JB, et al. Radiofrequency catheter ablation for the treatment of human type I atrial flutter: identification of a critical zone in the reentrant circuit by endocardial mapping techniques. Circulation. 1992;86:1233–40.
3. Cosio FG, Lopez-Gil M, Giocolea A, Arribas F, Barroso JL. Radiofrequency ablation of the inferior vena cava–tricuspid valve isthmus in common atrial flutter. Am J Cardiol. 1993;71:705–9.
4. Cabrera JA, Sanchez-Quintana D, Ho SY, Medina A, Anderson RH. The architecture of the atrial musculature between the orifice of the inferior caval vein and the tricuspid valve: the anatomy of the isthmus. J Cardiovasc Electrophysiol. 1998;9:1186–95.
5. Klimek-Piotrowska W, Hołda MK, Koziej M, Hołda J, Piątek K, Tyrak K, et al. Clinical anatomy of the cavotricuspid isthmus and terminal crest. PLoS One. 2016;11:e0163383.
6. Cabrera JA, Sanchez-Quintana D, Ho SY, Medina A, Wanguemert F, Gross E, et al. Angiographic anatomy of the inferior right atrial isthmus in patients with and without history of common atrial flutter. Circulation. 1999;99:3017–23.
7. Da Costa A, Faure E, Thévenin J, Messier M, Bernard S, Abdel K, et al. Effect of isthmus anatomy and ablation catheter on radiofrequency catheter ablation of the cavotricuspid isthmus. Circulation. 2004;110:1030–5.
8. Saoudi N, Cosio F, Waldo A, Chen SA, Iesaka Y, Lesh M, et al. Classification of atrial flutter and regular atrial tachycardia according to electrophysiologic mechanism and anatomic bases: a statement from a joint expert group from the Working Group of Arrhythmias of the European Society of Cardiology and the North American Society of Pacing and Electrophysiology. J Cardiovasc Electrophysiol. 2001;12:852–66.
9. Chugh A, Latchamsetty R, Oral H, Elmouchi D, Tschopp D, Reich S, et al. Characteristics of cavotricuspid isthmus-dependent atrial flutter after left atrial ablation of atrial fibrillation. Circulation. 2006;113:609–15.
10. Mittal S, Pokushalov E, Romanov A, Ferrara M, Arshad A, Musat D, et al. Long-term ECG monitoring using an implantable loop recorder for the detection of atrial fibrillation after cavotricuspid isthmus ablation in patients with atrial flutter. Heart Rhythm. 2013;10:1598–604.
11. Shah D, Haïssaguerre M, Takahashi A, Jaïs P, Hocini M, Clémenty J. Differential pacing for distinguishing block from persistent conduction through an ablation line. Circulation. 2000;102:1517–22.
12. Tada H, Oral H, Sticherling C, Chough SP, Baker RL, Wasmer K, et al. Double potentials along the ablation line as a guide to radiofrequency ablation of typical atrial flutter. J Am Coll Cardiol. 2001;38:750–5.
13. Hamdan MH, Kalman JM, Barron HV, Lesh MD. P-wave morphology during right atrial pacing before and after atrial flutter ablation—a new marker for success. Am J Cardiol. 1997;79:1417–20.
14. Shah DC, Takahashi A, Jaïs P, Hocini M, Peng JT, Clementy J, et al. Tracking dynamic conduction recovery across the cavotricuspid isthmus. J Am Coll Cardiol. 2000;35:1478–84.
15. Tsaï SF, Taï CT, Yu WC, Chen YJ, Hsieh MH, Chiang CE, et al. Is 8-mm more effective than 4-mm-tip electrode catheter for ablation of typical atrial flutter? Circulation. 1999;100:768–71.
16. Jaïs P, Shah DC, Haïssaguere M, Hocini M, Garrigue S, Le Metayer P, et al. Prospective randomized comparison of irrigated-tip versus conventional-tip catheters for ablation of common atrial flutter. Circulation. 2000;101:772–6.
17. Feld G, Wharton M, Plumb V, Daoud E, Friehling T, Epstein L, EPT-1000 XP Cardiac Ablation System Investigators. Radiofrequency catheter ablation of type 1 atrial flutter using large-tip 8- or 10-mm electrode catheters and a high-output radiofrequency energy generator: results of a multicenter safety and efficacy study. J Am Coll Cardiol. 2004;43:1466–72.
18. Ilg KJ, Kuhne M, Crawford T, Chugh A, Jongnarangsin K, Good E, et al. Randomized comparison of cavotricuspid isthmus ablation for atrial flutter using an open irrigation-tip versus a large-tip radiofrequency ablation catheter. J Cardiovasc Electrophysiol. 2011;22:1007–12.
19. Manusama R, Timmermans C, Limon F, Philippens S, Crijns HJ, Rodriguez LM. Catheter-based cryoablation permanently cures patients with common atrial flutter. Circulation. 2004;109:1636–9.
20. Andrew P, Hamad Y, Jerat S, Montenero A, O'Connor S. Approaching a decade of cryo catheter ablation for type 1 atrial flutter-a meta-analysis and systematic review. J Interv Card Electrophysiol. 2011;32:17–27.
21. Kuniss M, Vogtmann T, Ventura R, Willems S, Vogt J, Grönefeld G, et al. Prospective randomized comparison of durability of bidirectional conduction block in the cavotricuspid isthmus in patients after ablation of common atrial flutter using cryothermy and radiofrequency energy: the CRYOTIP study. Heart Rhythm. 2009;6:1699–705.
22. Miyazaki S, Takahashi A, Kuwahara T, Kobori A, Yokoyama Y, Nozato T, et al. Randomized comparison of the continuous vs point-by-point radiofrequency ablation of the cavotricuspid isthmus for atrial flutter. Circ J. 2007;71:1922–6.
23. Jacobsen PK, Klein GJ, Gula LJ, Krahn AD, Yee R, Leong-Sit P, et al. Voltage-guided ablation technique for cavotricuspid isthmus-dependent atrial flutter: refining the continuous line. J Cardiovasc Electrophysiol. 2012;23:672–6.
24. Pérez FJ, Schubert CM, Parvez B, Pathak V, Ellenbogen KA, Wood MA. Long-term outcomes after catheter ablation of cavo-tricuspid isthmus dependent atrial flutter: a meta-analysis. Circ Arrhythm Electrophysiol. 2009;2:393–401.

Uncommon Atrial Flutter

Yasushi Miyauchi

Keywords

Mitral surgery • Intra-atrial reentrant tachycardia • Biatrial surgical ablation • Maze • Entrainment

10.1 Introduction

A classical classification of regular atrial tachycardia had been based exclusively on the surface ECG, where differentiation of atrial tachycardia and atrial flutter depends on a rate cut-off around 240–250 min and the presence of isoelectric baselines in atrial tachycardia but not in atrial flutter. Uncommon atrial flutter is a classification from the surface ECG with the presence of continuous flutter wave which is not consistent with typical atrial flutter. In 2001, a joint ESC/NASPE expert consensus report updated the classification of regular atrial tachycardia that is based on the mechanisms [1]. The term macroreentrant tachycardia was proposed as a general mechanistic description for all reentrant tachycardia with a large central obstacle, no matter what the ECG pattern. Macroreentry can be based on surgical scars or other electrically silent areas of atrial myocardium, and the reentrant circuit often includes a slow conduction zone in the low-voltage area which makes the ECG pattern of atrial tachycardia with discrete P waves with isoelectric baselines. This chapter describes uncommon flutter as macroreentrant tachycardia outside the typical atrial flutter or other cavotricuspid isthmus-dependent flutter regardless of the ECG pattern. Uncommon flutter develops most frequently in patients following open-heart surgery such as surgical repair of congenital heart disease, mitral valve surgery, and biatrial surgical ablation of atrial fibrillation, but may occur without any history of surgical intervention [2].

Y. Miyauchi
Division of Cardiology, Department of Medicine, Nippon Medical School Chiba-Hokusou Hospital, 1715 Kamagari, Inzai, Chiba 270-1694, Japan
e-mail: miyauchi@nms.ac.jp

10.2 General Approach for Mapping and Ablation of Uncommon Flutter

It is difficult to speculate by the location of the reentrant circuit from an ECG pattern because the circuit often includes slow conduction zone that does not generate a large electrical activity, and recorded ECG pattern may reflect largely the activation outside the circuit. The circuit of uncommon flutter mostly depends on the atriotomy scar, and it is important to obtain information on the surgical interventions. A three-dimensional mapping system is essential for delineating the reentrant circuit and ablating the tachycardia. An activation pattern in the coronary sinus (CS) helps determining which chamber is mapped [3]. A distal to proximal CS activation pattern is specific for left atrial (LA) flutter. Chevron or reversed chevron CS activation pattern (activations recorded on both the proximal and the distal CS dipoles are latest or earliest, respectively) are also specific for LA flutter. On the other hand, a proximal to distal CS activation pattern can be both right and left atrial flutter. Entrainment technique further helps to determine the diagnosis of macroreentry and localizing the circuit (Fig. 10.1). Recent version of EnSite and Carto system have multi-polar electrode mapping function with automated point acquisition that enables quick evaluation of the global activation. Electrode size and inter-electrode spacing significantly affect the voltage and resolution of mapping [4]. Smaller electrodes with close inter-electrode spacing improve mapping resolution particularly in low-voltage area. When an activation map suggests reentry, entrainment pacing can be performed to confirm the location of the reentrant circuit. A consistent post-pacing interval at distant two or more sites exclusively rules out focal tachycardia with passive complex activation pattern

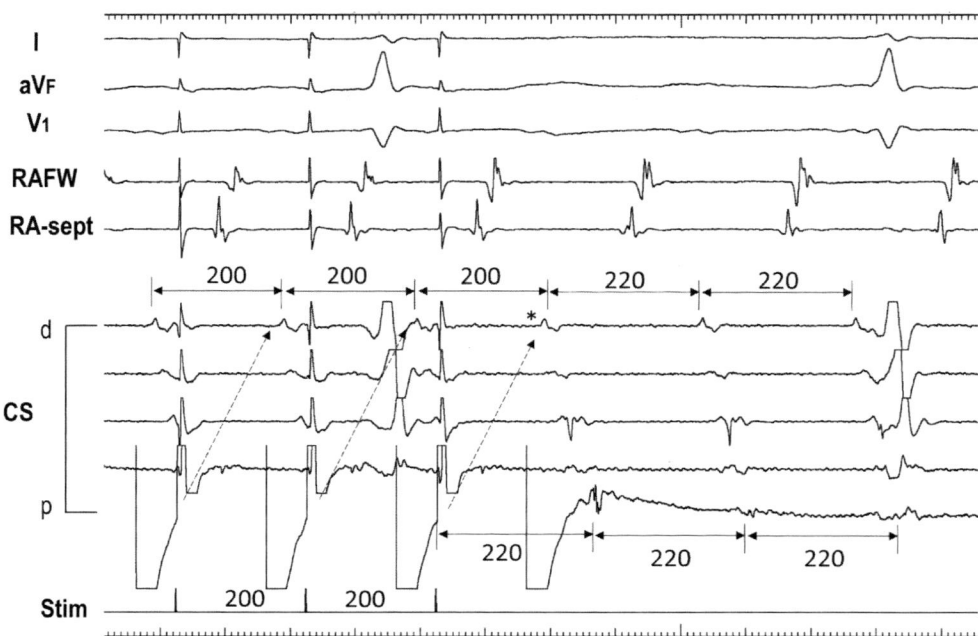

Fig. 10.1 Intracardiac recordings during entrainment pacing from proximal (p) coronary sinus (CS) dipole in a case with uncommon flutter. Distal to proximal activation of CS suggest left atrial origin. The post-pacing interval was identical to the tachycardia cycle length, suggesting that the p-CS is on the circuit. Further, activation interval of the distal (d) CS dipole (*asterisk*) identical to the pacing cycle length demonstrating orthodromic capture by the last pacing from the p-CS. These findings strongly suggest macroreentry which may occur in post-atriotomy flutter [5]. Ablation is performed to transect the identified isthmus. The conventional endpoint is its termination and non-inducibility of the tachycardia by atrial programmed pacing. Demonstration of bidirectional block across the isthmus may result in better outcome [6, 7].

10.3 Specific Substrates for Uncommon Flutter

10.3.1 Mitral Valve Surgery

Uncommon flutter occurs frequently after mitral valve surgery. The superior trans-septal approach, in which a right atriotomy is prolonged into the interatrial septum and the roof of the left atrium for excellent exposure of the complete mitral annulus and subvalvar apparatus [8], carries a higher risk of atrial tachycardia or flutter than the standard left atrial approach [9]. The superior trans-septal incision creates slow conduction between the atriotomy and the tricuspid annulus, predisposing incisional tachycardia and typical atrial flutter [10]. In our case series, 12 out of 15 patients with uncommon flutter after mitral valve surgery via superior trans-septal approach had incisional tachycardia rotating around the right atrial part of the incision (Fig. 10.2). Four patients exhibited dual loops of incisional reentry and cavotricuspid isthmus-dependent flutter. For this type of incisional reentry, creating an ablation lesion connecting the lower edge of the right atrial incision and inferior vena cava is most safe and efficacious [7]. Since the superior pathway from the sinoatrial node to the atrioventricular node is interrupted by the atriotomy extending superior part of the right and left atrium, an ablation targeting the interatrial septum may cause atrioventricular block. Ablation of the cavotricuspid isthmus should also be created since typical flutter is also frequent. Optimal end point for ablating incisional tachycardia after superior trans-septal approach is to establish the lines of block that can be recognized by characteristic patterns of activation in the lateral right atrial free wall [7]. Lateral conduction block after ablation is characterized by late-activated corridor in the anterolateral right atrial free wall (Fig. 10.3). Other possible circuit includes incisional tachycardia rotating around the septal and left atrial part of the incision. Focal atrial tachycardia may also develop [7, 10, 11].

Standard left atrial approach incising along the interatrial groove is less arrhythmogenic [9]. Although rare, incisional tachycardia may occur. In patients with concomitant tricuspid surgery with right atriotomy, incisional reentry around the right atriotomy scar may occur.

10.3.2 Biatrial Surgical Ablation of Atrial Fibrillation

Biatrial surgical ablation of atrial fibrillation (AF) such as maze procedure consists of isolation of all four pulmonary

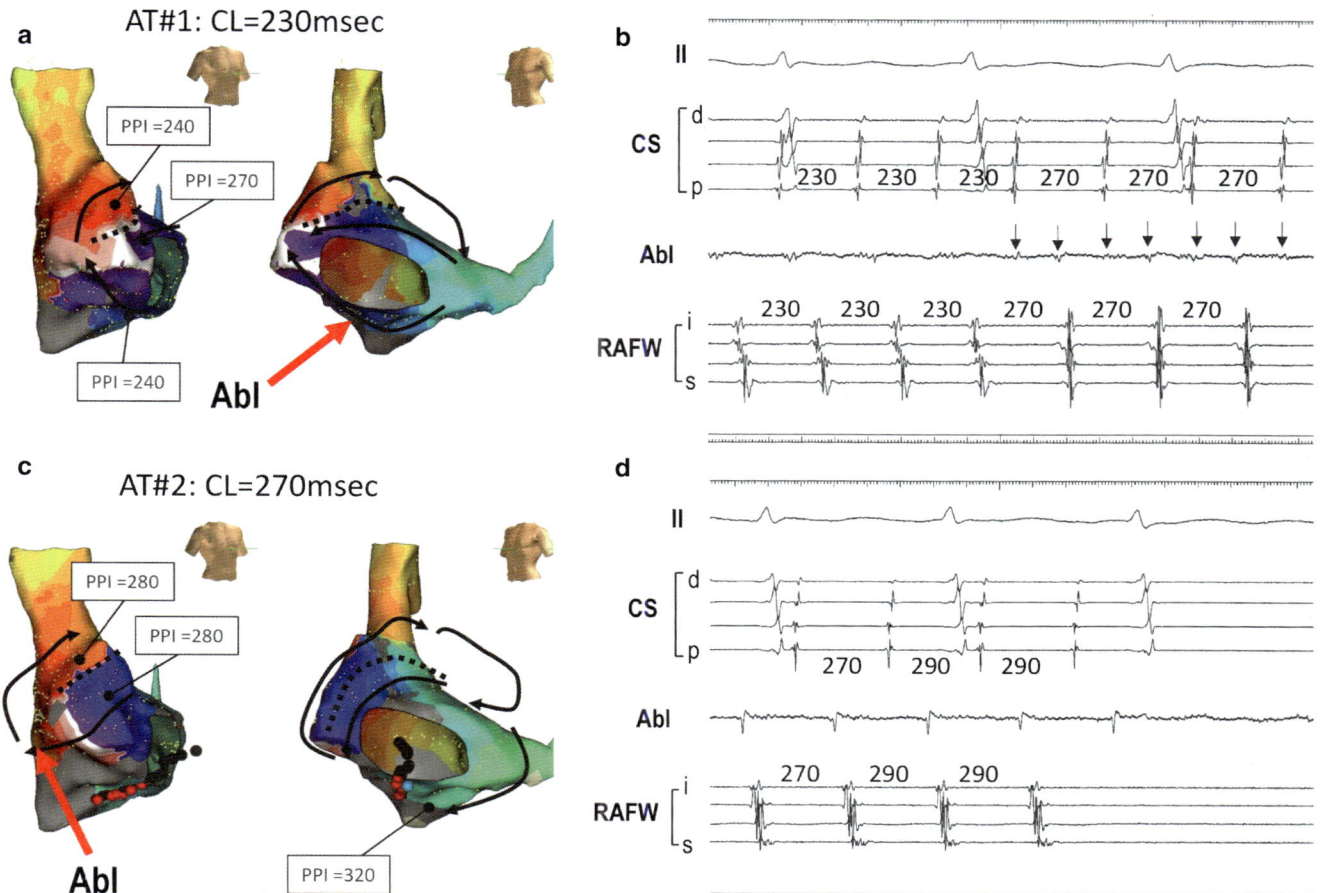

Fig. 10.2 Activation maps and intracardiac recordings in a patient with atrial tachycardia (AT) after mitral valve surgery via superior transseptal approach. (**a**) Activation map of the right atrium during AT#1, exhibiting a reentrant circuit involving the posterior part of the right atrial incision and the cavotricuspid isthmus. Post-pacing interval (PPI) was close to the tachycardia cycle length (CL) at the cavotricuspid isthmus and the posterior part of the right atrial incision, whereas that was longer than the tachycardia CL at the superior part of the tricuspid annulus. (**b**) Intracardiac recordings during radiofrequency application to the cavotricuspid isthmus for AT #1. Tachycardia CL prolonged from 230 to 270 ms with the local potential of the ablation catheter exhibiting double potentials (*arrows*), suggesting completion of the conduction block at the cavotricuspid isthmus and transition to different tachycardia (AT #2). (**c**) Activation maps of the right atrium during AT #2

veins (PVs) to prevent propagation of repetitive activations and multiple incisions on the right and left atria to block the reentrant activation [12]. The biatrial surgical ablation procedures have been reported to result in the emergence of regular atrial tachycardia or flutter [5, 13–18], in which the mechanism includes macroreentry and focal tachycardia. In our institute, radiofrequency catheter ablation was performed in 34 patients with atrial tachycardia or flutter that developed late after biatrial surgical ablation for atrial fibrillation [19]. The mechanisms of a total of 53 tachycardias were macroreentry in 30, a focal mechanism in 20, localized reentry in 1, and could not be determined in 2. The cause of the macroreentrant AT (uncommon flutter) was a residual conduction across a surgical lesion, most of which was located at the annular end of the mitral (N = 18) or tricuspid isthmus incision (N = 7) where radiofrequency or cryoablation was applied during the surgery. We did not find any gaps across the cut and sew lesions. The residual conduction at the mitral end of the posterior mitral isthmus incision resulted in peri-mitral flutter (Fig. 10.4) or macroreentry around the right pulmonary veins, depending on the design of the surgical lesion set. For this type of tachycardia, ablating inside the coronary sinus first is effective. The mitral annulus has several possible obstacles for both surgical and radiofrequency catheter ablation, including the muscular sleeve of the coronary sinus, ramus of the

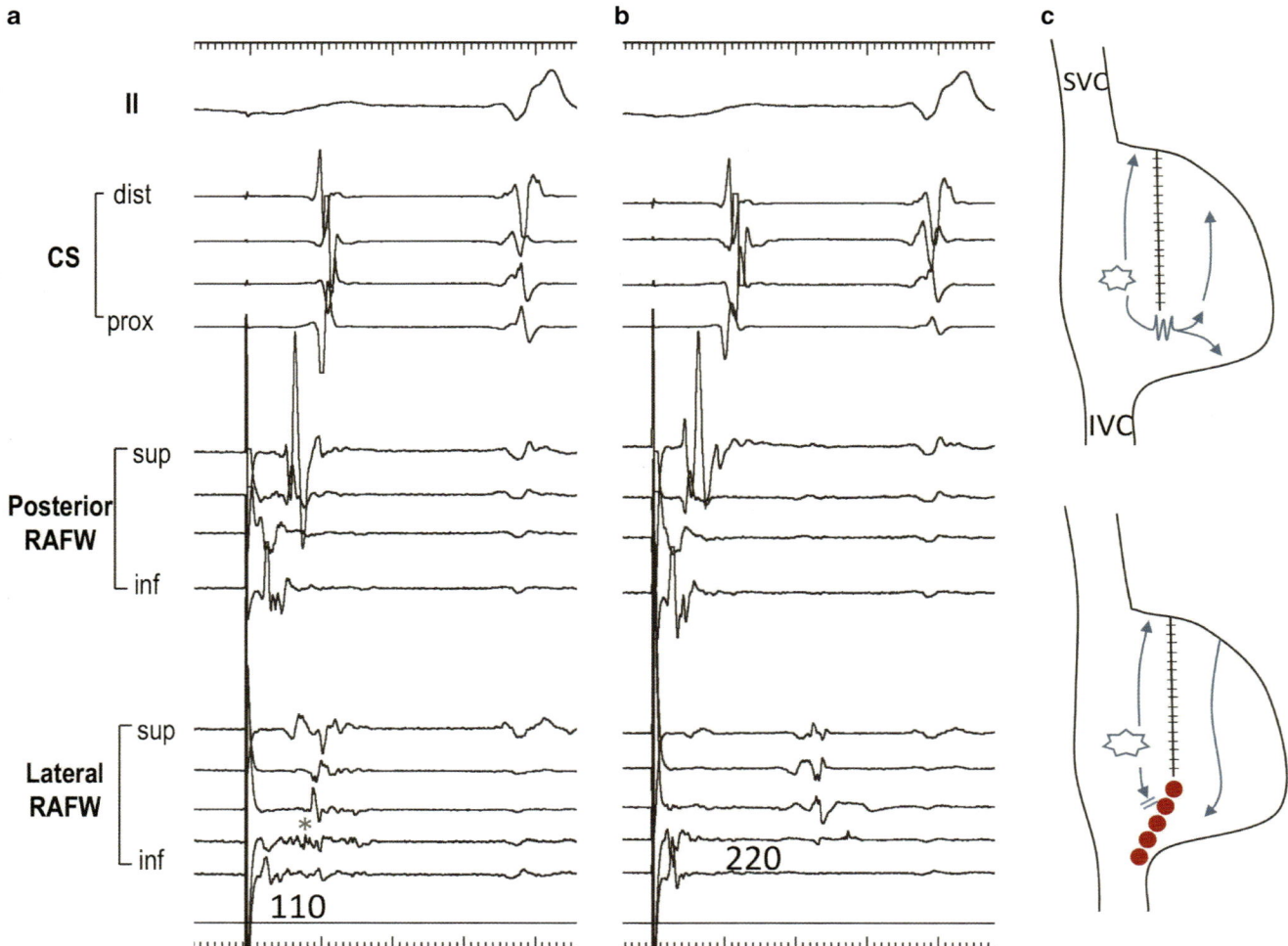

Fig. 10.3 Conduction block in the lateral wall after linear ablation of the right atrial wall (RAFW) between the atriotomy and inferior vena cava in a patient with incisional tachycardia following mitral valve surgery via superior trans-septal approach. (**a**) Lateral RAFW activation during posterior RAFW pacing before ablation. Electrogram at the site close to the lower edge of the atriotomy exhibits fractionated potential (*asterisk*) suggesting pre-existing slow conduction. (**b**) Lateral RAFW activation during posterior RAFW pacing after ablation of the lateral wall between the atriotomy and the inferior vena cava (IVC). Activation of the lateral RAFW markedly delayed. (**c**) Schematic interpretations of the wave front propagation in panels **a** and **b**. *CS* coronary sinus, *SVC* superior vena cava

circumflex coronary arteries, and thick adipose tissue around the atrioventricular groove [20, 21]. Since a part of the coronary sinus musculature sleeve is surrounded by dense adipose tissue, complete radiofrequency or cryoablation could not be easily achieved even when these were applied from both the endocardial and epicardial surface of the mitral annulus. In the case shown in Fig. 10.4, the local electrogram of the mitral annulus at the end of the posterior mitral isthmus incision exhibited low-voltage double potentials suggesting local conduction block (Fig. 10.4). In contrast, the local electrogram in the coronary sinus at the level of mitral isthmus incision exhibited a discrete potential in which the post-pacing interval was identical to the tachycardia cycle length (Fig. 10.4), suggesting participation of the coronary sinus musculature in the reentrant circuit. Radiofrequency application at the site successfully terminated the tachycardia and creation of bidirectional at this lesion. In 8 of 13 patients with this "CS first approach" had a successful elimination of the conduction gaps by ablation only in the coronary sinus. Radiofrequency applications to the gap or an alternative site to transect the circuit were successful in 26 out of 30 macroreentrant tachycardia. Even when the surgical lesion is complete and has no gap, focal atrial tachycardia may develop. Interestingly, focal atrial tachycardia may exhibit uncommon flutter like ECG pattern because of a complex activation pattern through the corridors made by several surgical lesions. The origin of the focal atrial tachycardia was distributed to the right atrial

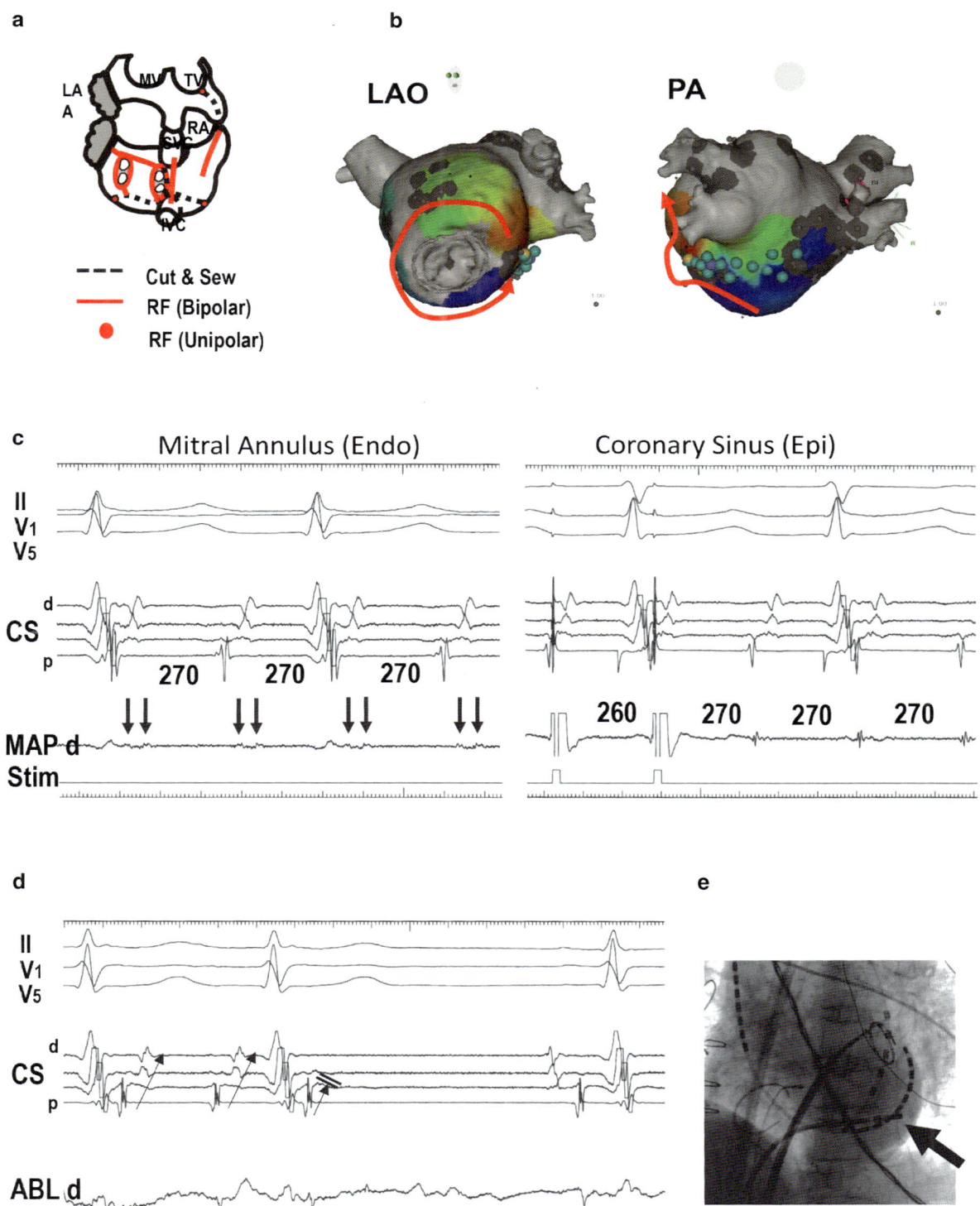

Fig. 10.4 Mechanism and treatment of uncommon atrial flutter in a patient after a biatrial surgical ablation of atrial fibrillation. (**a**) Schematics of the surgical lesion sets of the modified maze procedure. (**b**) Activation map of the left atrium during uncommon atrial flutter in left anterior oblique (LAO) and posteroanterior (PA) projection, showing counter-clockwise activation along the mitral annulus. Double potentials are recorded along the mitral isthmus incision (*green tag*). However, a residual conduction across the incision was detected at the mitral end of the incision. (**c**) Intracardiac signals during atrial flutter. The coronary sinus (CS) electrogram shows proximal to distal activation. Local electrogram at the mitral annulus (MAP d) where the mitral isthmus incision had been created exhibits low-voltage double potentials. On the other hand, the local electrogram in the CS at the level of the mitral isthmus incision exhibits a discrete potential where the post-pacing interval was identical to the tachycardia cycle length. (**d**) Termination of the tachycardia during radiofrequency applications in the CS. (**e**) Fluoroscopic image of the successful ablation site (*arrow*). RF indicates radiofrequency lesion

free wall, sinus node lesion, superior vena cava, interatrial septum, cavotricuspid isthmus, coronary sinus, and mitral annulus. Radiofrequency application to the earliest activation site of the focus was effective.

10.3.3 Surgical Repair of Congenital Heart Disease

Uncommon flutter occurs commonly after surgical repair of congenital heart disease (CHD) such as atrial septal defect repair, correction of tetralogy of Fallot, or Fontan procedures. Common mechanisms include incisional tachycardia rotating around the right atriotomy scar [22, 23] and reentry around the interatrial septal patch [24]. Uncommon flutter with these mechanisms is referred as "intra-atrial reentrant tachycardia." Coexistence of intra-atrial reentrant tachycardia with isthmus-dependent atrial flutter is common and may show an ECG pattern predictive of typical atrial flutter [23]. Three-dimensional mapping during the tachycardia combined with entrainment technique is quite useful in delineating the reentrant circuit and ablation in stable tachycardia. For transecting the reentrant circuit around the right atriotomy scar, making a linear lesion between the atriotomy scar and the anatomical obstacle such as inferior vena cava or tricuspid annulus is the most effective and safe approach.

For multiple or unstable tachycardia associated with complex substrate, the substrate-based approach, where the location of the critical isthmus is detected by a voltage map during sinus rhythm or atrial pacing may be effective [6]. Recent version of EnSite Precision® can make an activation map of a specific cycle length and activation pattern from a stored mapping information during unstable tachycardia.

10.4 Uncommon Flutter in Patients Without Obvious Structural Heart Disease

Macroreentrant atrial tachycardia based on a variety of substrates have been described in patients without previous surgery or catheter ablation [2, 25–29]. Cases of macroreentrant atrial tachycardia associated with spontaneous scaring in the LA was first described by Jais et al. [27], where three patients who had no prior cardiac surgery had posterior, anterior, or roof of the left atrium had associated macroreentrant atrial tachycardia. More recently, Fukamizu et al. reported six patients with macroreentrant atrial tachycardia originating from the left atrial anterior wall, where spontaneous scars were observed. The activation map showed a double loop around the scar and mitral annulus. Slow conduction at the critical isthmus between the scar and the mitral annulus was observed and ablation was effective. Zhang et al. also reported similar ten cases with macroreentrant tachycardia [28]. Successful ablation could be achieved at the isthmus between the scar and the anatomical obstacle (i.e., mitral annulus). Figure 10.5 demonstrates uncommon flutter in a case with dilated phase of hypertrophic cardiomyopathy without any previous ablation or surgery. Marrouche et al. reported 11 patients with left septal flutter rotating around the left septum prinum with a critical isthmus located between the pulmonary veins posteriorly or the mitral annulus anteriorly and the septum prinum [29]. Slow conduction in the left atrial septum due to antiarrhythmic drugs or atrial myopathy is thought to promote this tachycardia, and radiofrequency ablation from the septum prinum to the right inferior pulmonary vein or the mitral annulus is reported to be usually effective.

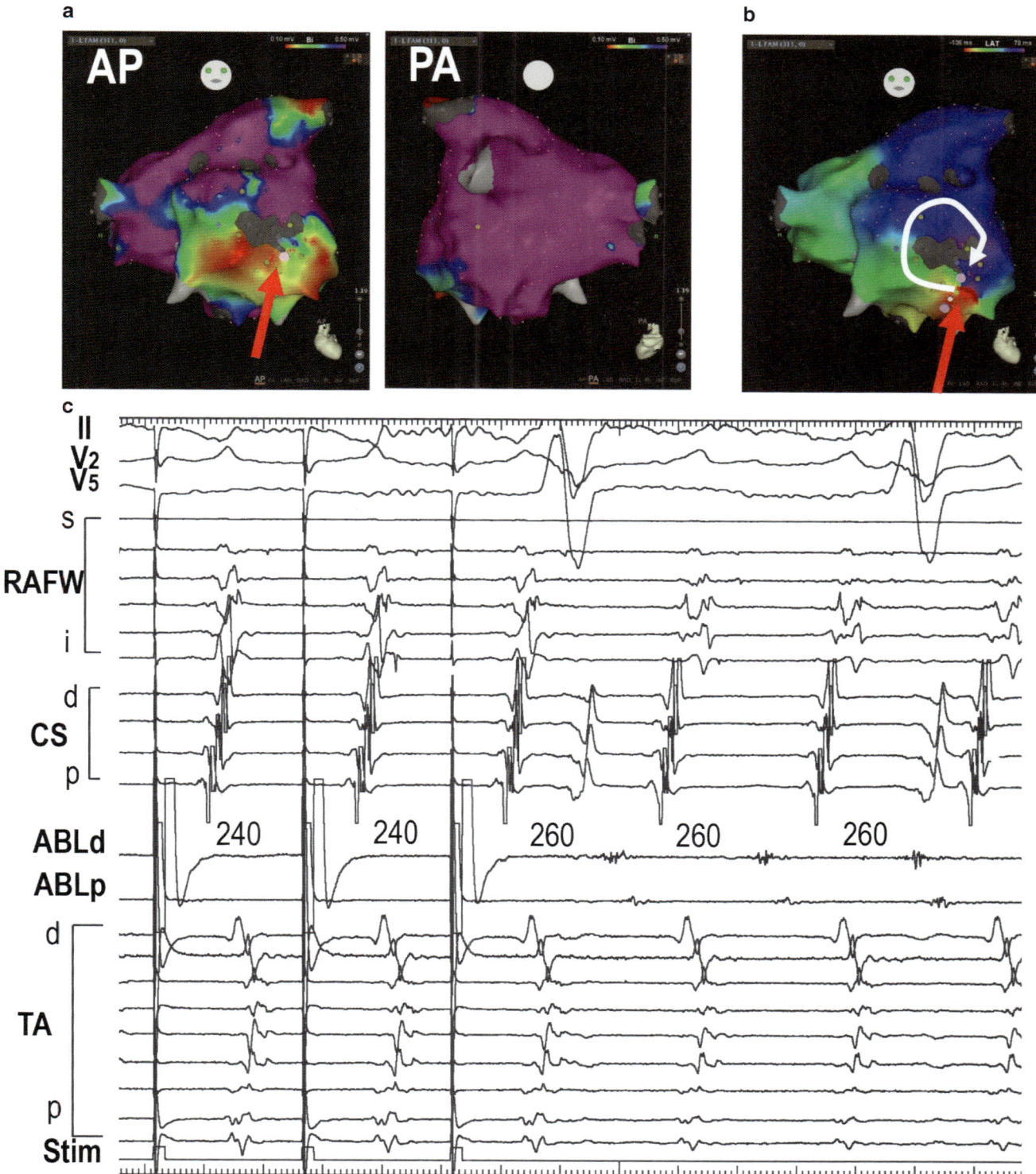

Fig. 10.5 Uncommon flutter in a case without previous surgery or ablation. (**a**) Voltage map of the left atrium. Bipolar voltage >0.5 mV is displayed in purple. *Gray* indicates dense scar with no detectable electrogram. A large low-voltage area is detected in the anterior wall. (**b**) Activation map during uncommon flutter demonstrates reentry around the dense scar in the left atrial anterior wall. (**c**) Intra-cardiac recordings during and following entrainment of the tachycardia from the successful ablation site (*arrows* in panels **a** and **b**). The local electrogram at the successful site (ABLd) exhibits low-voltage, fractionated potentials suggesting slow conduction, and the post-pacing interval was identical to the tachycardia cycle length. Radiofrequency application at this site terminated the tachycardia

References

1. Saoudi N, Cosio F, Waldo A, Chen SA, Iesaka Y, Lesh M, et al. A classification of atrial flutter and regular atrial tachycardia according to electrophysiological mechanisms and anatomical bases; a Statement from a Joint Expert Group from The Working Group of Arrhythmias of the European Society of Cardiology and the North American Society of Pacing and Electrophysiology. Eur Heart J. 2001;22(14):1162–82. https://doi.org/10.1053/euhj.2001.2658.
2. Fukamizu S, Sakurada H, Hayashi T, Hojo R, Komiyama K, Tanabe Y, et al. Macroreentrant atrial tachycardia in patients without previous atrial surgery or catheter ablation: clinical and electrophysiological characteristics of scar-related left atrial anterior wall reentry. J Cardiovasc Electrophysiol. 2013;24(4):404–12. https://doi.org/10.1111/jce.12059.
3. Pascale P, Shah AJ, Roten L, Scherr D, Komatsu Y, Jadidi AS, et al. Pattern and timing of the coronary sinus activation to guide rapid diagnosis of atrial tachycardia after atrial fibrillation ablation. Circ Arrhythm Electrophysiol. 2013;6(3):481–90. https://doi.org/10.1161/circep.113.000182.
4. Anter E, Tschabrunn CM, Josephson ME. High-resolution mapping of scar-related atrial arrhythmias using smaller electrodes with closer interelectrode spacing. Circ Arrhythm Electrophysiol. 2015;8(3):537–45. https://doi.org/10.1161/circep.114.002737.
5. Takahashi K, Miyauchi Y, Hayashi M, Iwasaki YK, Yodogawa K, Tsuboi I, et al. Mechanisms of postoperative atrial tachycardia following biatrial surgical ablation of atrial fibrillation in relation to the surgical lesion sets. Heart Rhythm. 2016;13(5):1059–65. https://doi.org/10.1016/j.hrthm.2015.12.033.
6. Nakagawa H, Shah N, Matsudaira K, Overholt E, Chandrasekaran K, Beckman KJ, et al. Characterization of reentrant circuit in macroreentrant right atrial tachycardia after surgical repair of congenital heart disease: isolated channels between scars allow "focal" ablation. Circulation. 2001;103(5):699–709.
7. Kanagasundram AN, Baduashvili A, Liu CF, Cheung JW, Thomas G, Ip JE, et al. A novel criterion for conduction block after catheter ablation of right atrial tachycardia after mitral valve surgery. Circ Arrhythm Electrophysiol. 2013;6(1):39–47. https://doi.org/10.1161/circep.112.976340.
8. Berreklouw E, Ercan H, Schonberger JP. Combined superior-transseptal approach to the left atrium. Ann Thorac Surg. 1991;51(2):293–5.
9. Lukac P, Hjortdal VE, Pedersen AK, Mortensen PT, Jensen HK, Hansen PS. Atrial incision affects the incidence of atrial tachycardia after mitral valve surgery. Ann Thorac Surg. 2006;81(2):509–13. https://doi.org/10.1016/j.athoracsur.2005.07.083.
10. Lukac P, Hjortdal V, Pedersen AK, Jensen HK, Mortensen PT, Hansen PS. The superior transseptal surgical approach to mitral valve creates slow conduction. Pacing Clin Electrophysiol. 2006;29(7):719–26. https://doi.org/10.1111/j.1540-8159.2006.00425.x.
11. Roberts-Thomson KC, Kalman JM. Right septal macroreentrant tachycardia late after mitral valve repair: importance of surgical access approach. Heart Rhythm. 2007;4(1):32–6. https://doi.org/10.1016/j.hrthm.2006.09.032.
12. Cox JL, Jaquiss RD, Schuessler RB, Boineau JP. Modification of the maze procedure for atrial flutter and atrial fibrillation. II. Surgical technique of the maze III procedure. J Thorac Cardiovasc Surg. 1995;110(2):485–95.
13. Golovchiner G, Mazur A, Kogan A, Strasberg B, Shapira Y, Fridman M, et al. Atrial flutter after surgical radiofrequency ablation of the left atrium for atrial fibrillation. Ann Thorac Surg. 2005;79(1):108–12. https://doi.org/10.1016/j.athoracsur.2004.06.063.
14. Henry L, Durrani S, Hunt S, Friehling T, Tran H, Wish M, et al. Percutaneous catheter ablation treatment of recurring atrial arrhythmias after surgical ablation. Ann Thorac Surg. 2010;89(4):1227–1231.; discussion 31–2. https://doi.org/10.1016/j.athoracsur.2010.01.042.
15. Kobza R, Kottkamp H, Dorszewski A, Tanner H, Piorkowski C, Schirdewahn P, et al. Stable secondary arrhythmias late after intraoperative radiofrequency ablation of atrial fibrillation: incidence, mechanism, and treatment. J Cardiovasc Electrophysiol. 2004;15(11):1246–9. https://doi.org/10.1046/j.1540-8167.2004.04356.x.
16. Chun KR, Bansch D, Ernst S, Ujeyl A, Huang H, Chu H, et al. Pulmonary vein conduction is the major finding in patients with atrial tachyarrhythmias after intraoperative maze ablation. J Cardiovasc Electrophysiol. 2007;18(4):358–63. https://doi.org/10.1111/j.1540-8167.2007.00771.x.
17. Trumello C, Pozzoli A, Mazzone P, Nascimbene S, Bignami E, Cireddu M, et al. Electrophysiological findings and long-term outcomes of percutaneous ablation of atrial arrhythmias after surgical ablation for atrial fibrillationdagger. Eur J Cardiothorac Surg. 2016;49(1):273–80. https://doi.org/10.1093/ejcts/ezv034.
18. Wazni OM, Saliba W, Fahmy T, Lakkireddy D, Thal S, Kanj M, et al. Atrial arrhythmias after surgical maze: findings during catheter ablation. J Am Coll Cardiol. 2006;48(7):1405–9. https://doi.org/10.1016/j.jacc.2006.05.061.
19. Takahashi Y, Takahashi A, Miyazaki S, Kuwahara T, Takei A, Fujino T, et al. Electrophysiological characteristics of localized reentrant atrial tachycardia occurring after catheter ablation of long-lasting persistent atrial fibrillation. J Cardiovasc Electrophysiol. 2009;20(6):623–9. https://doi.org/10.1111/j.1540-8167.2008.01410.x.
20. Castella M, Garcia-Valentin A, Pereda D, Colli A, Martinez A, Martinez D, et al. Anatomic aspects of the atrioventricular junction influencing radiofrequency Cox maze IV procedures. J Thorac Cardiovasc Surg. 2008;136(2):419–23. https://doi.org/10.1016/j.jtcvs.2008.03.049.
21. Wittkampf FH, van Oosterhout MF, Loh P, Derksen R, Vonken EJ, Slootweg PJ, et al. Where to draw the mitral isthmus line in catheter ablation of atrial fibrillation: histological analysis. Eur Heart J. 2005;26(7):689–95. https://doi.org/10.1093/eurheartj/ehi095.
22. Lukac P, Pedersen AK, Mortensen PT, Jensen HK, Hjortdal V, Hansen PS. Ablation of atrial tachycardia after surgery for congenital and acquired heart disease using an electroanatomic mapping system: which circuits to expect in which substrate? Heart Rhythm. 2005;2(1):64–72. https://doi.org/10.1016/j.hrthm.2004.10.034.
23. Akar JG, Kok LC, Haines DE, DiMarco JP, Mounsey JP. Coexistence of type I atrial flutter and intra-atrial re-entrant tachycardia in patients with surgically corrected congenital heart disease. J Am Coll Cardiol. 2001;38(2):377–84.
24. Delacretaz E, Ganz LI, Soejima K, Friedman PL, Walsh EP, Triedman JK, et al. Multi atrial maco-re-entry circuits in adults with repaired congenital heart disease: entrainment mapping combined with three-dimensional electroanatomic mapping. J Am Coll Cardiol. 2001;37(6):1665–76.
25. Ouyang F, Ernst S, Vogtmann T, Goya M, Volkmer M, Schaumann A, et al. Characterization of reentrant circuits in left atrial macroreentrant tachycardia: critical isthmus block can prevent atrial tachycardia recurrence. Circulation. 2002;105(16):1934–42.
26. Fiala M, Chovancik J, Neuwirth R, Nevralova R, Jiravsky O, Sknouril L, et al. Atrial macroreentry tachycardia in patients without obvious structural heart disease or previous cardiac surgical or catheter intervention: characterization of arrhythmogenic substrates, reentry circuits, and results of catheter ablation. J Cardiovasc Electrophysiol. 2007;18(8):824–32. https://doi.org/10.1111/j.1540-8167.2007.00859.x.
27. Jais P, Shah DC, Haissaguerre M, Hocini M, Peng JT, Takahashi A, et al. Mapping and ablation of left atrial flutters. Circulation. 2000;101(25):2928–34.
28. Zhang J, Tang C, Zhang Y, Han H, Li Z, Su X. Electroanatomic characterization and ablation outcome of nonlesion related left atrial macroreentrant tachycardia in patients without obvious structural heart disease. J Cardiovasc Electrophysiol. 2013;24(1):53–9. https://doi.org/10.1111/j.1540-8167.2012.02426.x.
29. Marrouche NF, Natale A, Wazni OM, Cheng J, Yang Y, Pollack H, et al. Left septal atrial flutter: electrophysiology, anatomy, and results of ablation. Circulation. 2004;109(20):2440–7. https://doi.org/10.1161/01.cir.0000129439.03836.96.

Adenosine-Sensitive Atrial Tachycardia

Hiroshige Yamabe

Keywords
Atrial tachycardia · Entrainment · Mapping · Reentry

Abbreviation

AT   Atrial tachycardia
AV   Atrioventricular
EAAS Earliest atrial activation site
HB   His bundle

11.1 Adenosine-Sensitive Atrial Tachycardia Originating from the Vicinity to the Atrioventricular Node

11.1.1 Historical Background and Electrophysiologic Feature

Adenosine-sensitive atrial tachycardia (AT) originating from the vicinity to the atrioventricular (AV) node has been first reported by Iesaka et al. [1]. They demonstrated that there may be an entity of adenosine-sensitive AT probably due to focal reentry within the AV node or its transitional tissues without involvement of the AV nodal pathways. Since AT is sensitive to adenosine and verapamil, Ca-channel-dependent tissue is suggested to be involved in the reentry circuit. They also showed that this AT can be ablated without disturbing AV nodal conduction from the right atrial septum. Subsequently, Lai et al. also reported 6 patients with AT near the AV nodal region [2]. Their ATs were successfully eliminated by the radiofrequency energy application which was delivered to the earliest atrial activation site (EAAS) vicinity to the AV node; however, they emphasized the potential risk of inadvertent AV block. Regarding the mechanism of these ATs, they speculated that AT was due to reentry because induction and reset return cycle length showed an increasing pattern with progressive coupling prematurity [2]. Frey et al. examined 16 patients with AT origination from the AV nodal region [3]. Mapping the both right and left atrial septum revealed that EAAS was observed at the right side in ten patients and at the left side in the remaining six patients. Thus, they concluded that mapping of both sides of the interatrial septum is required prior to the ablation of focal AT originating from the vicinity of the AV node [3]. Ouyang et al. mapped the non-coronary aortic cusp in nine patients with focal AT near the His bundle (HB) region in whom the five of nine patients were previously failed ablation cases by the right-sided approach [4]. Mapping in atria demonstrated that the earliest atrial activation was located at the HB region, whereas mapping in the non-coronary aortic cusp demonstrated that an earliest atrial activation preceded the atrial activation at the HB by 12.2 ± 6.9 ms and was anatomically located supero-posterior to the HB site in all nine patients [4]. Radiofrequency energy application to the EAAS in the non-coronary aortic cusp terminated the AT in all patients [4]. Since His potential was not observed at the successful ablation site in the non-coronary aortic cusp, they suggested that mapping the non-coronary aortic cusp in focal AT near the HB region is a safe alternative approach and can improve the clinical outcome [4]. Their AT was also sensitive to adenosine and

H. Yamabe, M.D., Ph.D., F.J.C.C
Department of Cardiovascular Medicine, Graduate School of Medical Sciences, Kumamoto University, 1-1-1 Honjo, Kumamoto City 860-8556, Japan
e-mail: yyamabe@kumamoto-u.ac.jp

reproducibly induced and terminated by atrial stimulation in all patients. Therefore, they suggested the tachycardia mechanism was due to either micro-reentry or trigger activity [4]. Das et al. reported the usefulness of non-coronary cusp ablation in peri-AV nodal AT [5]. Radiofrequency ablation in the non-coronary aortic cusp was successful in seven patients but not in the remaining three patients and required left atrial septal ablation [5]. Their result indicates that the non-coronary sinus is not the only effective site of ablation, but there is variable location of the AT origin, as reported previously [3, 6].

11.1.2 Tachycardia Circuit and Its Mechanism

Regarding the substrate of this form of AT, a calcium channel-dependent substrate is suggested to be involved in the reentry circuit because verapamil and adenosine triphosphate were both effective in terminating tachycardia. A calcium channel-dependent tissue, such as part of AV node or transitional cells surrounding the AV node has been suggested as the substrate of this form of AT. However, less information exists regarding the anatomic tachycardia circuit of this verapamil-sensitive AT originating from the vicinity of the AV node. To define the anatomic tachycardia circuit of this form of AT, we examined whether atrial tissue within the Koch's triangle, including the AV nodal conduction system, is involved in the circuit [7]. For this purpose, a single extrastimulus was delivered during tachycardia to ten sites of the intra-atrial septum in ten patients with the verapamil-sensitive AT originating from the AV node vicinity [7]. We found that the tachycardia circuit of verapamil-sensitive AT does not involve atrial tissue within the Koch's triangle extending from the HB site to posteroinferior CSOS. Furthermore, we have shown that the AV conduction system does not participate in the tachycardia circuit of this form of AT. Calcium channel-dependent tissue located close to the AV node but not the AV conducting system was suggested to form the substrate of verapamil-sensitive AT originating from the vicinity of the AV node [7]. In this study, tachycardia was induced and terminated by atrial rapid and extrastimulus pacing. An inverse relation of tachycardia induction and resetting was also observed in all patients. In addition, concealed entrainment was shown in all patients. Furthermore, manifest entrainment was demonstrated in two of ten patients in whom rapid atrial pacing was attempted from multiple sites of the atrium during tachycardia. These findings suggest that the mechanism of verapamil-sensitive AT originating from the vicinity of the AV node is due to reentry.

11.1.3 Demonstration of Reentry Circuit and Appropriate Ablation Site

The exact boundaries of the reentry circuit have not been convincingly defined. Therefore, we subsequently elucidated the exact anatomical tachycardia circuit of this AT using the entrainment pacing technique [8]. The slow conduction area of the reentry circuit of this form of AT is quite similar to that of the AV nodal reentrant tachycardia. Previously, Satoh et al. reported that orthodromic capture of the earliest atrial electrogram at HB site by coronary sinus pacing during AV nodal reentrant tachycardia indicates the absence of upper common pathway in AVNRT [9]. This finding also indicates that entrance site of the reentry circuit exists distinct from the exit site, suggesting the presence of slow conduction area between entrance and exit [9]. Based on their finding, we postulated that demonstration of manifest entrainment can be used as the tool to define the reentry circuit of verapamil-sensitive AT arising from the AV node vicinity. If manifest entrainment with the orthodromic capture of the EAAS is demonstrated, then the pacing site is considered to be proximal to the slow conduction area [10]. We first identified such a site proximal to the slow conduction area and then delivered radiofrequency energy to a site located between the pacing site and the EAAS (Fig. 11.1).

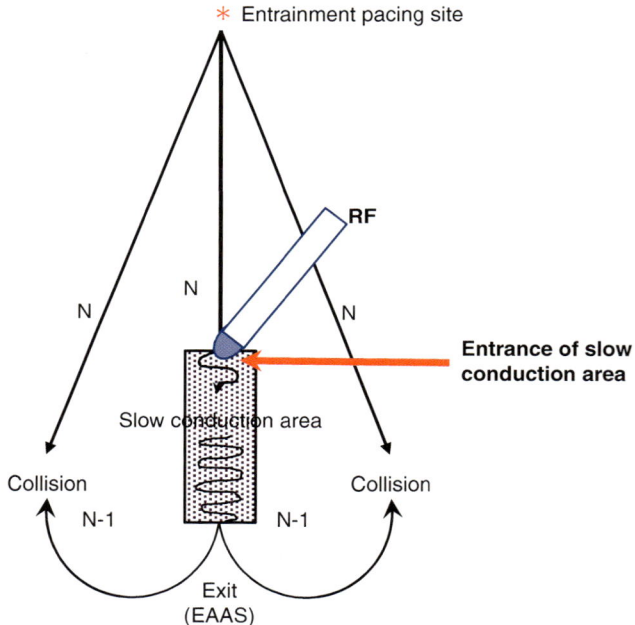

Fig. 11.1 Schematic drawing which shows the method to identify the entrance of the slow conduction area of the reentry circuit using the manifest entrainment method and catheter ablation technique. *RF* radiofrequency energy

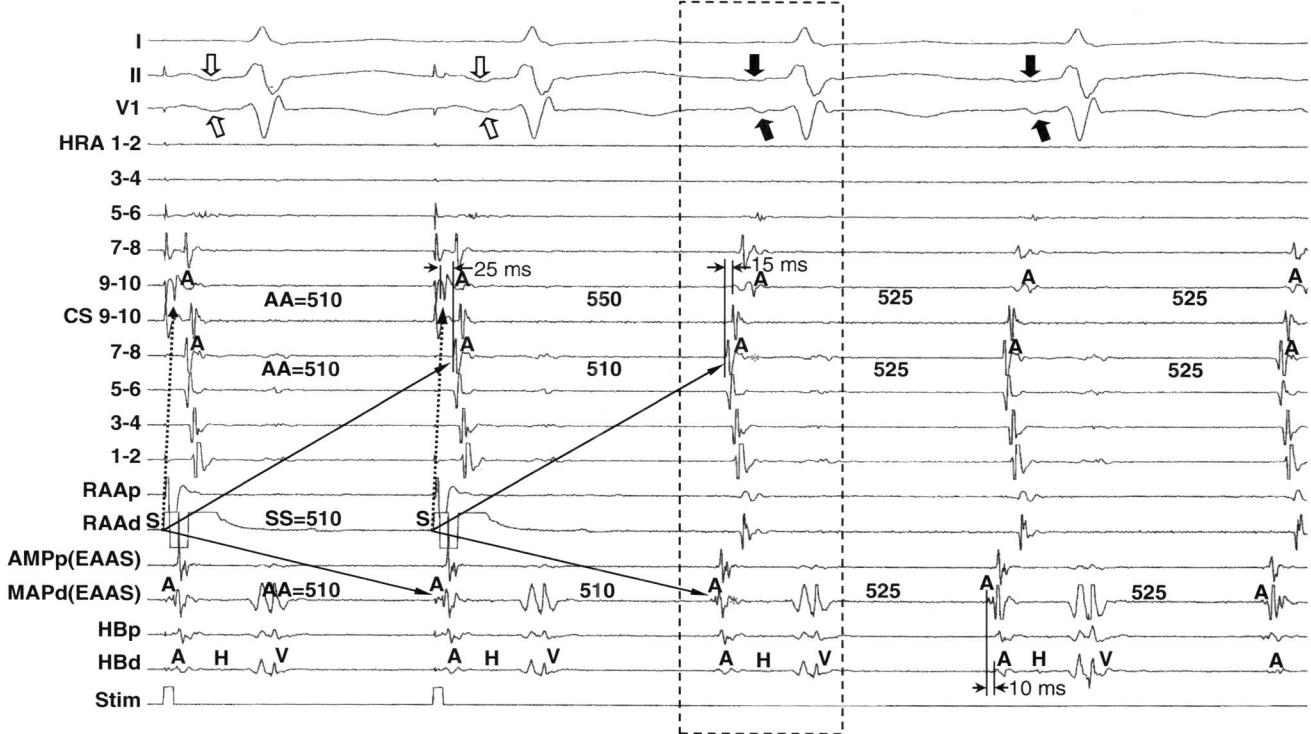

Fig. 11.2 Tracing during manifest entrainment by rapid atrial pacing delivered during tachycardia from the right atrial appendage (RAA) in a patient with AT originating from the AV node vicinity in whom the earliest atrial activation site (EAAS) was observed close to the His bundle site. The electrocardiographic leads I, II, and V1, and electrograms recorded at high right atrium (HRA), coronary sinus (CS), and His bundle (HB) position are shown. *MAP* mapping catheter, *Stim* stimulation

Our study hypothesis is that if AT is terminated during the radiofrequency energy application, this ablation site is on the reentry circuit, most likely at the entrance of the slow conduction area (Fig. 11.1). With the uses of these entrainment pacing and radiofrequency energy application techniques, we attempted to clarify the mechanism of verapamil-sensitive AT, focusing on the location of the slow conduction area [8]. Manifest entrainment associated with the orthodromic capture of the EAAS was demonstrated in all 17 patients [8]. Furthermore, radiofrequency energy delivery to the site, 10.1 ± 2.8 mm away from the EAAS, terminated AT immediately after the onset of delivery (2.9 ± 1.0 s) [8]. Figure 11.2 shows the tracing during manifest entrainment by the pacing delivered from the right atrial appendage. During pacing, the EAAS and coronary sinus region were orthodromically captured, but the high right atrial region was antidromically captured. Surface P-wave morphology shows the constant fusion during pacing. (Fig. 11.2). AT termination was obtained by radiofrequency energy application delivered 9 mm proximal to the EAAS in the direction of entrainment pacing site, suggesting that this site is located at the entrance of the slow conduction area of the reentry circuit (Fig. 11.3). Figure 11.4 shows the tracing during radiofrequency energy application to the entrance of reentry circuit. The atrial electrogram at the successful ablation site was observed 20 ms later than that at the HB site. Furthermore, unipolar electrogram shows the rS morphology, suggesting that this site is away from the EAAS. However, AT was terminated immediately after the onset of energy delivery, suggesting that this site is located on the entrance of the reentry circuit (i.e., entrance of the slow conduction area). Figure 11.5 shows the summary of the relative location of the EAAS, successful ablation site and entrainment pacing site in all patients. AT was successfully terminated by the radiofrequency energy application which was delivered to the site proximal to the EAAS in the direction of entrainment pacing site in all patients (Fig. 11.5) [8]. Since the successful ablation site located more distant from the HB site than the EAAS (12.4 ± 2.9 vs 6.4 ± 1.9 mm; $P < 0.0001$), application of radiofrequency energy to the entrance of the reentry circuit is an alternative and safer therapeutic option than targeting the EAAS [8].

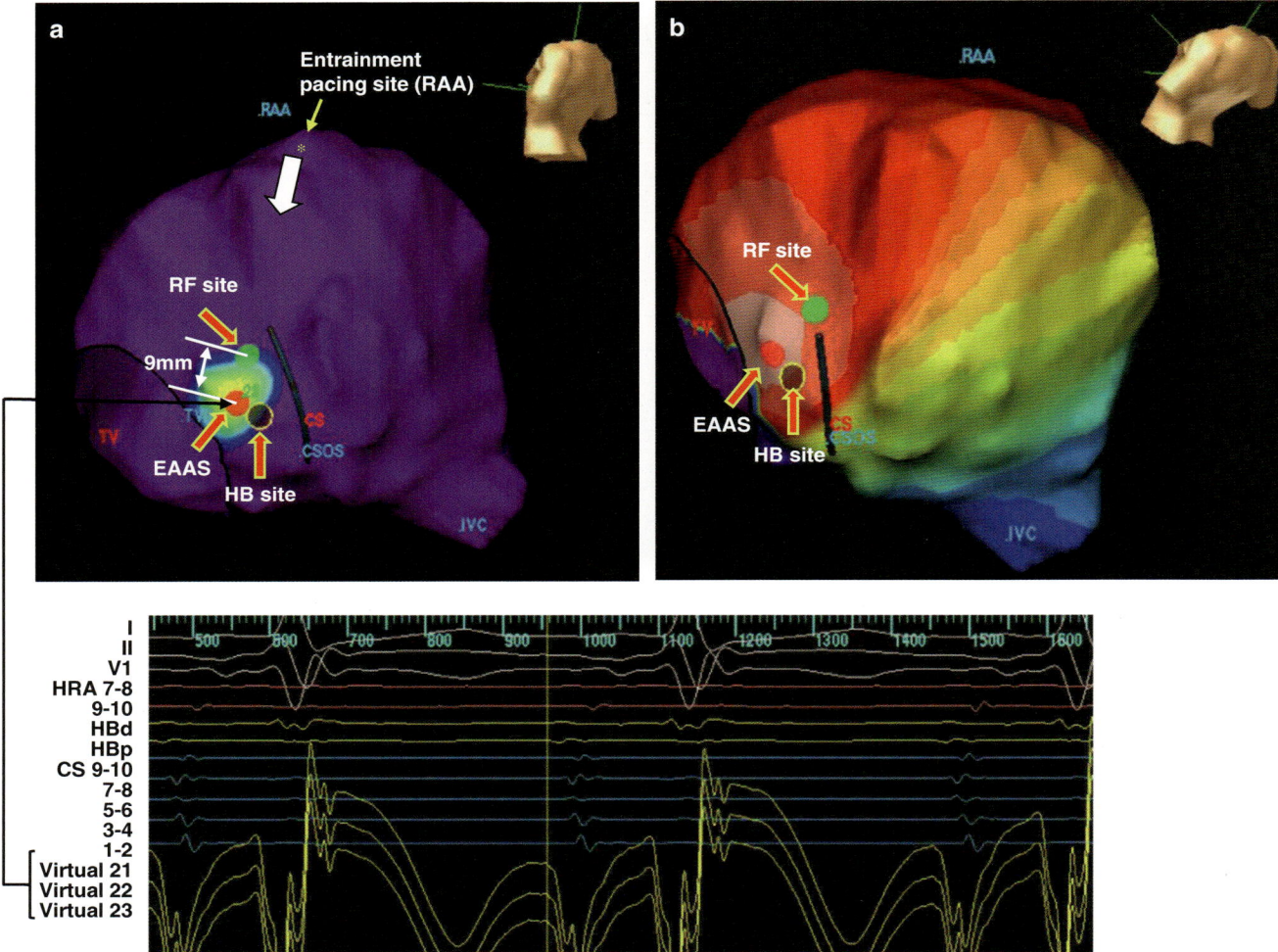

Fig. 11.3 *Top:* Isopotential map at the atrial tachycardia (AT) onset (**a**) and isochronal map during AT (**b**) in the same patient as in Fig. 11.2. *Asterisk*: pacing site at the right atrial appendage (RAA) where the manifest entrainment was demonstrated (Entrainment pacing site). RF site: radiofrequency ablation site. *Bottom:* virtual unipolar electrogram at the earliest atrial activation site (EAAS) at AT onset. See Fig. 11.2 for abbreviations

11.2 Adenosine-Sensitive Atrial Tachycardia Originating from the Atrioventricular Annulus Other than the AV Node Vicinity

11.2.1 Historical Background and Electrophysiologic Feature

Previous studies reported that the AV annulus provides an anatomic substrate for focal AT [11–14]. Tada et al. reported 12 patients with focal AT arising from the tricuspid annulus [11]. Although adenosine sensitivity was documented, they suggested that AV annulus provides the preferable AT origin. They also suggest reentry as the underlying mechanism in 11 of 12 patients [11]. Morton et al. reported nine patients with focal AT arising from the tricuspid annulus though underlying mechanism and adenosine sensitivity were not mentioned [12]. Matsuoka et al. reported five patients with focal AT originating not only from the tricuspid annulus but also from the mitral annulus [13]. Their ATs were terminated by the small dose of adenosine triphosphate. Since AT was induced and terminated by the atrial extra-stimulation, they suggested micro-reentry involving the cells with nodal-type action potentials around the AV annuli [13]. Iwai et al. also reported adenosine-sensitive focal AT arising from the tricuspid annulus and indicated that sensitivity to adenosine suggest focal origin [14]. In the 18 patients with verapamil-sensitive AT, we have compared the electrophysiologic characteristics between ATs originating from the AV node vicinity ($n = 10$) and those arising from the AV annulus other than the AV node vicinity ($n = 8$) [15]. We have shown that this form of AT in which a calcium channel-dependent substrate is involved arises not only from the vicinity of the AV node but also along the AV annulus with common

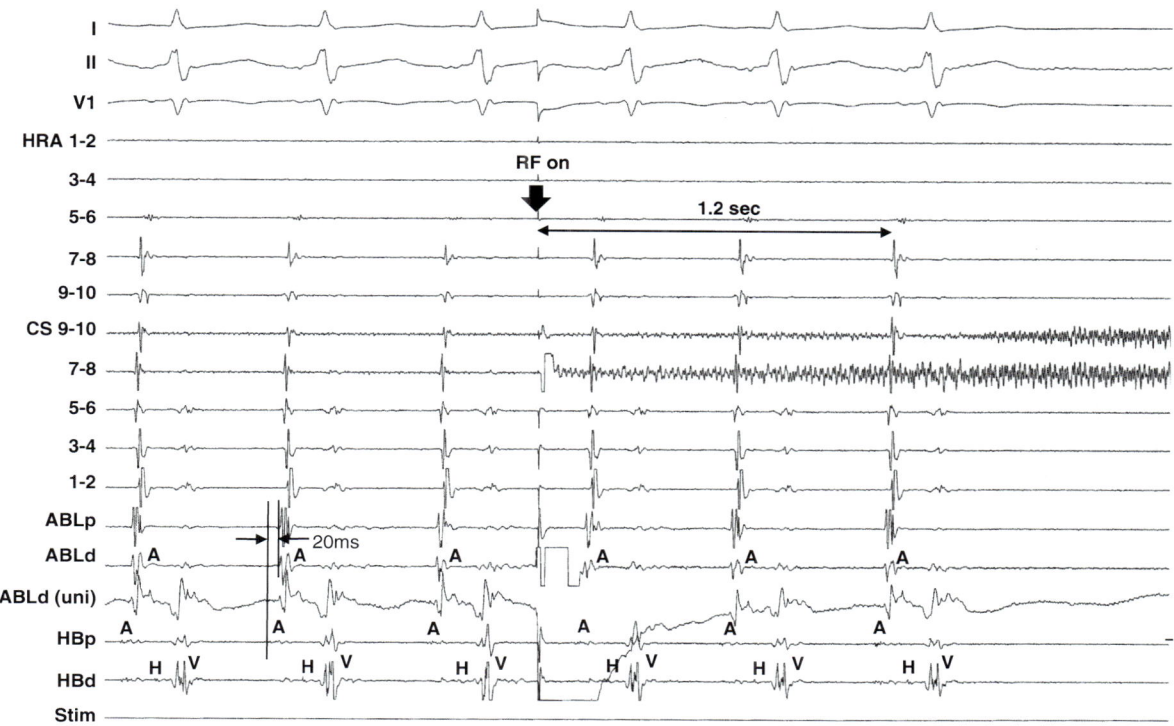

Fig. 11.4 Tracing during radiofrequency energy ablation. *RF* radiofrequency, *Uni* unipolar electrogram. See Fig. 11.2 for abbreviations

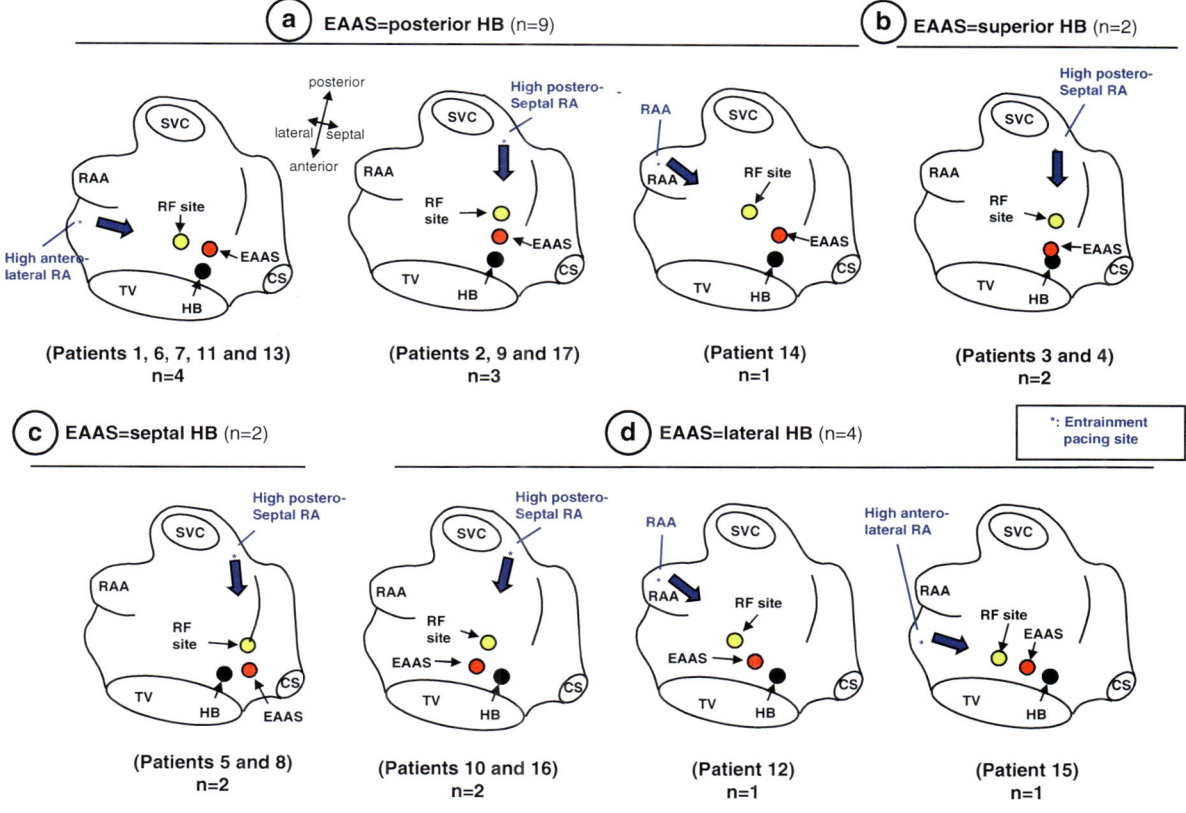

Fig. 11.5 Supero-inferior views of the right atrium showing the location of the earliest atrial activation site (EAAS), successful radiofrequency (RF) ablation site, and His bundle (HB) site. *Asterisk* indicates the pacing site from which the manifest entrainment was demonstrated (entrainment pacing site)

electrophysiologic characteristics [15]. Therefore, we have suggested the presence of a distinct entity of tachycardia more appropriately classified as verapamil-sensitive AV annular AT [15].

11.2.2 Mechanism of Tachycardia and Its Circuit

We examined the mechanism and tachycardia circuit of AT arising from the AV annulus other than the AV node vicinity in 23 patients [16]. For this purpose, we initially delivered rapid atrial pacing a rate 5 beats/min faster than the tachycardia rate during AT from multiple sites of the atrium whether the manifest entrainment of AT is demonstrable. When the manifest entrainment with orthodromic capture of the EAAS, the exit point from the area of the slow conduction area of the reentry circuit, is demonstrated, the pacing site is considered to be proximal to the slow conduction area of the reentry circuit [10]. After identification of a site proximal to the slow conduction area, radiofrequency energy was delivered to a site between the pacing site and the EAAS to identify the entrance of the slow conduction area of the reentry circuit in the same way as previously used for AT originating from the AV node vicinity [8]. Radiofrequency energy was delivered starting at a site 2 cm away from the EAAS in the direction of entrainment pacing site. Then application site was gradually advanced toward the EAAS until termination of tachycardia to define the entrance of slow conduction area of the reentry circuit. Manifest entrainment was demonstrated in all ATs [16]. The EAAS, distributed along the tricuspid annulus from 3- to 12-o' clock position, was orthodromically captured by pacing delivered from high anterolateral right atrium ($n = 6$), high anteroseptal right atrium ($n = 7$), high posteroseptal right atrium ($n = 3$), low anterolateral right atrium ($n = 6$), and coronary sinus ostium ($n = 1$) [16]. Radiofrequency energy delivery to the site, 10.4 ± 2.4 mm proximal to the EAAS where the atrial electrogram was observed 13.9 ± 5.7 ms later than the EAAS, terminated AT immediately after the onset of energy delivery (2.9 ± 1.1 s) [16]. Figure 11.6 shows the tracing during manifest entrainment by the pacing from the high anterolateral right atrium. The EAAS was in the 5-o' clock position of the tricuspid annulus in this patient. During pacing, not only EAAS but also coronary sinus region was orthodromically captured. In contrast, the atrial electrograms at the high right atrium [5–10] were captured antidromically during pacing. In addition, the surface P-wave morphologies in lead V1 during pacing (open arrow) were different from those during tachycardia (closed arrow), indicating fusion of surface P wave during pacing except for the last captured beat. All of these clearly demonstrate classic

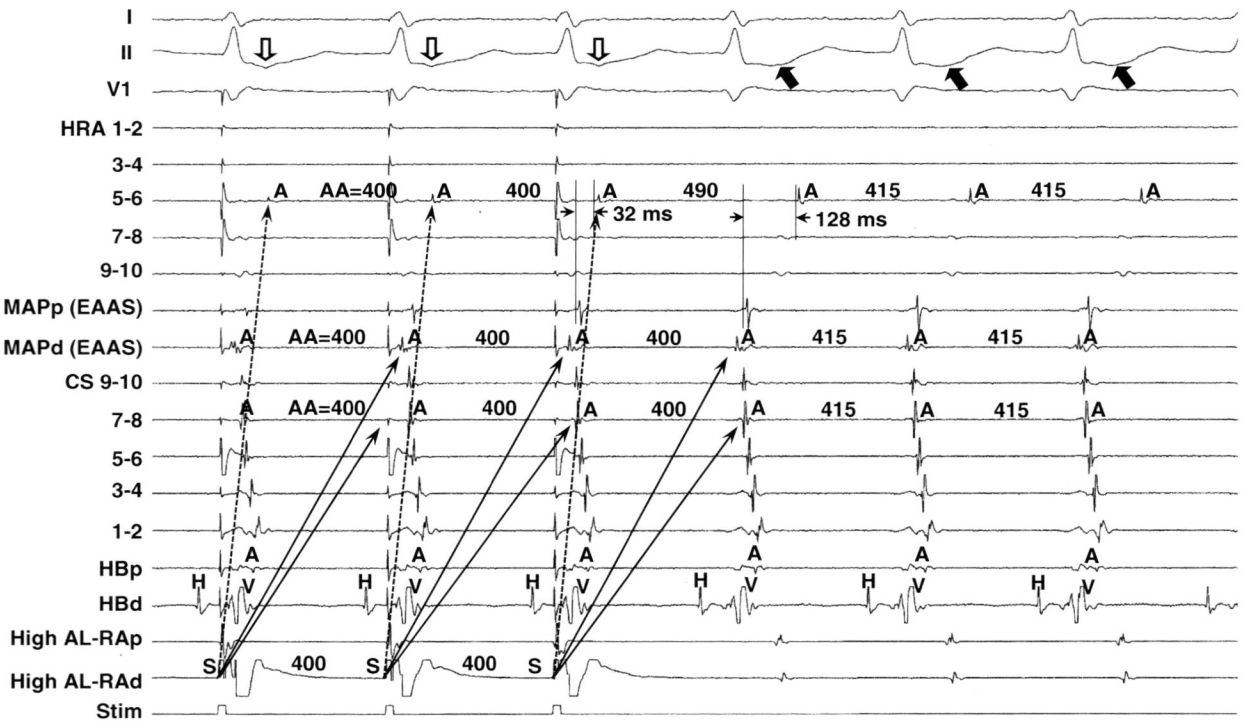

Fig. 11.6 Tracing during manifest entrainment by rapid atrial pacing delivered during tachycardia from the high anterolateral right atrium (AL-RA) in a patient with AT originating from the 5-o' clock position of the tricuspid annulus. See Fig. 11.2 for abbreviations

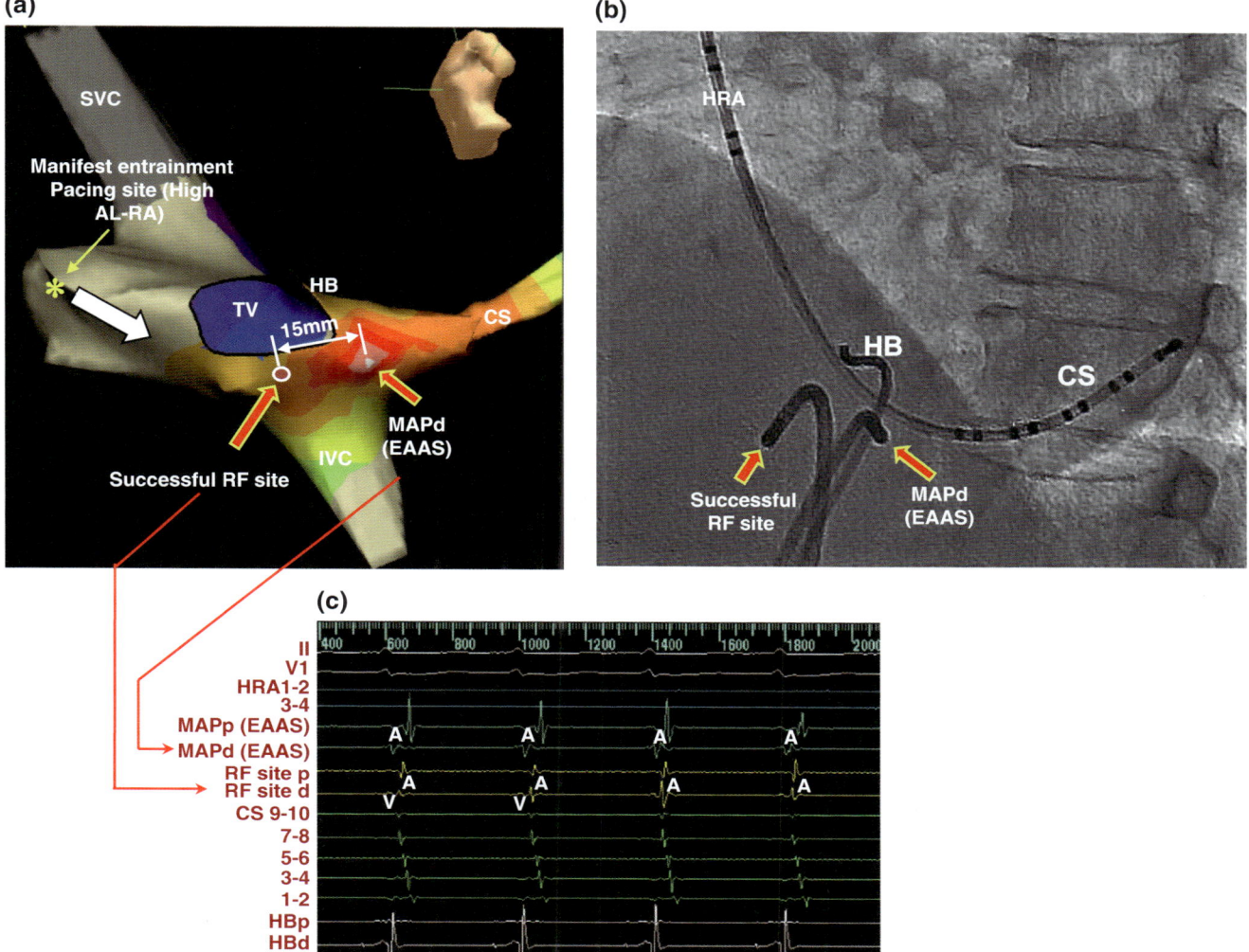

Fig. 11.7 Isochronal map during AT navigated by contact mapping (**a**), fluoroscopic image in the left anterior oblique view (**b**), and tracing during AT (**c**) in the same patient as in Fig. 11.6. *Asterisk*: pacing site at the high anterolateral right atrium (AL-RA) where the manifest entrainment was demonstrated (Manifest entrainment pacing site). The successful radiofrequency ablation (RF) site was located 15 mm lateral to the EAAS

entrainment. Figure 11.7 shows the locations of the EAAS, successful radiofrequency ablation site, and manifest entrainment pacing site in the same patient as shown in Fig. 11.6. Atrial activation appeared from the 5-o' clock position of the tricuspid annulus (i.e., EAAS; Fig. 11.7). Radiofrequency energy was delivered to the proximal portion of the EAAS in the direction of the high anterolateral RA from which the manifest entrainment was demonstrated. AT was terminated by the application of radiofrequency energy to a site 15 mm away from the EAAS (Fig. 11.7), suggesting that this site is located at the entrance of the slow conduction area of the reentry circuit. Figure 11.8 summarizes the location and the direction of the reentry circuit [16]. All tachycardia circuits were observed along the tricuspid annulus. The direction of the slow conduction area from the entrance (i.e., successful ablation site) to the exit (i.e., the EAAS) was clockwise in 13 patients and counterclockwise in the remaining ten patients (Fig. 11.8) [16].

Our study showed that the critical slow conduction area of the reentry circuit was located along the tricuspid annulus in all patients. Because verapamil and adenosine triphosphate were both effective in terminating the AT, a calcium channel-dependent tissue has been suggested to be involved in the reentry circuit [13, 15]. Indeed, cells with AV nodal or transitional-type action potentials have been shown to be present in the AV valve [17–19]. Anderson et al. also demonstrated AV node-like structures in normal adult hearts and suggested that they were remnants of specialized AV ring tissue [20]. These remnants were identified along the tricuspid annulus. More recently, McGuire et al. noted that a sleeve of AV nodal-type tissue, which responds to adenosine, was present around the tricuspid annulus [21, 22]. These

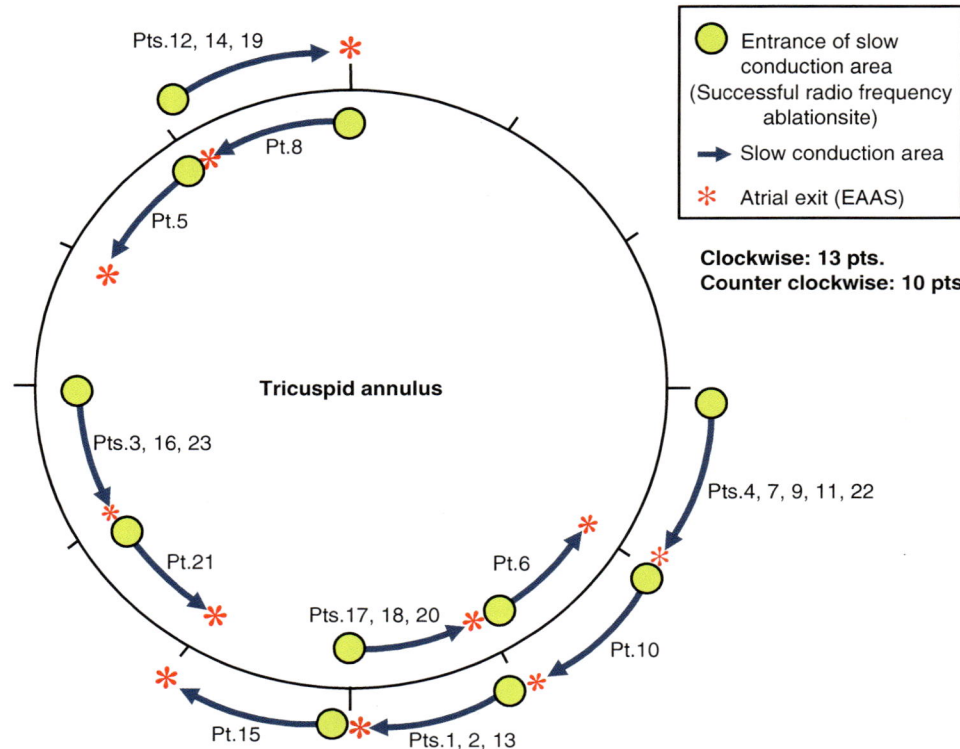

Fig. 11.8 Left anterior oblique view of the tricuspid annulus (TA) showing the location of atrial exit (*red asterisk*) and entrance of the slow conduction area (successful radiofrequency ablation site, *yellow circle*). *Blue arrow*, interposed between the entrance and exit of the AT, denotes the direction of wavefront propagation over the slow conduction area during tachycardia. *Pt* patient

histologic findings are consistent with the results of the present study and suggest the preferential location of a calcium channel-dependent slow conduction area of AT along the tricuspid annulus.

In the ATs originating from the vicinity of the AV node, we have demonstrated manifest entrainment and suggested that the underlying mechanism is due to small reentry involving a calcium channel-dependent slow conduction area [8]. We also showed that the distance from the entrance to the exit of the reentry circuit in verapamil-sensitive AT originating from the vicinity of the AV node was 10.1 ± 2.8 mm [8], which was comparable to the small dimension of the reentry circuit in the AT arising from the AV annulus other than the AV node vicinity (10.4 ± 2.4 mm). These findings suggest that verapamil-sensitive AT, which is organized as reentry, is distributed not only at the vicinity of the AV node but also along the AV annulus with similar electrophysiological features, indicating the presence of a much broader group of AT more appropriately classified as verapamil-sensitive AV annular reentrant AT.

References

1. Iesaka Y, Takahashi A, Goya M, Soejima Y, Okamoto Y, Fujiwara H, Aonuma K, Nogami A, Hiroe M, Marumo F, Hiraoka M. Adenosine-sensitive atrial reentrant tachycardia originating from the atrioventricular nodal transitional area. J Cardiovasc Electrophysiol. 1997;8:854–64.
2. Lai LP, Lin JL, Chen TF, Ko WC, Lien WP. Clinical, electrophysiological characteristics, and radiofrequency catheter ablation of atrial tachycardia near the apex of Koch's triangle. Pacing Clin Electrophysiol. 1998;21:367–74.
3. Frey B, Kreiner G, Gwechenberger M, Gössinger HD. Ablation of atrial tachycardia originating from the vicinity of the atrioventricular node: significance of mapping both sides of the interatrial septum. J Am Coll Cardiol. 2001;38:394–400.
4. Ouyang F, Ma J, Ho SY, Bansch D, Schmidt B, Ernst S, Kuck KH, Liu S, Huang H, Chen M, Chun J, Xia Y, Satomi K, Chu H, Zhang S, Antz M. Focal atrial tachycardia originating from the noncoronary aortic sinus: electrophysiological characteristics and catheter ablation. J Am Coll Cardiol. 2006;48:122–31.
5. Das S, Neuzil P, Albert CM, D'Avila A, Mansour M, Mela T, Ellinor PT, Singh J, Patton K, Ruskin JN, Reddy VY. Catheter ablation of peri-AV nodal atrial tachycardia from the noncoronary cusp of the aortic valve. J Cardiovasc Electrophysiol. 2008;19:231–7.
6. Marrouche NF, SippensGroenewegen A, Yang Y, Dibs S, Scheinman MM. Clinical and electrophysiologic characteristics of left septal atrial tachycardia. J Am Coll Cardiol. 2002;40:1133–9.
7. Yamabe H, Tanaka Y, Morihisa K, Uemura T, Enomoto K, Kawano H, Ogawa H. Analysis of the anatomical tachycardia circuit in verapamil-sensitive atrial tachycardia originating from the vicinity of the atrioventricular node. Circ Arrhythm Electrophysiol. 2010;3:54–62.
8. Yamabe H, Okumura K, Morihisa K, Koyama J, Kanazawa H, Hoshiyama T, Ogawa H. Demonstration of anatomical reentrant tachycardia circuit in verapamil-sensitive atrial tachycardia originating from the vicinity of the atrioventricular node. Heart Rhythm. 2012;9:1475–83.
9. Satoh M, Miyajima S, Koyama S, Ishiguro J, Okabe M. Orthodromic capture of the atrial electrogram during transient entrainment of atrioventricular nodal reentrant tachycardia. Circulation. 1993;88:2329–36.
10. Okumura K, Henthorn RW, Epstein AE, Plumb VJ, Waldo AL. Further observations on transient entrainment: importance of pacing site and properties of the components of the reentry circuit. Circulation. 1985;72:1293–307.

11. Tada H, Nogami A, Naito S, Suguta M, Nakatsugawa M, Horie Y, Tomita T, Hoshizaki H, Oshima S, Taniguchi K. Simple electrocardiographic criteria for identifying the site of origin of focal right atrial tachycardia. Pacing Clin Electrophysiol. 1998;21:2431–9.
12. Morton JB, Sanders P, Das A, Vohra JK, Sparks PB, Kalman JM. Focal atrial tachycardia arising from the tricuspid annulus: electrophysiologic and electrocardiographic characteristics. J Cardiovasc Electrophysiol. 2001;12:653–9.
13. Matsuoka K, Kasai A, Fujii E, Omichi C, Okubo S, Teramura S, Uchida F, Nakano T. Electrophysiological features of atrial tachycardia arising from the atrioventricular annulus. Pacing Clin Electrophysiol. 2002;25:440–5.
14. Iwai S, Markowitz SM, Stein KM, Mittal S, Slotwiner DJ, Das MK, Cohen JD, Hao SC, Lerman BB. Response to adenosine differentiates focal from macroreentrant atrial tachycardia: validation using three-dimensional electroanatomic mapping. Circulation. 2002;106:2793–9.
15. Yamabe H, Tanaka Y, Okumura K, Morikami Y, Kimura Y, Hokamura Y, Ogawa H. Electrophysiologic characteristics of verapamil-sensitive atrial tachycardia originating from the atrioventricular annulus. Am J Cardiol. 2005;95:1425–30.
16. Yamabe H, Okumura K, Koyama J, Kanazawa H, Hoshiyama T, Ogawa H. Demonstration of anatomic reentrant circuit in verapamil-sensitive atrial tachycardia originating from the atrioventricular annulus other than the vicinity of the atrioventricular node. Am J Cardiol. 2014;113:1822–8.
17. Paes de Carvalho A, de Almeida F. Spread of activity through the atrioventricular node. Circ Res. 1960;8:801–9.
18. Wit AL, Fenoglio JJ Jr, Wagner BM, Bassett AL. Electrophysiological properties of cardiac muscle in the anterior mitral valve leaflet and the adjacent atrium in the dog. Possible implications for the genesis of atrial dysrhythmias. Circ Res. 1973;32:731–45.
19. Wit AL, Fenoglio JJ Jr, Hordof AJ, Reemtsma K. Ultrastructure and transmembrane potentials of cardiac muscle in the human anterior mitral valve leaflet. Circulation. 1979;59:1284–92.
20. Anderson RH, Davies MJ, Becker AE. Atrioventricular ring specialized tissue in the normal heart. Eur J Cardiol. 1974;2:219e230.
21. McGuire MA, de Bakker JM, Vermeulen JT, Opthof T, Becker AE, Janse MJ. Origin and significance of double potentials near the atrioventricular node. Correlation of extracellular potentials, intracellular potentials, and histology. Circulation. 1994;89:2351–60.
22. McGuire MA, de Bakker JM, Vermeulen JT, Moorman AF, Loh P, Thibault B, Vermeulen JL, Becker AE, Janse MJ. Atrioventricular junctional tissue. Discrepancy between histological and electrophysiological characteristics. Circulation. 1996;94:571–7.

Focal Atrial Tachycardia

Kazuhiro Satomi

Keyword

Atrial tachycardia • Ablation • Abnormal automaticity • Triggered activity • Localized reentry

12.1 Introduction

Focal atrial tachycardia (AT) is defined as a supraventricular tachycardia with a P wave before the QRS, the so-called long RP tachycardia. AT accounts for 5–15% of adults with supraventricular tachycardias undergoing electrophysiological studies [1]. Recently, focal AT sometimes develops after atrial fibrillation (AF) ablation or from non-PV foci triggers of AF.

The activation pattern exhibits a centrifugal activation from a small area (focus or origin of tachycardia). The identification of the origin of focal AT is usually easy if the tachycardia is stably sustained. But mapping and ablation are sometimes difficult in non-sustained AT or multi-foci AT.

12.2 The Characteristics of Focal AT

Focal AT has three forms of mechanisms: abnormal automaticity, triggered activity, and micro (or localized) reentry. Although the precise definition of a particular AT may be difficult in clinical circumstances, understanding their basic principle can help with the therapeutic decisions.

The warm-up phenomenon is characterized as a progressively increasing cycle length at the onset of the tachycardia facilitated by adrenergic activity, and it is the typical form with abnormal automaticity. In abnormal automaticity, the tachycardia is also suppressed by over drive pacing.

Triggered activity is the mechanism involving cardiac cell after depolarizations and depends on the prior depolarization. This form of AT is induced by programmed stimulation, and commonly by constant pacing facilitated by catecholamines.

Micro (or localized) reentry also demonstrates a centrifugal activation pattern during the tachycardia. Instead of a point source, a small area (less than 2 cm) harbors the entire cycle length of the reentrant tachycardia in localized reentry. The electrical activity covering almost the entire cycle length of the tachycardia can be recorded by using multipolar catheters, such as the Pentaray (Biosense Webstar Inc., Irvine, CA, USA) or Afocus II (St Jude Medical Inc, Minnetonka, MN, USA). Localized reentry has been reported as an iatrogenic tachycardia after AF ablation. Recently, aggressive RF applications for AF, such as linear lesions or electrogram-guided ablation during AF, cause a conduction delay or conduction gap, resulting in localized reentry (Fig. 12.1).

Regardless of the mechanism of focal AT, the target of the ablation is the earliest activation site during the tachycardia. If the tachycardia is stable, the identification of the target site is not difficult. The most common sites of origin of autonomic tachycardias are along the crista terminalis, atrial appendage, triangle of Koch, pulmonary veins, and coronary sinus (CS). Mapping should be preferentially performed at the predominant area if the tachycardia is not sustained or hard to induce (it frequently occurs with abnormal automaticity).

K. Satomi, M.D., Ph.D.
Department of Cardiology, Tokyo Medical University,
6-7-1 Nishi-shinjuku, Shinjuku, Tokyo 160-0023, Japan
e-mail: ksatomi@tokyo-med.ac.jp

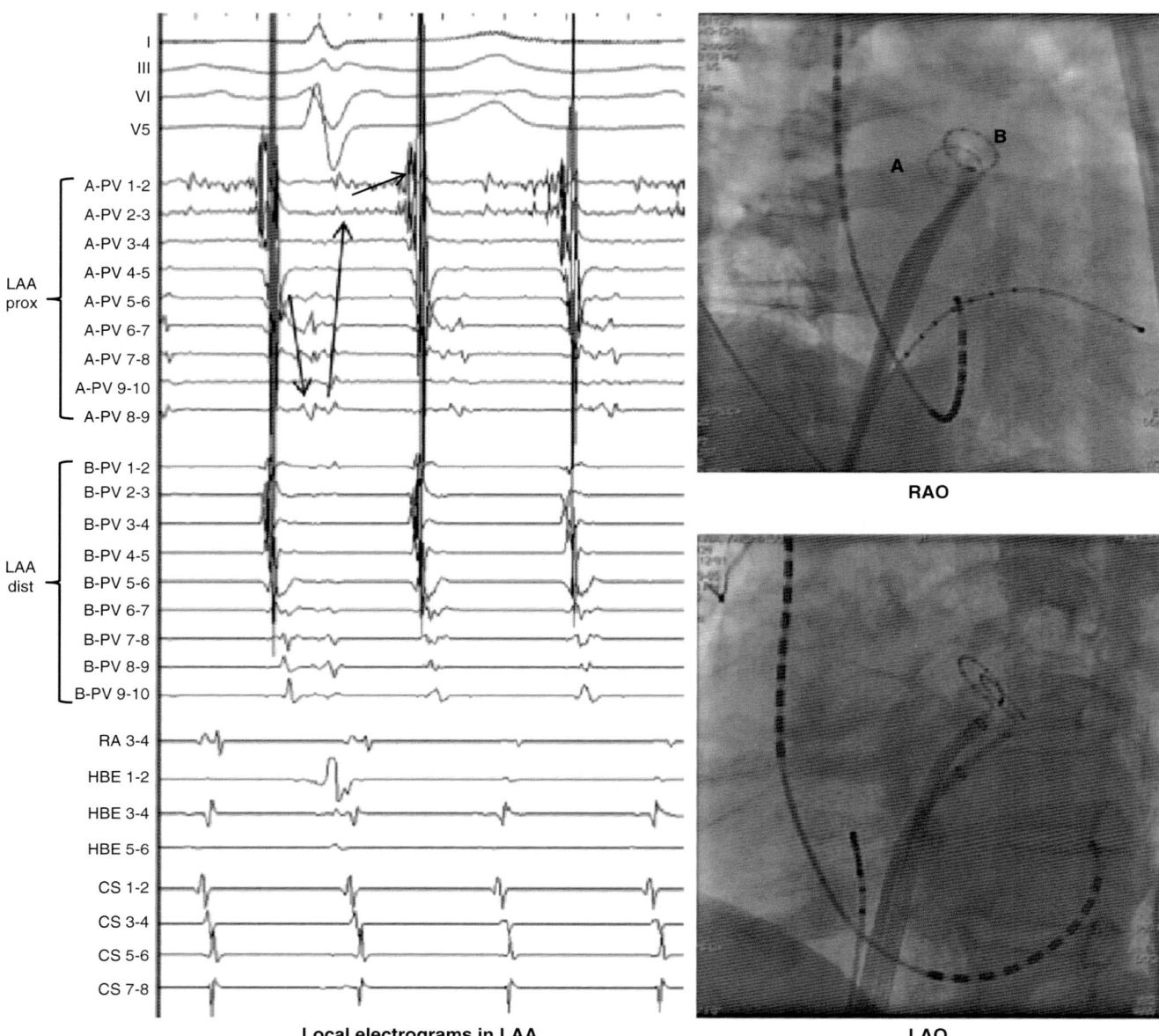

Fig. 12.1 Localized reentry. The *right panel* indicates the surface ECG and intracardiac electrogram during AT. The *left panel* shows the catheter location in RAO and LAO view of the fluoroscopy. Two circumferential catheters locate within proxysmal (LAA prox, A) and distal LAA (LAA dist, B). The electrical activity covers almost the entire cycle length of the tachycardia by the LAA prox (allows). *CS* coronary sinus, *RA* right atrium, *HBE* His electrogram

12.3 Patient Management Before the Ablation

12.3.1 Interrupted Anti-arrhythmic Drugs

The onset of focal AT with abnormal automaticity is related to autonomic nervous activation. The incidence and duration of the tachycardia exhibit a circadian and day-to-day variation. If the tachycardia becomes silent, the induction is sometimes difficult even by programmed stimulation in the catheter laboratory or by a catecholamine injection. Therefore, catheter ablation should be considered during the active phase of the tachycardia.

Anti-arrhythmic drugs, including beta-adrenergic antagonists, should be withdrawn at least 1 week before the ablation. If patients have a specific trigger of the tachycardia, such as alcohol consumption or a lack of sleep, similar loads of those triggers can be asked of the patients the day before the ablation. For the same reason, it is better to avoid sedation during the procedure for at least the start of the procedure.

12.3.2 Interpretation of an AT Focus by the ECG

The P wave configuration analyzed by the 12 lead ECG during AT provides important information to localize the location of the AT origin (Table 12.1). Leads aVL and V1 are most useful to distinguish between LA and RA origins. Positive or biphasic P waves in aVL predict a right atrial focus with a sensitivity of 88% and specificity of 79%. A positive P wave in lead V1 predicts a left atrial focus with a sensitivity of 100% [2, 3]. Leads II, III, and aVF may help differentiate a superior (positive P wave) from an inferior focus (negative P wave). Hachiya et al. reported that negative or flat P waves in V1 indicate a focal AT from the LA septum or anterior mitral annulus (MA). The initial negative deflection in lead V1 may be caused by the relatively anterior position of both the MA and septum [4]. A narrow P wave compared to sinus rhythm (SR) is also useful to suggest a septal origin of the AT. The simultaneous activation of both atria causes a narrow P wave compared to that during SR. In exceptional cases, positive P waves in lead V1 and negative P waves in leads II, III, and aVL are related origins from the ostium of the CS and even from the RA. This type of P wave is also observed during the fast-slow type of atrioventricular node reentrant tachycardia.

Aggressive RF applications such as linear lesions in the LA and CFAE ablation, MAZE operations, and congenital heart diseases make it more difficult to predict the focal origin due to conduction delays in the atrium and the complicated atrial activation. In most cases, the P wave cannot be clearly observed during the AT due to the overlap of the P wave with the QRS. Ventricular stimulation or ventricular extrastimulation is useful to unmask the P waves (Fig. 12.2).

12.4 Practical Approach to Catheter Ablation

12.4.1 AT Induction

The catheters are generally located in the HRA, His, and CS. With abnormal automaticity, programmed stimulation, such as

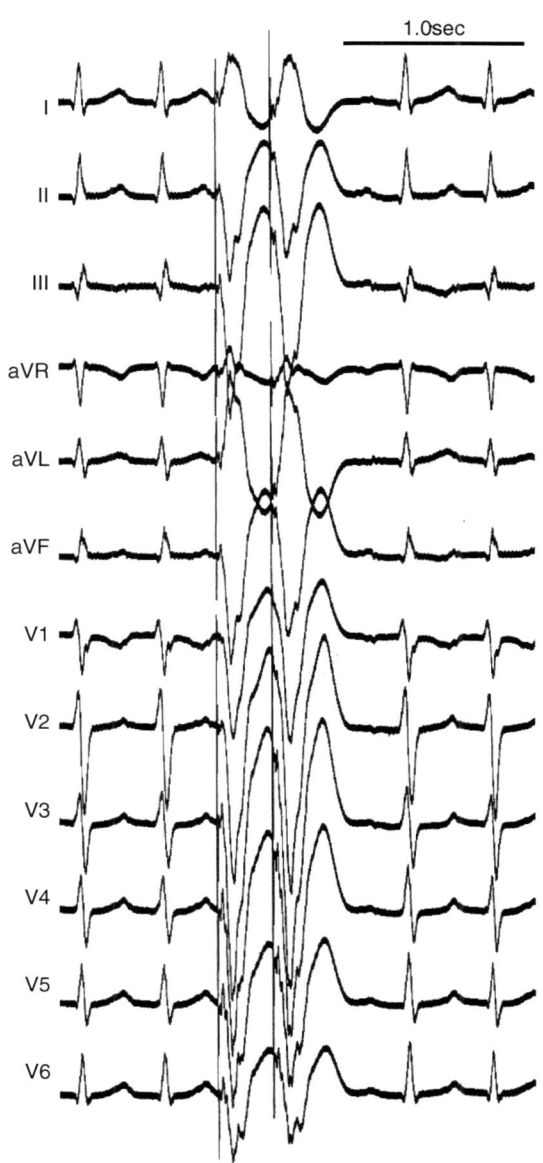

Fig. 12.2 Twelve-lead ECG showing the P-wave morphology during an atrial tachycardia. The P wave was unmasked from the ventricular repolarization during the tachycardia by ventricular extrastimuli

Table 12.1 P wave morphology during focal atrial tachycardia

Site of origin	ECG lead											
	I	II	III	aVR	aVL	aVF	V1	V2	V3	V4	V5	V6
Superior CT	+	+	+	−	+	+	−	−	−	−	−	−
Inferior CT	+	−	−	−	+	−	−	−	−	−	−	−
RAA	+	+	+	−	iso	+	−	−	−	−	−	iso,−,+
Peri-nodal	+	−	−	+	+	−	−/+, iso	−	−	−	−	−
CSOS	iso,+	−	−	+	+	−	−/+, +	−/+,−	−	−	−	−
CS dis	−, iso	−	−	+	+/−,+/iso	−	+	+	+,−	−	−	−
RSPV	+	+	+	−	+	+	+	+	+	+	+	+
LSPV	−, iso	+	+	−	−	+	+	+	+	+	+	+
LAA	−	+	+	iso, −	−	+	+	+	+	+	+	+

CS coronary sinus *CT* crista terminalis, *LAA* left atrial appendage, *LSPV* left superior pulmonary vein, *RAA* right atrial appendage, *RSPV* right superior pulmonary vein, *iso* isoelectric

extrastimulation or burst pacing, are usually not effective for inducing tachycardias. If pacing cannot induce the tachycardia, drug administration is subsequently performed. An isoproterenol injection is administered for sympathetic stimulation and neostigmine for cholinergic stimulation. Ephedrine is an α-agonist and increases the blood pressure resulting in the stimulation of baroreceptors followed by parasympathetic stimulation as a negative feedback. Additionally, some ATs are observed during the "washout phase" of isoproterenol. The handgrip test also is useful for AT related to sympathetic stimulation.

Once the tachycardia is induced, the atrial refractory period shortens, then the tachycardia will be easily induced. After AF is induced by aggressive burst pacing and terminated by cardioversion, spontaneous AT can subsequently be induced.

12.4.2 The Efficacy of Multipolar Catheters and the Ensite Array

The reentrant circuit or origin of the AT has the potential risk of changing during mapping due to catheter manipulation, stimulation during entrainment, or the RF application. The 3D mapping systems such as CARTO (Biosense Webstar Inc.), Ensite (St Jude Medical Inc.), and Rhythmia (Boston scientific Inc., Marlborough, MA, USA) are useful to visually identify the AT focus, especially during stable sustained ATs. A misdiagnosis of the AT focus can occur by missing a change in the AT activation sequence during the 3D mapping. Multi-electrode catheters should be placed and careful observation is necessary to identify any sudden change in the activation sequence.

The Ensite Array (St. Jude Medical Inc.) has the advantage of being able to locate the origin of non-sustained ATs or premature atrial complexes (PACs). This device can analyze the focus and activation sequence with only a single extra beat. The accuracy of the location information depends on the distance from the catheter to the endocardial mapping area. Therefore, the array should be located as close as possible to the AT focus. Simultaneous mapping in both atria is impossible with this system. The prediction of the AT focus before ablation by the ECG is quite important to deploy the Ensite Array into the appropriate site (Fig. 12.3).

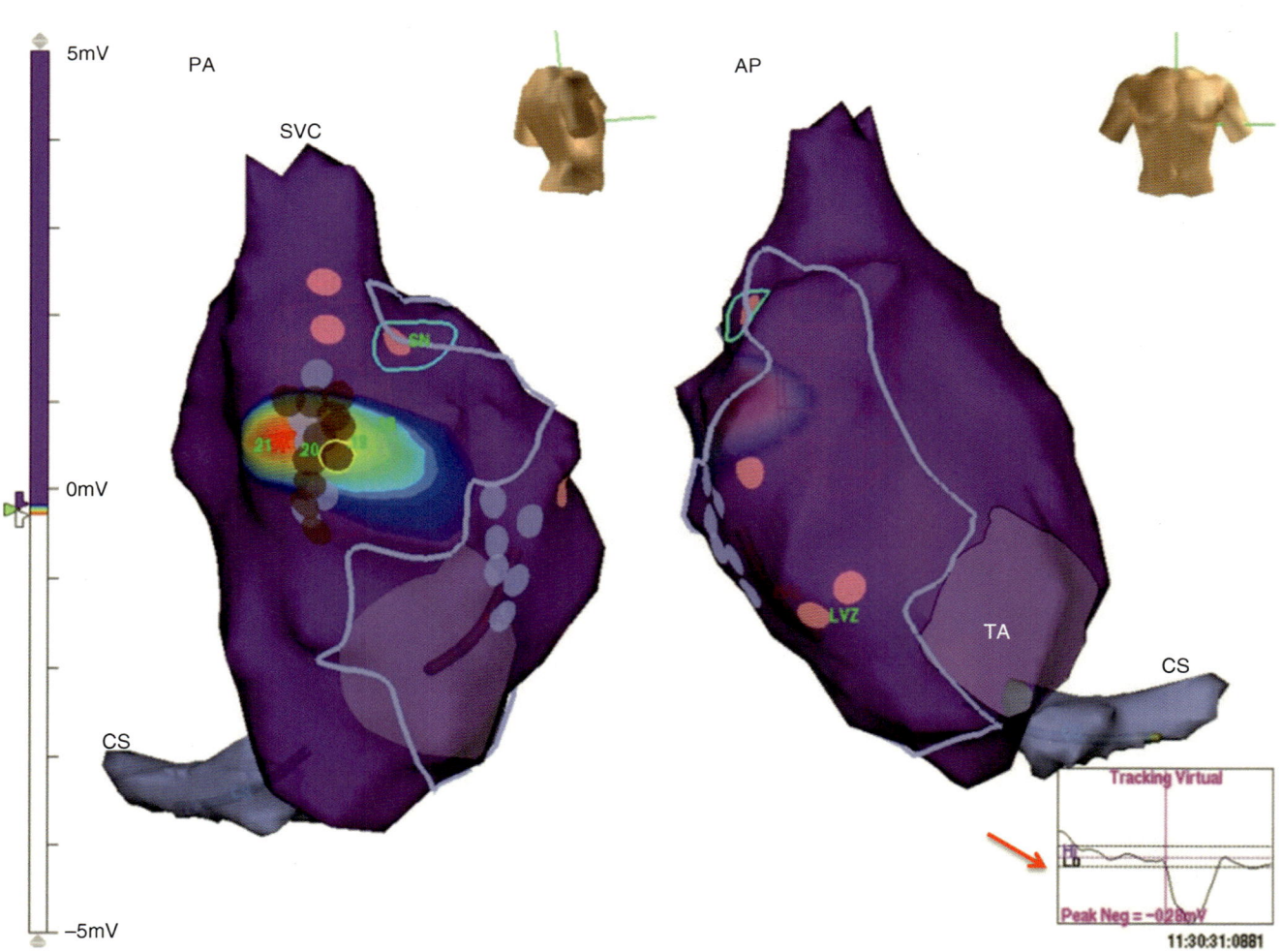

Fig. 12.3 Activation mapping during an AT demonstrated by the Ensite array. The figures show the activation map of the RA during the AT in the PA and AP views. The earliest activation site is demonstrated in the RA mid-posterior wall, indicated by a red color, and propagating with a centrifugal pattern. The virtual unipolar electrogram, "Tracking Virtual" indicates the QS pattern at the earliest activation site. *AP* anterior posterior view, *CS* coronary sinus, *PA* posterior anterior view, *RA* right atrium, *SVC* superior vena cava, *TA* tricuspid annulus

12.4.3 The Ideal Local Potential for a Successful Ablation

The 3D mapping system shows the centrifugal activation pattern during focal ATs, but is not specific for a successful ablation. The earliest activation site demonstrates a relatively wide area in the 3D mapping system. Careful consideration of the local potentials is required to decide the optimal ablation site. The initial deflection of the bipolar electrograms is the onset of the activation of the local area. The earliest local activation time is compared to the onset of the P wave. The sites with a local activation ranging from 20 to 60 ms prior to the P wave onset are targeted for ablation. Often, the electrograms at the earliest site will be fractionated. The distal unipolar electrogram exhibiting the earliest rapid negative QS deflection identifies the site of the impulse formation (Fig. 12.4).

12.4.4 Pace Map and Activation Sequence Mapping

If AT is not sustained or is difficult to induce, pace mapping or paced activation sequence mapping can be useful. The paced P wave morphology is then compared with the P wave during the tachycardia. This technique has the limitation of requiring clear P waves on the 12 lead ECG undisturbed by the QRS or T wave. If one of the origins, pacing at that site should demonstrate a similar activation pattern to that recorded in the right and left atria during the tachycardia (Fig. 12.5).

12.5 Ablation

Once mapping identifies the optimal site, 25–30 W of radiofrequency energy are delivered for 30–60 s. Irrigated tip catheters are useful for ATs arising from the appendage with

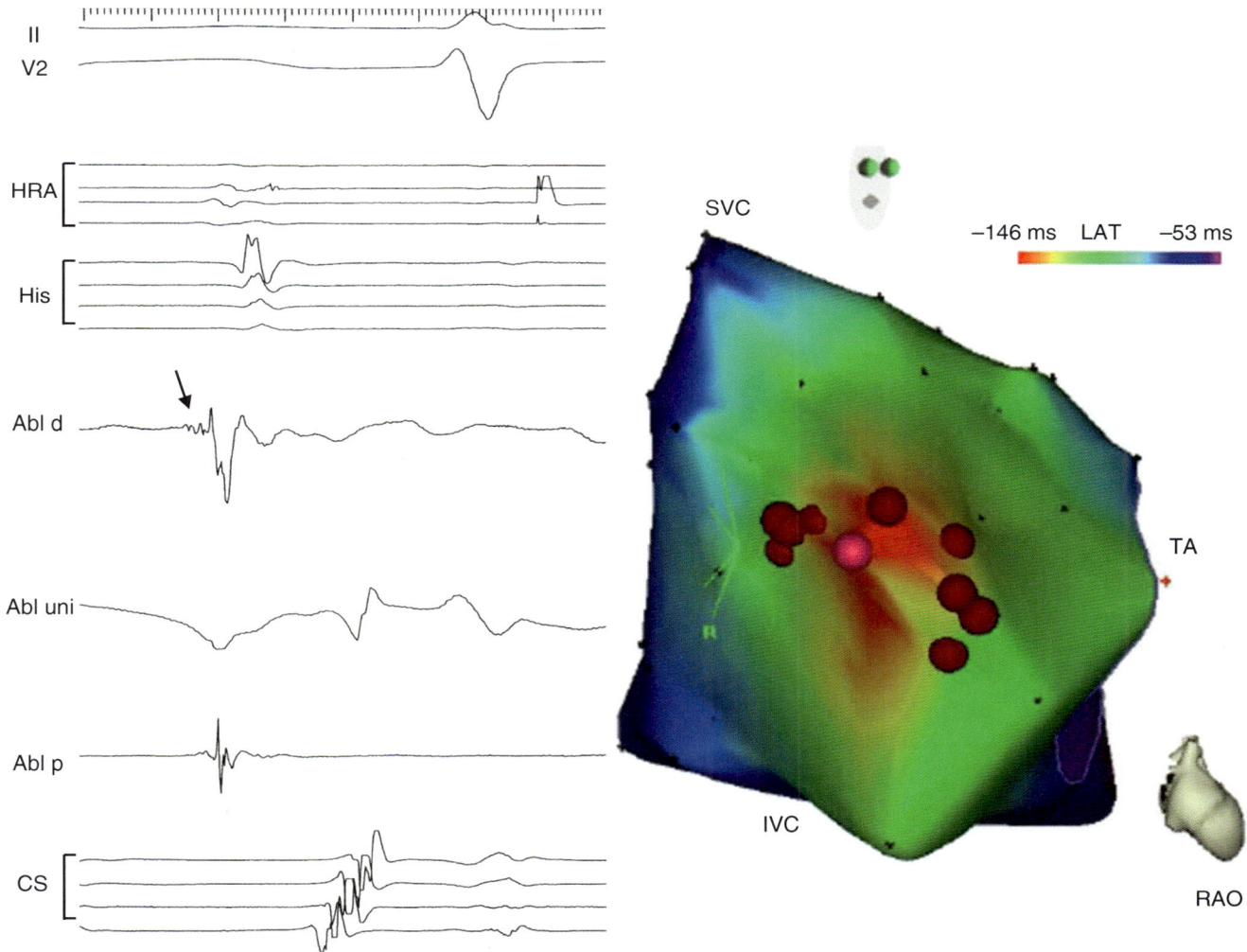

Fig. 12.4 The local electrogram is the focus of AT. The left figure shows the body surface ECG and intracardiac electrode during AT. The allow indicates the local electrogram at the earliest activation site with fractionated electrogram. The right figure is the activation map by Electroanatomical map during AT, indicating that the earliest site is RA free wall. Abl d: Ablation distal, Abl p Ablation proxsymal, CS: Coronary Sinus, HRA: high right atrium, IVC: inferior vena cava, SVC: superior vena cava, TA tricuspid annulus

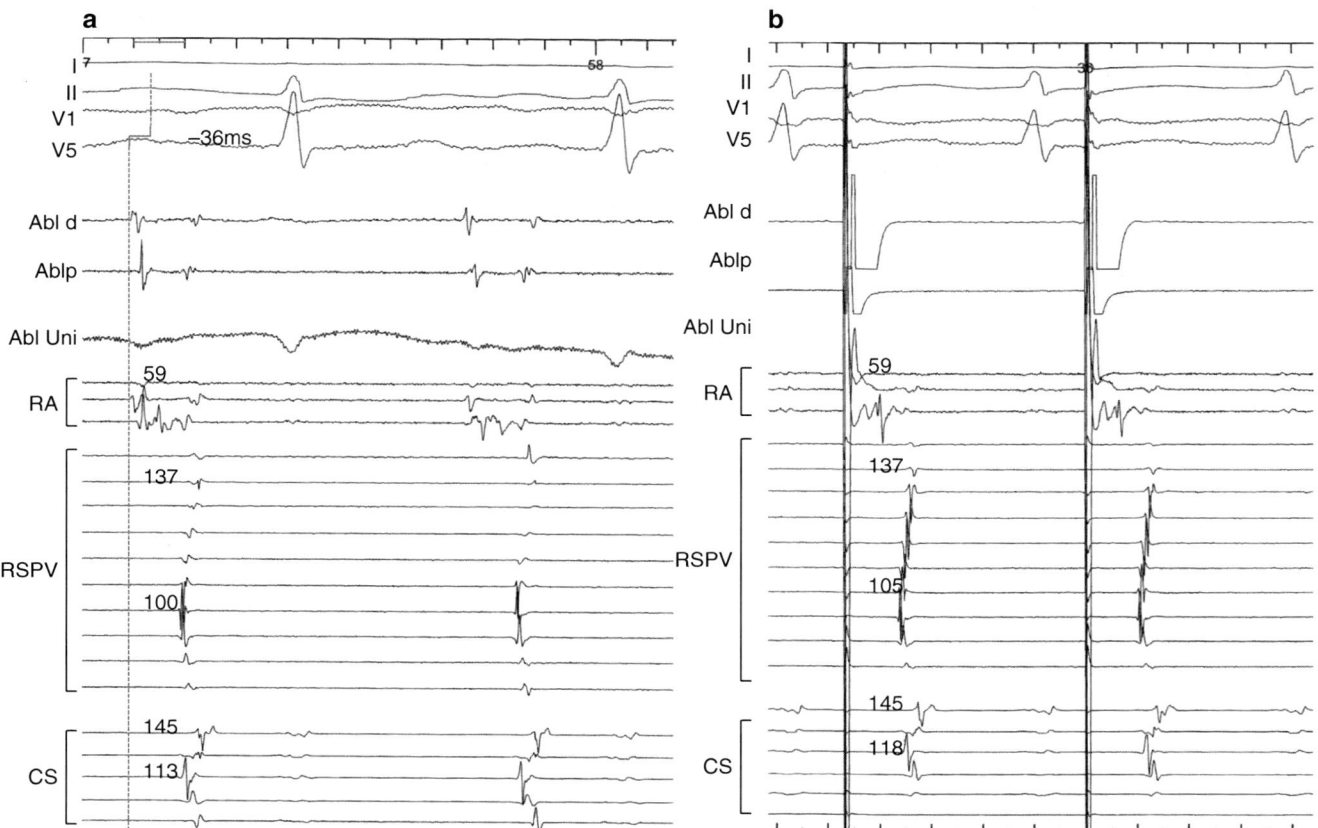

Fig. 12.5 The activation sequence mapping. The figures showed intracardiac recording of the earliest activation site during AT (**a**) and constant pacing at the same place (**b**). The activation times compared to the onset of P wave were shown in several leads. The activation time of each electrogram is similar between AT and pacing, indicating that this site is the focus of AT. *CS* coronary sinus, *RA* right atrium, *RSPV* right superior pulmonary vein

thick tissue and low blood flow. The contact force sensor is also useful for achieving an adequate lesion formation and preventing a perforation of the myocardial wall.

Focal AT has a quick response to the RF application even at remote areas around the earliest activation site, but will easily be recurrent. Bonus applications around the termination site should be related to a better outcome. The catheter stability at the atrioventricular annulus is unstable, and long sheaths or deflectable sheaths provide an effective RF application.

Mechanical bump is defined as the termination of a tachycardia due to catheter manipulation. The induction of an AT is sometimes difficult after mechanical bump and causes recurrence after the session. Careful manipulation of the catheter is required in the area around the earliest activation site.

Acceleration of the tachycardia before termination and termination within 10 s suggest a successful ablation site. A successful ablation is verified by the non-inducibility of the AT. If isoproterenol is necessary for the induction prior to the ablation, it should be used again during the re-induction attempts to confirm the success.

Catheter ablation of focal AT has been reported to have success rates between 77% and 100% [5]. Therefore, ablation is indicated for all symptomatic patients who have symptoms despite medical therapy.

12.6 Complications

A specific complication during focal AT ablation is injury to the sinus node or AV node. The surrounding tissue of the sinus node or AV node is the predominant area for focal AT. Before ablation, an accurate localization of the sinus node or HIS electrogram recording site should be performed during SR. The location tags using the 3D map may be useful to recognize the SN or AVN during ablation. The long sheath or deflectable sheath is quite powerful tool to stabilize the ablation catheter for avoid injury of sinus node or AV node. Intravenous isoproterenol administration sometimes is performed for the induction of AT, but the continuous use of isoproterenol causes a hyper-contraction of the ventricles and a worse stability of the ablation catheter. Before the ablation, titration of the isoproterenol should be considered.

References

1. Roberts-Thomson KC, Kistler PM, Kalman JM. Focal atrial tachycardia I: clinical features, diagnosis, mechanisms, and anatomic location. Pacing Clin Electrophysiol. 2006;29(6):643–52.
2. Tang CW, Scheinman MM, Van Hare GF, Epstein LM, Fitzpatrick AP, Lee RJ, et al. Use of P wave configuration during atrial tachycardia to predict site of origin. J Am Coll Cardiol. 1995;26(5):1315–24.
3. Kistler PM, Roberts-Thomson KC, Haqqani HM, Fynn SP, Singarayar S, Vohra JK, et al. P-wave morphology in focal atrial tachycardia: development of an algorithm to predict the anatomic site of origin. J Am Coll Cardiol. 2006;48(5):1010–7.
4. Hachiya H, Ernst S, Ouyang F, Mavrakis H, Chun J, Bänsch D, et al. Topographic distribution of focal left atrial tachycardias defined by electrocardiographic and electrophysiological data. Circ J. 2005;69(2):205–10.
5. Badhwar N, Lee B, Scheinman M, Olgin J. Mapping of focal right atrial and coronary sinus tachycardia. In: Shenasa M, Hindricks G, Borggrefe M, Breithardt G, Josephson M, editors. Cardiac mapping. 4th ed. West Sussex: Wiley-Blackwell; 2013. p. 367–79.

Catheter Ablation of Atrial Tachycardia Following Catheter and Surgical Ablation of Atrial Fibrillation

Hiroshi Nakagawa and Warren M. Jackman

Keywords

Catheter ablation • Atrial fibrillation • Atrial tachycardia • Surgical ablation

13.1 Introduction

Atrial tachycardia (AT) occurs frequently during and after catheter or surgical ablation of atrial fibrillation (AF) [1–15]. The mechanism of AT may be focal (automaticity or microreentry) or macroreentry (Fig. 13.1) [1, 4–7, 9, 13, 15], and differentiation of the AT mechanism is critical for successful ablation. For a focal AT, ablation should be targeted at the site of earliest atrial activation. In contrast, for a macroreentrant AT, atrial activation exhibits a continuous pattern and there is no earliest or latest activation. Therefore, ablation should be targeted at an isolated narrow arrhythmogenic channel located between two scars (Fig. 13.1), or if an isolated channel cannot be identified, by linear ablation between two anatomical barriers.

Complex arrhythmogenic substrates for these ATs are produced by areas of fibrosis (scar) and conduction block resulting from underlying disease and injury from prior catheter or surgical ablation of AF. The intracardiac electrograms in the scared myocardium exhibit low amplitude potentials with multiple components or fractionated electrograms, requiring great care (or sophisticated algorithms) in assigning the correct activation time ("annotation") to accurately identify the circuit and a successful ablation target in these patients [9, 16].

Macroreentrant AT occurs in patients with dilated, severely scared right or left atria. Macroreentrant AT may be identified either by overdrive pacing to test for entrainment or by electroanatomical mapping. However, limitations of entrainment pacing for mapping include: (1) in patients with extensive previous ablation, local conduction delay and block may produce artificially long post-pacing intervals, masking the circuit location; (2) localizing circuits by entrainment pacing leads to the use of a long linear ablation lesion (such as across the mitral isthmus, i.e., "mitral isthmus line" or across the left atrial roof between the right and left superior pulmonary veins, i.e., "roof line"), rather than locating a narrow arrhythmogenic channel between scars, which is easier to ablate and may have better long-term success; (3) failure of pacing capture may occur at sites within the arrhythmogenic channel, incorrectly suggesting dense scar and losing an optimal ablation site; and (4) pacing for entrainment may terminate the AT or change it to another AT.

When using electroanatomical mapping, macroreentrant AT is defined by the recording of continuous atrial activation ("head meets tail") with a total activation time equal to the tachycardia cycle length [9, 16]. The substrate for macroreentrant AT is a large heterogeneous atrial scar with surviving myocardial bundles bounded by two or more dense scars, forming protected conduction channels ("arrhythmogenic channels"). During electroanatomical mapping (recorded during AT, sinus rhythm, or atrial pacing), the heterogeneous atrial scar is manifested by a large area of low bipolar voltage (≤ 0.5 mV). The dense scars are identified as areas without a recordable atrial potential (usually ≤ 0.02–0.03 mV), dissociated atrial potentials, or as lines of double atrial potentials signifying conduction block. The reentrant impulse propagates through one or more of the arrhythmogenic channels between dense scars, and depending on the size of the circuit, may remain confined to the heterogeneous

H. Nakagawa, M.D., Ph.D. (✉) • W.M. Jackman, M.D.
Heart Rhythm Institute and Department of Medicine,
University of Oklahoma Health Sciences Center, 1200 Everett
Drive (TUH-6E-103), Oklahoma City, OK 73104, USA
e-mail: hiroshi-nakagawa@ouhsc.edu

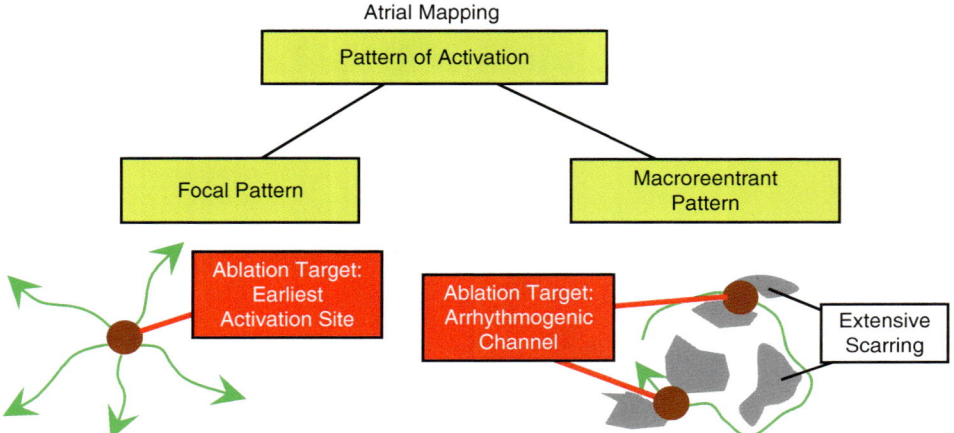

Fig. 13.1 The mechanism of atrial tachycardia (AT) based on atrial activation patterns. For a focal AT, atrial activation exhibits a centrifugal pattern and ablation should be targeted at the site of earliest atrial activation. Macroreentrant AT exhibits a continuous activation (head meets tail) and the total activation time is equal to the tachycardia cycle length. The substrate for macroreentrant AT is a large heterogeneous atrial scar with surviving myocardial bundles bounded by two or more dense scars, forming protected conduction channels ("arrhythmogenic channels"). The optimal ablation approach for macroreentry is to identify the narrow arrhythmogenic channel providing the critical component of the macroreentrant circuit and create a short linear lesion across the channel

scar (often in small macroreentrant circuits (2–3 cm in diameter) or may include relatively normal atrial myocardium in larger circuits [9, 16]).

13.2 Macroreentrant Left Atrial Tachycardia Following Catheter Ablation of Atrial Fibrillation

Macroreentrant left AT often results from arrhythmogenic channels created by catheter ablation of AF. During AF ablation, AF can organize into a stable AT or AT may become inducible after (when it was not inducible before) isolation of the pulmonary vein (PV) ostia in approximately 10% of patients [4]. These patients generally have other scars in the left atrium which contribute to the arrhythmogenic channels. Some of these macroreentrant left AT have a very short cycle length (160–200 ms), mimicking AF [9].

Most of the recent AF ablation approaches extend the ablation lesions posteriorly outside the PV ostia (to include much of the PV antrum), and some approaches for persistent AF include the addition of left atrial linear lesions [17–21]. The inducibility of macroreentrant AT may increase (up to 20–30%) with these approaches for two reasons [1–5, 9]. First, the larger areas of conduction block produced by PV antrum isolation facilitates reentry around the PVs and/or the mitral annulus. Second, the absence of complete conduction block in either the PV isolation lesions or linear lesions create narrow arrhythmogenic channels, which may support smaller and more complex macroreentrant circuits.

The pulmonary veins (PVs) provide anatomical obstacles in the left atrium, frequently supporting macroreentry with a large single loop propagating around either the left PVs, right PVs, or mitral annulus (Fig. 13.2). For ablation, a relatively long linear lesion is required between the isolated right and left PVs (or PV antra) and between the isolated PVs and the mitral annulus, if there is not a narrow channel between scars.

For reentry around the left PVs (Fig 13.3a), the linear lesion is usually created: (1) between the isolated left PVs and isolated right PVs (roof line); and (2) between the isolated left inferior PV and the mitral annulus (an area referred to as the "mitral isthmus") or along the anterior wall between the isolated left superior PV and mitral annulus, septal to the left atrial appendage. The greatest difficulty is creating complete conduction block near the mitral annulus due to conduction over the coronary sinus (CS) myocardium which is connected to the left atrium on both sides of the ablation line. Ablation within the CS is often required to achieve complete conduction block (Fig 13.3b). However, ablation within the CS is associated with a small risk of injury to the left circumflex coronary artery [22]. Placing the ablation line more superiorly within the mitral isthmus may reduce the likelihood of CS myocardium close to the mitral annulus, but this region of the mitral isthmus usually has greater voltage (thicker pectinate atrial myocardium) which often correlates with greater difficulty producing transmural lesions. Complete conduction block along the mitral isthmus can be

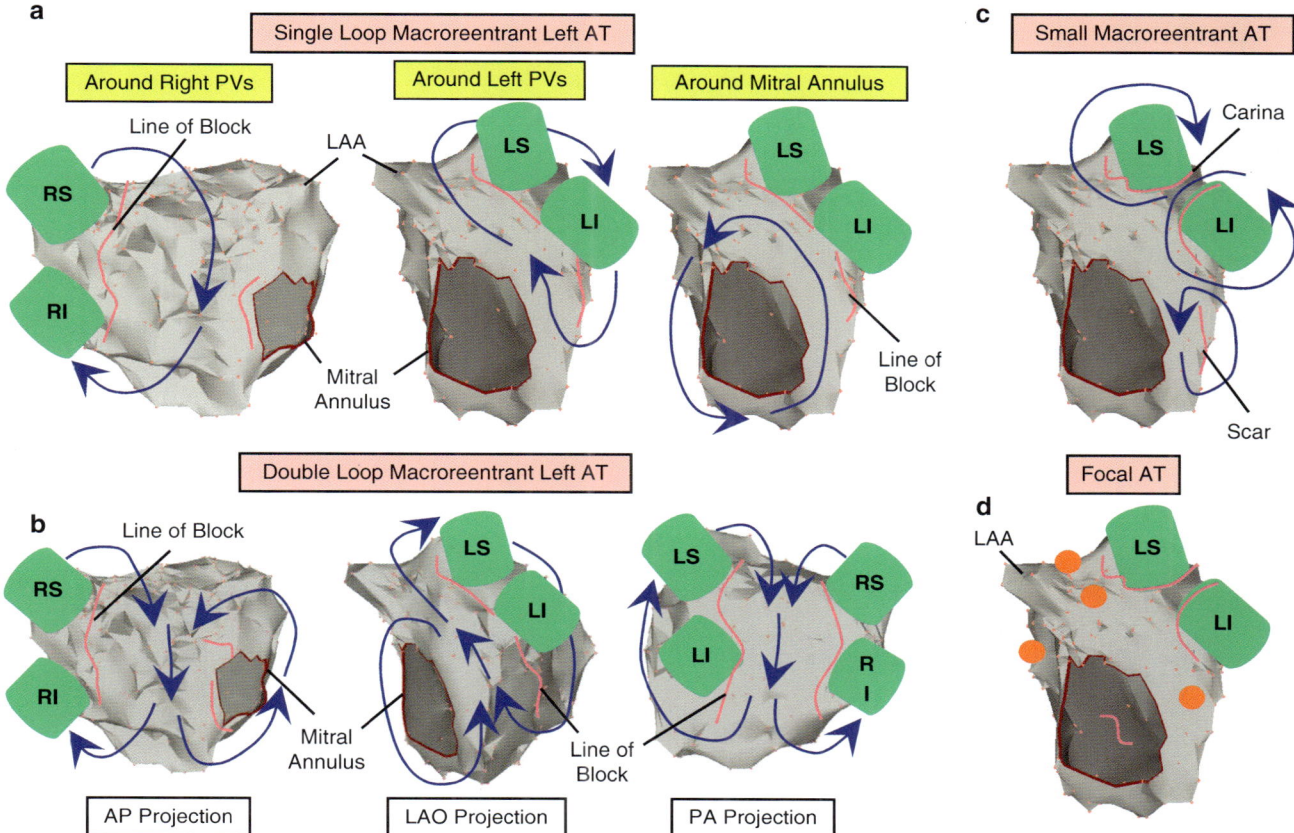

Fig. 13.2 Schematic representation of the location of the macroreentrant circuits and focal ATs. Single-loop large macroreentrant circuits (*blue arrows*) are represented in panel (**a**) and double-loop circuits (*blue arrows*) are represented in panel (**b**). (**c**) Small complex reentrant circuits, such as propagating through the "carina" (between the superior and inferior PVs) and around one PV, and reentry around a short linear lesion. (**d**) Common sites for focal left ATs (*orange tags*) after AF ablation are located at the region anterior to the right superior PV (not shown), the roof of the left atrium close to the superior base of the left atrial appendage, along the left atrial appendage ridge, and along the region of Marshall tract between the left inferior PV and the mitral annulus

verified during the distal CS pacing or pacing within the left atrial appendage by identifying a widely separated double atrial potentials along the ablation line and the reversed activation sequence within the CS (CS myocardium is activated from the proximal to the distal portions).

For reentry around the right PVs, the linear lesion between the isolated right and left PVs (Fig. 13.4) or between the isolated right PVs and the mitral annulus (anterior line) can be created. The anterior line is sometimes difficult to create complete conduction block due to the relatively long length and thick left atrial myocardium close to Bachmann's bundle. Another limitation in creating this ablation line is the difficulty in maneuvering an ablation catheter close to the transeptal site. After ablation, complete conduction block across the roof line or between the right PVs and mitral annulus can be confirmed by a repeat left atrial map during the left atrial appendage (LAA) pacing (Fig. 13.5).

For reentry around the mitral annulus, either of the linear lesions described above between the left or right PVs and the mitral annulus (mitral isthmus or anterior line) can be used. Selection of the location of the ablation line is based on the presence of a short isolated channel or on shorter length, lower voltage, location of the CS myocardium, and ease of catheter manipulation in that region.

Double-loop reentry is also common in patients after AF ablation. Reentrant circuits are located around the right or left PVs and around the mitral annulus or around the right PVs and around the left PVs (Figs 13.2b and Fig. 13.5). For double-loop reentry around the mitral annulus and either the right PVs or left PVs, a linear lesion between the isolated PVs forming one of the circuits and the mitral annulus elimi-

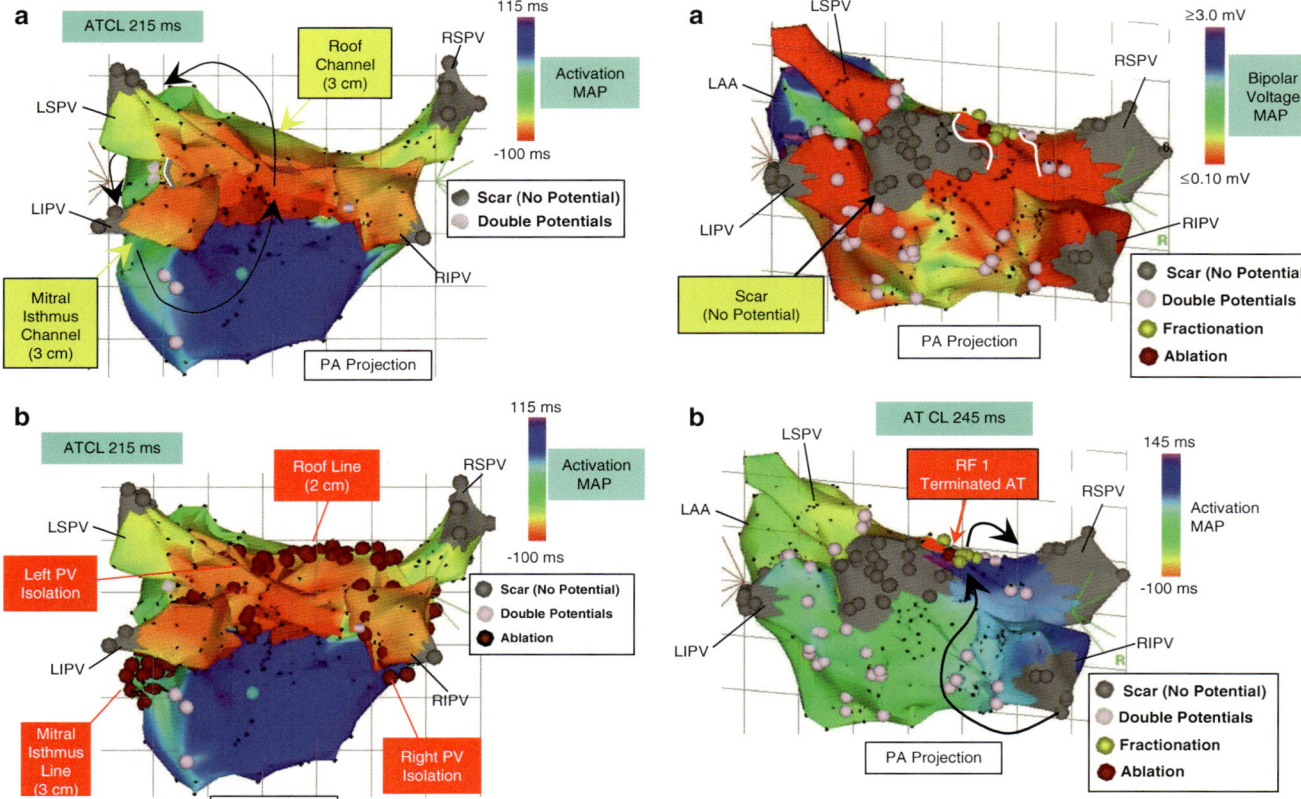

Fig. 13.3 Single-loop macroreentrant AT in a 50-year-old woman with paroxysmal AF (no previous AF ablation). (**a**). Before ablation, AF organized into a stable AT. High-density (413 mapped points) activation map during AT (cycle length ATCL-215 ms) in the posterior-anterior (PA) projection was obtained using a magnetic catheter maneuvering system (CARTO-RMT, Biosense Webster, Inc. and Epoch, Stereotaxis, Inc.) with a mapping time of 38 minutes and fluoroscopy time of only 3 sec, demonstrating a large macroreentrant circuit around the left PVs. Sites exhibiting double atrial potentials are marked by *pink tags* and sites with no potentials (scar) are marked by *gray tags*. (**b**). Spontaneous PV firing from the left superior PV disorganized the AT to AF, and then AF was terminated. Isolation of all four PVs was performed, follow by linear ablation across the mitral isthmus (3 cm in length) between the isolated LIPV and the mitral annulus (including ablation within the CS) and the roof between the isolated left superior PV (LSPV) and the isolated right superior PV (RSPV, 2 cm in length). After ablation, programmed atrial stimulation failed to induce either AT or AF

Fig. 13.4 Incessant single-loop macroreentrant AT in a 63-year-old man, 3 years following a catheter ablation procedure for AF, including PV antrum isolation and ablation of complex fractionated atrial potential (CFAE). (**a**). Bipolar voltage map (PA projection) during incessant AT showing markedly low voltage (red, <0.10 mV) with dense scars (no atrial potentials, *gray tags*), double atrial potentials (*pink tags*) and fractionated atrial potentials (*olive tags*) in the large areas surrounding the PVs and between the right and left PVs. PV potentials were recorded in all four PVs, indicating incomplete PV isolation. (**b**). High-density activation map (581 mapped points) in the PA projection during AT (cycle length CL 245 ms) obtained using a magnetic catheter maneuvering system (CARTO-RMT, Biosense Webster, Inc. and Epoch, Stereotaxis, Inc.) with 45 min mapping time and 2 sec fluoroscopy time, demonstrating a single-loop macroreentrant circuit around the right PVs (*black arrows*), propagating through a narrow channel (1.0 cm in width) located at the roof between the dense scar at the LSPV antrum and a line of block (double potentials) at the RSPV antrum. A single RF application within the narrow channel terminated the tachycardia

nates both circuits of the macroreentrant left AT (Fig. 13.5). For double-loop reentry around the right PVs and around the left PVs, a linear lesion between the isolated right PVs and left PVs will eliminate this tachycardia (Fig. 13.6). The choice between a superior location for the ablation line (connecting the right and left superior PVs) or an inferior/posterior location (connecting the right and left inferior PVs) is based on the presence of a short isolated channel or based on shorter length, lower voltage, and location of the esophagus (to reduce the risk of a left atrial-esophageal fistula, Fig. 13.6) [9]. Creating transmural necrosis is generally easier on the posterior wall (thinner wall thickness) than the anterior or superior left atrium. Using a 3.5 mm saline irrigated electrode, transmural necrosis in the posterior wall, identified by electrogram attenuation and development of double atrial potentials, is often achieved using RF power of ≤35 Watts. We generally limit RF power to 20–25 W (and ablation time) at sites close to the esophagus, while monitoring esophageal temperature.

Linear ablation between the isolated right and left PVs may facilitate macroreentry around the mitral annulus. Similarly, linear ablation between the mitral annulus and either the isolated right or left PVs may facilitate macroreen-

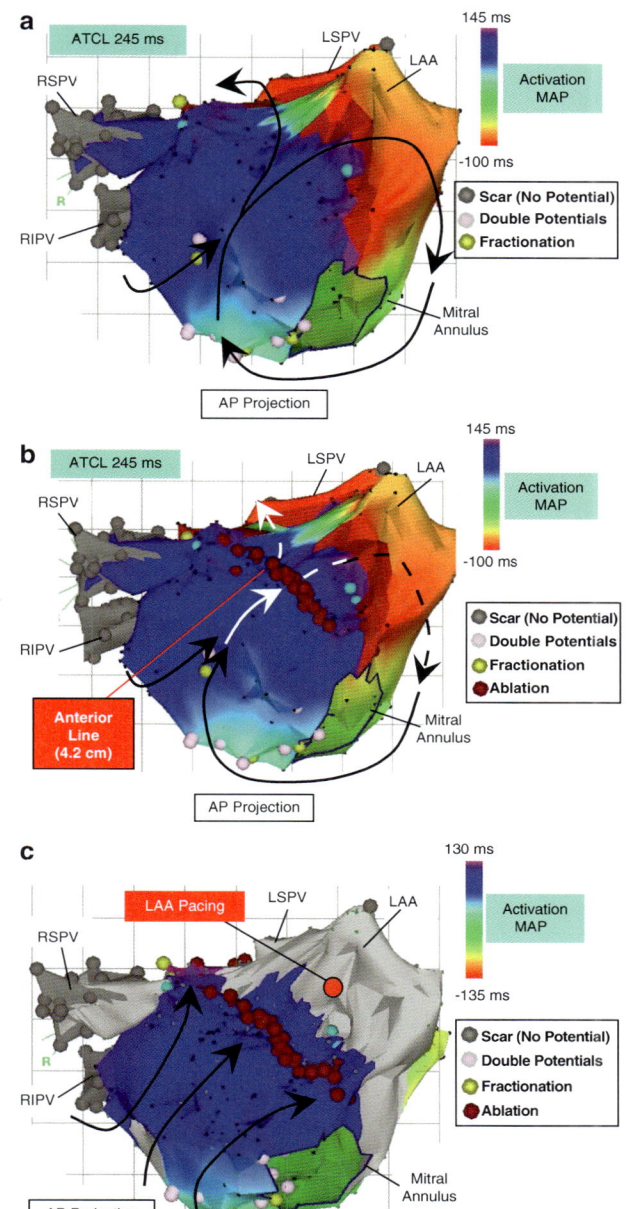

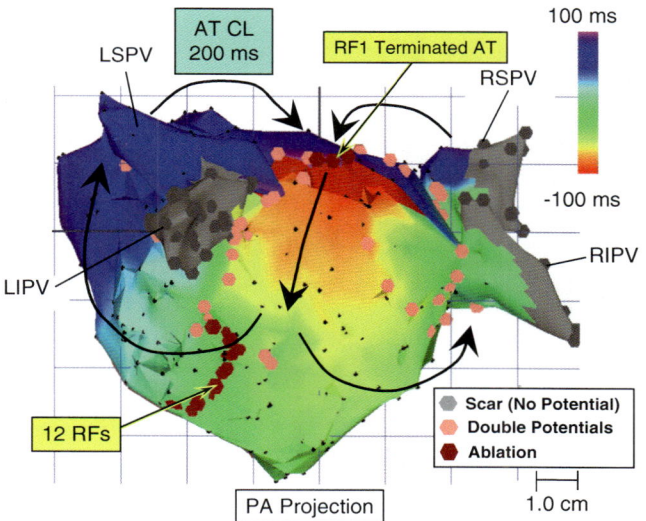

Fig. 13.6 Double-loop macroreentrant left AT in a 47-year-old man following two catheter ablation procedures for AF (PV isolation and roof line). Activation map in the PA projection demonstrating double-loop reentry (cycle length 200 ms) with macroreentrant circuits around the left PVs in the clockwise direction and around the right PVs in the counterclockwise directions (*bold black arrows*). Note the small, isolated channel in the prior roof line (gap in the line of double potentials marked by *pink tags*) between the right and left PVs. A single RF application was delivered in the center of the isolated channel, terminating the tachycardia. Six additional RF applications were delivered across the roof channel to ensure complete conduction block. Programmed atrial stimulation then induced two unmappable ATs. Another ablation line was created during CS pacing between the mitral annulus and a line of double atrial potentials extending inferiorly from the isolated LIPV using 12 RF applications (12 RFs), resulting in complete conduction block across the mitral isthmus. PV potentials were recorded in the RSPV, RIPV, and LSPV, and these three PVs were re-isolated

Fig. 13.5 Double-loop macroreentrant left atrial tachycardia with a wide common arrhythmogenic channel in a 63-old-year man following three catheter ablation procedures for AF, including PV antrum isolation and linear ablation along the left atrial roof. (**a**) Activation map in the anterior-posterior (AP) projection demonstrating double-loop macroreentrant AT (CL 245 ms) with reentry around the mitral annulus in the clockwise direction and around the right PVs in the counterclockwise direction. (**b**) A long linear ablation (4.2 cm in length) along an anterior line between the RSPV and the mitral annulus was created using a magnetic catheter maneuvering system terminated the AT. (**c**) Repeat activation map obtained following ablation during pacing from the left atrial appendage (LAA) at the cycle length of 600 ms. Activation below the ablation line is occurring in the septal-to-lateral direction with latest activation (purple area, 210 ms after the LAA pacing stimulus) approaching the ablation line, confirming complete conduction block across the ablation line. Additional ablation was also performed to produce complete conduction block along the roof line. Programmed atrial stimulation then failed to induce any form of AT

try around the left or right PVs, respectively. Therefore, the creation of two linear ablation lines may be recommended (between the right and left PVs and between the mitral annulus and the right or left PVs, Fig 13.3b and Fig. 13.6).

Smaller and complex macroreentrant circuits may not be eliminated by the empiric use of the two linear ablation lines described above. Conduction through the "carina" between the superior and inferior PVs often provides the arrhythmogenic channel for a small macroreentrant circuit (reentry around one PV, Fig. 13.7). Complete PV antrum isolation may prevent many of the small macroreentrant circuits. The small macroreentrant circuits involving the PV boundaries appear to occur more frequently when the criterion for successful circumferential ablation is a reduction in voltage within the ablated region rather than validating complete PV antrum isolation by the absence of potentials or the presence of dissociated atrial/PV potentials (Fig. 13.7) [3, 23]. Other small macroreentrant circuits may be located either around lesions for ablation of complex atrial fractionated electrograms (CFAE) or ablation of ganglionated plexi (GP) or between these lesions and PV isolation lesions or other anatomical obstacles [24].

13.3 Focal Atrial Tachycardia Following Catheter Ablation of Atrial Fibrillation

Focal AT also occurs following AF ablation. The most common sites for a focal AT are the region anterior to the right superior PV, the roof of the left atrium close to the superior base of the left atrial appendage, along the ridge between the appendage and left PVs, and along the region of Marshall tract between the left inferior PV and the mitral annulus [9]. These sites are located close to autonomic ganglinated plexi (GP), i.e., the anterior right GP, superior left GP and Marshall Tract GP, respectively, and therefore receive heavy autonomic innervation [25, 26]. Focal AT also occurs in the right atrium following AF ablation. The most common sites are along the crista terminalis, at the base of right atrial appendage, and the posterolateral right atrium, as well as within the superior vena cava (also heavily innervated areas) [25, 26].

We obtain a high-density left or right atrial map during a stable tachycardia because of the possibility of a focal atrial tachycardia or a small complex macroreentrant circuit. These two forms of tachycardia would not be expected to be eliminated by an empiric ablation line between the right PVs and left PVs or between the mitral annulus and either the right or left PVs.

13.4 Macroreentrant Left Atrial Tachycardia Following Surgical Ablation of Atrial Fibrillation

Macroreentrant left AT also occurs in patients following surgical ablation of AF. Unlike patients with macroreentrant left AT following catheter ablation, the posterior left atrial wall and PVs are usually isolated following the original Cox Maze operation using cut and sew techniques (Fig. 13.8) [27, 28]. Macroreentry most commonly propagates around the mitral annulus due to recovery of the surgical cryo-thermia lesions over the CS to complete the line to the mitral annulus [27, 28]. We prefer to use high-density electroanatomical mapping, as a small complex macroreentrant circuit may be present and an empiric ablation line between the isolated area (posterior wall and PVs) and the mitral annulus will fail to eliminate the tachycardia (Fig. 13.8). After surgical abla-

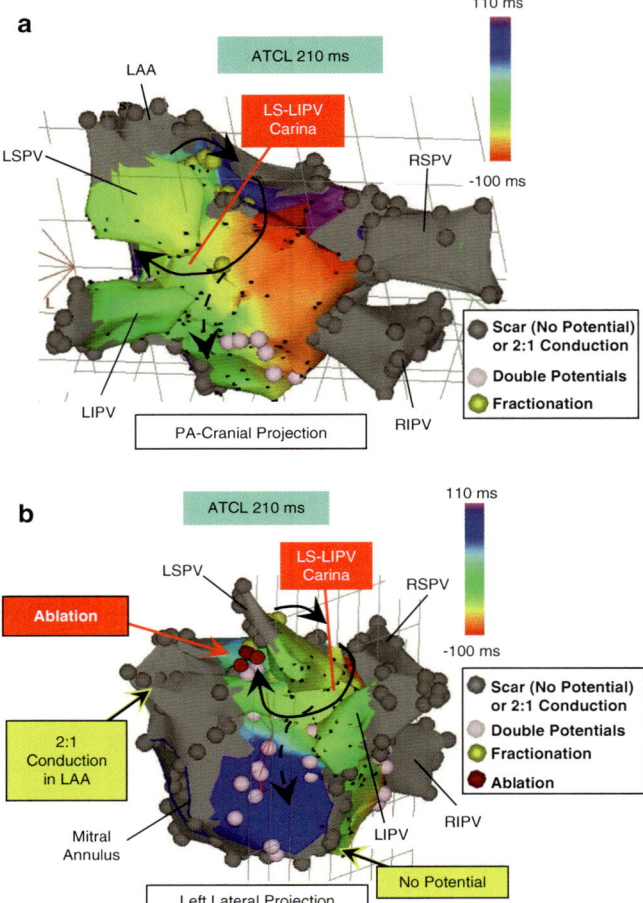

Fig. 13.7 Incessant small macroreentrant left AT in a 59-year-old man 9 months following the second catheter ablation procedure for AF. The first procedure was PV antrum isolation and the second procedure was CFAE ablation and a linear ablation across the mitral isthmus. Activation map during AT (cycle length, CL 210 ms) in the PA cranial projection (panel **a**) and in the left lateral projection (panel **b**), demonstrating a small circuit propagating through the carina between the LSPV and LIPV and around the LSPV (*bold black arrows*). During tachycardia, 2:1 conduction was observed in the left atrial appendage (shown in *gray*) and no atrial potential between the LIPV and the mitral annulus (*gray tags*), presumably resulting from the previous ablation procedures. A single RF application within the narrow channel between the isolated left atrial appendage and the LSPV terminated the AT. PV isolation was also performed for the reconnected LSPV and LIPV. After ablation, programmed atrial stimulation failed to induce AT or AF

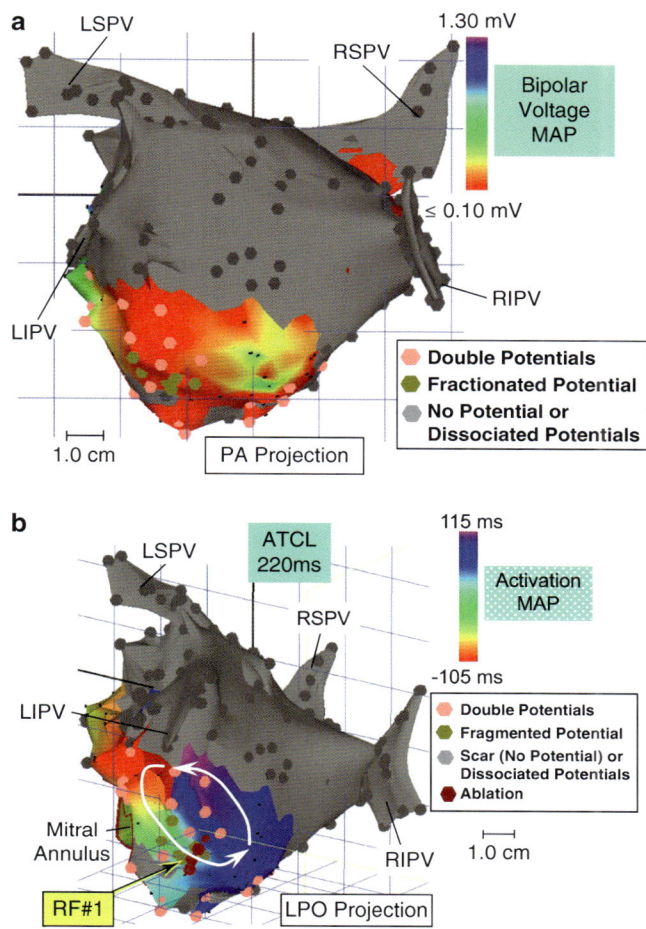

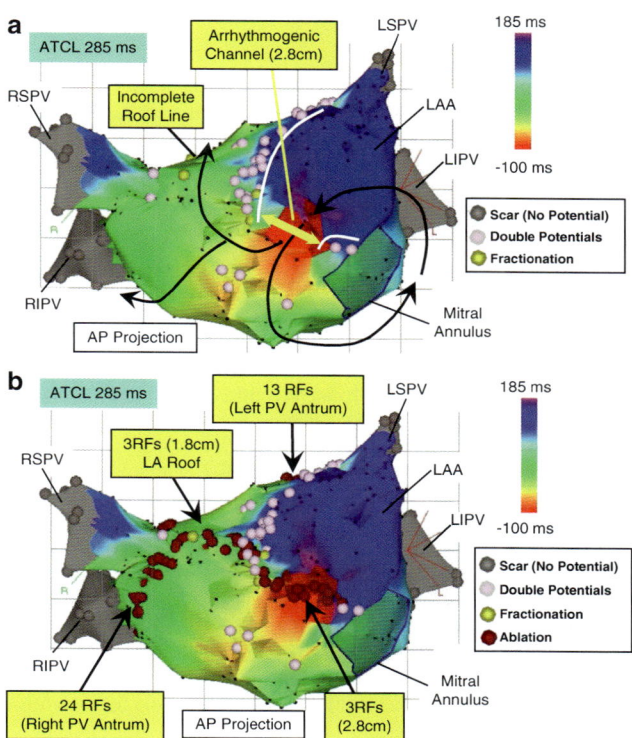

Fig. 13.8 Incessant small macroreentrant left AT in a 59-year-old man 11 months following surgical ablation of AF (Cox Maze III) and 7 months following an unsuccessful attempt at catheter ablation of the AT using two empiric linear left atrial lesions between the LIPV and mitral annulus (mitral isthmus line) and between the RSPV and mitral annulus. (**a**) Bipolar voltage map during incessant AT (cycle length 220 ms) in the PA projection, showing no potentials or dissociated potentials (*gray tags*) in all four PVs and the posterior left atrium surrounding the PVs. The remaining left atrium exhibited markedly low voltage (*red*, <0.10 mV) with double atrial potentials (*pink tags*) and fractionated atrial potentials (*olive tags*). (**b**) High-density activation map (left posterior oblique, LPO projection) within the markedly low voltage area inferior to the left inferior PV (LIPV) identified a small macroreentrant circuit propagating around a line of double potentials (*white arrows* around *pink tags*). The AT was terminated by the first RF application (RF#1) delivered within the narrow channel (1.5 cm in width, voltage only 0.05 mV) between the line of double potentials and a small scar adjacent to the mitral annulus. Three additional RF applications were delivered, producing complete conduction block cross the channel

Fig. 13.9 Incessant macroreentrant left AT in a 59-year-old man 7 months following surgical ablation of AF using a surgical bipolar RF clamp for PV isolation and a RF "pen" probe for linear lesions along the roof between the RSPV and the LSPV and an anterior line between the roof line to the mitral annulus. (**a**) Activation map (AP projection) during AT (cycle length 285 ms), demonstrating a macroreentrant circuit around the mitral annulus in the counterclockwise direction with an arrhythmogenic channel (2.8 cm in width) formed by a gap in the anterior line (*yellow allow* between the *pink tags*). (**b**) Three RF applications across the channel terminated the tachycardia. Three RF applications were required to close a gap (1.8 cm in width) in the roof line (LA Roof). Twenty-four RF applications around the right PV antrum and 13 RF applications around the left PV antrum were required to isolate all 4 PVs. Programmed atrial stimulation then failed to induce any AT or AF

tion of AF using bipolar RF clamps for PV isolation or linear lesions produced by surgical epicardial ablation (RF or cryothermia), reconnection of PV activity and conduction gaps along the linear lesions may support macroreentrant ATs (Fig. 13.9) [29–32].

Conflicts of Interest H. Nakagawa and W.M. Jackman are consultants for Biosense Webster, Inc.

References

1. Gerstenfeld EP, Callans DJ, Dixit S, et al. Mechanisms of organized left atrial tachycardias occurring after pulmonary vein isolation. Circulation. 2004;110:1351–7.
2. Mesas CE, Pappone C, Lang CC, et al. Left atrial tachycardia after circumferential pulmonary vein ablation for atrial fibrillation: electroanatomic characterization and treatment. J Am Coll Cardiol. 2004;44:1071–9.
3. Pappone C, Manguso F, Vicedomini G, et al. Prevention of iatrogenic atrial tachycardia after ablation of atrial fibrillation: a prospective randomized study comparing circumferential pulmonary vein ablation with a modified approach. Circulation. 2004;110:3036–42.
4. Chugh A, Oral H, Lemola K, Hall B, et al. Prevalence, mechanisms, and clinical significance of macroreentrant atrial tachycardia during and following left atrial ablation for atrial fibrillation. Heart Rhythm. 2005;2:464–71.
5. Gerstenfeld EP, Callans DJ, Sauer W, et al. Reentrant and nonreentrant focal left atrial tachycardias occur after pulmonary vein isolation. Heart Rhythm. 2005;2:1195–202.
6. Haissaguerre M, Hocini M, Sanders P, et al. Catheter ablation of long-lasting persistent atrial fibrillation: clinical outcome and mechanisms of subsequent arrhythmias. J Cardiovasc Electrophysiol. 2005;16:1138–47.
7. Chae S, Oral H, Good E, et al. Atrial tachycardia after circumferential pulmonary vein ablation of atrial fibrillation: mechanistic insights, results of catheter ablation, and risk factors for recurrence. J Am Coll Cardiol. 2007;50:1781–7.
8. Gerstenfeld EP, Dixit S, Bala R, et al. Surface electrocardiogram characteristics of atrial tachycardias occurring after pulmonary vein isolation. Heart Rhythm. 2007;4:1136–43.
9. Nakagawa H, Jackman WM, Yokoyama K, et al. Catheter ablation of macro- reentrant right and left atrial tachycardias. In: Wilber DJ, Packer DL, Stevenson WG, editors. Catheter ablation of cardiac arrhythmias: basic concepts and clinical applications. 3rd ed. Carlton, VIC: Blackwell Futura; 2008. p. 192–217.
10. Veenhuyzen GD, Knecht S, O'Neill MD, et al. Atrial tachycardias encountered during and after catheter ablation for atrial fibrillation. Pacing Clin Electrophysiol. 2009;32:393–8.
11. Steven D, Seiler J, Roberts-Thomson KC, et al. Mapping of atrial tachycardias after catheter ablation for atrial fibrillation: use of bi-atrial activation patterns to facilitate recognition of origin. Heart Rhythm. 2010;7:664–72.
12. Rostock T, Drewitz I, Steven D, et al. Characterization, mapping, and catheter ablation of recurrent atrial tachycardias after stepwise ablation of long-lasting persistent atrial fibrillation. Circ Arrhythm Electrophysiol. 2010;3:160–9.
13. Sawhney N, Anousheh R, Chen W, Feld GK. Circumferential pulmonary vein ablation with additional linear ablation results in an increased incidence of left atrial flutter compared with segmental pulmonary vein isolation as an initial approach to ablation of paroxysmal atrial fibrillation. Circ Arrhythm Electrophysiol. 2010;3:243–8.
14. Pascale P, Shah AJ, Roten L, et al. Pattern and timing of the coronary sinus activation to guide rapid diagnosis of atrial tachycardia after atrial fibrillation ablation. Circ Arrhythm Electrophysiol. 2013;6:481–90.
15. Barbhaiya CR, Kumar S, Ng J, Tedrow U, Koplan B, John R, Epstein LM, Stevenson WG, Michaud GF. Overdrive pacing from downstream sites on multielectrode catheters to rapidly detect fusion and to diagnose macroreentrant atrial arrhythmias. Circulation. 2014;129:2503–10.
16. Nakagawa H, Shah N, Matsudaira K, et al. Characterization of reentrant circuit in macroreentrant right atrial tachycardia after surgical repair of congenital heart disease: isolated channels between dense scars allow "focal" ablation. Circulation. 2001;103:699–709.
17. Jais P, Hocini M, Hsu L, et al. Technique and results of linear ablation at the mitral isthmus. Circulation. 2004;110:2996–3002.
18. Hocini M, Jais P, Sanders P, et al. Techniques, evaluation, and consequences of linear block at the left atrial roof in paroxysmal atrial fibrillation. Circulation. 2005;112:3688–96.
19. Knecht S, Hocini M, Wright M, et al. Left atrial linear lesions are required for successful treatment of persistent atrial fibrillation. Eur Heart J. 2008;29:2359–66.
20. Ouyang F, Ernst S, Vogtmann T, et al. Characterization of reentrant circuits in left atrial macroreentrant tachycardia: critical isthmus block can present atrial tachycardia recurrence. Circulation. 2002;105:1934–42.
21. Sawhney N, Anand K, Robertson CE, et al. Recovery of mitral isthmus conduction leads to the development of macro-reentrant tachycardia after left atrial linear ablation for atrial fibrillation. Circ Arrhythm Electrophysiol. 2011;4:832–7.
22. Takahashi Y, Jais P, Hocini M, et al. Acute occlusion of the left circumflex coronary artery during mitral isthmus linear ablation. J Cardiovasc Electrophysiol. 2005;16:1–4.
23. Pappone C, Oreto G, Rosanio S, et al. Atrial electroanatomic remodeling after circumferential radiofrequency pulmonary vein ablation: efficacy of an anatomic approach in a large cohort of patients with atrial fibrillation. Circulation. 2001;103:2539–44.
24. Nademanee K, McKenzie J, Kosar E, et al. A new approach for catheter ablation of atrial fibrillation: mapping of the electrophysiologic substrate. J Am Coll Cardiol. 2004;43:2044–53.
25. Nakagawa H, Scherlag BJ, Patterson E, et al. Pathophysiologic basis of autonomic ganglionated plexi ablation in patients with atrial fibrillation. Heart Rhythm. 2009;6:S26–34.
26. Stavrakis S, Nakagawa H, Po SS, et al. The role of the autonomic ganglia in atrial fibrillation. J Am Coll Cardiol. 2015;1-2:1–13.
27. Cox JL, Schuessler RB, D'Agostino HJ Jr, et al. The surgical treatment of atrial fibrillation. III. Development of a definitive surgical procedure. J Thorac Cardiovasc Surg. 1991;101:569–83.
28. Cox JL, Ad N. The importance of cryoablation of the coronary sinus during the maze procedure. Semin Thorac Cardiovasc Surg. 2000;12:20–4.
29. Edgerton JR, Jackman WM, Mack MJ. Minimally invasive pulmonary vein isolation and partial automatic denervation for surgical treatment of atrial fibrillation. J Interv Card Electrophysiol. 2007;20:89–93.
30. Lockwood D, Nakagawa H, Peyton MD, et al. Linear left atrial lesions in minimally invasive surgical ablation of persistent atrial fibrillation: techniques for assessing conduction block across surgical lesions. Heart Rhythm. 2009;6:S50–63.
31. Gaynor SL, Diodato MD, Prasad SM, et al. A prospective, single-center clinical trial of modified Cox maze procedure with bipolar radiofrequency ablation. J Thorac Cardiovasc Surg. 2004;128:535–42.
32. Edgerton JR, Jackman WM, Mack MJ. A new epicardial lesion set for minimal access left atrial maze: the Dallas lesion set. Ann Thorac Surg. 2009;88:1655–7.

Part V

Catheter Ablation of Atrial Fibrillation

Pulmonary Vein Isolation: Radiofrequency Energy

14

Teiichi Yamane

Keywords
Atrial fibrillation • PV isolation • Radiofrequency • Adenosine

14.1 Introductory Remarks

It is well accepted that atrial fibrillation (AF) requires both a trigger and a substrate that maintains AF. Several attempts of linear ablation in the right or left atrium using radiofrequency energy (RF) in the 1990s were unsuccessful due to the lack of ablation at the triggers. The historical observation that AF is frequently triggered by ectopic, rapidly firing atrial foci located predominantly in the pulmonary veins (PVs) amounted to a paradigm shift in the ablative treatment of AF [1]. Although the initial ablation target was the focal trigger itself in the PV, the limitation and dangers of this strategy were quickly noted: high recurrence rates due to multiple PV triggers and a high incidence of PV stenosis [2].

The most commonly employed ablation strategy today is the electrical isolation of the PVs by ablating the PV antrum around the right and left PV ostia, which can influence both the trigger and substrate of AF [3]. Mounting evidence suggests that PVs play critical roles not only as triggers but also as perpetuators of AF, partly due to the microreentry localized at the PV-left atrium (LA) junction [4]. In contrast to the traditional "random reentry hypothesis" of AF in the whole atrium, a "venous wave hypothesis" has been proposed as a more practical mechanism of AF occurrence and perpetuation [5].

14.2 Definition of PV Isolation

The term "PV isolation" has been used to describe the electrical isolation of the PV myocardium from the adjacent LA. Its current wide acceptance and popularity are based on the demonstration of a pathophysiological mechanism and a clear-cut endpoint under sinus rhythm. Although the electrical isolation of the PVs can be assessed in a variety of ways with various tools, the most commonly employed method involves a circular mapping catheter (CMC) [6]. A CMC can be deployed to the ostium/antrum of the PV to record the local potential of the PV muscles. PV isolation is an electrophysiological endpoint defined as the stable absence of any conduction into the PVs from the LA (entrance block) as well as in the opposite direction from the PV to the LA, confirmed using pacing techniques in the PV (exit block) [7].

In the mid-2000s, discussions were held concerning the necessity of PV isolation. Some authors reported the importance of the electrical isolation of PVs from the left atrium [6], while others showed sufficient efficacy of RF around the PV, even when PV-LA conduction persisted [7]. Mounting evidence that most recurrences of AF following ablation were derived from the reconduction of isolated PVs [8] has underscored the principal importance of the electrical isolation of PVs as a cornerstone of AF ablation [3].

14.3 Circumferential and Segmental PV Isolation

Historically, PV isolation started with the segmental isolation of individual PV ostia from the LA using a CMC [6]. However, over the past decade, the methodology used to achieve PV isolation has evolved from an electrophysiologically guided

T. Yamane, M.D., Ph.D., F.H.R.S.
Division of Cardiology, Department of Internal Medicine,
The Jikei University School of Medicine, 3-25-8 Nishi-shinbashi,
Minato-ku, Tokyo 105-8461, Japan
e-mail: yamanet1@aol.com

segmental ostial catheter ablation (SOCA) approach to a more anatomically guided circumferential pulmonary vein ablation approach (CPVA), generally using electroanatomical mapping systems [7, 8].

In the segmental PV isolation method, longitudinal fibers of finger-like extensions that bridge the LA-PV muscle conduction are segmentally targeted with detailed mapping using a CMC. One factor that may have led to the wider use of the CPVA is the fact that the SOCA may be associated with an increased risk of PV stenosis. In addition, several early studies suggested that the CPVA might provide better outcomes in the prevention of AF recurrence (Fig. 14.1a) [9]. However, at least one study has shown a better outcome with the SOCA than the CPVA with respect to the AF-free survival (Fig. 14.1b) [10], and very importantly, the total outcome of the SOCA was better than that of the CPVA in a Worldwide Survey (albeit not to a significant degree) [11].

We previously reported the feasibility and high efficacy of segmental antral PV isolation, targeting the more atrial portion of the longitudinal fibers bridging the PV and LA using a larger-size CMC [12]. However, there has been no definitive, prospective, randomized study on this issue with an acceptable duration of follow-up that convincingly proves one method superior to another in the outcome of PV isolation. Although over the past decade, in parallel with the development of three-dimensional mapping systems, more anatomical PV isolation (CPVA) has become much more popular than the traditional EP-guided approach (SOCA), it would be prudent to perform the minimal amount of ablation necessary to eliminate AF, under both electrophysiological and anatomical guidance.

14.4 Current Strategy of RF-PV Isolation in Japan

Since the initial development of PV isolation by Haissaguerre et al. [6], various techniques have been developed, all requiring the same energy (RF) for the same purpose (to isolate the PV and its surrounding areas from the LA). Under the current guideline of the Japanese Circulation Society (JCS), four representative techniques are recommended for PV isolation, as follows (Fig. 14.2) [13]:

(a) Known as circumferential PV ablation (CPVA), circumferential PV isolation (CPV ISOLATION), or wide-area circumferential ablation (WACA), both the ipsilateral superior and inferior PVs are isolated by an encircling continuous ablation line located at the border between the PV antrum and the LA wall at the posterior junction and on the border between the anterior PV edges and surrounding tissue, including the anterior junction [8].

(b) Known as extensive encircling PV isolation (EEPVI), the method is similar to that of panel (a), but the ipsilateral PVs are isolated together by linear RF application at the posterior LA wall and segmental RF application at the anterior wall [14]. This method can be applied by monitoring the ablation site and intra-PV electrograms and is evaluated using an ablation catheter together with two Lasso catheters positioned in both ipsilateral PVs. In this method, both ipsilateral PVs are usually disconnected spontaneously, resulting in AF-free rates of 86% and 94% without and with antiarrhythmic agents (AADs), respectively.

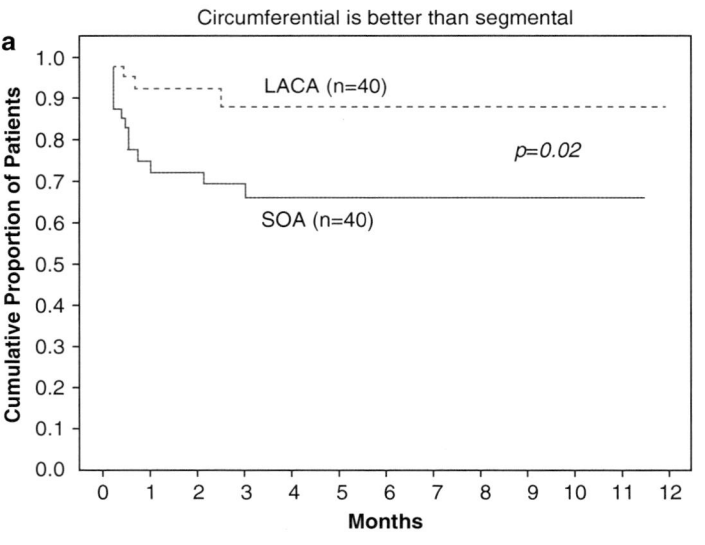
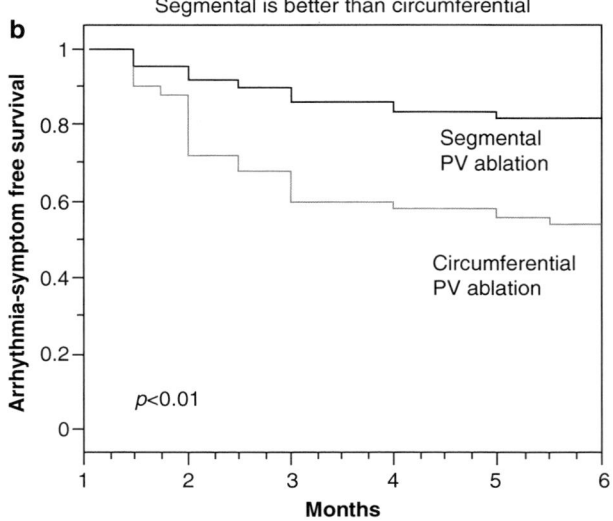
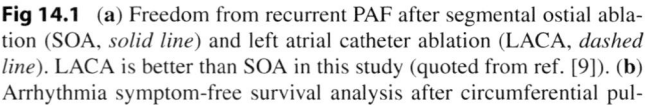

Fig 14.1 (a) Freedom from recurrent PAF after segmental ostial ablation (SOA, *solid line*) and left atrial catheter ablation (LACA, *dashed line*). LACA is better than SOA in this study (quoted from ref. [9]). (b) Arrhythmia symptom-free survival analysis after circumferential pulmonary vein ablation (CPVA, *dashed line*) and segmental pulmonary vein ablation (SOA, *solid line*). SOA is better than CPVA in this study (quoted from ref. [10])

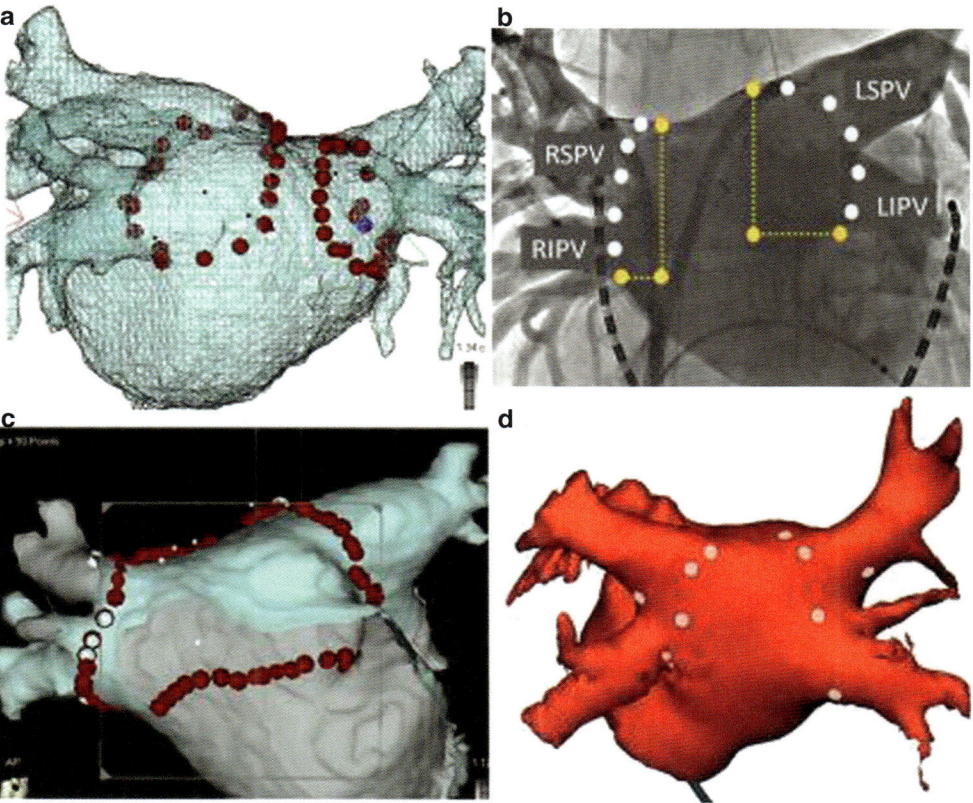

Fig 14.2 Current strategy of RF-PV isolation in Japan. (**a**) Circumferential PV ablation (CPVA), (**b**) Extensive encircling PV isolation (EEPVI), (**c**) BOX isolation, (**d**) Segmental PV antrum isolation

(c) Known as BOX isolation, the posterior LA (including all PVs) is electrically isolated by a single ablation line drawn at the anterior portion of the ipsilateral PVs, and the linear ablation of the LA roof as well as the LA bottom is performed [15]. Complete isolation of the posterior LA is achieved in 90% of cases, resulting in an AF-free rate of 95% without AAD (all paroxysmal AF cases, after a mean of 1.1 procedures).

(d) Known as segmental PV antral isolation, segmental RF (without making a linear ablation line) based on the circumferential PV antrum mapping (under guidance of a large CMC) to identify the electrical breakthrough between the LA and PVs is used to electrically isolate the individual PVs at their antrum, resulting in an AF-free rate of 92.7% in patients with paroxysmal AF (including 12% of cases with AAD) [12].

Regardless of the manner of PV isolation, similar efficacies and safeties have been reported, particularly for paroxysmal AF cases.

14.5 Obtaining Durable PV Isolation with RF

It has largely been established that in most AF recurrences, particularly in paroxysmal AF cases, PV reconnection is nearly always related to recurrence following RF ablation [8]. Since reconnection of the PV occurs through the half-killed myocardium in the LA-PV antral region, we need to improve the region permanence to ensure durable PV isolation. Several methods of accomplishing this have been suggested, including the adenosine method and the pacing on the line method.

14.5.1 Contact Force-Guided RF Ablation

It is well recognized that a major determinant of lesion size during RF application is the electrode-tissue interface contact force (CF) [16]. However, operators currently face a fundamental trade-off: if the contact is insufficient, the lesion will be smaller and likely to recover subsequently, whereas if contact is excessive, there will be greater risk of a steam pop, cardiac perforation, and thrombus formation. Recent improvements in catheter design have made it possible to measure the CF [16]. In the TOCCATA study [17], the authors observed a low CF (<10 g) in 35% of all RF applications around the PVs, all of which experienced a recurrence of AF during follow-up, while 80% of cases with a CF > 20 g were free of AF. Kimura et al. compared the number of residual gaps following circumferential RF applications around the ipsilateral PVs between CF-guided and non-guided cases in a prospective, randomized fashion [18]. The mean CF was significantly greater (5.9 ± 4.5 g and 11.1 ± 4.3 g, $p < 0.001$), and the number of residual gaps was significantly less (2.8 ± 1.9 vs 6.3 ± 3.0, $p < 0.001$) in the CF group than in the non-CF group. More recently, the force-time integral with color variations in three-dimensional mapping has been widely used in many ablation laboratories.

14.5.2 Adenosine Triphosphate (ATP) Method

Adenosine has been shown to temporarily restore PV connection in up to 30% of cases after the achievement of isolation via the hyperpolarization of half-killed ablated tissue [19]. Additional RF application at sites of reconnection has been shown to improve the subsequent long-term freedom from AF recurrence in several reports [20]; however, conflicting results with adenosine methods have also been observed [21]. A recent meta-analysis by McLellan et al. [22] aggregating data from nine studies showed that the use of adenosine to assess dormant conduction and guide additional targeted ablation was associated with a significant decrease in AF recurrence after PV isolation, while those with reconnection tended to have an increased risk of AF recurrence, despite additional ablation.

Recently, a few prospective randomized studies evaluated the usefulness of adenosine/ATP in improving the outcome of PV isolation. In the ADVICE study [23], 284 (53%) of 534 patients who had PV reconnection with adenosine after isolation were randomly assigned to either additional ablation to eliminate dormant conduction ($n = 147$) or to no further ablation ($n = 137$). As a result, additional adenosine-guided ablation improved the freedom from symptomatic atrial tachyarrhythmias (69.4% vs. 42.3%), with an absolute risk reduction of 27.1% (Fig. 14.3). Furthermore, the outcome in the additional ablation group was even better than in those without dormant conductions.

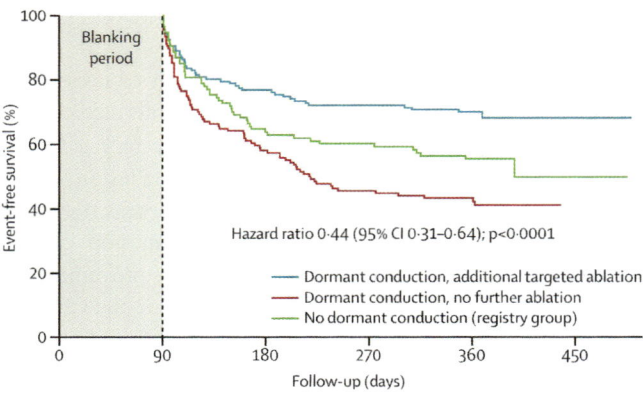

Fig 14.3 ADVICE trial: Freedom from symptomatic atrial tachyarrhythmia after a single ablation procedure (primary endpoint). The hazard ratio is for the comparison between dormant conduction, additional targeted ablation versus dormant conduction, no further ablation (quoted from ref. [23])

In contrast, in the UNDER-ATP study [24], 1112 and 1001 AF patients (paroxysmal, persistent or long-lasting AF) were randomly assigned to received ATP-guided and conventional (non-ATP-guided) PV isolation, respectively, and the outcomes of ablation were compared between the groups. ATP-provoked dormant conduction appeared in 307/1112 (27.6%) patients, and the additional RF ablation eliminating dormant conduction resulted in no significant difference in the AF-free ratio compared with the conventional ablation group. Given that the above two randomized studies were based on different patient populations and different study protocols, it is difficult to simply compare these outcomes and draw conclusions about the usefulness of adenosine/ATP during ablation. However, the differences in the basic ablation method (EP-guided or anatomical PV isolation) and the prevalence of dormant conduction (53% vs. 27.6% in ADVICE and UNDER-ATP, respectively) are closely related to the positive/negative results of these studies. The usefulness of the adenosine method after PV isolation is still controversial, and further evidence on this issue is required.

14.6 Acute, Mid- and Long-Term Efficacies of PV Isolation

The efficacy of AF catheter ablation in previously published manuscripts has varied, largely due to heterogeneous patient populations and different definitions of success among operating institutions. More recent publications have clarified the classification of the patient population (e.g., paroxysmal or chronic form) and determined the success a certain time after the final procedure, with mention of the AAD requirement. With these criteria, the cure rate without AAD in paroxysmal AF is around 85% to 95% after approximately 1.5 ablation procedures [4, 8, 12, 14]. The success rate is generally lower in chronic AF than in paroxysmal AF, at approximately 70–85% [25].

Although the acute effect of PV isolation in eliminating paroxysmal AF is already well established, another issue is its very-long-term effects. A few reports have described very-long-term follow-up observations of patients (>5 years). A Bordeaux group described the follow-up data in a mixed paroxysmal and persistent AF population, showing a sinus maintenance rate of only about 30% after a single procedure, which increased to over 60% with multiple ablation procedures [26]. They also revealed the slow but steady decline of 8.9% per year in the arrhythmia-free survival even after multiple procedures. A report by a Hamburg group showed similar data in paroxysmal AF cases, with a 46.6% success rate after a single procedure and 79.5% success rate with multiple procedures

[27]. In contrast to these disappointing data, another study reported hopeful data showing an approximately 3% late recurrence rate if patients were in sinus rhythm for the first year after ablation [28]. It is now largely accepted that both the short- and long-term efficiency of ablation are closely related to the degree of durability and perfection of PV isolation.

14.7 Effect of PV Isolation on Persistent AF

In contrast to ablation for paroxysmal AF, it has been suggested that in persistent AF, the PVs are less important for the pathophysiology, and other ablation procedures targeting atrial substrates are necessary in addition to PV isolation. In the past decade, it has been believed that more aggressive ablations with multiple targets, including the PV, complex electrograms (CFAEs), linear ablation and GP, would result in better outcomes for the suppression of persistent AF [25, 29]. However, a recent large-scale randomized trial including 589 patients revealed no reduction in the rate of recurrent AF when either linear ablation or ablation of CFAEs was performed in addition to PV isolation (Fig. 14.4) [30]. In a very recent meta-analysis report as well, the addition of CFAE ablation or linear ablation offered no significant improvement in the arrhythmia-free survival in comparison with PV isolation alone. Furthermore, these substrate ablations are associated with increases in both the procedural and fluoroscopy times. Of note, the optimum ablation strategy for persistent AF is currently unclear, but the importance of PV isolation in suppressing persistent AF as well as paroxysmal AF is now being reevaluated.

14.8 Complications of PV Isolation with RF

As with any kind of invasive procedure, catheter ablation for AF carries associated risks of complications; however, given the nature of AF ablation, the overall complication rates are relatively low [31]. Although the incidence of complications differs among institutions, the current estimated risks have been reported in a global survey. Of note, some complications (e.g., PV stenosis) that were not infrequent became much less common depending on recent advances in certain procedures [11, 32].

In that global survey (2005) [32], major complications were reported to occur in 4.5% of patients, including death in 0.15% and esophageal fistula in 0.04%. Among other major complications, cardiac tamponade accounted for 1.31%, stroke for 0.23%, transient ischemic attack for 0.71%, and PV stenosis requiring surgical or percutaneous dilatation for another 0.29% of all procedures.

In a newer global survey (2010) [11], the incidence of PV stenosis dropped to less than half of that in the previous survey, while the rates of most other complications were similar between the two surveys. We need to recognize the current complication rate of PV isolation since recent advances in novel technologies (e.g., cryoballoons and laser balloons) are changing the incidence of complications involved in PV isolation. AF ablation is being adopted to larger extent in patients with more advanced disease and more comorbidities. This may explain the lower-than-expected success rates but similar complication rates despite improvements in techniques and equipment.

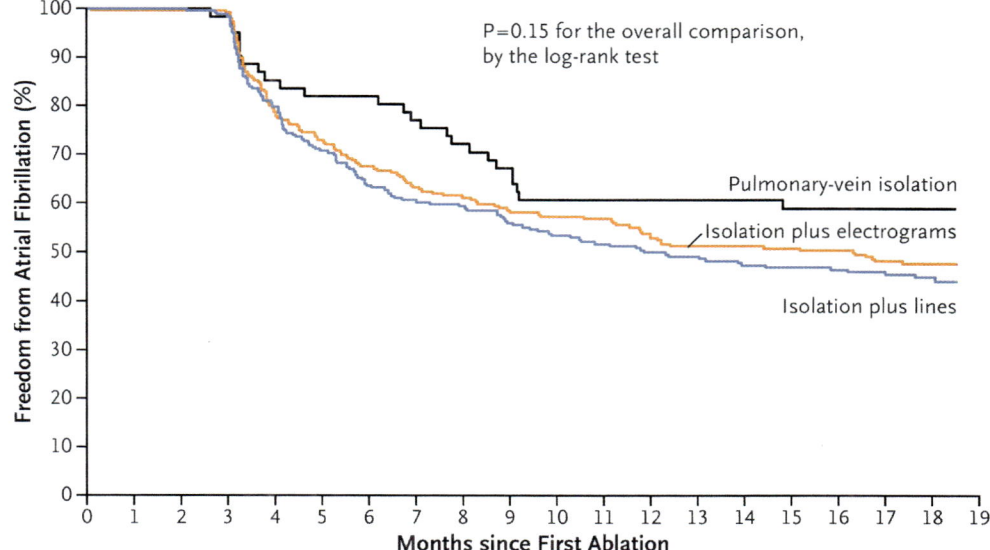

Fig 14.4 Kaplan–Meier estimates of freedom from documented atrial fibrillation after a single procedure, with or without the use of antiarrhythmic medications (no significant differences between groups). Isolation plus electrograms denotes ablation with pulmonary vein isolation plus additional ablation of complex fractionated electrograms; isolation plus lines refers to ablation with pulmonary vein isolation plus additional linear ablation (quoted from ref. [30])

14.8.1 Thromboembolic Events

Stroke is one of the most serious complications in the early phase of AF ablation and can cause sequelae in most cases. The introduction of irrigated catheters and the use of early and aggressive heparinization have significantly reduced the risk of cerebrovascular events related to the procedure. An activated clotting time (ACT) of more than 300 s and the continuous administration of warfarin throughout the procedure without low-molecular-weight heparin bridging help to reduce the incidence of stroke and transient ischemic attacks with no significant increase in the rates of bleeding complications [33]. More recently, the safety and efficacy of the periprocedural use of direct oral anticoagulants (DOACs) in patients undergoing catheter ablation has received focus, and evidence is mounting that, despite variations in the action of drugs, DOACs—whether interrupted or not—are associated with equal risks of stroke or TIA and major bleeding complications compared with uninterrupted vitamin K antagonists in catheter ablation of AF [34–36].

14.8.2 Esophageal Injury/Esophageal Fistula

Atrio-esophageal fistula formation is a rare but lethal complication related to AF catheter ablation. Patients with esophageal injury/fistula can present with a variety of signs and symptoms, such as a fever, appetite loss, chest pain, neurological disorder (consciousness loss, convulsion, hemiparesis), and hematemesis [37]. Since early surgical repair, if necessary, is mandatory to increase the chance of surviving in these patients, a rapid diagnosis is required. The most useful diagnostic tool is a chest CT scan, while endoscopy should be avoided due to the high risk of worsening the damage to the esophageal wall [37]. To prevent this lethal complication, it is common to use esophageal inner-temperature-monitoring with esophageal prove and to titrate the RF application at the areas of the LA posterior wall close to the esophagus [38]. However, monitoring the esophageal inner wall temperature can never be a fundamental/perfect method of avoiding esophageal damage from RF. Another simple method of prevention is to avoid unnecessary RF application close to esophagus. As mentioned in Sects. 14.3 and 14.4, antral PV isolation can be achieved by segmental RF application without making a linear lesion around the PV along the esophagus [12], which can reduce the number of RF applications to the esophageal region to isolate PVs.

14.8.3 PV Stenosis

PV stenosis is reported to occur in 1–3% of patients after RF catheter ablation for AF [31]. With the development of three-dimensional mapping systems and extraostial ablation strategies, the actual incidence of PV stenosis has dropped to <1% [31, 39]. However, since these values are based on symptomatic cases, the true incidence of PV stenosis will always be underestimated.

The clinical symptoms of PV stenosis vary from asymptomatic to highly symptomatic with a persistent cough, exertional dyspnea, chest pain, hemoptysis, and recurrent pulmonary infarction. In patients with symptomatic and severe PV stenosis, interventional procedures, such as balloon angioplasty and stent implantation, have been performed with symptomatic improvement; however, the incidence of re-stenosis is relatively high [40].

Although PV stenosis is a rare complication of point-by-point RF ablation as mentioned above, it is garnering more attention with the widespread application of cryoballoon PV isolation. Although cryothermal energy has theoretically been shown to be safer than conventional RF, concerns have been raised regarding the 3.1% incidence of PV stenosis reported in the STOP-AF trial [41] and the reported cases of severe PV stenosis requiring angioplasty [42].

References

1. Haïssaguerre M, Jaïs P, Shah DC, et al. Spontaneous initiation of atrial fibrillation by ectopic beats originating in the pulmonary veins. N Engl J Med. 1998;339:659–66.
2. Sesgadri N, Novaro GM, Prieto L, et al. Images in cardiovascular medicine: pulmonary vein stenosis after catheter ablation of atrial arrhythmias. Circulation. 2002;105:2571–2.
3. Calkins H, Kuck KH, Cappato R, et al. HRS/EHRA/ECAS expert consensus statement on catheter and surgical ablation of atrial fibrillation: recommendations for patient selection, procedural techniques, patient management and follow-up, definitions, endpoints, and research trial design. Europace. 2012;14:528–606.
4. Kumagai K, Ogawa M, Noguchi H, et al. Electrophysiologic properties of pulmonary veins assessed using a multielectrode basket catheter. J Am Coll Cardiol. 2004;16:2281–9.
5. Haïssaguerre M, Sanders P, Hocini M, et al. Pulmonary veins in the substrate for atrial fibrillation: the "venous wave" hypothesis. J Am Coll Cardiol. 2004;43:2290–2.
6. Haïssaguerre M, Shah DC, Jaïs P, et al. Electrophysiological breakthroughs from the left atrium to the pulmonary veins. Circulation. 2000;102:2463–5.
7. Pappone C, Rosanio S, Oreto G, et al. Circumferential radiofrequency ablation of pulmonary vein ostia: a new anatomic approach for curing atrial fibrillation. Circulation. 2000;102:2619–28.
8. Ouyang F, Bänsch D, Ernst S, et al. Complete isolation of the left atrium surrounding the pulmonary veins: new insights from the double Lasso technique in paroxysmal atrial fibrillation. Circulation. 2004;110:2090–6.
9. Oral H, Scharf C, Chugh A, et al. Catheter ablation for paroxysmal atrial fibrillation: segmental pulmonary vein ostial ablation versus left atrial ablation. Circulation. 2003;108:2355–60.
10. Karch MR, Zrenner B, Deisenhofer I, et al. Freedom from atrial tachyarrhythmias after catheter ablation atrial fibrillation: a randomized comparison between 2 current ablation strategies. Circulation. 2005;111:2875–80.
11. Cappato R, Calkins H, Chen SA, et al. Updated worldwide survey on the methods, efficacy, and safety of catheter ablation for human atrial fibrillation. Circ Arrhythm Electrophysiol. 2010;3:32–8.

12. Yamane T, Date T, Kanzaki Y, et al. Segmental pulmonary vein antrum isolation using the "Large-size" Lasso catheter in patients with atrial fibrillation. Circ J. 2007;5:753–60.
13. Guidelines for indications and procedural techniques of catheter ablation (JCS: Japanese Circulation Society 2012) (in Japanese) http://www.jcirc.or.jp/guideline/pdf/JCS2012_okumura_h.pdf
14. Takahashi A, Iesaka Y, Takahashi Y, et al. Electrical connections between pulmonary veins: Implication for ostial ablation of pulmonary veins in patients with paroxysmal atrial fibrillation. Circulation. 2002;105:2998–3003.
15. Kumagai K, Muraoka S, Mitsutake C, et al. A new approach for complete isolation of the posterior left atrium including pulmonary veins for atrial fibrillation. J Cardiovasc Electrophysiol. 2007;18:1047–52.
16. Yokoyama K, Nakagawa H, Shah DC, et al. Novel contact force sensor incorporated in irrigated radiofrequency ablation catheter predicts lesion size and incidence of steam pop and thrombus. Circ Arrhythm Electrophysiol. 2008;1:354–62.
17. Kuck KH, Reddy VY, Schmidt B, et al. A novel radiofrequency ablation catheter using contact force sensing: TOCCATA study. Heart Rhythm. 2012;9:18–23.
18. Kimura M, Sasaki S, Owada S, et al. Comparison of lesion formation between contact force-guided and non-guided circumferential pulmonary vein isolation: a prospective, randomized study. Heart Rhythm. 2014;11:984–91.
19. Datino T, Macle L, Qi XY, et al. Mechanisms by which adenosine restores conduction in dormant canine pulmonary veins. Circulation. 2010;121:963–72.
20. Matsuo S, Yamane T, Date T, et al. Reduction of AF recurrence after pulmonary vein isolation by eliminating ATP-induced transient venous re-conduction. J Cardiovasc Electrophysiol. 2007;18:704–8.
21. Miyazaki S, Kuwahara T, Kobori A, et al. Impact of adenosine-provoked acute dormant pulmonary vein conduction on recurrence of atrial fibrillation. J Cardiovasc Electrophysiol. 2012;23:256–60.
22. McLellan AJA, Kumar S, Smith C, et al. The role of adenosine following pulmonary vein isolation in patients undergoing catheter ablation for atrial fibrillation: a systematic review. J Cardiovasc Electorophsiol. 2013;24:742–51.
23. Macle L, Khairy P, Weerasooriya R, et al. Adenosine-guided pulmonary vein isolation for the treatment of paroxysmal atrial fibrillation: an international, multicentre, randomised superiority trial. Lancet. 2015;386:672–9.
24. Kobori A, Shizuta S, Inoue K, et al. Adenosine triphosphate-guided pulmonary vein isolation for atrial fibrillation: the UNmasking Dormant Electrical Reconduction by Adenosine TriPhosphate (UNDER-ATP) trial. Eur Heart J. 2015;36:3276–87.
25. Brooks AG, Stiles MK, Laborderie J, et al. Outcomes of long-standing persistent atrial fibrillation ablation: a systematic review. Heart Rhythm. 2010;7:835–46.
26. Weerasooriya R, Khairy P, Litalien J, et al. Catheter ablation for atrial fibrillation: are results maintained at 5 years of follow-up? J Am Coll Cardiol. 2011;57:160–6.
27. Ouyang F, Tilz R, Chun J, et al. Long-term results of catheter ablation in paroxysmal atrial fibrillation: lessons from a 5-year follow-up. Circulation. 2010;122:2368–77.
28. Fichtner S, Czudnochowsky U, Hessling G, et al. Very late relapse of atrial fibrillation after pulmonary vein isolation: incidence and results of repeat ablation. PACE. 2010;33:1258–63.
29. Haïssaguerre M, Sanders P, Hocini M, et al. Catheter ablation of long-lasting persistent atrial fibrillation : critical structures for termination. J Cardiovasc Electrophysiol. 2005;16:1125–37.
30. Verma A, Jiang CY, Betts TR, et al. STAR AF II InvestigatorsApproaches to catheter ablation for persistent atrial fibrillation. N Engl J Med. 2015;372:1812–22.
31. Gupta A, Perera T, Ganesan A, et al. Complications of catheter ablation of atrial fibrillation: a systematic review. Circ Arrhythm Electrophysiol. 2013;6:1082–8.
32. Cappato R, Calkins H, Chen SA, et al. Worldwide survey on the methods, efficacy, and safety of catheter ablation for human atrial fibrillation. Circulation. 2005;111:1100–5.
33. Wazni O, Beheiry S, Fahmy T, et al. Atrial fibrillation ablation in patients with therapeutic international normalized ratio: comparison of strategies of anticoagulation management on the periprocedural period. Circulation. 2007;116:2531–4.
34. Wu S, Yang YM, Zhu J, et al. Meta-analysis of efficacy and safety of new oral anticoagulants compared with uninterrupted vitamin K antagonists in patients undergoing catheter ablation for atrial fibrillation. Am J Cardiol. 2016;117:926–34.
35. Okumura K, Aonuma K, Kumagai K, et al. Efficacy and safety of rivaroxaban and warfarin in the perioperative period of catheter ablation for atrial fibrillation: outcome analysis from a prospective multicenter registry study in Japan. Circ J. 2016;80: 2295–301.
36. Murakawa Y, Nogami A, Shoda M, et al. Nationwide survey of catheter ablation for atrial fibrillation: the Japanese catheter ablation registry of atrial fibrillation (J-CARAF)—a report on periprocedural oral anticoagulants. J Arrhythm. 2015;31:29–32.
37. Chavez P, Messerli FH, Casso Dominguez A, et al. Atrioesophageal fistula following ablation procedures for atrial fibrillation: systematic review of case reports. Open Heart. 2015;2:e000257.
38. Kuwahara T, Takahashi A, Kobori A, et al. Safe and effective ablation of atrial fibrillation: importance of esophageal temperature monitoring to avoid periesophageal nerve injury as a complication of pulmonary vein isolation. J Cardiovasc Electrophysiol. 2009;20:1–6.
39. Inoue K, Murakawa Y, Nogami A, et al. National survey of catheter ablation for atrial fibrillation: the Japanese Catheter Ablation Registry of Atrial Fibrillation (J-CARAF). J Arrhythm. 2013;29:221–7.
40. Holmes DR Jr, Monahan KH, Packer D, et al. Pulmonary vein stenosis complicating ablation for atrial fibrillation: clinical spectrum and interventional considerations. JACC Cardiovasc Interv. 2009;2:267–76.
41. Packer DL, Kowal RC, Wheelan KR, et al. Cryoballoon ablation of pulmonary veins for paroxysmal atrial fibrillation: first results of the North American Arctic Front (STOP AF) pivotal trial. J Am Coll Cardiol. 2013;61:1713–23.
42. Tokutake K, Tokuda M, Ogawa T, et al. Pulmonary vein stenosis after second-generation cryoballoon ablation for atrial fibrillation. Heart Rhythm Case Rep. 2017;3(1):36–9.

Pulmonary Vein Isolation: Cryoballoon Ablation

Kaoru Okishige

Keywords
Cryoballoon • Atrial fibrillation • Phrenic nerve palsy

15.1 Introduction Remarks

In the treatment of patients with atrial fibrillation (AF), the foremost goal of catheter ablation is achieving permanent electrical isolation of the pulmonary veins (PVs). The most commonly used source for electrical isolation of the PVs has been radiofrequency (RF) energy, and a linear RF lesion surrounding the antrum of the PVs has been performed using point-by-point applications [1, 2]. Various ablation technologies are being developed that aim to standardize the PV isolation procedure-foremost among these being balloon ablation catheters. The largest global experience with such a technology involves cryoballoon. Although the freezing technique has recently become a widespread ablation tool, the mechanisms of the hypothermic tissue injury have not yet been well described.

Cryothermy as an ablation energy source offers several distinct advantages when compared to the current standard of care. As a freezing energy source, Halocarbon 502 (Freon) was initially used, and then later changed to AZ-20, and currently nitrous oxide is being used. While RF energy results in hyperthermic cellular injury through a combination of coagulation and tissue necrosis, the objective of cryothermal ablation is to freeze the tissue in a discrete and focused fashion in order to destroy cells in a precisely targeted area [3]. This chapter reviews exploring the biophysics of cryoballoon ablation.

15.2 The Anatomy and Physiology of the Cryoballoon

The presently available cryoballoon catheter is the Arctic Front Advance catheter (Medtronic CryoCath Technologies. Inc., Minneapolis) (Fig. 15.1). This system consists of a steerable 10.5-Fr catheter with a distally mounted polyurethane and polyester balloon and is introduced to the left atrium via a 15-Fr deflectable delivery sheath (FlexCath, Medtronic) (Fig. 15.2) and connected to an external CryoConsole (Medtronic CryoCath Technologies) (Fig. 15.3), which houses the coolant. The cryoballoon catheter contains (1) an intake lumen (injection tube) that permits the injection of cryo-refrigerant to the inner balloon; (2) an exhaust lumen to facilitate its removal; (3) a central lumen that permits a guidewire to pass through to position and/or support a small-diameter circular diagnostic catheter for monitoring the PV potentials (Achieve, Medtronic) (Fig. 15.4); (4) a thermocouple on the central shaft near the proximal end of the balloon to facilitate inner balloon temperature monitoring; and (5) a dual pull-wire mechanism integrated into the handle of the catheter that facilitates catheter deflection. Of note, a constant vacuum is applied between the inner and outer balloon to ensure the absence of cryo-refrigerant leakage into the systemic circulation in the event of a breach in the integrity of the inner balloon as a safety system.

K. Okishige
Heart Center, Yokohama-City Bay Red Cross Hospital,
3-12-1 Shinyamashita, Naka-ku, Yokohama, Kanagawa
231-8682, Japan
e-mail: okishige@yo.rim.or.jp

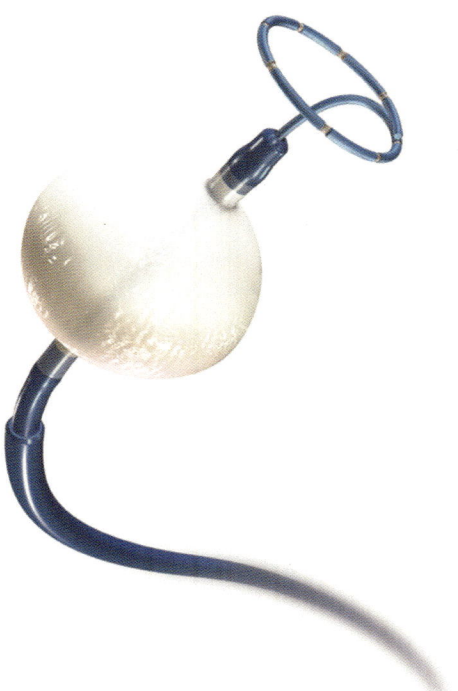

Fig. 15.1 The cryoballoon (Arctic Front Advance, Medtronic) and circular mapping catheter (Achieve, Medtronic)

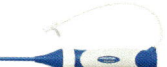

Fig. 15.2 A deflectable long guiding sheath (FlexCath Advance, Medtronic)

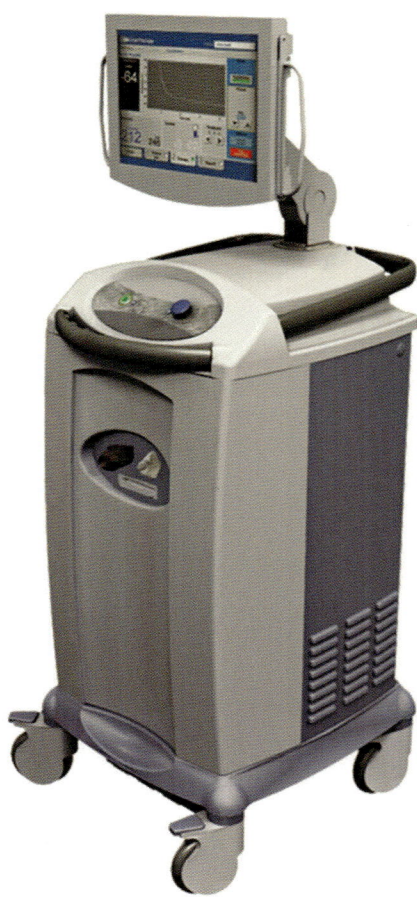

Fig. 15.3 A picture of the console for cryoenergy delivery, and monitoring the procedural parameters (CryoConsole, Medtronic)

The ablation procedure is performed through the delivery of pressurized cryo-refrigerant (nitrous oxide) to the distal aspect of the inner balloon via an ultrafine injection tube. When the refrigerant enters the distal inner balloon it undergoes a liquid-to-gas phase change, and the cryo-refrigerant is further pressurized through a restriction tube maximizing the temperature drop to −80 °C via the Joule-Thomson effect. The cryo-ferrigerant then absorbs heat from the surrounding tissue before returning to the console through a lumen maintained under vacuum.

15.3 Lesion Formation with the Cryoballoon

The cryoballoon application provides injurious effects based on the generation of hypothermia at the balloon-tissue interface and can be divided into three sequential stages: (1) the freeze/thaw phase, (2) hemorrhagic-inflammatory phase, and (3) replacement fibrous phase.

1. Progressive cooling can form ice crystals exclusively in the extracellular space at temperatures below −15 °C, and ice crystal formation occurs exclusively in the intracellular space below −40 °C. Ice crystal formation triggers an extracellular hypertonic state relative to the intracellular space. In order to reestablish an osmotic equilibrium, a compensatory egress of water occurs from the intracellular to extracellular space with a subsequent cellular shrinkage. This newly established osmotic gradient facilitates a diffusion gradient between the extracellular and intracellular spaces resulting in a net movement of H+ ions out of the cells causing a reduction in the intracellular pH. An intracellular acidic state causes cellular protein damage, enzyme system impairment, and adverse effects on the lipoprotein components of the plasma membrane. Among the cytoplasmic components, the mitochondria are particularly sensitive and the first structure to suffer irreversible damage by hypothermia [4]. Microcirculatory failure subsequently occurs provoking endothelial layer destruction, interstitial edema,

15.4 Characteristics Peculiar to Cryofreezing Energy

15.4.1 Cryo-Adhesion

In contrast to the RF ablation system, the cryothermal ablation catheter is associated with a freeze-mediated catheter adhesion to the target tissue. The catheter stability provoked by catheter-tissue attachment precipitates an efficacious ablation in technically challenging regions where contact of the ablation catheter is difficult to maintain. RF ablation might be applied not only to the target tissue, but also surrounding non-target tissue because of cardiac and respiratory motion. In contrast, the increased catheter stability with the cryothermal ablation would be expected to reduce any collateral damage to nearby critical structures such as the normal conduction system and epicardial coronary arteries. When RF energy is applied for ventricular tachycardia (VT), catheter stability can be expected during sustained VT. However, the tip of the ablation catheter might shift once the VT is terminated and the normal ventricular contraction resumes. Therefore, we might not be able to continue delivering sufficient RF energy at the target site for a sufficient duration. In contrast, the cryofreezing ablation catheter can continue to stay at the target site throughout the entire duration of the cryoablation even though normal ventricular contractions are resumed after a successful ablation procedure.

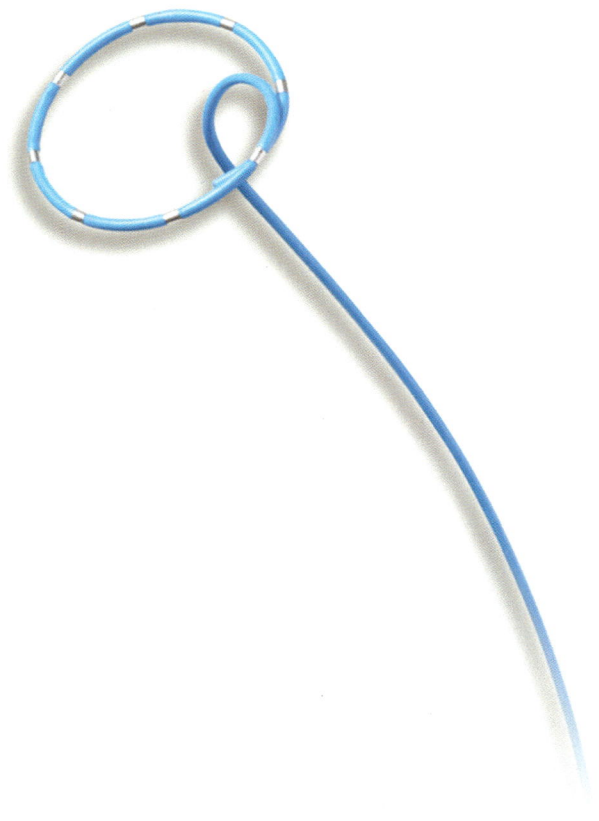

Fig. 15.4 The circular mapping catheter (Achieve, Medtronic)

15.4.2 Ice-Mapping

Cryofreezing energy has an obligatory reversible tissue inhibition preceding irreversible tissue destruction. Mild cryothermy has the capability to assess the safety and efficacy of a potential ablation lesion site dynamically and prospectively. The duration of the freezing with relatively warmer tissue temperatures (−10 to −25 °C) is associated with the degree of permanent cellular damage, whereas, extreme freezing with the tissue temperature reaching colder than −50 °C results in instantaneous permanent tissue injury. The efficacy of ice-mapping is the use of milder freezing temperatures and shorter ablation times to enable the assessment of the clinical effects at the target site. The safety-mapping is the use of this mild temperature to confirm that the target site does not have any adverse clinical outcomes. It is important to recognize that ice-mapping does not always guarantee the complete freedom from irreversible effects when ice-mapping does not provoke any adverse effects. The hypothermic wavefront spreads centrifugally from the catheter tip to the surrounding tissue [6, 7]. Vigilant monitoring must be maintained when treating critical substrates such as the perinodal region because tissues not initially affected have the

platelet aggregation, microthrombi, and vascular congestion and obliteration. This status results in the cessation of the blood flow and subsequent ischemia. During the thawing phase, rewarming of the tissue induces a hyperemic vascular response and intra- and extracellular ice crystal fusion into larger ice masses resulting in cellular destruction.

2. When the microcirculation is restored, tissue edema ensues. The fluid from the melted ice crystals traverses the damaged microvascular endothelial cells provoking ischemic necrosis. Whereas the central region subjected to the coldest freezing temperature undergoes direct cellular damage, the surrounding microvascular injury results in the extension of the tissue destruction.

3. Replacement of the cells by fibrosis and apoptosis ensues near the periphery of the frozen tissue after the hemorrhagic and inflammatory period. During the subsequent weeks, these processes culminate in the generation of a mature lesion, which has a distinct, well-circumscribed central region of dense fibrosis surrounded by a narrow border zone of variable cellular death [5].

potential to undergo irreversible injury as the cryolesion continues to expand during the cryoablation.

There are two methods for ice-mapping; "classic" ice-mapping and "dynamic" ice-mapping. "Classic" ice-mapping is to freeze the tissue at a temperature of −30 °C for shorter than 60 s, and "dynamic" ice-mapping is to freeze the tissue at a temperature of −80 °C for shorter than 10 s. These two methods of ice-mapping are able to avoid any irreversible injury to the cardiac tissue and provoke transient effects.

15.4.3 Lesion Characteristics

When a focal cryothermal ablation catheter is applied to the myocardium, it histologically demonstrates dense, homogeneous fibrosis that is well demarcated from the normal myocardium [7, 8]. The lesion created by a cryoenergy application exhibits the preservation of the ultrastructural integrity, and this aspect of the cryolesion theoretically is associated with a lower risk of myocardial perforation, esophageal injury, and aneurysmal dilation [3, 8, 9]. In addition, the cryolesion should be expected to be less arrhythmogenic and have a lower incidence of venous or arterial stenosis [8, 9].

The cryothermal ablation lesion exhibits minimal endothelial surface disruption and a lesser degree of platelet and coagulation cascade activation compared to RF ablation [10, 11]. The hyperthermic ablation system, such as RF energy, creates a lesion whose extent is positively correlated with the thrombus bulk, whereas the cryoablation lesion dimensions are not predictive of the overlying thrombus volume. These differences contribute to a less thrombogenic nature of the cryofreezing lesion [3, 11, 12]. The configuration of the cryothermal lesion by a focal catheter is similar to that created by an RF application (hemi-spherical configuration), and the lesion created by cryofreezing has a comparable depth and configuration to RF energy (Fig. 15.5).

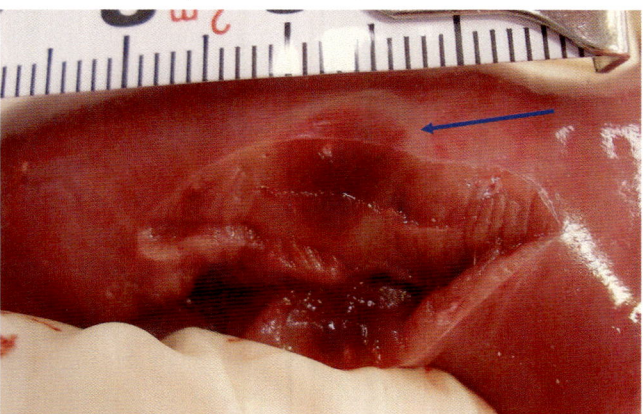

Fig. 15.5 Macroscopic view of the lesion created in the ventricular myocardium of a porcine heart

15.4.4 Clinical Symptoms During Freezing

When RF energy is applied to the posterior left atrium, inside the coronary sinus, or cavotricuspid isthmus, patients are apt to complain of pain through direct stimulation of the cardiac sensory nerves. This patient discomfort requires increased sedation or a decrease in the RF energy titration. In contrast, cryoablation does not provoke any sense of discomfort such as pain or heartburn [13, 14].

Pison et al. performed a clinical study as follows: twenty consecutive patients with symptomatic AF underwent cryoballoon ablation without sedation. Headaches were evaluated before, 150 s after the start, and after the first cryoapplication in each PV using a visual representation of a head for the exact location of the headache, a numerical rating scale (NRS) for measuring the pain intensity, and short-form McGill pain questionnaire (MPQ) for a qualitative analysis of the pain. The results were that in the majority (80%) of the patients with AF treated by balloon cryoablation, frontal headaches occurred during the cryoapplication. There was no correlation between the temperature reached during the cryoballoon freeze and the intensity of the perceived headache (the intensity of the perceived headache was not related to the temperature reached 150 s after the start of the cryoballoon freeze [$P = 0.81$]). Cryoablation of the first PV, irrespective of its location, was significantly more painful than that with cryoablation of the other three PVs [15]. The precise etiology of the headaches occurring during cryoballoon ablation is still unclear. As a possible explanation, the following have been proposed: vagal nerve stimulation in the mediastinum during freezing and hypothermia induced cerebral vasospasms [16]. Of note, this headache is transient, and we may explain that the possible headaches are a transient phenomenon during cryofreezing during the course of the cryoballoon ablation.

15.4.5 Safety of the Coronary Arteries

RF energy applications within the coronary sinus are required for various kinds of tachycardias and have been associated with venous injury, delayed fibrosis/stenosis [17], acute and subacute venous thromboses, and collateral damage to the esophagus and adjacent coronary arteries. In contrast, preclinical studies of catheter-based cryoablation have suggested a lower incidence of vascular injury, reduced propensity for thromboses, and lower risk of coronary artery injury/stenosis when cryoablation is performed within or adjacent to the coronary sinus [18, 19].

We performed an animal experiment in order to investigate this issue. When an RF ablation catheter with a 6 mm tip was applied just on the coronary artery, an acute coronary occlusion was provoked, which could be ascertained by intracardiac echocardiography as shown in Figs. 15.6 and 15.7.

Fig. 15.6 Coronary angiography of the porcine heart during the radiofrequency (RF) energy application right on the coronary artery. *Left panel*: An RF energy application was delivered right on the coronary artery. *Right panel*: Angiography obtained immediately after the RF application right on the coronary artery. A significant stenotic lesion is identified

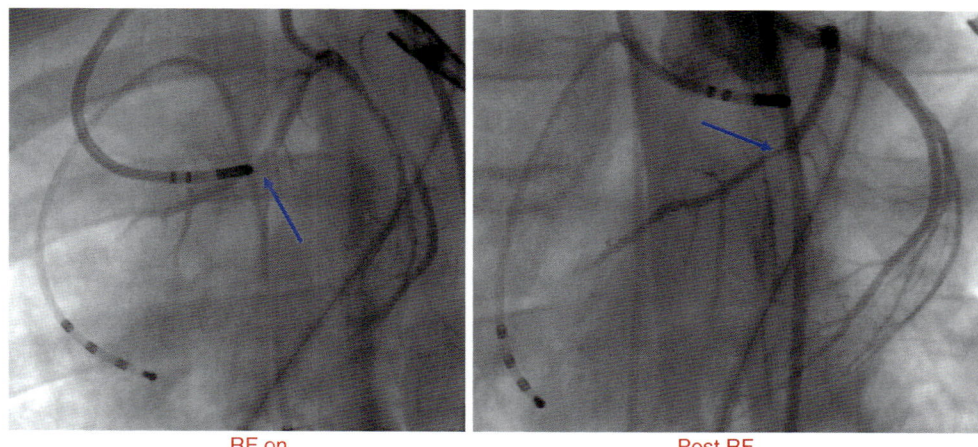

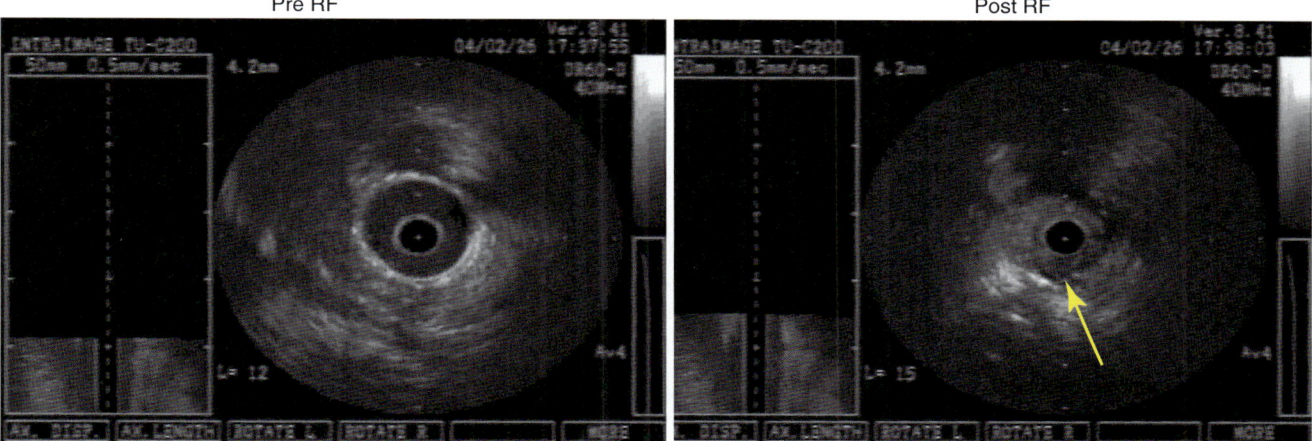

Fig. 15.7 Intracardiac echocardiography findings recorded immediately after an RF energy application right on the coronary artery. An acute occlusion of the coronary artery is recognized as shown by the *arrow*

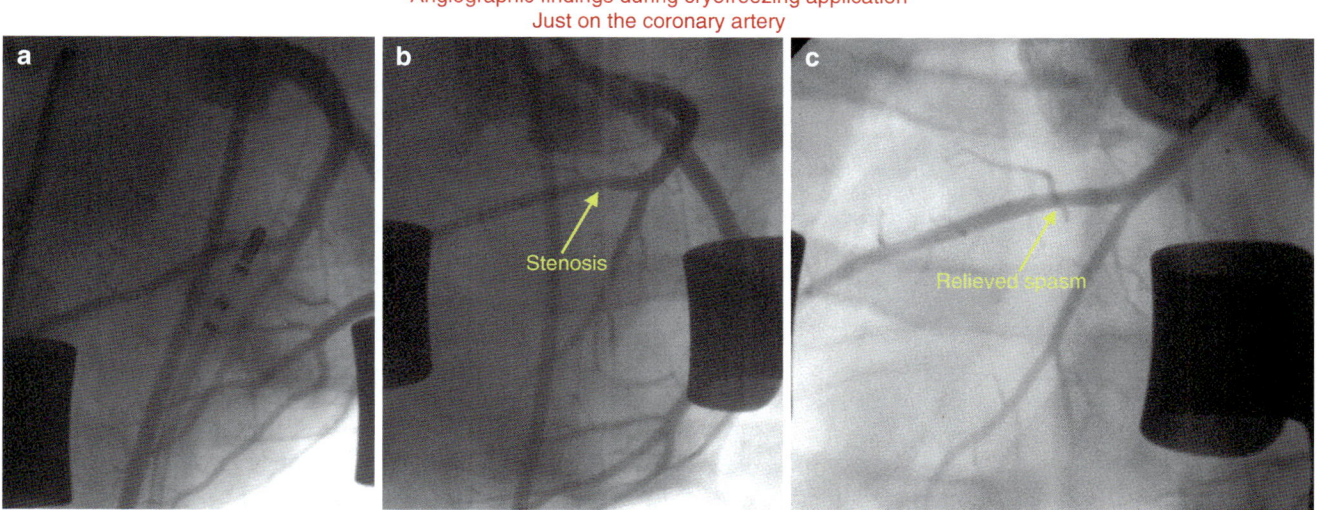

Fig. 15.8 Coronary angiography during a cryoenergy application right on the coronary artery. (**a**) A cryoenergy application was performed right on the coronary artery. (**b**) Coronary angiography was performed immediately after cryoenergy application, which showed significant stenosis. (**c**) After the intracoronary administration of nitrates, the stenotic lesion of the coronary artery was abolished. It meant that the coronary stenosis was due to coronary spasms rather than organic stenosis

When a focal cryoablation catheter with a 6 mm tip was applied in an identical fashion to the RF catheter, significant acute coronary stenosis was induced, however, that significant stenosis could be resolved by an intracoronary administration of nitrates as shown in Fig. 15.8. We repeated this trial fifteen times, and exactly the same phenomenon was observed, and it meant that a cryofreezing application just on the coronary artery can provoke coronary vasospasms, which are easily resolved by appropriate treatment, such as the administration of nitrates, without provoking any disastrous irreversible lesion formation. This aspect of cryofreezing might be very useful in the case of an epicardial application of cryoablation for a ventricular tachycardia whose arrhythmogenic focus is located very close to the coronary arteries. In addition, coronary arterial injury can be avoided when focal cryoablation is performed at a site very close to the left circumflex coronary artery on the mitral annulus in the case of AF ablation.

15.5 Clinical Results of Cryofreezing Ablation

15.5.1 Atrial Tachycardia (AT)

For a post-ablation atrial tachycardia (AT) occurring after performing a PVI, cryoablation was performed with a 6-mm tip catheter (Freezor Max, Medtronic, Minneapolis), and the cryoablation was started at the earliest excitation site on the lateral free wall of the right atrium, which was detected by a NavX 3-D mapping system. The atrial electrogram recorded by the cryoablation catheter preceded the onset of the P wave by 35 ms, and when the tip of the cryoablation catheter had frozen to −30 °C for 30 s, this AT terminated within 5 s. However, electrical stimulation to induce this AT was repeated, and this AT could be induced again ("ice-mapping") (Fig. 15.9). The cryofreezing temperature setting was further lowered to −80 °C for 3–4 min, resulting in the complete

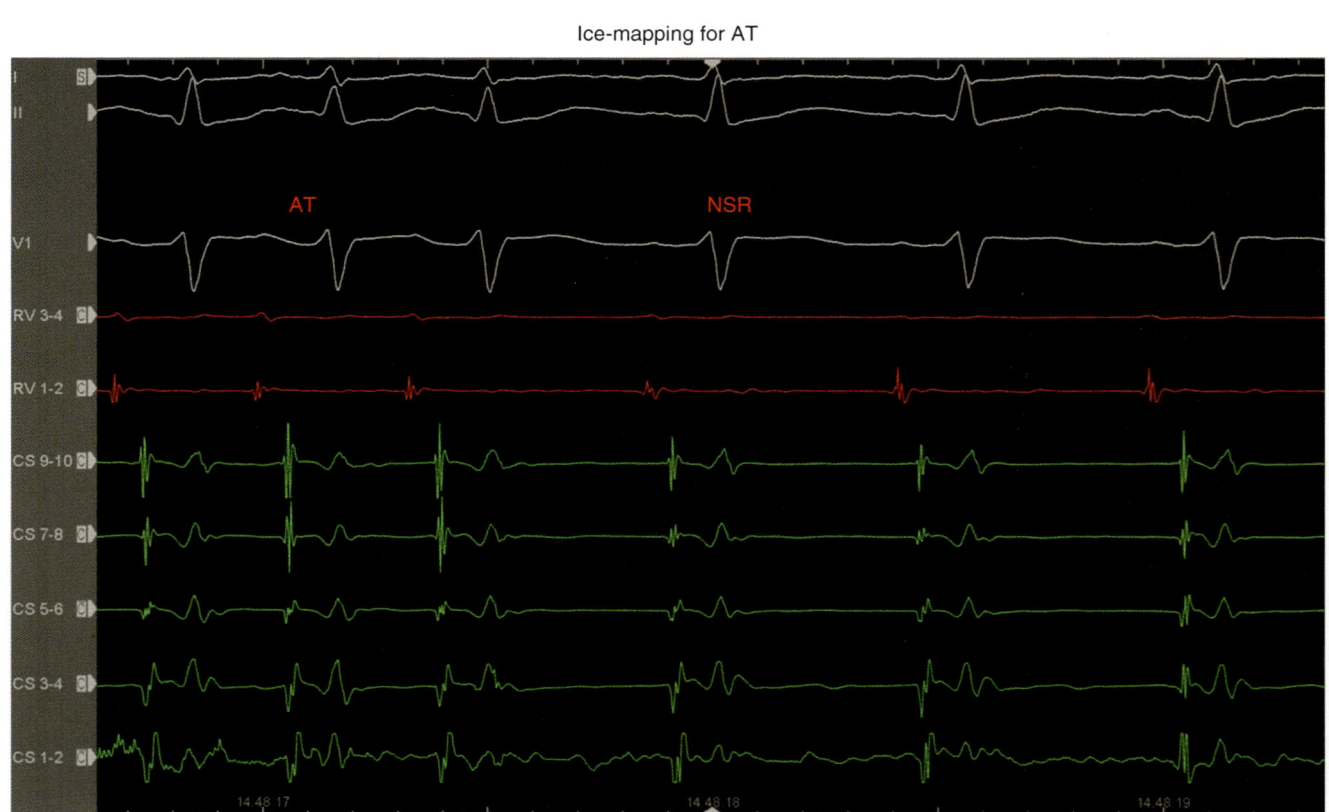

Fig. 15.9 Intracardiac electrograms during ice-mapping of an atrial tachycardia (AT). Cryofreezing at a temperature of −30 °C was able to terminate this AT, however, it was still inducible after rewarming

elimination of the arrhythmogenic tissue of this AT. Due to the milder injurious effects of the cryofreezing on the cardiac tissue, we were able to perform at least three or four cryoenergy applications.

15.5.2 Atrial Fibrillation

15.5.2.1 Advantage of the Cryoballoon for AF

The use of cryothermal energy has several potential advantages over RF energy.

1. Freezing mediated catheter adhesion results in increased catheter stability contributing to avoiding collateral damage to nearby structures [3].
2. Cryoablation can create well-demarcated homogeneous lesions that are less arrhythmogenic compared to RF lesions [20].
3. Mature lesions created by cryoablation demonstrate the preservation of the tissue ultrastructural integrity [21].
4. Lesions created by cryoablation result in minimal endocardial surface disruption and are less thrombogenic than those produced by RF energy [22].
5. Cryoablation leads to less patient discomfort and lower dosing requirements for conscious sedation when compared to RF [23].

Recent studies have confirmed the efficacy of RF catheter ablation of arrhythmogenic foci in the PVs as treatment for paroxysmal AF [24]. In addition, electrical isolation of the PVs responsible for the focal arrhythmogenic activity triggering AF is possible using a technique of circumferential ostial ablation or limited ostial ablation guided by a circumferential electrode catheter mapping in order to identify the point of entry of atrial muscle fibers into the PVs [25]. Balloon-based ablation systems potentially offer a simpler and faster means of achieving the PVI. Compared to other balloon-based ablation technologies (radiofrequency balloon and endoscopic laser), the cryoballoon is less direction dependent, as the refrigerant jet inside the balloon is directed to produce a lower ablation temperature in a large circular zone. Therefore, cryoballoon ablation may be expected to isolate the muscular PV sleeve as well as the observed PV antrum [26].

15.5.2.2 Cryoballoon Ablation Procedure

One transseptal puncture is made using a Brockenbrough technique to introduce a 15 Fr deflectable sheath (FlexCath, Medtronic). Rotational angiography of the left atrium (LA) is performed to identify the LA-PV anatomy. A microcircular mapping catheter (Achieve, Medtronic) is intro-

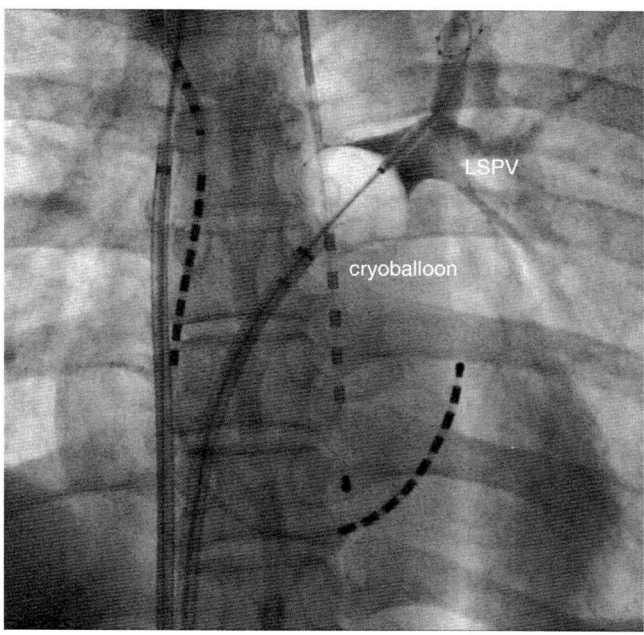

Fig. 15.10 The contrast medium (diluted 1:1 ratio with saline) was injected into the pulmonary vein (PV) through the central lumen of the cryoballoon catheter to obtain the PV angiogram. When complete occlusion by the cryoballoon was obtained, contrast medium retention was observed as shown in this figure

duced into the central lumen of a 28-mm cryoballoon (Arctic Front, Advance, Medtronic). The cryoballoon is introduced into the LA via the FlexCath, and the Achieve catheter can be used as a "guidewire." Using the "over-the-wire" technique with the FlexCath, the cryoballoon is guided to each PV ostium. Contrast medium (diluted 1:1 ratio with saline) is injected into each PV through the central lumen of the cryoballoon catheter to obtain the PV angiogram (Fig. 15.10). Prior to the balloon inflation, the Achieve is placed in the PV to record the PV potentials. The cryoballoon is then inflated and advanced toward the PV ostium. When the cryoballoon is docked on the tissue, the diluted contrast medium is injected from the lumen of the balloon catheter to evaluate the exact position of the balloon in relation to the LA-PV junction and determine the extent of vein occlusion with the cryoballoon. Successful occlusion of each vein is achieved when a selective contrast medium injection demonstrates total retention. Complete occlusion by the cryoballoon is preferable for a successful PVI [27]; however, the PVI can be accomplished in spite of the existence of a slight leakage of contrast medium. The following reasons are proposed: (1) the diameter of the cryoballoon is enlarged by 1.5 mm after starting the freezing, and (2) the leakage is crystallized after freezing and that itself occludes the leakage.

"Pull-Down" Technique

The inferior aspect of each PV is apt to provoke leakage of contrast medium despite effort to occlude the PVs by the cryoballoon. In those kinds of cases, the "pull-down" maneuver is useful to occlude the inferior aspect of the PVs. When the balloon temperature reaches approximately −10 °C, the balloon has to be pulled down to occlude the PVs. A pull-down technique involves waiting for the balloon to adhere to the superior aspect of the targeted vein followed by catheter and shaft deflection to pull the balloon downward, so as to achieve contact with the inferior portion of the vein, thereby eliminating the inferior gap [27].

Each cryolesion is delivered with a target time of 180–240 s depending on the physician's discretion. Premature lesion termination is performed if there is evidence of impending phrenic nerve damage.

15.5.2.3 Endpoint of the Ablation Procedure

The ablation endpoint is the complete isolation of all PVs. Following each application of cryoenergy, the circular mapping catheter is used to assess the electrical isolation, and an accurate placement of the mapping catheter is mandatory for the correct interpretation of the ablation results. An additional "bonus" delivery of cryoenergy cannot always guarantee the complete success of the PVI [28]. Thirty minutes after the termination of the ablation energy application, intravenous isoproterenol is administered, and all PVs are reassessed with the circular mapping catheter. Preservation of the electrical isolation of all PVs is the endpoint of the cryoballoon ablation procedure.

Adenosine triphosphate at a dose of 20 mg is administered in a bolus fashion to identify any dormant conduction (DC) after accomplishing the PVI. In a previous study DC was revealed in eight patient (3.7%) after ATP injections [29]. Touch-up ablation using RF energy has to be performed to eliminate dormant conduction to improve the success rate for preserving the PVI and preventing AF recurrence.

15.5.2.4 Adverse Events

Phrenic Nerve Injury

The most common complication is phrenic nerve palsy (PNP), and the overall incidence is 6.38% including persistent PNP of 4.73% [30]. PNP occurs in a much higher proportion of procedures that use 23-mm cryoballoons compared to 28-mm cryoballoons (12.37% vs. 3.53%, $P = 0.001$) [30]. PNP most often complicates the ablation of the right superior PV, however, left-sided PNP can also be provoked in 2% according to our clinical experience of more than 600 cases.

Compound Motor Action Potentials (CMAPs)

Cryoablation of the right-sided PVs is associated with a significant incidence of phrenic nerve injury (PNI) with a rate reaching as high as 11% [31]. PNI with cryoenergy may range from transient impairment injury to permanent phrenic nerve palsy. Many investigators tried to find a reliable predictor of PNI, and electromyography of the diaphragm has been commonly used to provide useful diagnostic information about the phrenic nerve function [32]. Compound motor action potential (CMAP) has been utilized, which are the recordings of the summated muscle potential waveforms produced by the stimulation of the phrenic nerve. A reduction in the diaphragmatic CMAP amplitude successfully predicts diaphragmatic paralysis, and recording CAMP during cryoballoon ablation using standard surface electrodes at the time of the phrenic nerve stimulation has been performed [33]. The majority of the PNI cases have occurred in the right-sided PN, however, left-sided PNI can occur during cryoballoon ablation [34]. CMAP recordings can be obtained using two leads: a standard surface right or left arm ECG electrode is positioned 5 cm above the xiphoid, and left and right arm ECG electrodes are positioned 16 cm along the right and left costal margin (Fig. 15.11). A quadripolar electrode is advanced into the left or right side subclavian vein, and the phrenic nerve is paced continuously during each application of cryoenergy at 40–50 bpm, using an output just

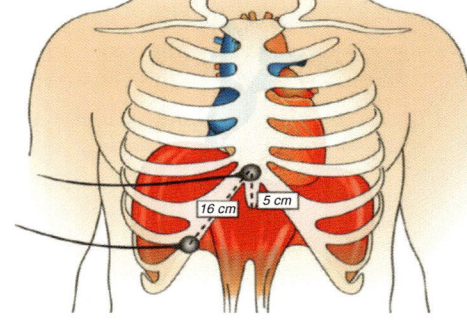
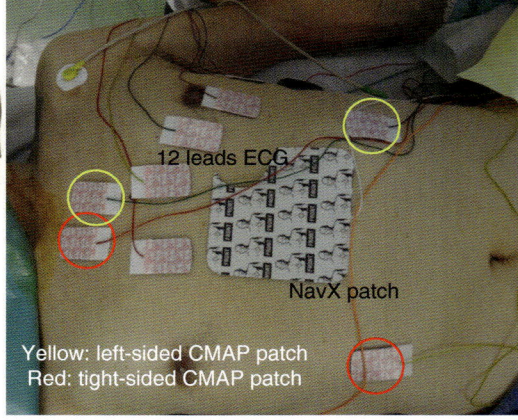

Fig. 15.11 Surface electrode placement for recording the diaphragmatic compound action motor potentials. The central arm surface electrode is placed 5 cm above the xiphoid and right and left arm surface electrodes are placed 16 cm from the xiphoid along the costal margin

above the pacing threshold by 10–20% in order to recognize the PNI in its early stage [34]. The CMAP signals can be amplified using a bandpass filter setting between 0.5 and 100 kHz and recorded on a NavX system (St. Jude Medical Inc., Minneapolis). The stability of the pacing is important in order to assess any injury to the phrenic nerve by cryoablation. The administration of a paralytic agent is also essential because it may inhibit phrenic nerve capture. In addition to CMAP recordings, the phrenic nerve function is also assessed continuously during cryofreezing by palpation of the diaphragmatic excursions. The maximum CMAP amplitude is measured from peak to peak at baseline and during each cryoablation application at 10 s intervals. Cryofreezing has to be prematurely terminated when either the diaphragmatic excursions decrease on palpation or the average amplitude of the CMAP is decreased by more than 30% compared to the prefreezing value [35].

PV Stenosis

PV stenosis is a rare complication in the PVI procedure using cryoballoon, and this condition should be taken into account when dyspnea, pulmonary infiltration, or hemoptysis appears after the PV ablation of AF [36, 37]. We observed a significant PV stenosis in 1.1% of 280 study patients including one serious case of PV stenosis (Fig. 15.12, 15.13), and we were able to identify the left atrial size as a reliable predictor of PV stenosis using an adjusted multivariate analysis (Fig. 15.14).

Esophageal Injury

Although the PV isolation by a cryoballoon is overall regarded as a safe ablation strategy, it can still pose a significant threat to the adjacent structures such as the esophagus, phrenic nerve, and vagus nerves. An atrioesophageal fistula (AEF) is the most devastating and feared complication, prompting different strategies to image, protect, and avoid injury to the esophagus. **Three** cases of an AEF as a complication of cryoballoon pulmonary vein isolation at three different institutions with two different generations of cryoballoons have been reported [38]. Temperature monitoring of the esophagus may be helpful to identify potentially dangerous lesions, but additional studies are warranted to define safer levels of esophageal temperature drops during cryoenergy deliveries when the esophageal proximity is an issue. This would possibly lead to an earlier detection if any symptoms occur after ablation. Recent data have shown that 19% of patients undergoing cryoablation with the second-generation balloon demonstrate esophageal lesions on endoscopy, with a luminal esophageal temperature of less than 12 °C exhibiting a 100% sensitivity [39].

Several temperature levels of the esophagus measured by a thermo-probe inserted into the esophagus for the prevention of esophageal injury have been advocated; however, no reliable value has been determined during cryoballoon applications for a PVI. At our institution, we prematurely terminate the cryofreezing when the esophageal temperature

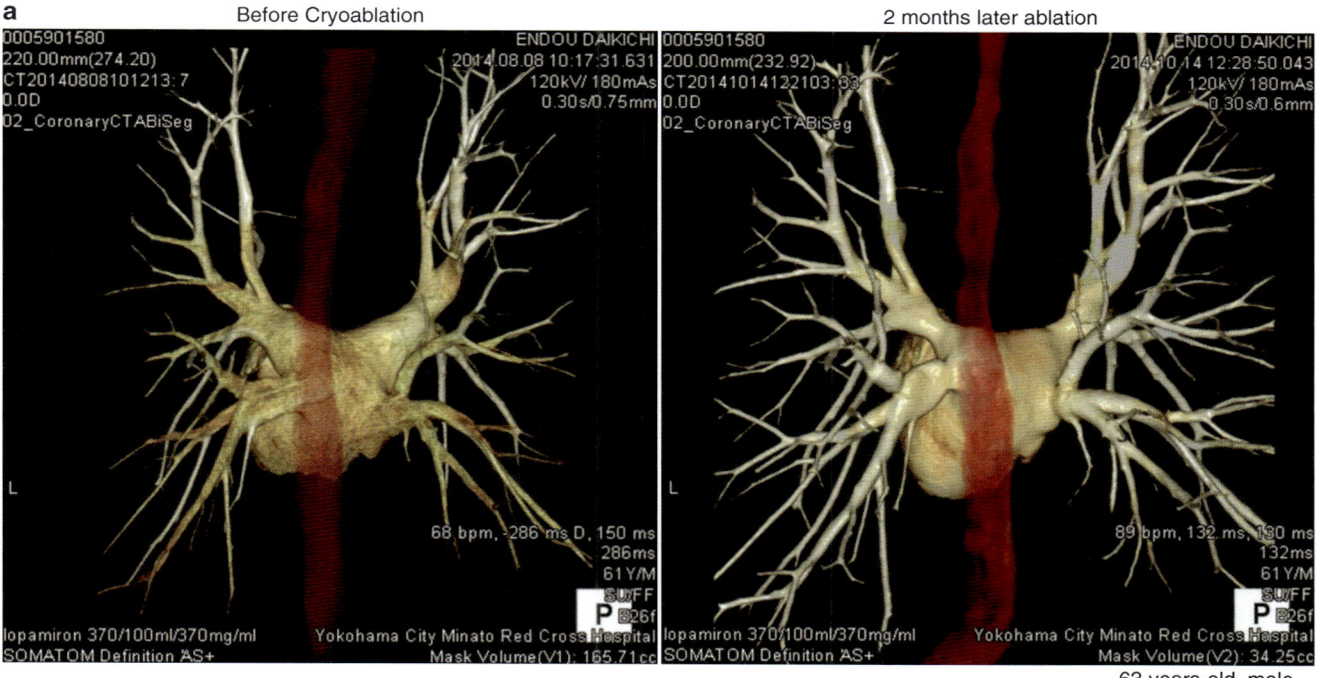

Fig. 15.12 (a) 3D-CT images obtained in the control (*left panel*) and 2 months after the cryoablation procedure. Mild to moderate stenosis of the PVs were recognized. (b) 3D-CT images recorded at 6 and 13 months after the cryoablation procedure. The stenotic lesions of the PVs became increasingly more serious with the progression of time after the cryoablation procedure

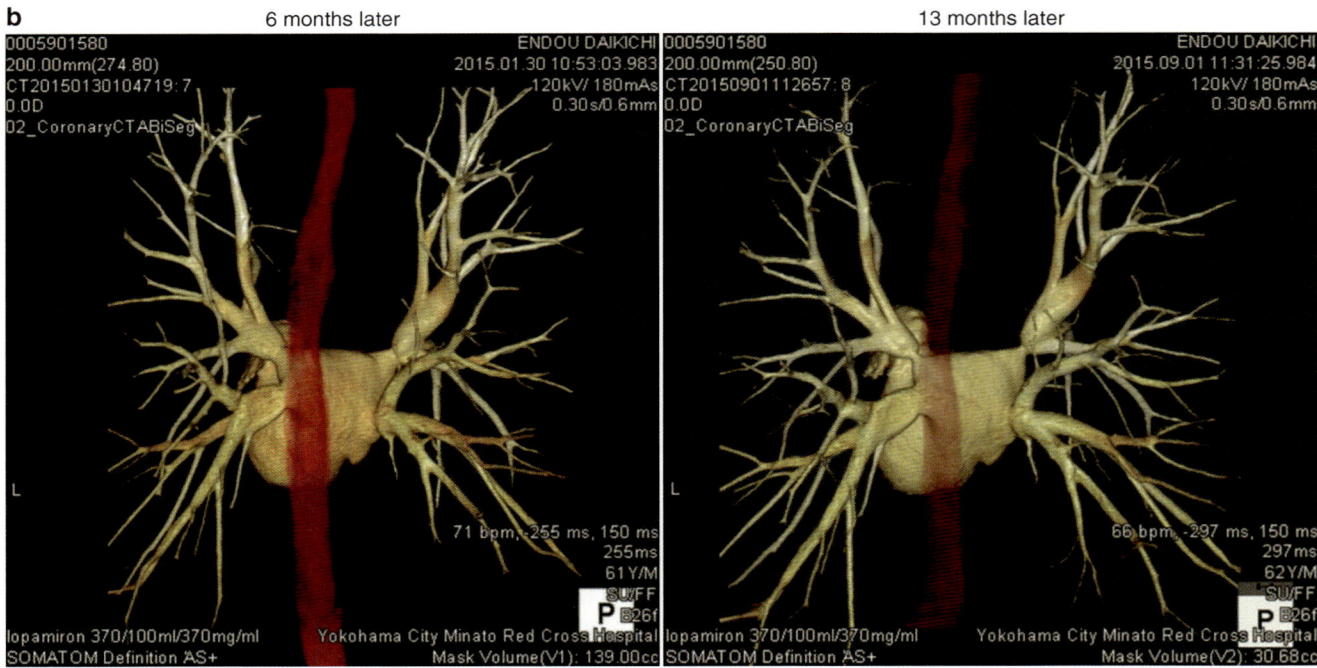

Fig. 15.12 (continued)

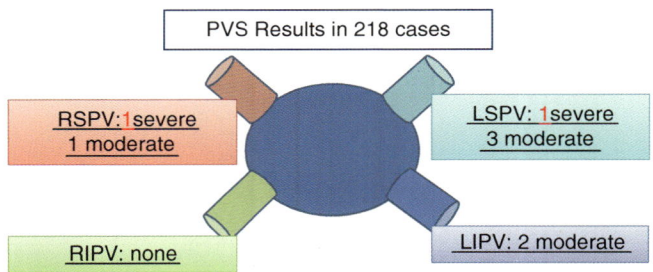

Fig. 15.13 The incidence of PV stenosis in each PV in our study patients after performing cryoballoon ablation for a PVI

Association between LA size and incidence of the PVS (Multiple Logistic Regression Analysis in 535 Study Subjects)			
Variables	Odds ratio	95%CI	P value
Left atrium diameter (1mm decrease)	1.3	1.07–1.71	<0.01

The dependent variable was PVS. This analysis included total freezing time, minimum temperature, freezing cycles, Troponin I value, Oval index of PV and left atrium diameter.)

Fig. 15.14 The left atrial size was identified as a reliable predictor of PV stenosis using an adjusted multivariate analysis

drops below 10 °C although no supporting data for this procedure exist.

When using the cryoballoon, forward pressure is placed on the cryoballoon to occlude the target PV ensuring circumferential contact with the left atrium. This forward pressure is achieved with both direct catheter pressure and by buttressing the outer steerable sheath (FlexCath, Medtronic) against the cryoballoon. This maneuver distorts the left atrium and may push it toward the esophagus, possibly enhancing the likelihood of cryothermal injury.

Thrombotic Events

With the open-irrigated RF catheter, the AF ablation procedure may cause cerebral silent ischemic lesions in up to 11–14% of cases [40]. A recent report demonstrated that the incidence of silent cerebral thrombolic lesions after cryoballoon application was 5.6%, whereas irrigated RF energy applications caused these ischemic events in 8.3%; however, there was no significant difference between the two groups [40].

We reported silent cerebral ischemic events in approximately 20% even though appropriate anticoagulation (ACT was maintained longer than 300 s) was undertaken during the ablation procedure and perioperative period [41]. In general, cryofreezing energy is able to preserve the endothelial tissue, which has an important antithrombotic role. Therefore, a lower incidence of thromboembolic events might be expected in cryoenergy ablation cases. Extracorporeal balloon inflation for the complete exclusion of the air entrapped in the balloon, as well as continuous flushing with heparinized saline during ablation procedure, would be recommended for the prevention of embolic adverse events.

References

1. Haissaguerre M, Jais DC, Garrigue S, Takahashi A, Lavergne T, Hocini M, Peng JT, Roudaut R, Clementy J. Electrophysiological end point for catheter ablation of atrial fibrillation from multiple pulmonary venous foci. Circulation. 2000;101:1409–17.
2. Marrouche NF, Dresing T, Cole C, Bash D, Saad E, Kizysztof B, Pavia SV, Schweikert R, Saliba W, Abdul-Karim A, Pisano E, Fanelli R, Tchou P, Natale A. Circular mapping and ablation of the pulmonary vein for treatment of atrial fibrillation: impact of different catheter technologies. J Am Coll Cardiol. 2002;40:464–74.
3. Khairy P, Dubuc M. Transcatheter cryoablation part I: preclinical experience. Pacing Clin Electrophysiol. 2008;31:112–20.
4. Andrade JG, Dubuc M, Guerra PG, Macle L, Mondesert B, Rivard L, Roy D, Talagic M, Thibault B, Khairy P. The biophysics and biomechanics of cryoballoon ablation. PACE. 2012;35:1162–8.
5. Andrade JG, Khairy P, Dubuc M. Catheter cryoablation: biology and clinical uses. Circ Arrhythm Electrophysiol. 2013;6:218–27.
6. Gage AA, Baust J. Mechanisms of tissue injury in cryosurgery. Cryobiology. 1998;37:171–86.
7. Gage AA, Guest K, Montes M, Caruana JA, Whalen DA Jr. Effects of varying freezing and thawing rates in experimental cryosurgery. Cryobiology. 1985;22:175–82.
8. Klein GJ, Harrison L, Ideker RF, Smith WM, Kasell J, Wallace AG, Gallagher JJ. Reaction of the myocardium to cryosurgery: electrophysiology and arrhytyhmogenic potential. Circulation. 1979;59:364–72.
9. Feld GK, Yao B, Reu G, Kudaravalli R. Acute and chronic effects of cryoablation of the pulmonary veins in the dogs as a potential treatment for focal atrial fibrillation. J Interv Card Electrophysiol. 2003;8:135–40.
10. Hochlozer W, Schlittenhardt D, Arenz T, Stockinger J, Weber R, Burkle G, Kalusche D, Trenk D, Neumann FJ. Platelet activation and myocardial necrosis in patients undergoing radiofrequency and cryoablation of isthmus-dependent atril flutter. Europace. 2007;9:490–5.
11. Sarabanda AV, Bunch TJ, Johnson SB, Mahapatra S, Milton MA, Leite LR, Bruce GK, Packer DL. Efficacy and safety of circufferential pulmonary vein isolation using a novel cryothermal balloon ablation system. J Am Coll Cardiol. 2005;46:1902–12.
12. Gaita F, Leclercq JF, Schumacher B, Scaglione M, Toso E, Halimi F, Schade A, Froehner S, Ziegler V, Sergi D, Cesarani F, Blandino A. Incidence of silent cerebral thromboembolic lesions after atrial fibrillation ablation may change according to technology used: comparison of irrigated radiofrequency, multipolar nonirrigated catheyter and cryoablation. J Cardiovasc Electrophysiol. 2011;22:961–8.
13. Collins NJ, Barlow M, Varghese P, Leitch J. Cryoablation versus radiofrequency ablation in the treatment of atrial fibrillation trial (CRAAFT). J Interv Card Electrophysiol. 2006;16:1–5.
14. Lowe MD, Meara M, Mason J, Grace AA, Murgartroyd FD. Catheter cryoablation of supraventricular arrhythmias; a painless alternative to radiofrequency energy. PACE. 2003;26:500–3.
15. Pison L, Peeters P, Blaauw Y, Vernooy K, Kumar N, Philippens S, Crijns HJ, Vlaeyen J, Schoenen J, Timmermans C. Headache during cryoballoon ablation for atrial fibrillation. Europace. 2015;17:898–901.
16. Schmoker JD, Terrien C III, McPartland KJ, Boyum J, Wellman GC, Trombley L. Cerebrovascular response to continuous cold perfusion and hypothermic circulation arrest. J Thorac Cardiovasc Surg. 2009;137:459–64.
17. Nakamura T, Okishige K, Aoyagi H, Yamashita M, Kawaguchi N, Katoh N, Yamauchi Y. Incidence of cerebral ischemia detected by cerebral mri after pulmonary vein isolation using the second generation cryoballoon. Europace. 2017;19:1681–88.
18. Aoyama H, Nakagawa H, Pitha JV, Khammar GS, Chandrasekaran K, Matsudaira K, Yagi T, Yokoyama K, Lazzara R, Jackman WM. Comparison of cryothermal and radiofrequency current in safety and efficacy of catheter ablation within the canine coronary sinus close to the left circumflex coronary artery. J Cardiovasc Electrophysiol. 2005;16:1218–26.
19. Skanes AC, Jones DL, Teefy P, Guiraudon C, Yee R, Krahn AD, Klein GJ. Safety and feasibility of cryothermal ablation within the mid- and distal coronary sinus. J Cardiovasc Electrophysiol. 2004;15:1319–23.
20. Khairy P, Chaubert P, Lehmann J, Lambert J, Macle L, Tanguay JF, Sirois MG. Lower incidence of thrombus formation with cryoenergy versus radiofrequency catheter ablation. Circulation 2003;107:2045–2050 catheter ablation for atrial fibrillation. J Cardiovasc Electrophysiol. 2007;18:642–6.
21. Ripley KL, Gage AA, Olsen DB, Van Vleet JF, Lau CG, Tse HF. Tome course of esophageal lesion after catheter ablation with cryothermal and radiofrequency ablation: Implication for atrioesophageal fistula formation after catheter ablation for atrial fibrillation. J Cardiovasc Electrophysiol. 2007;18:642–6.
22. Sarabanda AV, Bunch TJ, Johnson SB, Mahapatra S, Milton MA, Leite LR, Bruce GK. Efficacy and safety of circumferential pulmonary vein isolation using a novel cryothermal balloon ablation system. J Am Coll Cardiol. 2005;46:1902–12.
23. Lowe MD, Meara M, Mason J, Grace AA, Murgatroyd FD. Catheter cryoablation of supraventricular arrhythmias: a painless alternative to radiofrequency energy. PACE. 2003;26:500–3.
24. Jais P, Haissaguerre M, Shah DC, Chouairi S, Gencel L, Hocini M. A focal source of atrial fibrillation treated by discrete radiofrequency ablation. Circulation. 1997;95:572–6.
25. Tada H, Oral H, Greenstein R, Pelosi F Jr, Knight BP, Strickberger SA, Morady F. Differentiation of atrial and pulmonary vein potentials recorded circumferentially within pulmonary veins. J Cardiovasc Electrophysiol. 2002;13:118–23.
26. Ouyang F, Ernst S, Chun J. Electrophysiological findings during ablation of persistent atrial fibrillation with electroanatomic mapping and double Lasso catheter technique. Circulation. 2005;112:3038–48.
27. Ahmed H, Neuzil P, Skoda J, D'Avila A, Donaldson DM, Laragy MC, Reddy VY. The permanency of pulmonary vein isolation using a balloon cryoablation catheter. J Cardiovasc Electrophysiol. 2010;21:731–7.
28. Chun KRJ, Furnkranz A, Koster I, Metzner A, Tonnis T, Wohlmuth P, Wissner E, Schmidt B, Ouyang F, Kuck KH. Two versus one repeat feeze-thaw cycles after cryoballoon pulmonary vein isolation: the ALSTER EXTRA pilot study. J Cardiovasc Electrophysiol. 2012;23:814–9.
29. Okishige K, Yamashita M, Aoyagi H, Kawaguchi N, Katoh N, Nakamura T, Yamauchi Y, Keida K, Sasano T, Hirao K. Characteristics of dormant pulmonary vein conduction induced by adenosine triphosphate in patients with atrial fibrillation undergoing cryoballoon ablation. J of Cardiol (in press).
30. Andrade JG, Khairy P, Guerra PG, Deyell MW, Rivard L, Macle L, Thibault B, Talajic M, Roy D, Dubuc M. Efficacy and safety of cryoballoon ablation for atrial fibrillation: a systemic review of published studies. Heart Rhythm. 2011;8:1444–51.
31. Defaye P, Kane A, Chaib A, Jacon P. Efficacy and safety of pulmonary veins isolation by cryoablation for the treatment of paroxysmal and persistent atrial fibrillation. Europace. 2011;13:789–95.
32. Lakhani M, Saiful F, Parikh V, Goyal N, Bekheit S, Kowalski M. Recordings of diaphragmatic electromyograms during cryoballoon ablation for atrial fibrillation accurately predict phrenic nerve injury. Heart Rhythm. 2014;11:369–74.
33. Franceschi F, Dubuc M, Guerra PG, Khairy P. Phrenic nerve monitoring with diaphragmatic electromyography during cryoballoon ablation for atrial fibrillation: the first human application. Heart Rhythm. 2011;8:1068–71.

34. Andrie RP, Schrickel JW, Nickenig G, Lickfett L. Left phrenic nerve injury during cryoballoon ablation of the left superior pulmonary vein. PACE. 2012;35:e334–6.
35. Okishige K, Aoyagi H, Kawaguchi N, Katoh N, Yamashita M, Nakamura T, Kurabayashi M, Suzuki H, Asano M, Gotoh K, Shimura T, Yamauchi Y, Kanazawa T, Sasano T, Hirao K. Novel method for earlier detection of phrenic nerve injury during cryoballoon applications for electrical isolation of pulmonary veins in patients with atrial fibrillation. Heart Rhythm. 2016;13:1810–6.
36. Lakhani M, Satiful F, Parikh V, Goyal N, Bekheit S, Kowalski M. Recordings of disphragmatic electromyograms during cryoballoon ablation for atrial fibrillation accurately predict phrenic nerve injury. Heart Rhythm. 2014;11:369–74.
37. Miyazaki S, Ichihara N, Iesaka Y. Pulmonary vein stenosis after cryoablation using 28-mm second-generation balloon. J Cardiovasc Electrophysiol. 2015;26:570–1.
38. Kawasaki R, Gauri A, Elmouchi D, Duggal M, Bhan A. Atrioesophageal fistula complicating cryoballoon pulmonary vein isolation for paroxysmal atrial fibrillation. J Cardiovasc Electrophysiol. 2014;25:787–92.
39. Furnkranz A, Bordignon S, Schmidt B, Behmig M, Behmer MC, Bode F, Schulte-Hahn B, Nowak B, Dignaβ AU, Chun JK. Luminal esophageal temperature predicts esophageal lesions after second generation cryoballoon pulmonary vein isolation. Heart Rhythm. 2013;10:789–93.
40. Gaita F, Leclercq JF, Schumacher B, Scaglione M, Toso E, Halimi F, Schade A, Froehner S, Ziegler V, Sergi D, Cesarani F, Blandino A. Incidence of silent cerebral thromboembolic lesions after atrial fibrillation ablation may change according to technology used: comparison of irrigated radiofrequency, multipolar nonirrigated catheter and cryoballoon. J Cardiovasc Electrophysiol. 2011;22:961–8.
41. Nakamura T, Okishige K, Kanazawa T, Yamashita M, Kawaguchi N, Kato N, Aoyagi H, Yamauchi Y, Sasano T, Hirao K. Incidence of silent cerebral infarctions after catheter ablation of atrial fibrillation utilizing the second generation cryoballoon. Europace. 2017;19:1681–8.

Radiofrequency HotBalloon Ablation

Hiroshi Sohara

Keywords
Atrial fibrillation • Radiofrequency hot balloon ablation • Compliancy

16.1 Introduction

The conventional point-by-point radiofrequency (RF) ablation is helpful as a treatment for paroxysmal atrial fibrillation (PAF) [1, 2]. However, there are various AF triggers in many different areas of heart (PV, PV antrum, posterior wall of the left atrium, superior vena cava, atrial septum, and coronary sinus). It takes a huge effort and techniques to treat AF with a conventional tip catheter because its lesion size at one shot is only a few millimeters. Also, complications occur at a certain rate [3].

In this regard, we assumed that a balloon catheter would enable a wide circumferential lesion by one-shot RF energy and facilitate PVI.

Development of radiofrequency HotBalloon catheter started from 2000 [3, 4]. We conducted a Single-Center, Investigator-Initiated Clinical Study [5, 6], and then took two steps forward by PMDA (Japan Pharmaceutical and Medical Devices Agency) Clinical Trials: a Three-Center Pilot Study [7], and a Prospective, Randomized, Multi-Center Pivotal Study at 17 sites [8]. Japan market approval for the HotBalloon catheter was obtained in November, 2015.

This chapter summarizes the characteristics of this elastic and compliant balloon, control measures to prevent specific complications, some of the results of Japan PMS (Post-Marketing Surveillance), and future perspectives.

H. Sohara, M.D., Ph.D.
Osaki Hospital, The Heart Rhythm Center, Tokyo Heart Center, 5-4-12 Kitashinagawa, Shinagawa-ku, 141-0001 Tokyo, Japan
e-mail: hysohara@uranus.dti.ne.jp

16.2 About HotBalloon Catheter

The HotBalloon catheter system incorporates a coil electrode that delivers radiofrequency energy and a temperature sensor in the center of the elastic balloon. The physician inflates the balloon injecting a mixture of saline and contrast medium. Injecting 10–20 mL of the solution allows inflation of the balloon from 26 to 33 mm (it can be inflated up to 35 mm when balloon membrane is tightly fit with PV tissue). Most of the radiofrequency energy delivered is used to heat the solution filled in the balloon.

16.2.1 Heat Conduction from the Balloon Surface

Keeping the temperature of the coil electrode at 70 °C makes the whole balloon surface temperature at 62–65 °C, which heats the balloon contacted tissue by heat conduction. Radiofrequency energy is not delivered directly to the intramyocardial tissue and thus the tissue temperature remains below 60 °C, which minimizes damage to adjacent organs. It is contrastive to the conventional point-by-point ablation catheter that makes it difficult to predict deep intramyocardial tissue temperature due to resistance heating and cooling effect by blood flow (Fig. 16.1).

16.2.2 Uniform Temperature Inside of the Balloon

The extracorporeal agitation pump constantly agitates the solution in the balloon to uniformly maintain the whole balloon surface temperature. That system enables this catheter to create a uniform circumferential lesion at PVs.

Fig. 16.1 Principle of heating

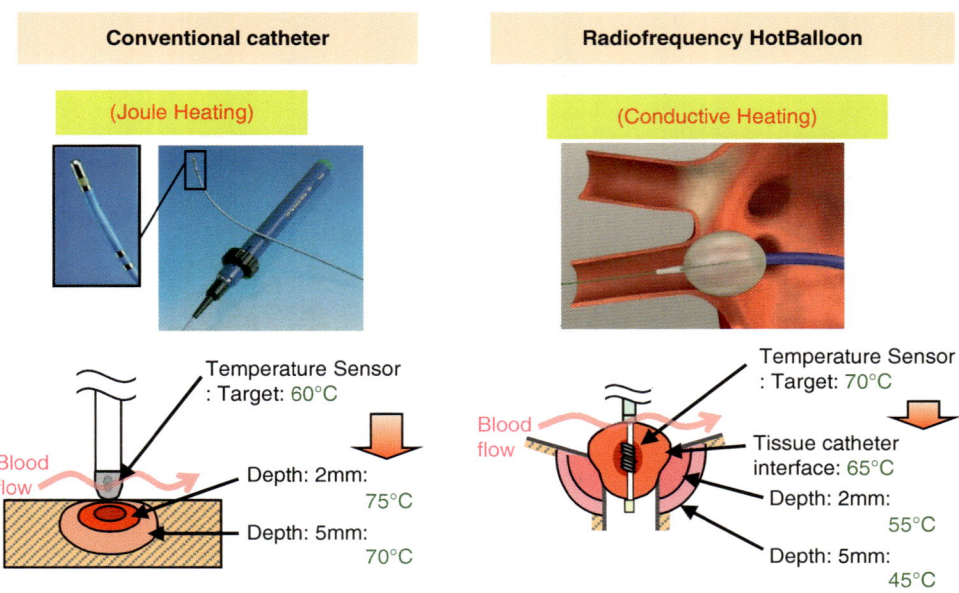

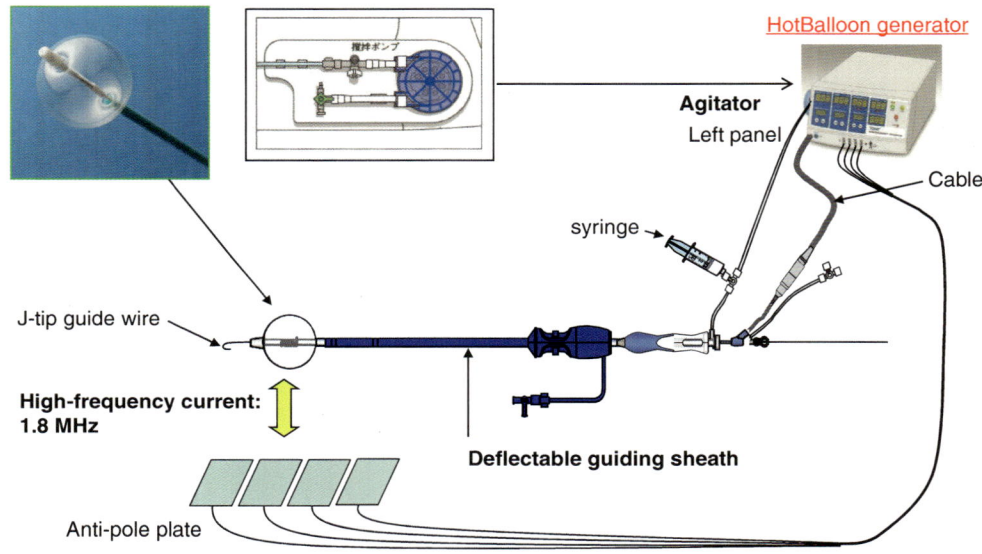

Fig. 16.2 HotBalloon System

16.2.3 High-Compliant Balloon

The elastic and compliant balloon is suitable for tight fit with a diverse configuration of PV shapes, having little anatomical limitation at a variety of ablation strategies.

16.3 Balloon Structure

In the center of the balloon, there is a coil electrode for radiofrequency delivery and a temperature sensor (Fig. 16.2). The balloon is inflated by filling with an ionic solution (mixture of normal saline and contrast medium). When radiofrequency energy passes between the coil electrode and the return electrodes pad on patient's back, the radiofrequency currents concentrate around the coil electrode creating Joule heat which makes the solution in the balloon heated. Meanwhile, agitation energy from the extracorporeal agitation pump mixes the solution inside the balloon, maintaining uniformly the entire balloon surface temperature.

16.4 Target Temperature and Ablation Time

The target temperature was carefully determined based on results in many nonclinical bench test, such as animal experiments and phantom tests, and also on our clinical experience in Investigator-Initiated Clinical study (Table 16.1).

16.5 Clinical Outcome

In our single-center study experience, consecutive 463 patients (PAF: 272, Persistent AF: 81, Longstanding persistent AF: 110) underwent "Balloon-based box isolation" (electrical isolation of four PVs + LA posterior wall isolation using HotBalloon [5]). After an average of 3.6 year (44 months) of follow-up, normal sinus rhythm rate for single procedure (chronic success) was seen in 70%, 67%, and 44% of patients, respectively [6].

In the Prospective, Randomized, Multi-Center PMDA Clinical Trial in 17 sites in Japan, normal sinus rhythm rate was 59% in HotBalloon ablation patients after *12 months*. This effectiveness outcome was significantly superior compared with those of drug treatment as a control arm [8].

16.6 How to Prevent Potential Risks of Complications Using HotBalloon Catheter

16.6.1 PV Stenosis

In the Multi-Center Clinical Trial, seven (5.2%) patients had significant PV stenosis (>70% at CT). All those cases of PV stenosis were found to be caused by insufficient injection of the solution into the balloon (appropriate amount: 10 mL, stenosis cases: 5–8 mL). That made the compliant balloon move into too distal PV (Fig. 16.3). To prevent PV stenosis, it is necessary to inflate the balloon more proximally (at antrum) and to confirm fluoro image frequently where the balloon is positioned during ablation. Today, it is recommended to inflate the balloon larger than 30 mm in diameter and at more proximal (antral) area.

16.6.2 Phrenic Nerve Paralysis

Of 463 cases in single-center study, three patients had phrenic nerve paralysis, and one of them was chronic. There were no cases of phrenic nerve paralysis in the Three-Center PMDA Pilot Trial [8] in Japan. In Multi-Center PMDA Clinical Trial, there were five (3.7%) cases of phrenic nerve paralysis but all of them were transient [8]. Phrenic nerve paralysis can be avoided by SVC high-power pacing to confirm diaphragm movement capture (at 30–40 ppm) during right superior PV ablation. If diaphragm movement capture becomes difficult, the physician only should immediately stop ablation and move the balloon. As the phrenic nerve runs along left and right cardiac border at AP view, positioning the balloon not beyond the cardiac border (i.e., inflating balloon at Antrum) is important.

16.6.3 Esophageal Injury

In our earlier single-center study (*n* = 288), we successfully avoided esophageal injury by monitoring its temperature and injecting cooling fluid (5–10 mL each time) to keep it below

Table 16.1 Ablation setting in the multi center clinical trial

Ablation target		Set temperature and ablation time
Right superior PV	1. Ostium	70 °C × 2 min
	2. Antrum (closer to roof)	70 °C × 2 min 30 s
	3. Antrum (closer to carina)	70 °C × 2 min 30 s
Right inferior PV	4. Ostium	65 °C × 1 min 45 s
	5. Antrum	70 °C × 2 min 30 s
Left superior PV	6. Ostium	70 °C × 3 min
	7. Antrum	70 °C × 3 min
	8. Antrum (closer to carina)	70 °C × 3 min
Left inferior PV	9. Ostium	68 °C × 2 min
	10. Antrum (closer to bottom)	70 °C × 2 min 30 s

PV Stenosis in multicenter clinical trial

	Case 1	Case 2	Case 3
	LIPV Ostium	RSPV Ostium	RIPV Ostium
Transparent image	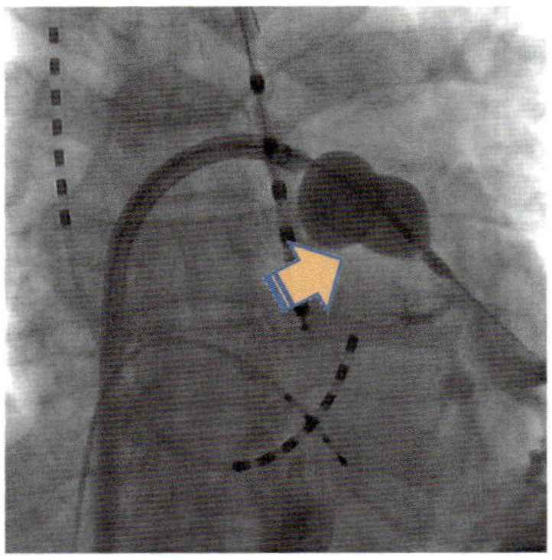	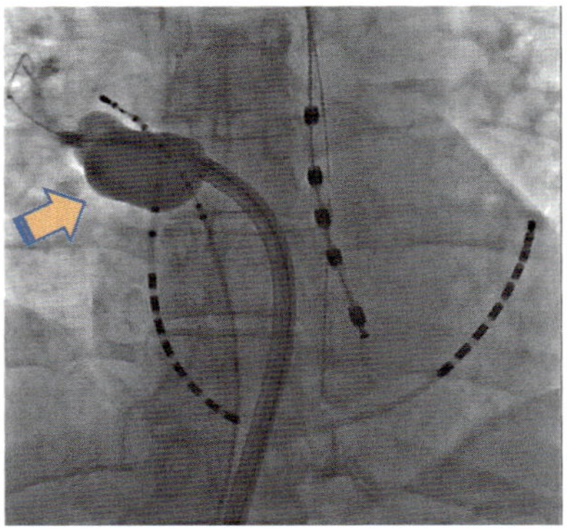	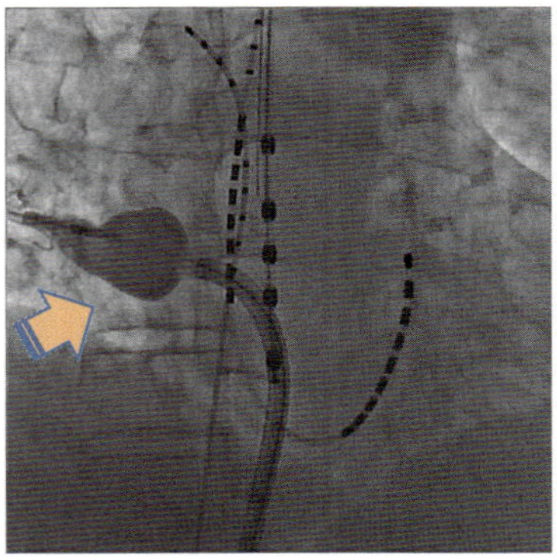
Condition	Balloon injection volume: 8.0 mL Maximum RF Generator Temperature setting: 68°C Ablation time: 2:00	Balloon injection volume: 8.0 mL Maximum RF Generator Temperature setting: 70°C Ablation time: 1:01	Balloon injection volume: 6.0 mL Maximum RF Generator Temperature setting: 65°C Ablation time: 1:45

Fig. 16.3 The characteristics of PV stenosis in multicenter clinical trial in Japan

39 °C as needed during ablation [9]. Based on this experience, the above method was strongly recommended in later PMDA clinical trials. As a result, there were no cases of damages to esophagus in the Multi-Center Clinical Trial. Since there was some events of Aspiration pneumonia when diluted contrast medium was used as cooling fluid, using only water or normal saline may be recommended as the safest way. In addition, water drainage through gastric tube every several times of cooling is recommended to prevent aspiration.

The Left Inferior PV (LIPV) is often close to the esophagus. The physician should not continue ablation without monitoring esophagus temperature or without injection of cooling fluid. In fact, severe esophagus ulcer occurred frequently when cooling fluid was not injected until the esophagus temperature rose to 43 °C [9].

There were no gastric dysmotility due to pyloric spasm which is sometimes reported in conventional radiofrequency ablation (point-by-point method).

16.7 How to Use Radiofrequency HotBalloon

16.7.1 Assess the Structure of Left Atrium and PVs

3D-CT is used to assess the diameter of each PV, particular anatomical structure (left common PV, inferior common PV), and approximate position and course of esophagus and phrenic nerve.

In our hospital, we insert two 5-Fr sheaths (RV, RA), a 4-Fr sheath (arterial line), and an 8.5-Fr SL0 sheath (intracardiac echocardiography) into the left groin. Then, the guiding sheath for HotBalloon ("TRESWALTZ": Fig. 16.2) and an 8-Fr SL0 sheath are inserted into the right groin. Both sheaths are placed in the LA by single transseptal puncture method. After positioning SL0 sheath into LSPV and TRESWALTZ into RSPV, PV venography is conducted under RV Burst pacing (180–200 ppm). At this time, the physician should confirm each visualized PV branch.

Then the physician determines in which branch the guidewire for Hot Balloon should be advanced. The pre-procedure 3D-CT image should not be cut from Lab screen because it is also used to confirm PV branches.

16.7.2 Right Superior PV (RSPV) Ablation

Ablation temperature × ablation time: 70 °C × 2.5 to 3.0 min (depend on the balloon diameter) (Table 16.2).

The physician may start from LSPV, which however sometimes causes sinus arrest due to vagal response and decrease in blood pressure due to temporary atrioventricular block. In that case, the procedure should be discontinued. Therefore, we usually start from RSPV.

As already mentioned in the paragraph on phrenic nerve paralysis, the physician should perform ablation positioning the balloon inside the cardiac border because phrenic nerve runs down along left and right cardiac border at AP view. The balloon should be inflated with a minimum of 10–12 mL of the solution. Stimulation of the phrenic nerve from SVC should be performed under high-power pacing of 15 V and held on frequency of 30–40 ppm to confirm phrenic nerve capture during ablation. If the high-power pacing does not capture phrenic nerve during ablation, the physician should immediately stop energy delivery then inflate the balloon bigger to move it to more antral position.

Although it has been also reported that C-MAP is effective for prevention of phrenic nerve paralysis [10], there has been no case of phrenic nerve paralysis with this pacing method in our hospital.

16.7.3 Right Middle PV (RMPV) Ablation (Fig. 16.4)

Ablation temperature × ablation time: 70 °C × 2.0–3.0 min (Table 16.2).

After ablation at RSPV Antrum, the physician advances guidewire more distal into the same branch of RSPV and use its action-reaction force to pull the balloon down to Carina area and make the strong contact between balloon surface and RMPV ostium. In case of large RMPV, guidewire is advanced inside and ablation is performed in the same way as RSPV.

Table 16.2 New concept of HotBalloon ABL post-marketing surveillance

Ablation target		Set temperature and ablation time
Right superior PV	1. Antrum	70 °C × 2.5–3.0 min
	2. Carina	70 °C × 2.5–3.0 min
Right inferior PV	3. Antrum	68–70 °C × 2.0 min
	4. Bottom	70 °C × 2.5 min (case by case)
Left superior PV	5. Antrum	70 °C × 3.5–4.0 min
	6. Carina	70 °C × 2.5–3.0 min (Carina area)
		70 °C × 2.5–3.0 min (Roof area)
Left inferior PV	7. Antrum	68–70 °C × 2.0–2.5 min
	8. Bottom	68–70 °C × 2.0–2.5 min (case by case)

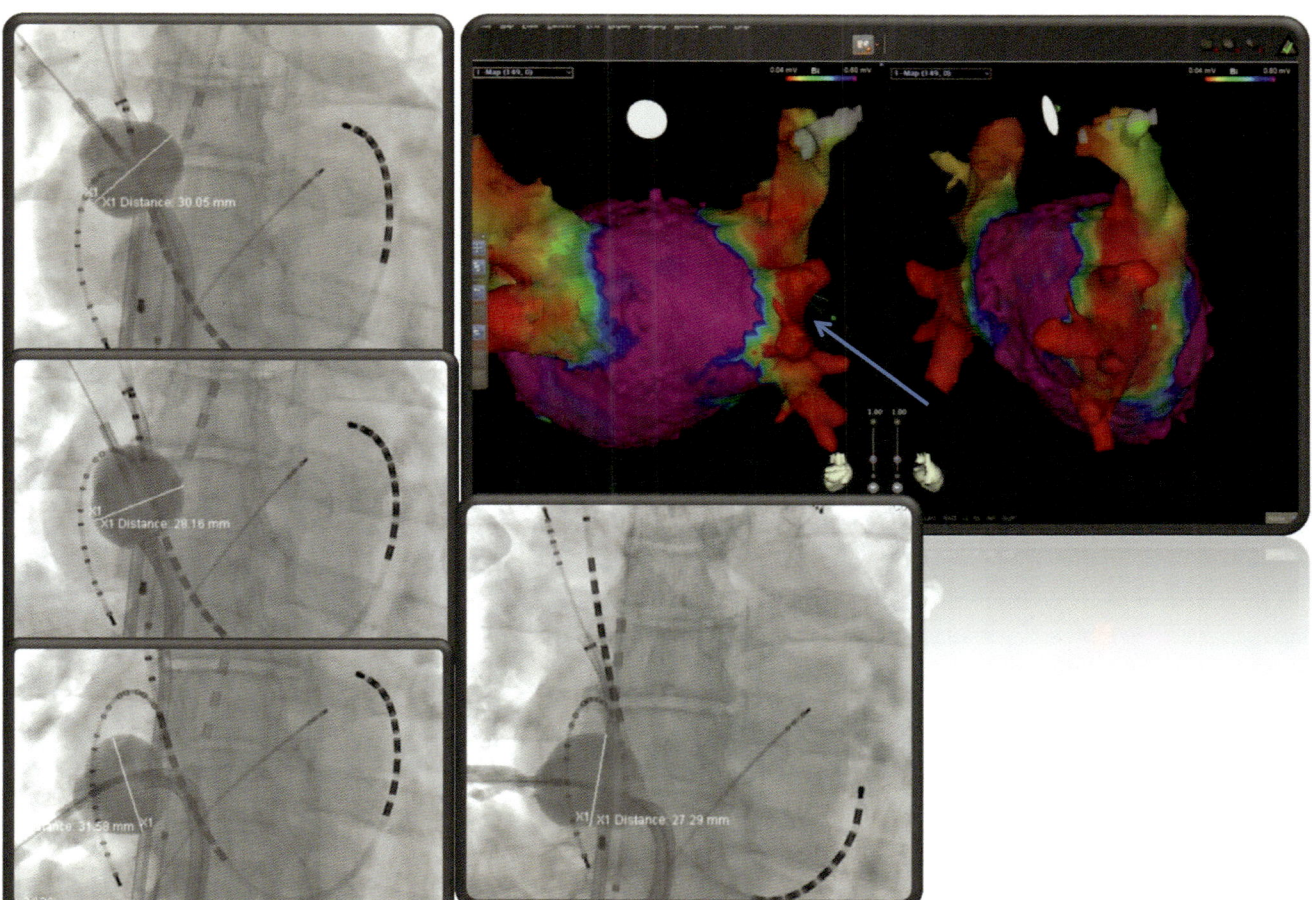

Fig. 16.4 Ablation for RMPV and RIPV

16.7.4 Right Inferior PV (RIPV) Ablation
(Fig. 16.4)

Ablation temperature × ablation time: 68 or 70 °C × 2.0 min (Table 16.2).

In the Multi-Center clinical trials, we conducted ablation at 65 °C × 1 min 45 sec positioning the balloon slightly inside the PV. Now, from a standpoint of prevention of PV stenosis, we focus on ablation with the balloon inflated with 10–12 mL (30 mm in diameter) of solution, placing it as proximal side as possible. We select either of 68 or 70 °C based on the thickness of myocardial sleeves and the balloon diameter assessed at pre-procedure CT. On the basis of the results of our Single-Center clinical study that AF tends to recur on the bottom side of RIPV [6], we hold guidewire position as inserted into PV and pull down the guiding sheath.

16.7.5 Left Superior PV (LSPV) Ablation
(Table 16.2)

16.7.5.1 Case of Normal Shape (LSPV Narrows Smoothly Toward the Left Atrium)
Ablation temperature × ablation time: 70 °C × 3.0 min (3.5–4.0 min when the balloon diameter is >30 mm).

In the past clinical trials, PV stenosis occurred in a patient ablated with the insufficiently inflated balloon inserted too distal (almost one third of the balloon into the PV). From this experience, we make sure to inflate the balloon with 11–13 mL of the solution to insert only one third of the balloon into the PV. Inflating as much as possible can prevent it from misplacement into too distal PV.

16.7.5.2 Case if LSPV Has Tubular Shape (Branching from Distal Part (Fig. 16.5))
This type of LSPV requires some technique. The balloon is inflated to 30 mm as shown above and ablation is performed for 3.5–4 min. Then, if the electric potential remains, the guidewire is advanced again into the lower branch of LSPV and the balloon is inflated to the extent that balloon tip part such as only one third of the balloon can be inserted inside of PV. With ring electrode catheter placed into the same PV, ablation is conducted at 70 °C for 3 min.

Most of gap tends to remain at anterior inferior area of LSPV. Therefore, the ring mapping catheter should be placed consciously inside of PV so that the balloon does not contact firmly to superior area of LSPV, in other words, to prevent excessive ablation. PV potential usually disappears around the first 30 s of effective ablation (Fig. 16.6 white arrow).

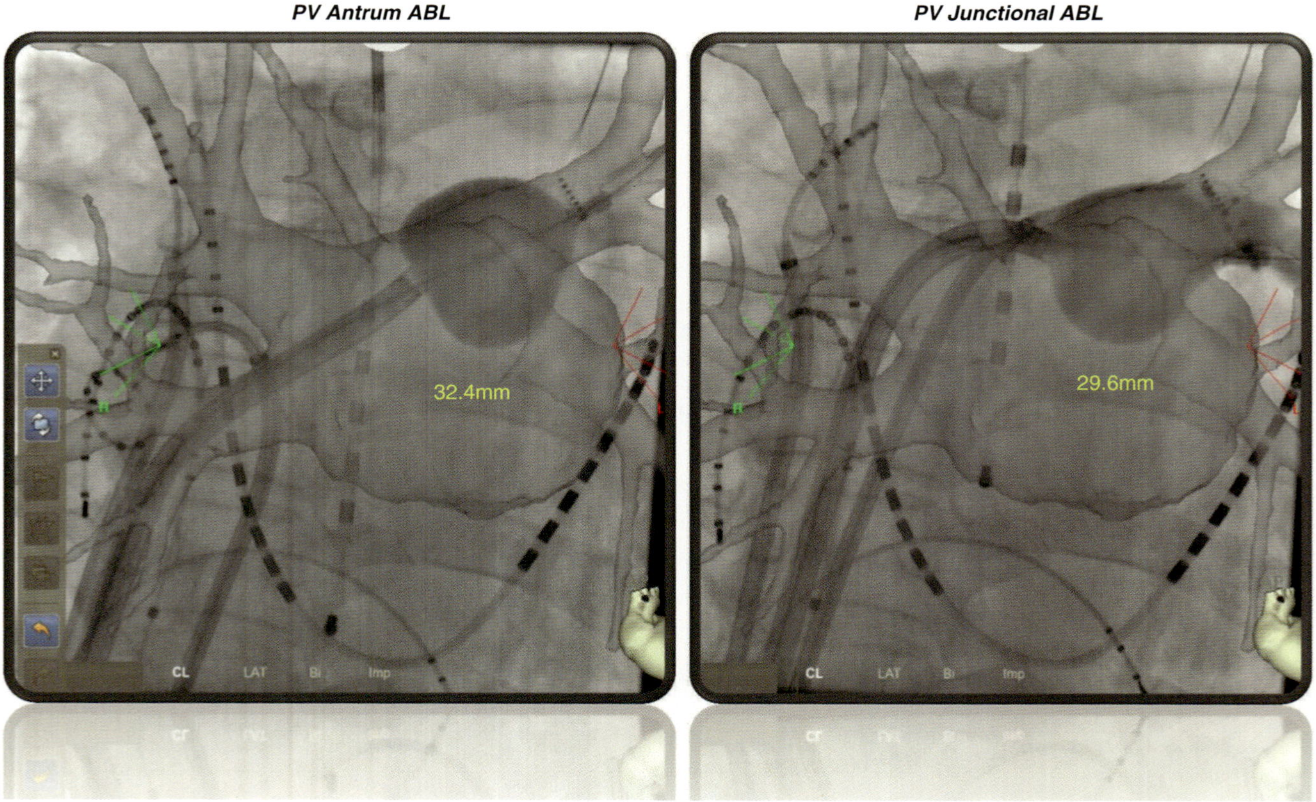

Fig. 16.5 New approach for LSPV

Fig. 16.6 PVI is available during real-time monitoring PV potentials

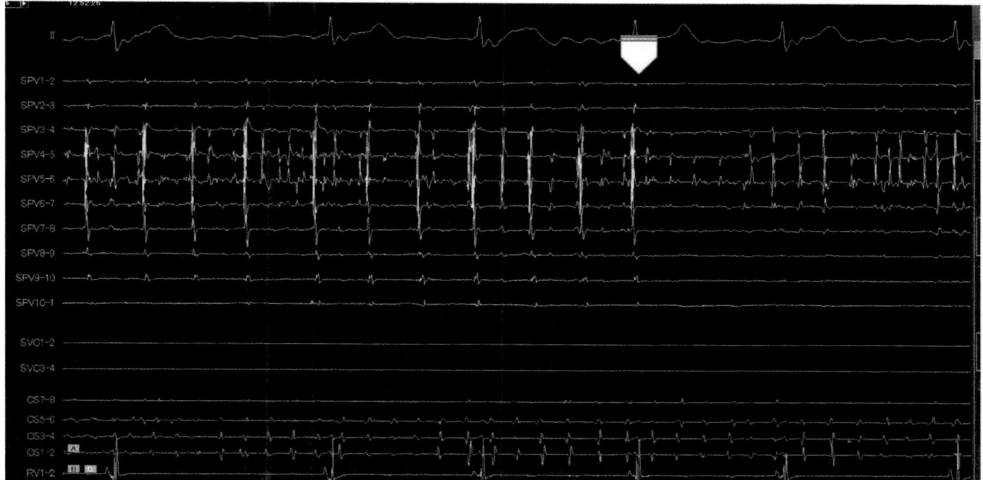

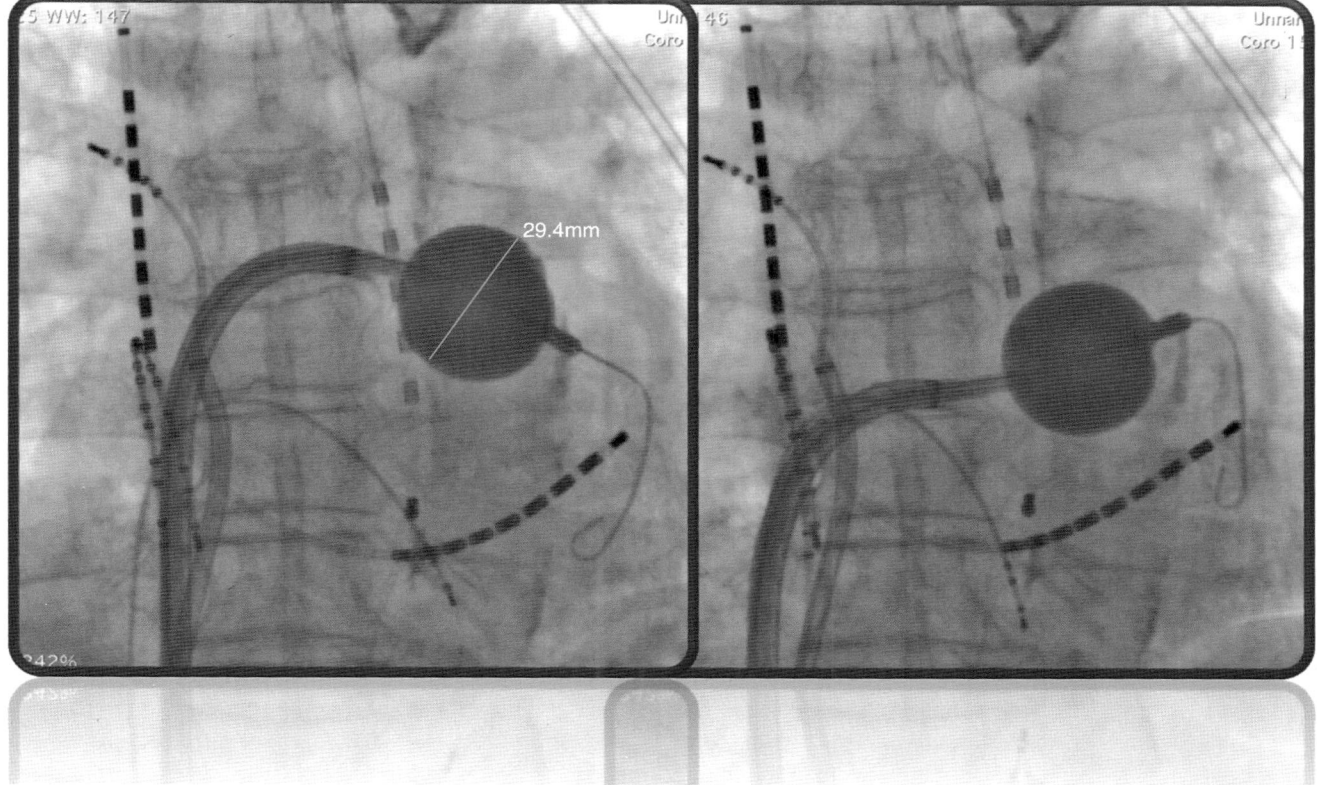

Fig. 16.7 RF delivery for LIPV (balloon position)

16.7.6 Left Inferior PV (LIPV) Ablation
(Fig. 16.7) (Table 16.2)

In the clinical trials, we had standardized on ablation at 68 °C for 2 min with the balloon inflated up to 26–28 mm and positioned at the PV ostium or near the inside. But today we perform ablation at 70 °C for 2–3 min with the balloon inflated to 30 mm and placed as close as possible to PV antrum to minimize the risk of PV stenosis. In this strategy, it is important to ablate additionally at 70 °C for 2–3 min pulling down the balloon to lower wall (bottom) of LIPV same as RIPV ablation.

16.8 Particular Anatomical Structure

16.8.1 Left Common PV

The diameter of the common PV trunk is often over 30 mm. However, as the myocardial sleeves of the PV is comparatively thin, PVI is gained with relative ease by advancing the guidewire into superior or inferior branch and then by pressing the balloon inflating it to approximate 33 mm.

16.8.2 Dilated RIPV

While pressing the balloon against the large RIPV over 25 mm in diameter requires a special attention. If we would press the insufficiently inflated balloon leads to slip into too distal in PV and can be cause of PV stenosis. The HotBalloon, with its compliance, can be inflated to 28 to 33 mm and allows effective ablation at more antral area from PV ostium (Figs. 16.8 and 16.9).

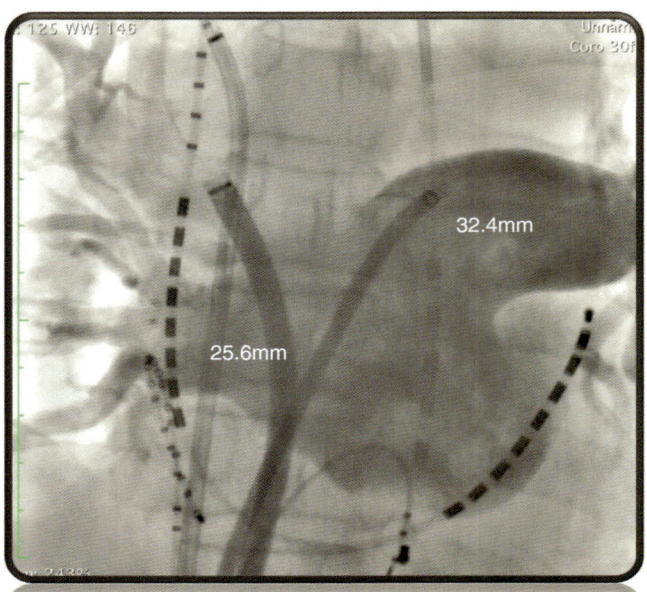

Fig. 16.8 Dilated RIPV and Lt common PV (venography)

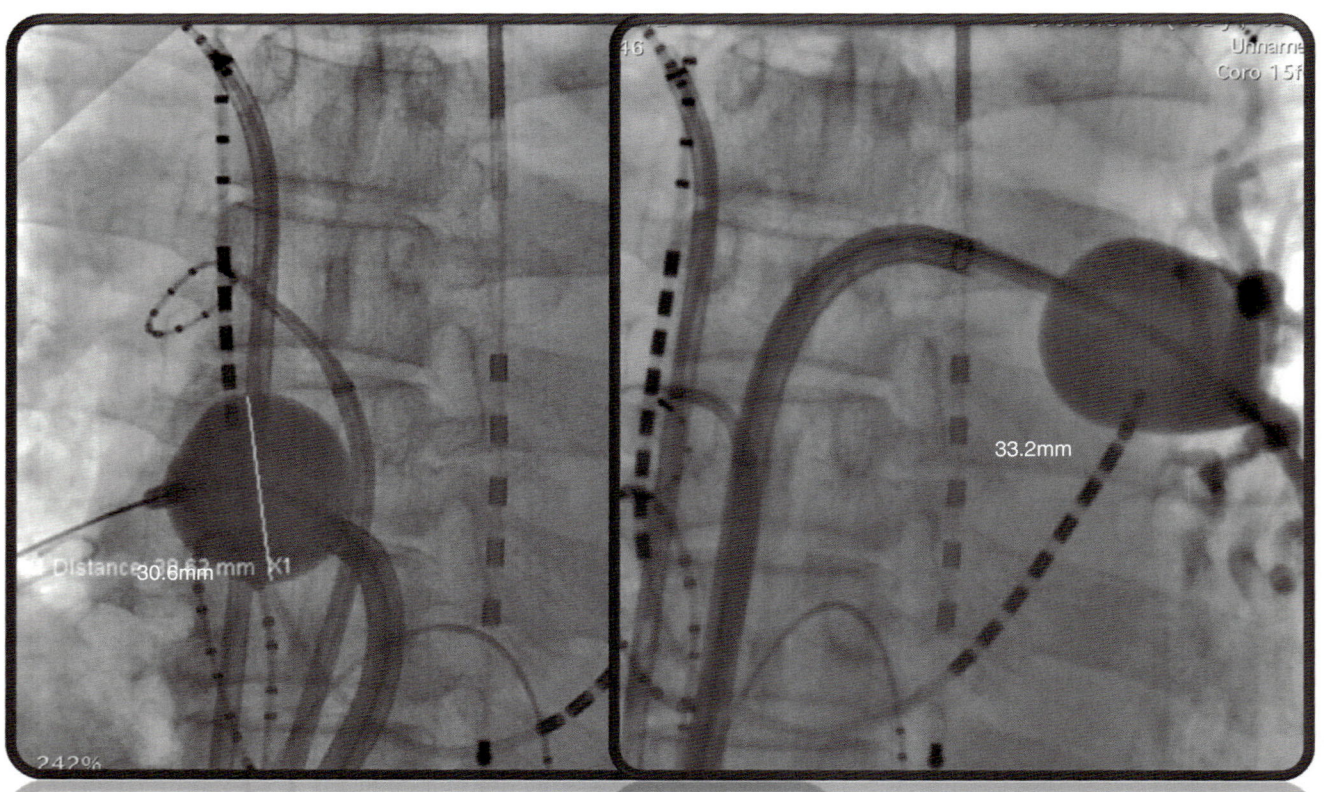

Fig. 16.9 Dilated RIPV and Lt common PV (balloon position)

16.8.3 Residual Gap

In some patients, gap may remain even though the physician attempted the standard ablation mentioned above. Especially, it appears more commonly at anterior/lower area of LSPV, and bottom area of RIPV and LIPV. In that case, the ring mapping catheter is firstly placed into the PV along with superior site already ablated (no need of further ablation). The ring catheter shaft prevents the balloon from contacting this area. Secondly, the guidewire is advanced into inferior branch of the same real-time monitoring PV potentials. Thirdly, the inflated balloon is pressed against PV so that one third of the balloon can be inserted inside and then RF energy is delivered. Typical ablation time is 2–3 min in total. Most of PVI is achieved within first 30 s of ablation (Figs. 16.5, 16.6, 16.10, and 16.11).

16.9 New Treatment Method

Monitoring PV potential during energy delivery (Figs. 16.10 and 16.11).

In this method, PVI is performed while real-time monitoring changes of PV potential with the ring mapping catheter inserted inside the same PV. The physician can see changes of activation sequence between Left Atrial(LA) and PVs, check if the direction of balloon compression is appropriate or not, and predict the effective ablation time for PV ((like a time to effect (TTE) predictable for PV reconnection)) [11]. There is no obvious malfunction at heated part of ring catheter shaft (which positioned close to balloon membrane), compared to non-heated part. Moreover, this method will be unsuitable for short PV including "early branch."

16.10 Future Tasks Found in Japan Post-marketing Surveillance and Perspectives

16.10.1 Learning Curve for Acute Success Rate Only Using HotBalloon

PMDA approval, many new physicians started to use HotBalloon catheter at recommended target ablation temperature and time. However, their PVI acute success rate

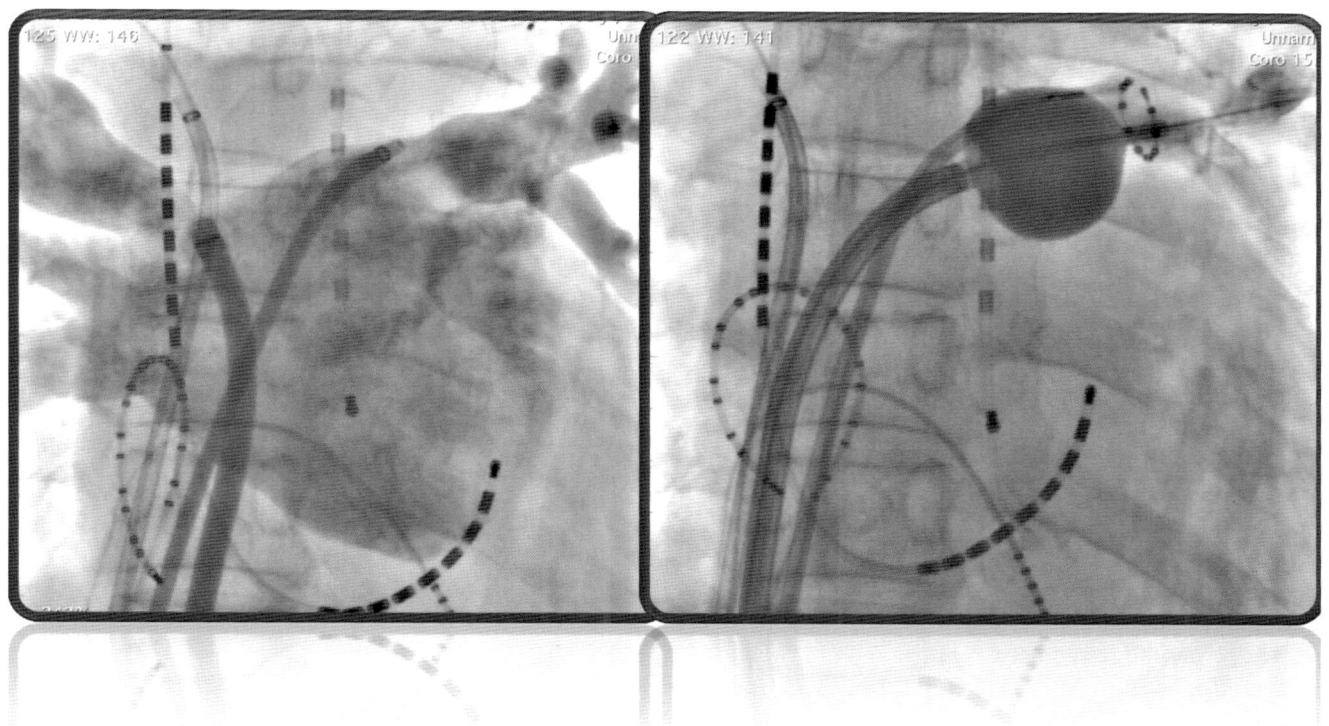

Fig. 16.10 PVI during real-time monitoring of PVP case 1: LSPV

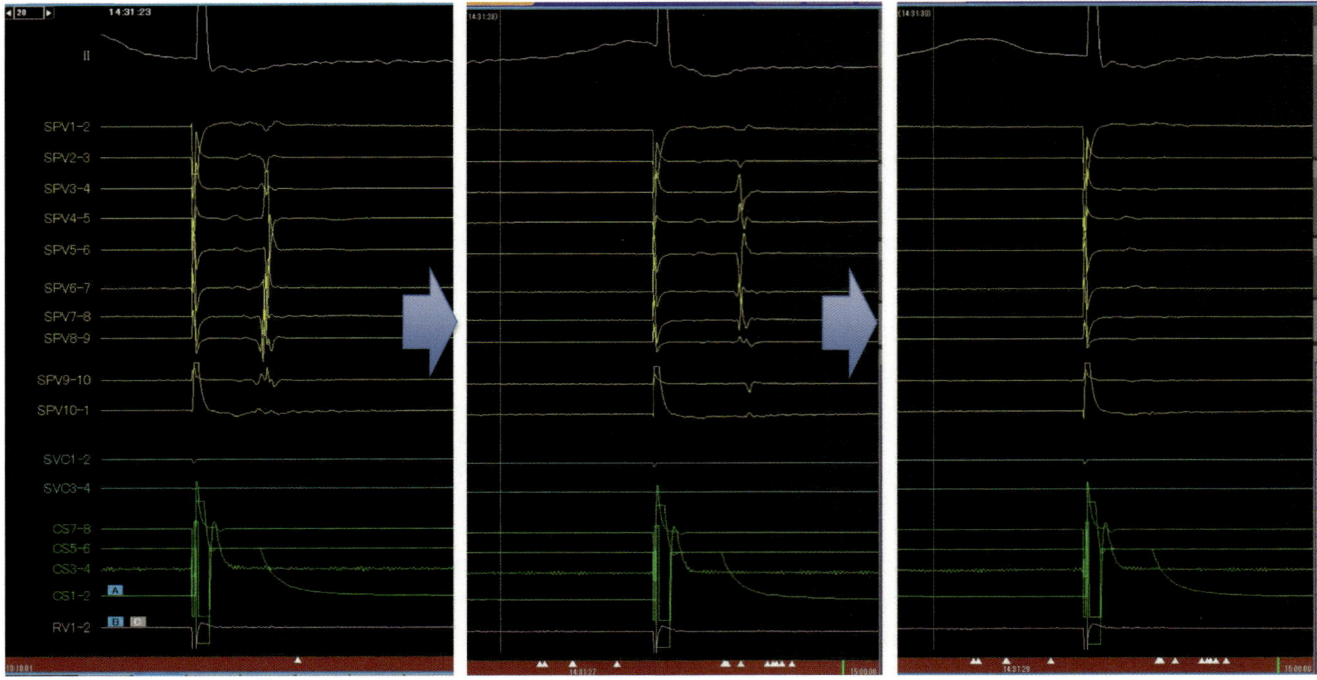

Fig. 16.11 PVI during real-time monitoring of PVP case 1: LSPV

with "HotBalloon only" is still not high as we experienced in multicenter pivotal trial. It often requires additional "touch up" ablation at some gaps by conventional, single tip point-by-point ablation catheter within the single procedure.

This has two possible causes:

16.10.1.1 Insufficient Power Control Sometimes Occurs at Radiofrequency Generator

During energy delivery, radiofrequency power is automatically controlled by its software to maintain set temperature. Power control is up to 150 W. In our experience, from 60 to 120 W seems to be the most appropriate for effective heating of the central coil electrode. In that case, it does not take long time to reach the set temperature. However, the generator sometimes take long time to reach the preset temperature and its keeping power at ablation temperature zone rises only 40 W. Besides, energy delivery sometimes gets started before the temperature reaches to the set value and its keeping power becomes high (120–150 W). We consider these may be caused by ineffective agitation of inner fluid of the balloon due to viscosity of contrast medium. Our examination showed that lowering the dilution rate (reducing viscosity) of contrast medium in the solution for balloon inflation from 50% to 33% (the proportion of contrast medium to normal saline = 1:2) increases the power to more than 40 W. Enhancing mixing function may enable power up regardless of dilution rate. Improving the function of the agitation pump is now under development.

16.10.1.2 Relationship Between Balloon Diameter and Temperature of Balloon Surface

We have been advocating ablation with well-inflated balloon on reflection of associated PV stenosis risk in clinical trials. However, the surface temperature of the balloon greater than 30 mm is found to decline slightly (about 2 °C) compared with that of the smaller-sized balloon. Therefore, with bigger balloon size, the original target ablation time in clinical trials (2–3 min per single burn) might have been insufficient. For effective ablation with bigger balloon size, this is manageable by increasing ablation time to 3.5–4 min at 70 °C for LSPV and to 2–3 min at 70 °C for RSPV considering depth of ablated tissue. Regarding RIPV and LIPV, we make sure to ablate for 2–2.5 min with set temperature of 68 and 70 °C, respectively, depending on the balloon diameter. Moreover, during RIPV and LIPV ablation, it is important to conduct additional ablation (for 2–3 min) dragging the balloon from PV antrum to more antral bottom area at the same set temperature, based on the Yamaguchi's reports that gap is likely to remain in the bottom of RIPV and LIPV [6]. Importantly no severe PV (especially in RIPV, LIPV) stenosis as long as ablation in this setting.

16.10.2 Balloon Catheter Shaft Needs Improvement

During the ablation treatment, the balloon catheter shaft slightly softens up with increasing balloon temperature and sometimes it seems to us difficult to hold the balloon. In that case, it requires pressing the guiding sheath (TRESWALTZ) slightly to the proximal end of the balloon to the extent that it would not affect the inner fluid agitation. For the future, some improvement to strengthen the catheter shaft would be needed (including embedment of a braided mesh).

16.10.3 Guiding Sheath (TRESWALTZ Steerable Sheath) Needs Improvement

TRESWALTZ is deflectable to a single direction. The flushing port (side port) of TRESWALTZ is on opposite side of that direction. It is the opposite side of that on normal sheaths, which may confuse the physician to manipulate deflection.

Besides, the guiding sheath sometimes has twisted kink when physician rotate it to place the balloon at appropriate position. In that case, it may become difficult to hold the guiding sheath and to compress the balloon to PVs.

And its outer diameter is larger (17 Fr.) than the other similar devices. For the future, downsizing improvement is to be planned.

16.11 Concluding Remarks

16.11.1 Advantages and Future of Radiofrequency HotBalloon Catheter

As mentioned above, the radiofrequency HotBalloon catheter has elastic balloon with high compliance. It enables contact to a variety of PV sizes and shapes with few anatomical limitations that occur in patients ablated with standard methods. In other words, it brings tailor-made treatments adjusting finely to PVs which anatomical structure is completely different in every case.

No other treatment device is so helpful as the HotBalloon catheter, as long as the physician keeps in mind that he/she never advance it too distal in PVs and prevent its misplacement too distal in PVs with well-inflated balloon positioned as just before PV (PV antrum) as possible.

For the future, we hope next generation device having "impedance monitoring censor" at balloon. It will enable physicians to understand the impedance change of the site of PV-Balloon contact and changes in the tissues so that we can modify set temperature and time more appropriately (by tracking the impedance change that is likely to reflect patient-by-patient tissue characteristics, myocardial thickness, and the volume of myocardial sleeves).

If there will be an option for temperature setting (currently up to only 70 °C) that makes it possible to gain sufficient lesion depth more certainly and safely, more effective and safer treatment will be feasible.

The HotBalloon catheter has just come into the world. There is a lot of room for improvement. The Cryoballoon catheter took years to release its second generation.

We sincerely hope that the second- and third generation of HotBalloon will be developed resolving each tasks mentioned above and thereby to contribute even more to treatment of catheter ablation for AF.

References

1. Natale A, Raviele A, Arentz T, Calkins H, Chen SA, Haïssaguerre M, et al. Venice Chart international consensus document on atrial fibrillation ablation. J Cardiovasc Electrophysiol. 2007;18:560–80.
2. Calkins H, Brugada J, Packer DL, Cappato R, Chen SA, Crijns HJ, et al. HRS/EHRA/ECAS expert consensus statement on catheter and surgical ablation of atrial fibrillation: recommendations for personnel, policy, procedures and follow-up. A report of the Heart Rhythm Society (HRS) Task Force on catheter and surgical ablation of atrial fibrillation. Heart Rhythm. 2007;4:816–61.
3. Tanaka K, Satake S, Saito S, Takahashi S, Hiroe Y, Miyashita Y, et al. A new radiofrequency thermal balloon catheter for pulmonary vein isolation. J Am Coll Cardiol. 2001;38:2079–86.
4. Satake S, Tanaka K, Saito S, Tanaka S, Sohara H, Hiroe Y, et al. Usefulness of a new radiofrequency thermal balloon catheter for pulmonary vein isolation: a new device for treatment of atrial fibrillation. J Cardiovasc Electrophysiol. 2003;14:609–15.
5. Sohara H, Takeda H, Ueno H, Oda T, Satake S. Feasibility of the radiofrequency hot balloon catheter for isolation of the posterior left atrium and pulmonary veins for the treatment of atrial fibrillation. Circ Arrhythm Electrophysiol. 2009;2:225–32.
6. Yamaguchi Y, Sohara H, Takeda H, Sohara H, Takeda H, Ueno H, et al. Long-term results of radiofrequency hot balloon ablation in patients with paroxysmal atrial fibrillation: safety and rhythm outcomes. J Cardiovasc Electrophysiol. 2015;26:1298–306.
7. Sohara H, Satake S, Takeda H, Yamaguchi Y, Toyama H, Kumagai K, et al. Radiofrequency hot balloon catheter ablation for the treatment of atrial fibrillation: a 3-center study in Japan. J Arrhythm. 2013;29(1):20–7.
8. Sohara H, Ohe T, Okumura K, Naito S, Hirao K, Shoda M, et al. HotBalloon ablation of the pulmonary veins for paroxysmal AF: a multicenter randomized trial in Japan. J Am Coll Cardiol. 2016;68:2747–57.
9. Sohara H, Satake S, Takeda H, Yamaguchi Y, Nagasu N. Prevalence of esophageal ulceration after atrial fibrillation ablation with the hot balloon ablation catheter: what is the value of esophageal cooling? J Cardiovasc Electrophysiol. 2014;25:686–92.
10. Miyazaki S, Hachiya H, Taniguchi H, Nakamura H, Ichihara N, Usui E, et al. Prospective evaluation of bilateral diaphragmatic electromyograms during cryoballoon ablation of atrial fibrillation. J Cardiovasc Electrophysiol. 2015;26(6):622–8.
11. Aryana A, Mugnai G, Singh SM, Pujara DK, Asmundis CD, Singh SK, et al. Procedural and biophysical indicators of durable pulmonary vein isolation during cryoballoon ablation of atrial fibrillation. Heart Rhythm. 2016;13:424–32.

Catheter Ablation of Posterior LA Isolation: Box Isolation

Koichiro Kumagai

Keywords

Atrial fibrillation • Pulmonary vein • Posterior left atrium • Box isolation

17.1 Introduction

A recent consensus of world-renowned experts in atrial fibrillation (AF) ablation states that the pulmonary vein (PV) isolation is a cornerstone of catheter ablation of AF. To prevent PV stenosis, most operators have moved toward ablation away from the PV ostium toward the level of the antrum [1–3]. The antrum blends into the posterior wall of the left atrium (LA). To encompass as much of the PV structure as possible, ablation needs to be performed around the entire antrum, along the posterior LA wall [3]. Both PVs and the posterior LA are developed from the sinus venosus, where there are many pacemaker cells with spontaneous rhythmic activity in the early embryonic heart [4]. The discrete site of high-frequency periodic activity is localized most often to the posterior LA, including the PV during AF in sheep hearts [5]. Non-PV foci originated mainly from the PV ostium or from the posterior LA [6], and the posterior LA and the LA roof serve as a substrate for maintenance of AF in the patients with AF [7, 8]. It has been proposed that the surgical procedures for isolating the posterior LA and PVs could cure AF in 93% of patients with lone AF [9]. These findings support that isolation of not only PVs but also the whole posterior LA can result in a much better cure rate in the patients with paroxysmal and persistent AF. Therefore, we developed a new approach for complete isolation of the posterior LA including all PVs, namely *Box isolation* [10] (Fig. 17.1).

K. Kumagai, M.D.
Heart Rhythm Center, Fukuoka Sanno Hospital,
3-6-45, Momochihama, Sawara-ku, Fukuoka 814-0001, Japan
e-mail: kumagai@kouhoukai.or.jp

17.2 Advantages of Box Isolation

A big difference between the box isolation and extensive two by two PV isolation is line design of the posterior LA. The total length of two horizontal lines in box isolation is usually shorter than two vertical lines in two by two continuous circular lesions (Fig. 17.2). Although total length of lines in the box isolation is shorter than the extensive PV isolation, the box isolation can isolate the posterior LA wider than two by two continuous circular lesions. Thus, box the isolation can minimize lesions and maximize success rate.

Additional linear ablation across the LA roof and mitral valve isthmus has been proposed as a strategy to improve outcomes in AF ablation. However, a recent randomized clinical study found no reduction in the rate of recurrent AF when linear ablation (roof and mitral isthmus lines) was performed in addition to PV isolation in patients with persistent AF [11]. In this study, complete conduction block across both lines was achieved in 74% of patients in the group receiving PV isolation plus lines [11]. Mitral isthmus line is generally more difficult to create conduction block compared with roof or floor line. Therefore, box isolation may be easier than mitral isthmus line for additional ablation in patients with persistent AF.

Previous studies have addressed the importance of non-PV foci in both paroxysmal and persistent AF, which tend to be located at sites such as the posterior LA, the superior vena cava, crista terminalis, coronary sinus ostium, ligament of Marshall, left atrial appendage, and atrial septum [6, 12, 13]. Non-PV foci are sometimes difficult to identify and eliminate because sometimes only one ectopic beat initiates AF or non-PV foci cannot be reproducibly induced. Therefore, if an ectopic focus originates from the posterior LA, box isolation may be better than a focal ablation. When

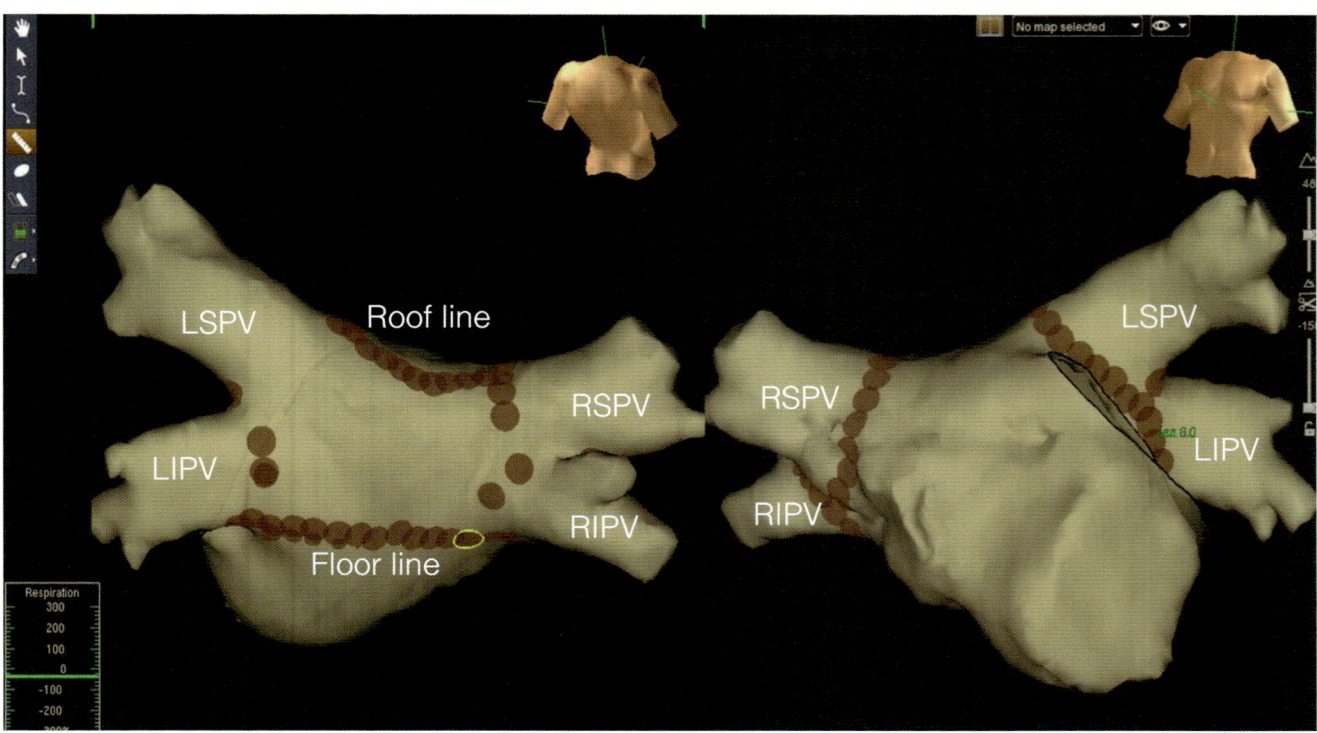

Fig. 17.1 Box isolation. *LSPV* left superior pulmonary vein, *LIPV* left inferior pulmonary vein, *RSPV* right superior pulmonary vein, *RIPV* right inferior pulmonary vein

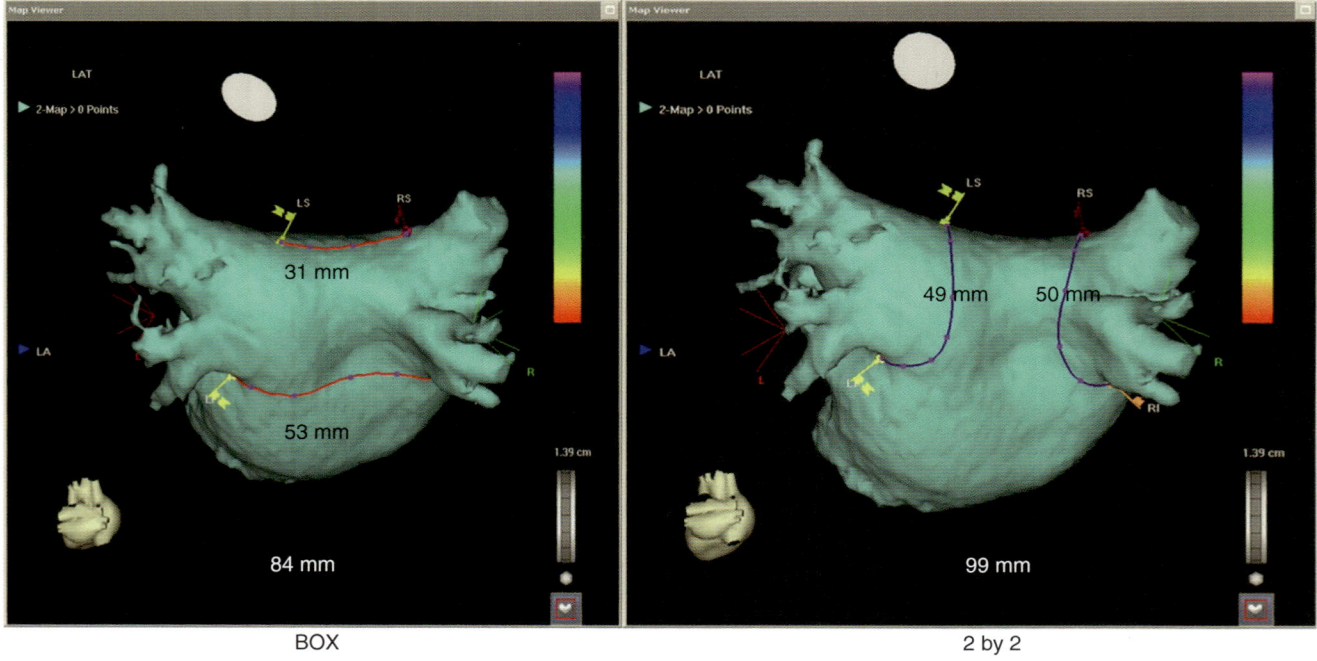

Fig. 17.2 A difference between box isolation and extensive two by two PV isolation in total length of lines. The total length of two *horizontal lines* in box isolation (84 mm) is shorter than two vertical lines in two by two PV isolation (99 mm)

non-PV foci could not be accurately mapped, box isolation may be effective because the posterior LA is the most common sites [6, 13].

17.3 Techniques and Endpoints of Box Isolation

Continuous lesions at the anterior portions of the ipsilateral superior and inferior PVs were initially created under guidance of a ring catheter and the 3D mapping system. Ablation was started at the superior wall and continued around the anterior and inferior venous perimeter. There was no vertical lesion line created at the posterior portions of the PVs along the esophageal aspect of the posterior LA. However, when PVs were not isolated by only anterior lines, segmental ablation at the breakthrough points was performed. After complete isolation of all PVs was created, ablation of the LA roof was then performed by creating a contiguous line of ablation lesions joining the superior PVs. Finally, ablation of the LA floor was performed by creating a contiguous line of ablation lesions joining the inferior PVs to isolate the posterior LA. The operator should pay attention to ablation of the esophageal aspect of the floor line by decreasing the power and duration of radiofrequency energy application. Therefore, we monitor the luminal esophageal temperature with a catheter in the esophagus at a close to the tip of the ablation catheter. During the ablation at the posterior LA close to the esophagus, the ablation was performed at a maximum power of 20 W and a temperature of 40 °C. If the esophageal temperature was higher than 40 °C, RF applications were interrupted.

Entrance block of the box lesion is confirmed by lack of potentials in box during AF or sinus rhythm (Fig. 17.3). Exit block of the box lesion is confirmed during sinus rhythm. Gaps along the ablation lines are detected and closed using high output (10 V) pacing through the ablation catheter [14] (Fig. 17.4). With lack of LA capture, the line is considered as complete at this location. In case of LA capture, a gap is suspected and radiofrequency energy is delivered simultaneously while pacing from the tip of the ablation catheter. The endpoint of box isolation is defined as bidirectional conduction block that is both lack of potentials in box and lack of LA capture [14]. Although exit block may not always be performed, this is important to prevent a recurrence of gap-related atrial flutter.

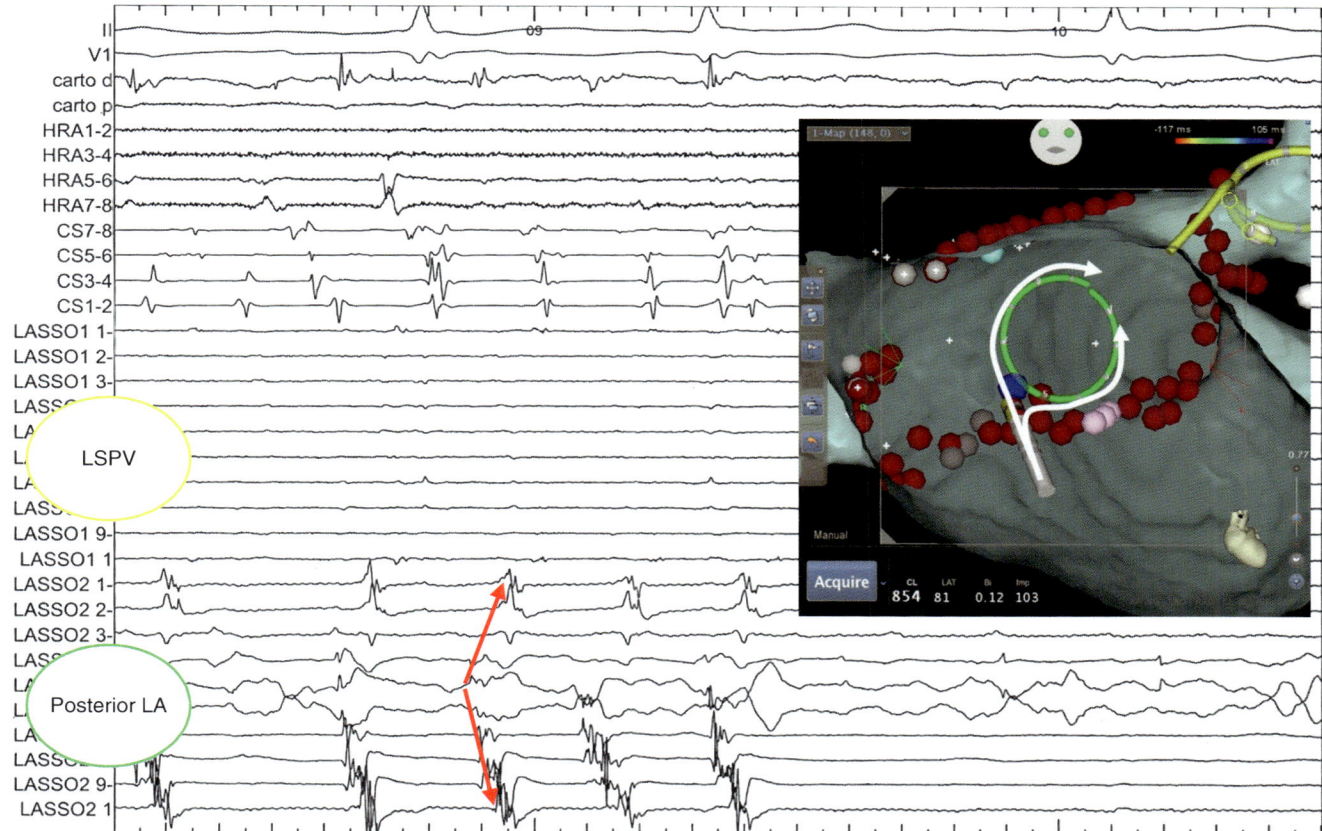

Fig. 17.3 Entrance block of the box lesion. Lasso 1 is positioned in LSPV (*yellow*) and Lasso 2 is positioned at the posterior wall within the box (*green*). Ablation of a gap at the mid floor line (Lasso #6) created the entrance block of the box lesion during AF

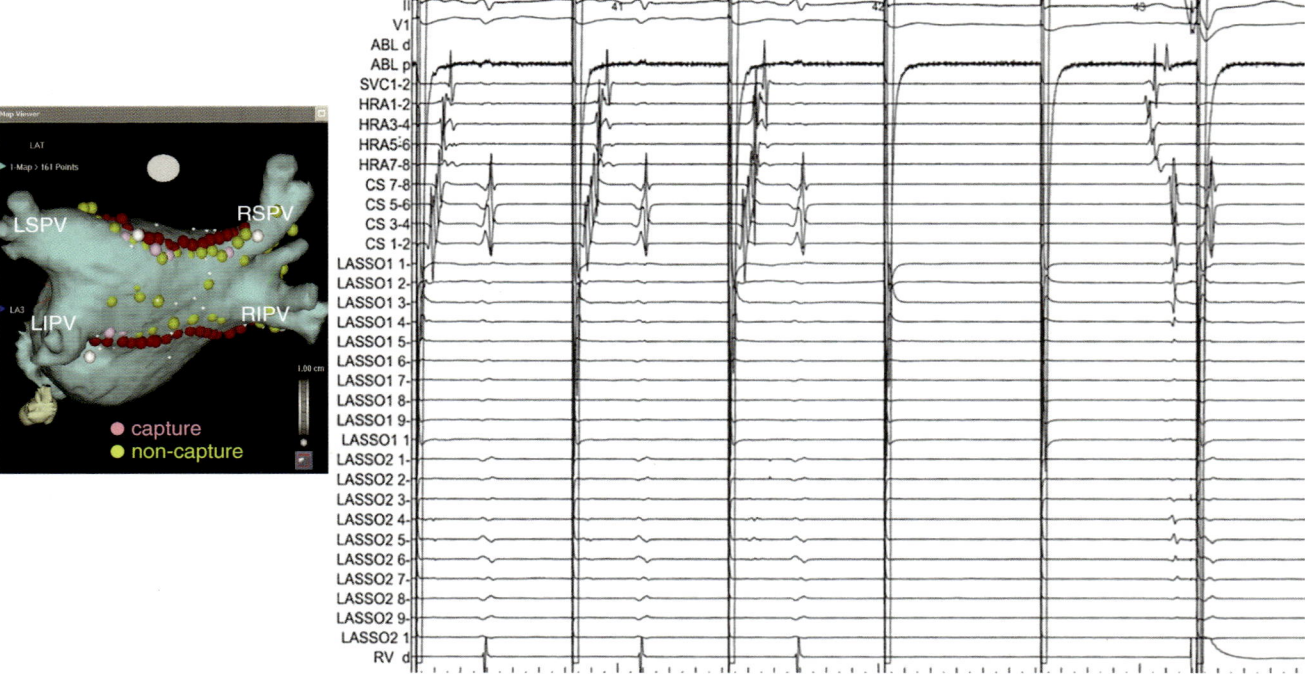

Fig. 17.4 Exit block of the box lesion. Left, during sinus rhythm, gaps along the ablation lines were detected and closed using high voltage (10 V) pace mapping through the ablation catheter. With lack of LA capture (*yellow*), the line was considered as complete at this location. In case of LA capture (*pink*), a gap was suspected and RF energy was delivered simultaneously while pacing from the tip of the ablation catheter. *Right*, ablation at the site with LA capture was continued until lack of LA capture

17.4 Clinical Outcomes

At our own institution, 513 patients including 353 with paroxysmal AF, 73 with persistent AF (<1 year, mean 5 ± 2 months), and 87 with longstanding persistent AF (>1 year, mean 5 ± 4 years) underwent box isolation. After a single procedure, AF recurred in 70 (20%) patients with paroxysmal AF, 20 (27%) patients with persistent AF, and 31 (36%) patients with longstanding persistent AF. A second procedure was performed in 39 (11%) patients with paroxysmal AF, 13 (18%) patients with persistent AF, and 26 (30%) patients with longstanding persistent AF, including atrial tachycardia or flutter in 3% of the patients. During second session, recovered conduction gaps along the lines were found in 88% of the patients and re-box isolation was performed. Additional ablation was performed in 74% of the patients, including superior vena cava isolation in 30%, mitral isthmus in 26%, focal atrial tachycardia in 24%, cavo-tricuspid isthmus in 20%, and gap-related flutter in 11%. After the follow-up period of 24 ± 8 months, 297 (84%) patients with paroxysmal AF, 58 (79%) patients with persistent AF, and 63 (72%) patients with longstanding persistent AF were free of AF without antiarrhythmic drugs.

17.5 Procedure Complications

Cardiac tamponade occurred in five patients (1.0%). This was managed by percutaneous drainage. One patient had homonymous hemianopsia. One patient had phrenic nerve injury, but recovered fully within three months. One patient had gastric hypomotility, but recovered fully within two weeks. No atrio-esophageal fistula, significant PV stenosis or procedure-related death occurred.

17.6 Impact of Box Isolation in Persistent AF

Some patients with paroxysmal AF may be undertreated with PV isolation alone and PV isolation is not enough for cure of persistent AF. Further modification of atrial substrate maintaining AF seems necessary in some patients. In the posterior LA, there are many arrhythmogenic substrates for AF, including the ganglionated plexi, reentries, triggers, and low-voltage areas [14, 15]. Box isolation can contain these abnormal substrates in the posterior LA and reduce the critical mass for maintenance of AF. Additional posterior LA isolation to PV isolation facilitates AF termination and non-inducibility (Fig. 17.5).

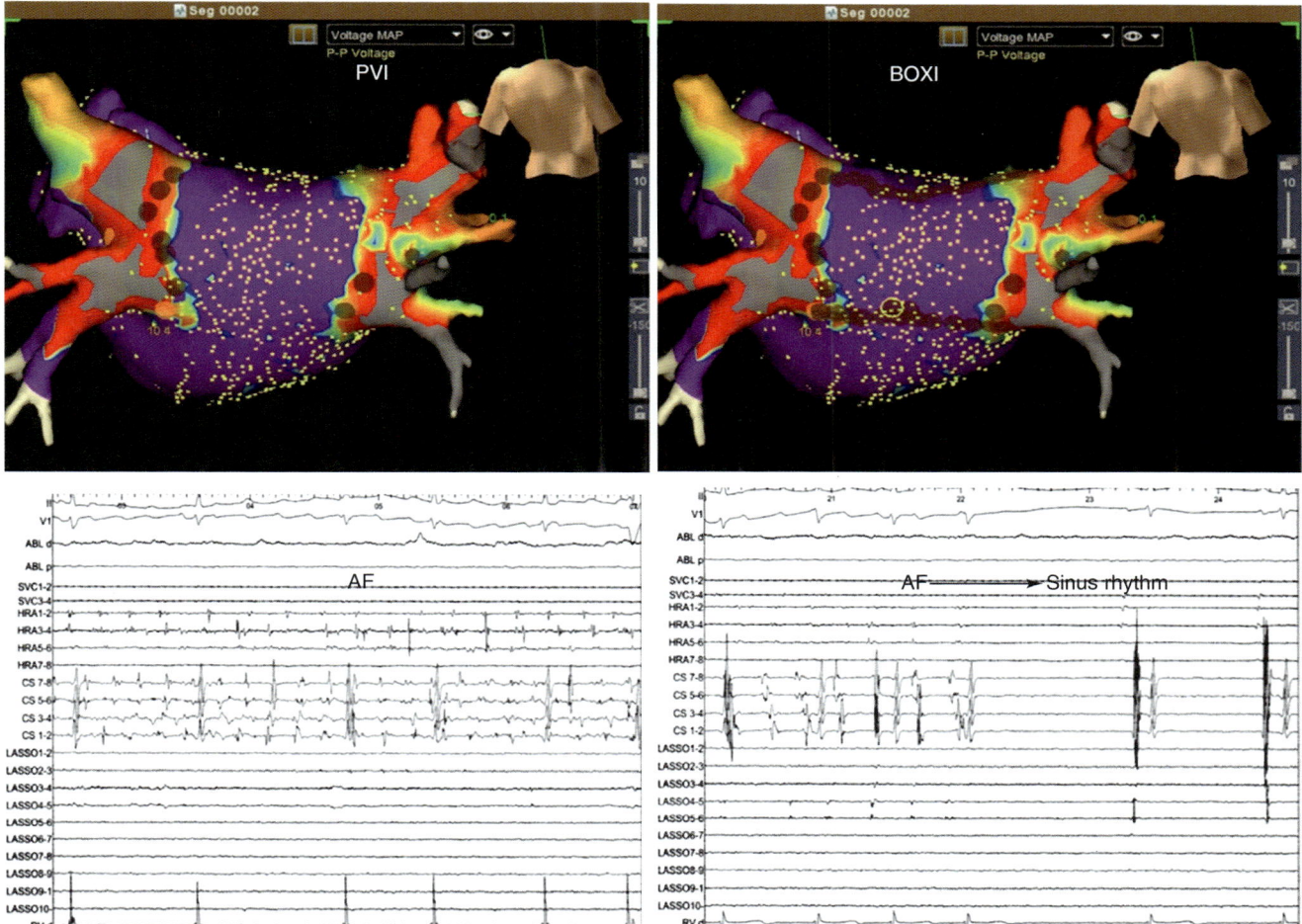

Fig. 17.5 Additional effects of posterior LA isolation to PV isolation. After PV isolation, AF still sustained (*left panel*) and was cardioverted. AF was re-induced by rapid atrial pacing, then roof and floor linear ablation isolating the posterior LA was subsequently performed during AF. AF terminated during posterior LA isolation (*right panel*). After posterior LA isolation, AF was no longer inducible

Previous studies reported that box isolation is an effective and safe treatment for paroxysmal or persistent AF [16–21]. A meta-analysis showed that box isolation reduced AF recurrence with comparable recurrence rates of atrial tachycardia/flutter, complications, and procedure time compared with PV isolation alone [21]. A prospective randomized clinical trial demonstrated that box isolation in addition to PV isolation plus linear lesions resulted in superior AF free survival compared with PV isolation plus linear lesions without deterioration of LA pump function in patients with persistent AF [22].

References

1. Yamane T, Date T, Kanzaki Y, et al. Segmental pulmonary vein antrum isolation using the "large-size" lasso catheter in patients with atrial fibrillation. Circ J. 2007;71:753–60.
2. Ouyang F, Bansch D, Ernst S, et al. Complete isolation of left atrium surrounding the pulmonary veins: new insights from the double-Lasso technique in paroxysmal atrial fibrillation. Circulation. 2004;110:2090–6.
3. Verma A, Marrouche NF, Natale A. Pulmonary vein antrum isolation: intracardiac echocardiography-guided technique. J Cardiovasc Electrophysiol. 2004;15:1335–40.
4. Kamino K. Optical approaches to ontogeny of electrical activity and related functional organization during early heart development. Physiol Rev. 1991;71:53–91.
5. Mandapati R, Skanes A, Chen J, et al. Stable macroreentrant source as a mechanism of atrial fibrillation in the isolated sheep heart. Circulation. 2000;101:194–9.
6. Lim WS, Tai CT, Hsieh MH, et al. Catheter ablation of paroxysmal atrial fibrillation initiated by non-pulmonary vein ectopy. Circulation. 2003;107:3176–83.
7. Marcids V, Schilling RJ, Ho SY, et al. Characterization of left atrial activation in the intact human heart. Circulation. 2003;107:733–9.
8. Hocini M, Jais P, Sanders P, et al. Techniques, evaluation, and consequences of linear block at the left atrial roof in paroxysmal atrial fibrillation: a prospective randomized study. Circulation. 2005;112:3688–96.
9. Todd DM, Skanes AC, Guiraudon G, et al. Role of the posterior left atrium and pulmonary veins in human lone atrial fibrillation:

electrophysiological and pathological data from patients undergoing atrial fibrillation surgery. Circulation. 2003;108:3108–14.
10. Kumagai K, Muraoka S, Mitsutake C, et al. A new approach for complete isolation of the posterior left atrium including pulmonary veins for atrial fibrillation. J Cardiovasc Electrophysiol. 2007;18:1047–52.
11. Verma A, Jiang CY, Betts TR, et al. STAR AF II Investigators. Approaches to catheter ablation for persistent atrial fibrillation. N Engl J Med. 2015;372:1812–22.
12. Chang HY, Lo LW, Lin YJ, et al. Long-term outcome of catheter ablation in patients with atrial fibrillation originating from non-pulmonary vein ectopy. J Cardiovasc Electrophysiol. 2013;24:250–8.
13. Hayashi K, An Y, Nagashima M, Hiroshima K, et al. Importance of nonpulmonary vein foci in catheter ablation for paroxysmal atrial fibrillation. Heart Rhythm. 2015;12(9):1918–24.
14. Kumagai K. Catheter ablation of atrial fibrillation. State of the art. Circ J. 2011;75(10):2305–11.
15. Yamaguchi Y, Kumagai K, Nakashima H, et al. Long-term effects of box isolation on sympathovagal balance in atrial fibrillation. Circ J. 2010;74:1096–103.
16. Lim TW, Koay CH, See VA, et al. Single-ring posterior left atrial (box) isolation results in a different mode of recurrence compared with wide antral pulmonary vein isolation on long-term follow-up: longer atrial fibrillation-free survival time but similar survival time free of any atrial arrhythmia. Circ Arrhythm Electrophysiol. 2012;5(5):968–77.
17. Nalliah C, Lim TW, Bhaskaran A, et al. Posterior left atrial isolation for atrial fibrillation in left ventricular diastolic impairment is associated with better arrhythmia free survival. Int J Cardiol. 2015;184:674–9.
18. O'Neill L, Hensey M, Nolan W, et al. Clinical outcome when left atrial posterior wall box isolation is included as a catheter ablation strategy in patients with persistent atrial fibrillation. J Interv Card Electrophysiol. 2015;44(1):63–70.
19. Cutler MJ, Johnson J, Abozguia K, et al. Impact of voltage mapping to guide whether to perform ablation of the posterior wall in patients with persistent atrial fibrillation. J Cardiovasc Electrophysiol. 2016;27(1):13–21.
20. Roberts JD, Gerstenfeld EP. Concomitant isolation of the pulmonary veins and posterior wall using a box lesion set in a patient with persistent atrial fibrillation and variant pulmonary venous anatomy. Cardiovasc Electrophysiol Clin. 2016;8(1):145–9.
21. He X, Zhou Y, Chen Y, et al. Left atrial posterior wall isolation reduces the recurrence of atrial fibrillation: a meta-analysis. J Interv Card Electrophysiol. 2016;46:267–74.
22. Kim JS, Shin SY, Na JO, et al. Does isolation of the left atrial posterior wall improve clinical outcomes after radiofrequency catheter ablation for persistent atrial fibrillation?: A prospective randomized clinical trial. Int J Cardiol. 2015;181:277–83.

Isolation of Superior Vena Cava

Koji Higuchi

Keywords
Atrial fibrillation · Arrhythmogenic SVC · SVC isolation

18.1 Introduction

Since pulmonary veins (PVs) were found to be playing an important role in triggering atrial fibrillation (AF) [1], catheter ablation has been a promising method in the treatment of atrial fibrillation which potentially cure AF radically. The cornerstone procedure of AF ablation is the electrical isolation of PVs (PVI) from the left atrium (LA) by ablating PV antrum regions in the LA since ectopic beats initiating AF mostly originate from PVs. However, ectopic beats initiating AF also arise from non-PV foci; superior vena cava (SVC), LA posterior wall, crista terminalis, coronary sinus ostium, ligament of Marshall, and interatrial septum [2–5]. Approximately 20% of AF patients have non-PV foci although it differs according to clinical studies [2, 3, 5]. Of these sites, SVC is the most common source of ectopies which harbors approximately 30% of non-PV foci [3, 4, 6]. SVC often becomes an important target during AF ablation [6–8].

18.2 Embryogenesis, Histological Findings of SVC

18.2.1 Embryogenesis and Arrhythmogenicity of SVC Alike PVs

Right anterior cardinal vein is incorporated into the primitive right atrium to form a future SVC together with the right sinus horn. Right sinus horn forms the sinus venosus in the right atrium of the embryo which becomes a smooth part called the sinus venarum in the adult heart which is separated from the rest of the right atrium by a ridge of fibers called the crista terminalis. The sinus venosus also forms the SA node and the coronary sinus which contain cells of the cardiac conduction system.

PVs grow from the LA as the following process: a primitive vein sprouts out of the LA, which bifurcates twice to make four PVs that grow toward developing lungs. A plexus of veins is formed from lungs and will meet with the developing PVs out of the LA to establish a connection. As the LA develops, the common PV is progressively incorporated into the LA wall until all four PVs enter the posterior wall of the LA separately. The incorporated PVs form the smooth posterior wall of the LA, whereas the trabeculated portion of the LA occupy a more anterior part of the LA.

There are remnants of cardiac conduction system (pacemaker cell) in SVC and PVs, as in crista terminalis and coronary sinus from which atrial tachyarrhythmias frequently occur. Since these remnants in SVC and PVs can become arrhythmogenic foci triggering AF [9–11], treating AF triggers from SVC as well as PVs is important in catheter ablation of AF.

18.2.2 Histological Findings of SVC Myocardium

The postmortem study of Kholová et al. using 25 human autopsied hearts, the myocardial extension from RA to SVC was recognized in 19/25 SVCs (76%), and SVC-RA myocardial connection was discontinuous in most cases and circumferential in few cases, with the mean thickness of 1.2 ± 1.0 mm and a mean length of 13.7 ± 13.9 mm (maximum, up to

K. Higuchi, M.D.
Hiratsuka Kyosai Hospital, 9-11 Oiwake, Hiratsuka,
Kanagawa-Prefecture 254-8502, Japan
e-mail: khigu1013@gmail.com

47 mm) [12]. Heterogeneous fiber arrangements and degenerative changes of myocardium with penetrating fibrous tissue are often recognized in SVC myocardium, which could potentially form substrates for heterogeneity of electrical coupling and an arrhythmogenicity [12, 13].

18.3 Mechanism of Arrhythmogenicity in SVC

18.3.1 SVC as an Initiator of AF

Sicouri et al. [14] demonstrated in their study using canine SVC preparations that the late phase 3 early afterdepolarization (EAD) and the delayed afterdepolarization (DAD)-mediated extrasystoles as well as the abnormal automaticity may serve as triggers of AF, which were also observed in PV preparations. The exposure to isoproterenol, high calcium, or their combination amplified the extrasystoles by late phase 3 EAD and the DAD.

SVC-aorta ganglionated plexi (GP) is located in the medial SVC and aortic root, superior to the right pulmonary artery. SVC-aorta GP serves as a relay station between extrinsic and intrinsic cardiac autonomic nervous systems [15]. High-frequency stimulation of the SVC-aorta GP or acetylcholine injection into SVC-aorta GP can induce a significant shortening of the effective refractory period and subsequent AF originating from the SVC. These effects can be eliminated after the ablation of SVC-aorta GP [16]. These findings suggest that the SVC-aorta GP plays an important role in the initiation of AF from the SVC, especially in vagal AF.

18.3.2 SVC as a Perpetuator of AF

In the study of Higuchi et al. using a fluoroscopy and a 3D electro-anatomical mapping, myocardial extensions in the SVC of patients with SVC-related AF were significantly longer than those of patients without SVC-related AF (34.7 ± 4.4 mm, vs. 16.5 ± 11.4 mm, $P < 0.0001$). Some patients without SVC-related AF did not have any myocardial extensions in the SVC [8]. In a subset of SVC-related AF patients, the SVC fibrillation with passive conduction to right atrium (RA) is observed after initiation of AF from the SVC. SVC sometimes plays a role as a perpetuator of AF [17]. An example of intra-SVC fibrillation is shown in Fig. 18.1. A certain amount of myocardium in the SVC is essential to serve as a substrate of AF, not only as an initiator of AF [18]. Figure 18.2 shows the 3D electro-anatomical mapping which shows the myocardial extension in the SVC of a patient with a SVC-related AF. Note that the myocardial extension is recognized until 41.8 mm above the SVC-RA junction. Histological findings support that SVC can be a perpetuator (substrate) of AF [12, 13].

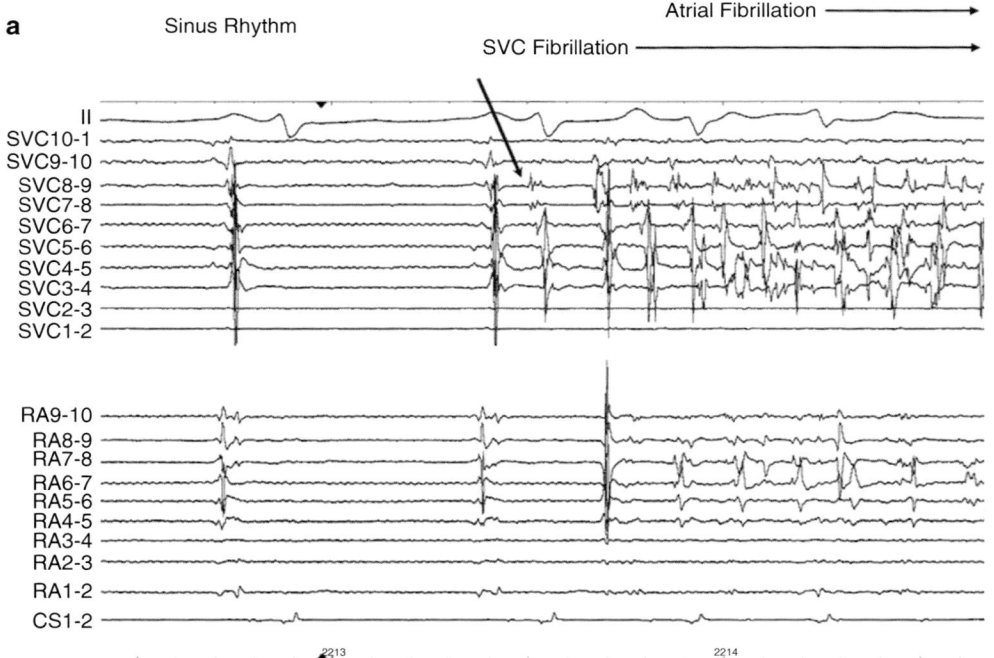

Fig. 18.1 A case of AF initiated from the SVC. Ectopic beats initiated a SVC fibrillation, and then AF started (**a**). Note the SVC fibrillation (tachycardia cycle length was 80–100 ms) with passive conductions to RA (**b**). SVC was an initiator and also a perpetuator of this AF. *SVC*, *RA* right atrium, *CS* coronary sinus, *ABL* ablation, *AF* atrial fibrillation

Fig. 18.1 (continued)

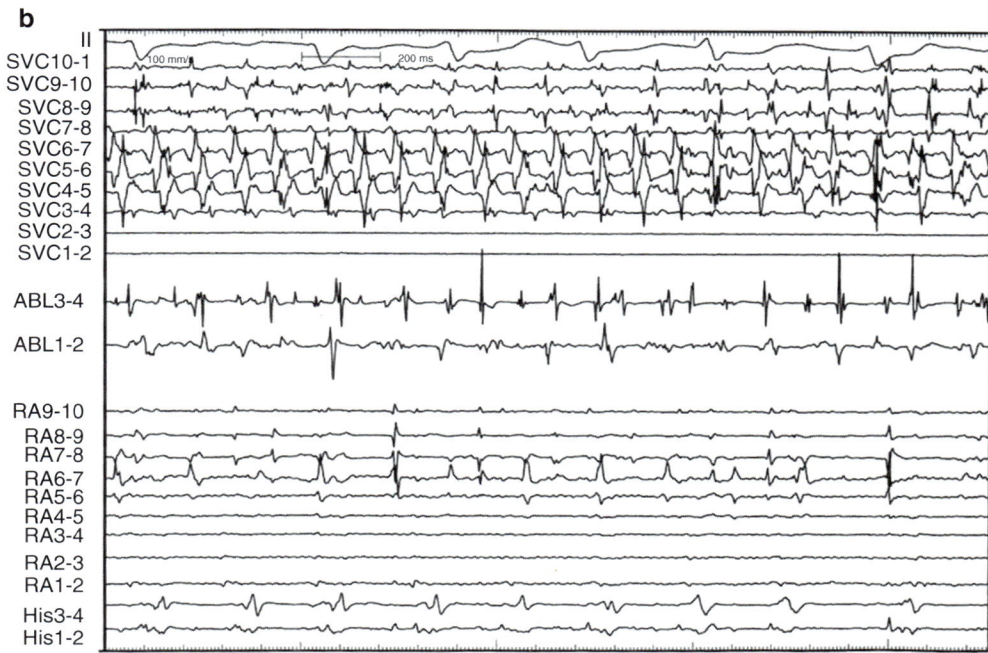

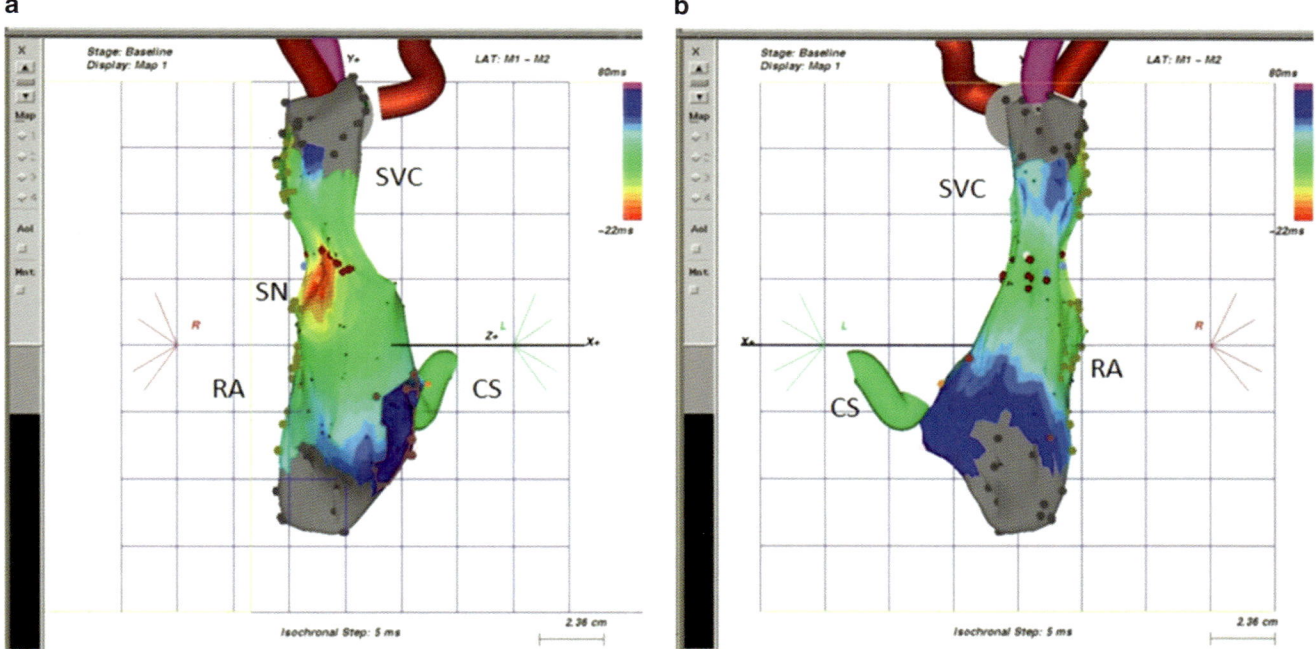

Fig. 18.2 Sinus activation by 3D electro-anatomical mapping of the SVC and the RA in a SVC-related AF patient (**a**: LAO view, **b**: RAO view). The earliest activation site indicates the location of sinus node. The SVC myocardial extension was recognized until 41.8 mm above the SVC-RA junction. *SVC* superior vena cava, *RA* right atrium, *CS* coronary sinus, *SN* sinus node, *LAO* left anterior oblique, *RAO* right anterior oblique

18.4 Induction of SVC Trigger and Procedure of SVC Isolation

18.4.1 SVC Trigger Induction

The basic maneuver to induce AF triggers is as follows: (1) Induce AF by high-frequency pacing from catheters placed in the RA, the coronary sinus, PVs, or SVC with intravenous infusion of isoproterenol (0.5–2 μg/min/kg) as necessary. (2) Recover sinus rhythm by electrical cardioversion. (3) Ectopic beats triggering AF can be recognized after cardioversion. Interestingly, in the study of Lin et al., only two patients had spontaneous SVC-AF. Eleven patients needed isoproterenol infusion with pacing-triggered ectopic beats to induce SVC-AF, and 15 patients had SVC-AF after electrical cardioversion of AF. It means that over 90% of SVC-AF needs isoproterenol infusion and/or pacing maneuver to be induced [2].. Similar finding was also reported in the experimental dog model, in which autonomic influences promoted spontaneous automaticity and triggered activity in SVC sleeves [14]. Thus, isoproterenol infusion, pacing maneuver, and cardioversion are often needed to recognize SVC triggers.

18.4.2 Procedure of SVC Isolation

Formerly, the arrhythmogenic focus inside the SVC was carefully examined under the guidance of a multipolar catheter or a basket catheter placed in the SVC, and focal ablation at arrhythmogenic foci in the SVC was performed [7]. The arrhythmogenic focus inside the SVC is located relatively far from the SVC-RA junction (Lin et al. 25.3 ± 9.7 mm, 29 ± 19.9 mm [2], Tsai et al. 19 ± 9.7 mm [7], Higuchi et al. 25.4 mm, 32.2 mm [8]). However, since arrhythmogenic foci can be multiple and SVC also has the role of maintaining AF (substrate of AF) same as PVs, the recent standard method is the electrical isolation of SVC (SVCI). SVCI can be obtained by ablating about 5 mm above the SVC-RA junction under the guidance of 3D electro-anatomical mapping and a circular mapping catheter placed above the SVC-RA junction. The SVC-RA junction should be defined "electrically" since the sinus node is located just beneath the SVC-RA junction. The SVC-RA junction can be defined by the presence of merged SVC and local RA potential recorded from a circular mapping catheter. Note the difference of electrical and anatomical SVC-RA junction (Fig. 18.3a). Sharp SVC potentials and far-field small RA potentials can be recognized when the circular mapping catheter is placed about 5 mm above the SVC-RA junction (Fig. 18.3b). The ideal SVCI line is just beneath the circular mapping catheter at that level. Usually, SVCI can be achieved by ablating the earliest activation of SVC potentials during sinus rhythm in a point-by-point fashion using a 3D electro-anatomical mapping, not by a circumferential ablation (Fig. 18.3c) [19]. The AF free survival 5 years after segmental SVCI was same as circumferential SVCI, which means that the segmental point-by-point ablation is sufficient for treating SVC-related AF [20]. SVCI is recommended to

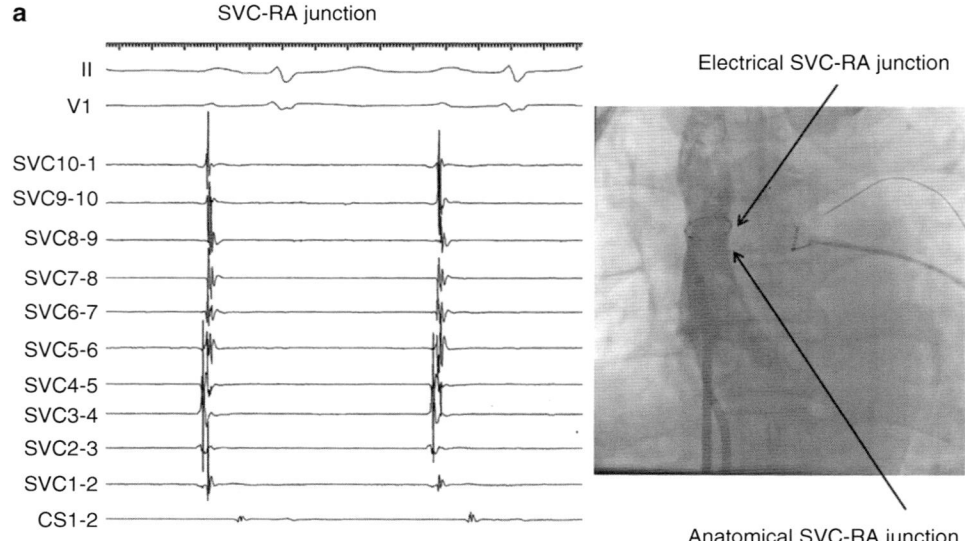

Fig. 18.3 (a) Local electrograms at the electrical SVC-RA junction. Sharp RA potentials at SVC 3–4, SVC 4–5 can be recognized. Note that anatomical SVC-RA junction is located far below the electrical SVC-RA junction. (b) SVC electrograms 5 mm above the SVC-RA junction. Sharp SVC potentials and far-field small RA potentials can be recognized. (c) 3D electro-anatomical mapping of SVC isolation. Gaps of ablation points can be seen from LAO and RAO view (see *arrows*). The *green point* indicates the successful point of SVC isolation at lateral wall of the SVC. *Blue points* indicate ablation points. The *broken line* is the electrical SVC-RA junction. *SVC* superior vena cava, *RA* right atrium, *LAO* left anterior oblique, *RAO* right anterior oblique

Fig. 18.3 (continued)

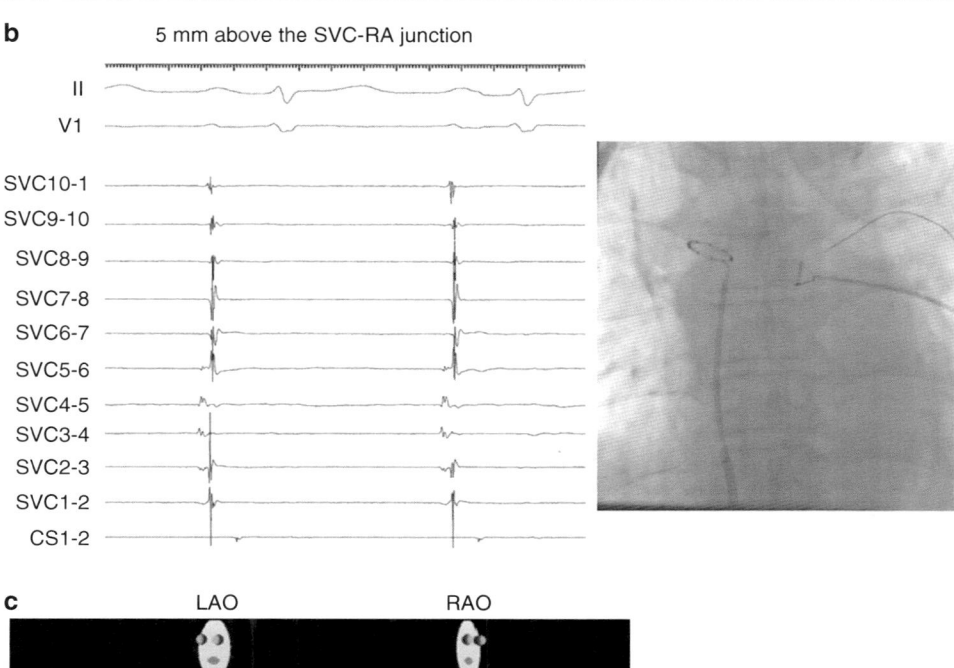

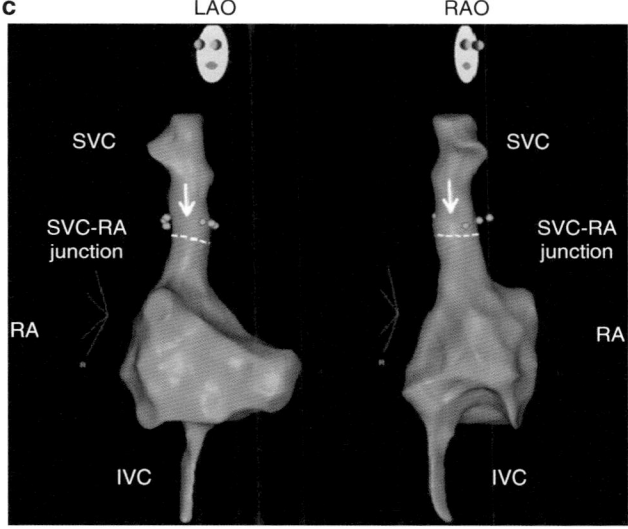

be started from the septal wall of SVC since serious complications such as right phrenic nerve injury (RFNI) mostly occurs at the lateral wall.

18.5 Possible Complications of SVC Isolation

Possible complications of SVCI and maneuvers to avoid complications are summarized in Table 18.1.

18.5.1 Right Phrenic Nerve Injury

RFNI is the most common complication. The right phrenic nerve is close to the SVC superiorly and adjacent to the lateral border of the entrance of the inferior vena cava to the right atrium inferiorly. While the right phrenic nerve is immediately adjacent to the anterolateral wall of the SVC, it veers posteriorly as it approaches the SVC-RA junction. RFNI often occurs during RF applications on the posterolateral aspect of the SVC, and it causes a right-side diaphragm paralysis. RFNI mostly recovers within one year [21], however, confirming not to capture the right phrenic nerve by a pacing maneuver should be performed before RF applications. Additionally, the movement of right diaphragm should be checked periodically using a fluoroscopy to detect RFNI as soon as possible. Compound motor action potential (CMAP), which is the monitor for detecting RFNI during cryoballoon ablation, is also a useful method in detecting RFNI in the early stage [22]. When ablating lateral wall of SVC, RF energy should be started from 20 W.

Table 18.1 Possible complications of SVCI: How to avoid

Possible complications	When does it occur?	How can we avoid?
Right phrenic nerve injury	Ablating lateral wall of SVC, especially at posterolateral side	1. Pacing maneuver prior to RF applications to detect phrenic nerve capture 2. Careful watching of the movement of right-side diaphragm by fluoroscopy 3. CMAP monitoring
Sinus node injury	Ablation close to SVC-RA junction, especially at anterolateral side	1. Careful definition of "electrical" SVC-RA junction 2. Immediately stop RF application when sinus arrest occurs 3. Exclude patients with pre-existing sinus node dysfunction by Holter ECG monitor, etc. in advance
SVC stenosis	Repeat and frequent ablation	1. Know the shape and the diameter of SVC prior to ablation by CT or contrast agent 2. Avoid RF application at narrow site of SVC 3. Point-by-point ablation, not circumferential

18.5.2 Sinus Node Injury

Sinus node injury is also a possible complication, which usually occurs if RF ablations are applied below the SVC-RA junction [23]. The SVC-RA junction should be determined carefully before RF applications, and the ablation line to create SVCI is about 5 mm above the "electrical" SVC-RA junction [24]. RF applications should be stopped immediately if sinus arrest is observed during ablation which indicates damages to the sinus node. Akoum et al. utilized late gadolinium enhancement MRI for detecting a pre-existing sinus node dysfunction by evaluating structural remodeling in the RA [25]. This modality can be used before performing SVCI for detecting patients with a pre-existing sinus node dysfunction, who may have a more potential risk of sinus node injury after ablations near the SVC-RA junction. Also, recent high density 3D activation mappings of RA and SVC using multi electrode catheters such as PentaRay® NAV Catheter (Biosense-Webster, Diamond Bar, CA, USA) would be useful to identify the sinus node, the SVC-RA junction, and the myocardial penetration into the SVC precisely prior to SVCI.

18.5.3 SVC Stenosis

SVC stenosis is sometimes recognized after RF application in the SVC. Callans et al. reported the SVC narrowing after conventional non-irrigated RF ablations at the SVC-RA junction in patients with inappropriate sinus tachycardia. In this study, local and circumferential swelling of the SVC, a progressive reduction in the SVC-RA junction by 24%, was observed using intracardiac echocardiography [26]. In a case report, severe narrowing of the SVC after SVCI using an open-irrigated RF catheter (25 W, ten times, 278 s, totally) was observed [27]. For PVs, extensive PVI at PV antrum area is the standard method to reduce the risk of PV stenosis and treat ectopies from PV ostia. On the other hand, since the sinus node is located just beneath the SVC-RA junction, SVCI should be performed "inside" the SVC, which is the major difference compared with PVI. RF energy should not be raised over 25 W (which is sufficient energy to achieve SVCI) to avoid SVC stenosis. Also, segmental point-by-point ablation (not circumferential) is recommended to avoid SVC narrowing.

18.6 Indication of SVCI

18.6.1 SVCI for Confirmed AF Trigger from SVC

Chang et al. reported the long-term outcome of ablation therapy in 68 patients with AF from SVC origins which were induced using isoproterenol infusions and cardioversions [20]. In this study, the rate of AF freedom was 85.3% at 1 year, 78.7% at 2 years, and 73.3% at 5 years after the initial ablation procedure. Patients with pure SVC-initiating AF presented a better outcome than those with coexisting PV triggers [5, 20].

18.6.2 Empiric SVCI

In a randomized control study in which patients were assigned into PVI only group or empiric SVCI + PVI group, the 1-year success rate after an initial ablation procedure was as follow: 77% vs. 90% in paroxysmal AF ($P = 0.04$), 74% vs. 80% ($P = 0.52$) in persistent AF, and 69% vs. 67% in permanent AF ($P = 0.77$). Empiric SVCI in addition to PVI has improved the outcome of AF ablation solely in patients manifesting paroxysmal AF, not in persistent or permanent AF [28]. Other non-randomized single center study also reported the efficacy of empiric SVCI in addition to PVI in paroxysmal AF patients [29]. On the other hand, another randomized prospective study comparing PVI only and empiric PVI + SVCI for paroxysmal AF did not find better outcome one year after initial AF ablation (PVI = 81%, PVI + SVCI = 86%; $P = 0.75$) [30].

18.6.3 Implication from Two Different Strategies

The effect of empiric SVCI in patients with persistent AF seems to be controversial. SVC-related AF often occurs in a

vagal paroxysmal AF supports this finding [31]. The rationale of empiric SVCI + PVI for paroxysmal AF is that an arrhythmogenic SVC can often be identified during the second or third procedures, not in the first AF ablation [4, 8, 17]. Another rationale is that the induction of SVC triggers is extremely time-consuming. However, in the study of Corrado et al., 16% of patients in empiric SVCI + PVI group could not accomplish SVCI because of the risk of phrenic nerve injury or "the absence of SVC sleeve" [28]. Therefore, empiric SVCI should be limited for paroxysmal AF with *"potentially arrhythmogenic SVC."*

18.6.4 Feature of Potentially Arrhythmogenic SVC

The ectopic focus of SVC is relatively far from the SVC-RA junction [2, 7, 8], and also long SVC myocardial extension is necessary for SVC to become a perpetuator of AF [17, 18]. In the study of Higuchi et al., patients with SVC which is over 30 mm length had significant SVC-related AF episodes. The length of SVC myocardial extension over 30 mm identified SVC-related AF with 100% sensitivity and 94% specificity [8]. Although it is still unclear regarding the true cut-off value of the length of SVC myocardial extension which have arrhythmogenicity and further studies are needed, it surely can be said that only SVC with long myocardial extension have arrhythmogenicity.

Conclusion

Because of the proximity of SVC-aorta GP to the SVC and the extension of myocardium in the SVC from the RA, SVC frequently becomes an important source of AF trigger. The procedure of SVCI is different from PVI in that SVCI should be performed "inside" the SVC from the SVC-RA junction to avoid sinus node injury. Empiric SVCI is useful, however, the efficacy would be limited for paroxysmal AF and for SVC with long myocardial extension which is potentially arrhythmogenic.

Acknowledgement There is no conflict of interest.

References

1. Haissaguerre M, Jais P, Shah DC, Takahashi A, Hocini M, Quiniou G, et al. Spontaneous initiation of atrial fibrillation by ectopic beats originating in the pulmonary veins. N Engl J Med. 1998;339(10):659–66.
2. Lin WS, Tai CT, Hsieh MH, Tsai CF, Lin YK, Tsao HM, et al. Catheter ablation of paroxysmal atrial fibrillation initiated by non-pulmonary vein ectopy. Circulation. 2003;107(25):3176–83.
3. Yamaguchi T, Tsuchiya T, Miyamoto K, Nagamoto Y, Takahashi N. Characterization of non-pulmonary vein foci with an EnSite array in patients with paroxysmal atrial fibrillation. Europace. 2010;12(12):1698–706.
4. Takigawa M, Takahashi A, Kuwahara T, Okubo K, Takahashi Y, Nakashima E, et al. Impact of non-pulmonary vein foci on the outcome of the second session of catheter ablation for paroxysmal atrial fibrillation. J Cardiovasc Electrophysiol. 2015;26(7):739–46.
5. Takigawa M, Takahashi A, Kuwahara T, Okubo K, Takahashi Y, Watari Y, et al. Long-term outcome after catheter ablation of paroxysmal atrial fibrillation: impact of different atrial fibrillation foci. Int J Cardiol. 2017;227:407–12.
6. Arruda M, Mlcochova H, Prasad SK, Kilicaslan F, Saliba W, Patel D, et al. Electrical isolation of the superior vena cava: an adjunctive strategy to pulmonary vein antrum isolation improving the outcome of AF ablation. J Cardiovasc Electrophysiol. 2007;18(12):1261–6.
7. Tsai CF, Tai CT, Hsieh MH, Lin WS, Yu WC, Ueng KC, et al. Initiation of atrial fibrillation by ectopic beats originating from the superior vena cava: electrophysiological characteristics and results of radiofrequency ablation. Circulation. 2000;102(1):67–74.
8. Higuchi K, Yamauchi Y, Hirao K, Sasaki T, Hachiya H, Sekiguchi Y, et al. Superior vena cava as initiator of atrial fibrillation: factors related to its arrhythmogenicity. Heart Rhythm. 2010;7(9):1186–91.
9. Blom NA, Gittenberger-de Groot AC, DeRuiter MC, Poelmann RE, Mentink MM, Ottenkamp J. Development of the cardiac conduction tissue in human embryos using HNK-1 antigen expression: possible relevance for understanding of abnormal atrial automaticity. Circulation. 1999;99(6):800–6.
10. Jongbloed MR, Mahtab EA, Blom NA, Schalij MJ, Gittenberger-de Groot AC. Development of the cardiac conduction system and the possible relation to predilection sites of arrhythmogenesis. ScientificWorldJournal. 2008;8:239–69.
11. Mommersteeg MT, Brown NA, Prall OW, de Gier-de Vries C, Harvey RP, Moorman AF, et al. Pitx2c and Nkx2-5 are required for the formation and identity of the pulmonary myocardium. Circ Res. 2007;101(9):902–9.
12. Kholova I, Kautzner J. Morphology of atrial myocardial extensions into human caval veins: a postmortem study in patients with and without atrial fibrillation. Circulation. 2004;110(5):483–8.
13. Yeh HI, Lai YJ, Lee SH, Lee YN, Ko YS, Chen SA, et al. Heterogeneity of myocardial sleeve morphology and gap junctions in canine superior vena cava. Circulation. 2001;104(25):3152–7.
14. Sicouri S, Blazek J, Belardinelli L, Antzelevitch C. Electrophysiological characteristics of canine superior vena cava sleeve preparations: effect of ranolazine. Circ Arrhythm Electrophysiol. 2012;5(2):371–9.
15. Chiou CW, Eble JN, Zipes DP. Efferent vagal innervation of the canine atria and sinus and atrioventricular nodes. The third fat pad. Circulation. 1997;95:2573–84.
16. Lu Z, Scherlag BJ, Niu G, Lin J, Fung KM, Zhao L, et al. Functional properties of the superior vena cava (SVC)-aorta ganglionated plexus: evidence suggesting an autonomic basis for rapid SVC firing. J Cardiovasc Electrophysiol. 2010;21(12):1392–9.
17. Miyazaki S, Takigawa M, Kusa S, Kuwahara T, Taniguchi H, Okubo K, et al. Role of arrhythmogenic superior vena cava on atrial fibrillation. J Cardiovasc Electrophysiol. 2014;25(4):380–6.
18. Nakamura T, Hachiya H, Yagishita A, Tanaka Y, Higuchi K, Kawabata M, et al. The relationship between the profiles of SVC and sustainability of SVC fibrillation induced by provocative electrical stimulation. Pacing Clin Electrophysiol. 2016;39(4):352–60.
19. Goya M, Ouyang F, Ernst S, Volkmer M, Antz M, Kuck KH. Electroanatomic mapping and catheter ablation of breakthroughs from the right atrium to the superior vena cava in patients with atrial fibrillation. Circulation. 2002;106(11):1317–20.
20. Chang HY, Lo LW, Lin YJ, Chang SL, Hu YF, Feng AN, et al. Long-term outcome of catheter ablation in patients with atrial fibrillation originating from the superior vena cava. J Cardiovasc Electrophysiol. 2012;23(9):955–61.
21. Bai R, Patel D, Di Biase L, Fahmy TS, Kozeluhova M, Prasad S, et al. Phrenic nerve injury after catheter ablation: should we worry about this complication? J Cardiovasc Electrophysiol. 2006;17(9):944–8.
22. Miyazaki S, Ichihara N, Taniguchi H, Hachiya H, Nakamura H, Usui E, et al. Evaluation of diaphragmatic electromyograms in radiofrequency ablation of atrial fibrillation: prospective study comparing

different monitoring techniques. J Cardiovasc Electrophysiol. 2015;26(3):260–5.
23. Ong MG, Tai CT, Lin YJ, Lee KT, Chang SL, Chen SA. Sinus node injury as a complication of superior vena cava isolation. J Cardiovasc Electrophysiol. 2005;16(11):1243–5.
24. Chen G, Dong JZ, Liu XP, Zhang XY, Long DY, Sang CH, et al. Sinus node injury as a result of superior vena cava isolation during catheter ablation for atrial fibrillation and atrial flutter. Pacing Clin Electrophysiol. 2011;34(2):163–70.
25. Akoum N, McGann C, Vergara G, Badger T, Ranjan R, Mahnkopf C, et al. Atrial fibrosis quantified using late gadolinium enhancement MRI is associated with sinus node dysfunction requiring pacemaker implant. J Cardiovasc Electrophysiol. 2012;23(1):44–50.
26. Callans DJ, Ren JF, Schwartzman D, Gottlieb CD, Chaudhry FA, Marchlinski FE. Narrowing of the superior vena cava-right atrium junction during radiofrequency catheter ablation for inappropriate sinus tachycardia: analysis with intracardiac echocardiography. J Am Coll Cardiol. 1999;33(6):1667–70.
27. Kuhne M, Schaer B, Osswald S, Sticherling C. Superior vena cava stenosis after radiofrequency catheter ablation for electrical isolation of the superior vena cava. Pacing Clin Electrophysiol. 2010;33(4):e36–8.
28. Corrado A, Bonso A, Madalosso M, Rossillo A, Themistoclakis S, Di Biase L, et al. Impact of systematic isolation of superior vena cava in addition to pulmonary vein antrum isolation on the outcome of paroxysmal, persistent, and permanent atrial fibrillation ablation: results from a randomized study. J Cardiovasc Electrophysiol. 2010;21(1):1–5.
29. Ejima K, Kato K, Iwanami Y, Henmi R, Yagishita D, Manaka T, et al. Impact of an empiric isolation of the superior vena cava in addition to circumferential pulmonary vein isolation on the outcome of paroxysmal atrial fibrillation ablation. Am J Cardiol. 2015;116(11):1711–6.
30. Wang XH, Liu X, Sun YM, Shi HF, Zhou L, Gu JN. Pulmonary vein isolation combined with superior vena cava isolation for atrial fibrillation ablation: a prospective randomized study. Europace. 2008;10(5):600–5.
31. Ghias M, Scherlag BJ, Lu Z, Niu G, Moers A, Jackman WM, et al. The role of ganglionated plexi in apnea-related atrial fibrillation. J Am Coll Cardiol. 2009;54(22):2075–83.

Catheter Ablation of Non-pulmonary Vein Foci

Yoshihide Takahashi

Keywords
Non-PV foci • Non-contact mapping • Isoproterenol • PLSVC • Ligament of Marshall

19.1 Introduction

Mapping of atrial fibrillation (AF) is challenging because of a chaotic atrial activation. Thus, the mechanism of AF remains to be elucidated. On the other hand, mapping of the initiating process of AF is feasible because the local activation time during the initiating beat can be determined. Haissaguerre et al. performed mapping of the initiating beat and discovered the role of the pulmonary veins (PVs) in the late 1990s [1]. In their first report of mapping initiating beats, it was described that a major source of the initiating beats came from the PVs, but a minority arose from non-PV regions. It was demonstrated that the presence of non-PV foci is associated with arrhythmia recurrence after catheter ablation, and the elimination of the non-PV foci improves the clinical outcome [2, 3]. Thus, mapping and ablation of non-PV foci is essential for the catheter ablation of AF.

19.2 Electrophysiological Characteristics

19.2.1 Provocation of Ectopic Beats

If ectopic beats constantly occur during the ablation procedure, the ectopic beats are readily mapped and successfully eliminated. However, that is not always the case.

Y. Takahashi, M.D.
The Department of Cardiovascular Medicine, Tokyo Medical and Dental University, Yushima 1-5-45, Bunkyo-ku, Tokyo 113-8510, Japan
e-mail: yoshihide_takahashi@oboe.ocn.ne.jp

Provocation of ectopic beats is usually required. The administration of isoproterenol is commonly used and effective in provoking ectopic beats. Particularly, foci in the ligament of Marshall are sensitive to the administration of isoproterenol [4]. Therefore, when ectopic beats occur after the administration of isoproterenol, mapping should be performed first in the coronary sinus (CS) and lateral the left atrium (LA).

Ectopic beats often occur after electrical cardioversion of spontaneous or induced AF. In patients in sinus rhythm, an administration of isoproterenol with a target heart rate of 120 bpm and atrial burst pacing with a cycle length of 250 ms down to 180 ms is performed to induce AF. After induction of AF, sinus rhythm is restored by electrical cardioversion. The administration of adenosine triphosphate is also effective in provoking ectopic beats. This test is effective to induce ectopic beats from the PVs and superior vena cava (SVC) rather than atrial foci. This may be associated with the sensitivity of the PV or SVC myocardium to autonomic modulation [5, 6].

The administration of adenosine triphosphate is commonly performed to identify any dormant conduction from the PVs. If ectopic beats occur during the administration of adenosine triphosphate, we firstly consider a conduction recovery between the PVs and LA or SVC foci. Additionally, we need to remember that catheter-induced ectopic beats are likely to occur during the above-mentioned provocation test due to the hyperdynamic state. A mapping catheter is often inserted from the jugular vein, which can cause catheter-induced ectopic beats during the administration of isoproterenol. When catheter-induced ectopic beats are suspected, the mapping catheter should be removed from the jugular vein.

19.2.2 Clinical Characteristics Associated with Non-PV Foci

If patients have arrhythmia recurrences with a persistent isolation of the PVs, non-PV foci are attributable to the recurrences. The risk factors associated with the presence of non-PV foci are a persistent form of AF, dilated LA, atrial fibrosis, and the presence of a low voltage area, suggesting a link between advanced atrial remodeling and non-PV foci. Sinus node dysfunction is also associated with non-PV foci [7]. This is plausible because sinus node dysfunction is associated with atrial remodeling [8, 9]. It is reported that patients with a history of hyperthyroidism are more likely to have non-PV foci, particularly from the ligament of Marshall [10]. In patients with a history of hyperthyroidism, the prevalence of foci in the ligament of Marshall is reported to be 7.1%.

Non-PV foci are commonly present in the atrial area displaying complex fractionated atrial electrograms (CFAE) during AF [11, 12]. It is also reported that ablation of non-PV foci terminates AF. Based on these reports, non-PV foci may play not only a triggering, but also a driving role in AF. This is reasonable when remembering the driving role of the PVs. Recently, mapping studies have demonstrated that AF is maintained by high-frequency activities arising from an atrial area/site, which are called a driver or source [13, 14]. It is not surprising that a focal AF driver acts as both an initiator and perpetuator, but this hypothesis remains to be proven. Mapping of ectopic beats requires restoration of sinus rhythm, but ectopic beats sometimes do not occur after restoration of sinus rhythm. Therefore, ablation targeting non-PV foci is optimal for an incessant type of AF.

19.3 Mapping

19.3.1 Distribution of Non-PV Foci

Non-PV foci are distributed in both atria. The most common source is the SVC. In the right atrium (RA), the crista terminalis is the most common source, followed by the interatrial septum, including the ostium of the CS. In the LA, common sources of ectopic beats are the CS, ligament of Marshall, posterior LA, LA appendage, and interatrial septum.

19.3.2 P-Wave Morphology

The opportunity to map non-PV foci is limited because ectopic beats infrequently occur and often initiate AF. The P-wave morphology of an ectopic beat allows us to quickly identify the location of the focus. However, trigger beats usually overlap with the preceding T-wave, and the P-wave morphology is often unidentifiable. A positive P-wave in lead V1 indicates a focus in the LA or crista terminalis, and a negative P-wave in lead V1 indicates an RA origin other than the crista terminalis. A negative P-wave in the inferior leads indicates the foci are in the CS, inferior LA, cavo-tricuspid isthmus, or inferior part of the interatrial septum. Of these areas, the ostium of the CS is associated with a "deep" negative P-wave in the inferior leads. Negative P-waves in the lateral leads indicate that the ectopic beat arises from the lateral LA or LA appendage. In general, ectopic beats arising from the interatrial septum are associated with a shorter P-wave duration and shorter PR interval compared to those arising from the lateral wall. However, the PR interval depends on the coupling interval as well. In patients with spontaneous or iatrogenic atrial scarring, including from prior linear ablation, the P-wave morphology may be misleading for the true location of foci due to intra-atrial conduction disturbances.

19.3.3 Contact Mapping

The location of non-PV foci is estimated by the P-wave morphology and activation sequence recorded by multi-electrode catheters. Multi-electrode catheters are usually deployed in the CS and RA, and the ablation catheter is deployed on the interatrial septum. This catheter position gives us an idea of whether non-PV foci arise from the LA or RA. For an accurate localization of the focus, a mapping catheter with 5-radiating splines (PENTARAY, Biosense-Webster) or a double loop catheter (AFocus II HD, St. Jude Medical) is commonly used in combination with a 3D navigation system (Fig. 19.1). However, these catheters cover a limited surface area, and it is necessary to map several sites to identify the focus. Thus, contact mapping is appropriate for cases with frequent ectopic beats. If a single ectopic beat initiates AF, multiple electrical cardioversions are required. When intracardiac electrical cardioversion is used, the defibrillation energy threshold is 5–20 J. Intracardiac electrical cardioversion minimizes post-shock body movements and is potentially less harmful to the myocardial tissue. In cases with infrequent ectopic beats or a frequent initiation of AF, non-contact mapping needs to be taken into consideration.

19.3.4 Non-contact Mapping

Because a non-contact mapping system enables the construction of an isopotential map of the entire chamber even during a single beat, such a system is useful for cases with infrequent ectopic beats or the immediate initiation of AF (Fig. 19.2). Ensite (St. Jude Medical) is a commercially available non-contact mapping system. In this system, far-field unipolar

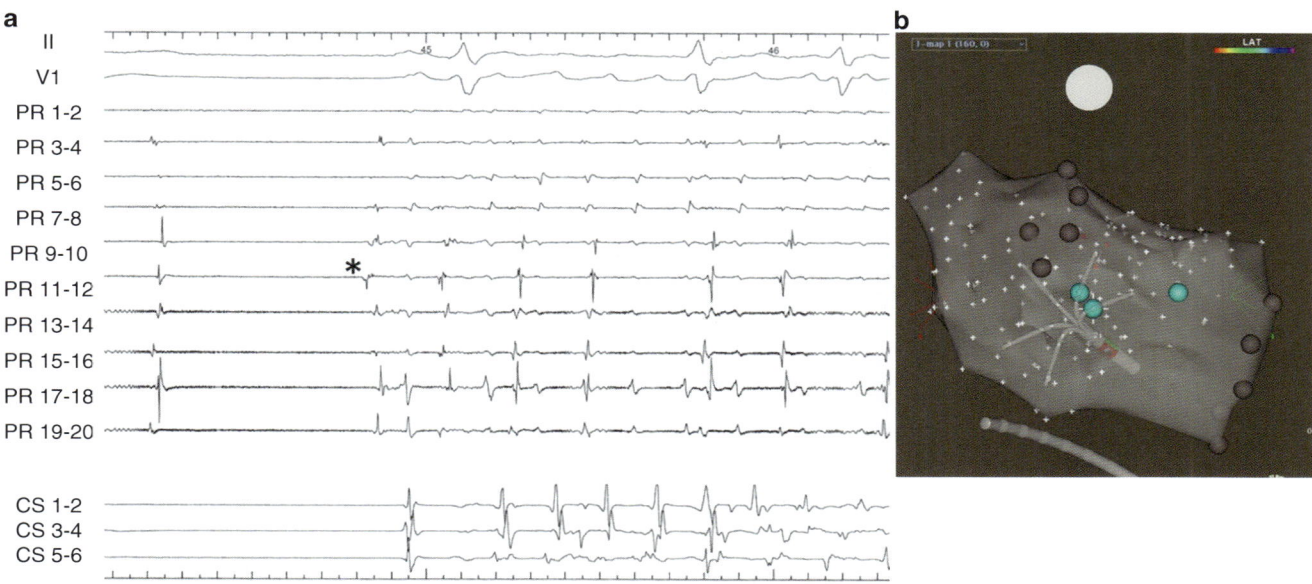

Fig. 19.1 Mapping of ectopic beats initiating atrial fibrillation using a multi-electrode mapping catheter with 5-radiating splines (PENTARAY). (**a**) Intracardiac electrograms demonstrating the earliest activation during the initiating beat (*asterisk*) are on one of the proximal electrodes [11, 12] of the mapping catheter. This suggests that the ectopic beats arise from near electrodes 11–12, and the activity propagates centrifugally to the periphery. (**b**) The posterior-anterior view of the CARTO system displays the mapping catheter. The *blue* and *gray tags* indicate the earliest activation site during the ectopic beats and scarring after the pulmonary vein isolation, respectively. *PR* PENTARAY, *CS* coronary sinus

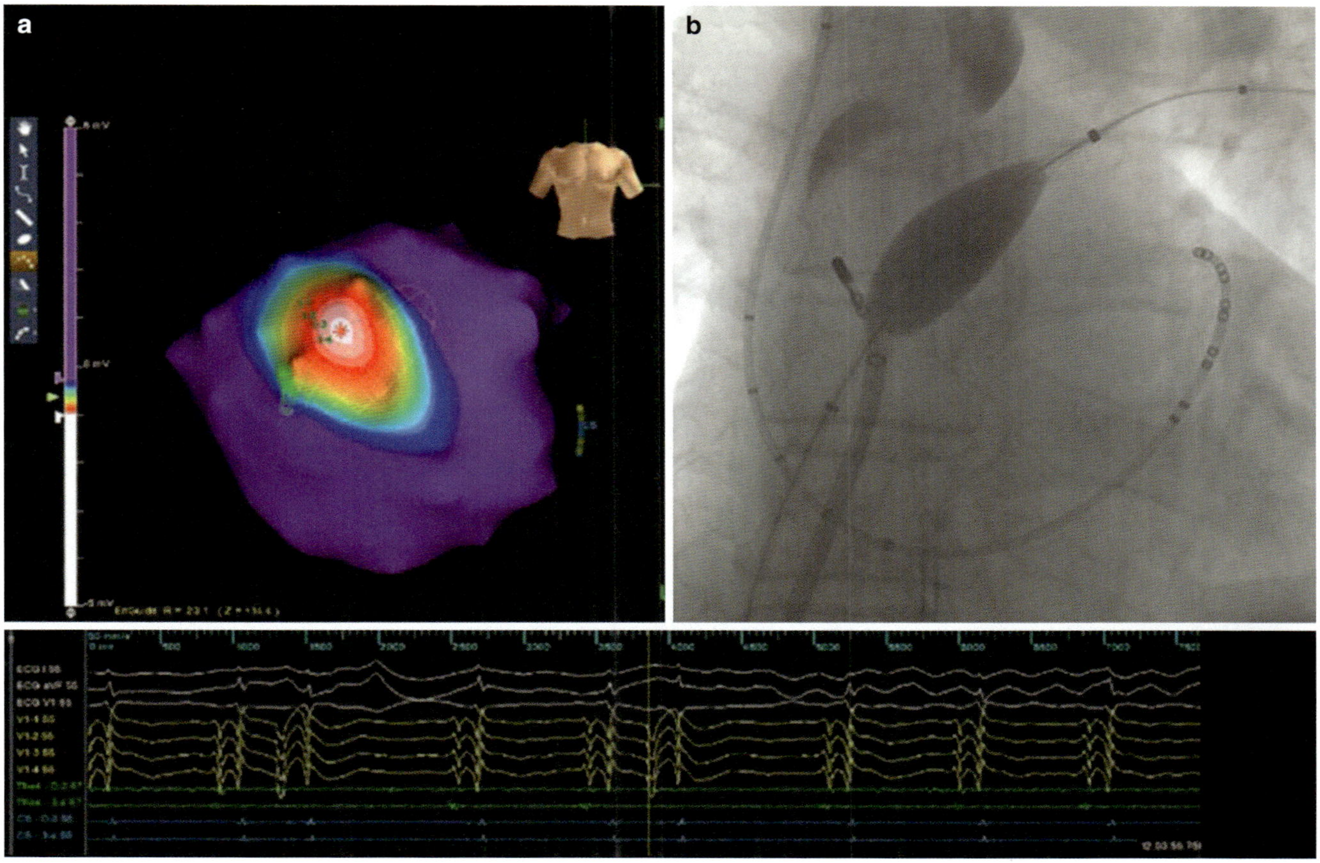

Fig. 19.2 Mapping of ectopic beats initiating atrial fibrillation using a non-contact mapping system (EnSite). (**a**) The Ensite system displays the ectopic focus in the anterior left atrium (*white color*). (**b**) An anterior–posterior fluoroscopic view of the EnSite Array catheter

electrograms are acquired for the creation of isopotential maps. The disadvantage of the non-contact mapping system is that far-field activity of the adjacent structures, such as the ventricle or appendage, masks the near-field activity. Thus, ectopic beats arising from the atrio-ventricular annulus are inappropriately mapped when the P-wave overlaps with the T-wave. In addition, the distance between the non-contact mapping catheter and endocardial surface is inversely related to the accuracy of the location and electrical information.

19.4 Catheter Ablation

19.4.1 LA Appendage

The LA appendage can be a source of ectopic beats initiating AF. However, focal ablation within the LA appendage often fails to eliminate ectopic beats. The use of an Ensite system is not so helpful for mapping within the LA appendage because the distance between the array and LA appendage is usually too far. Manipulation of the PENTARAY catheter within the LA appendage is difficult. In addition, ablation of the ectopic beats is challenging, due to the thickness of the pectinate muscle. Thus, isolation of the LA appendage is effective for the elimination of ectopic beats arising from the LA appendage [15]. Di Biase et al. reported that the isolation of the LA appendage is superior to focal ablation within the LA appendage in patients who have a source of AF or ectopic beats in the LA appendage [16]. In their report, isolation of the LA appendage was performed with the guidance of a circular mapping catheter deployed at the ostium of the LA appendage. In combination with PV isolation lesions, two linear lesions, an anterior line connecting the anterior mitral annulus and left superior PV and mitral isthmus line connecting the postero-lateral mitral annulus and left inferior PV isolate the LA appendage from the LA body. The LA appendage serves as not only a source of triggers, but also as an arrhythmia substrate, similar to the PVs and SVC [17]. This idea is supported also by the fact that arrhythmias continue within the LA appendage after isolation of this structure (Fig. 19.3).

Although the efficacy of an LA appendage isolation has been reported, this ablation technique should be performed with special concern because of the risk of thrombus formation in this structure after the isolation. Rillig et al. reported that 90% of patients continued on anticoagulation therapy after the LA appendage isolation, but 6% of the patients had strokes or transient ischemic attacks, and thrombus formation in the LA appendage was confirmed in 20% of the patients by transesophageal echocardiography during a median follow-up of 6.5 months [18]. The optimal ablation strategy for ectopic beats arising from the LA appendage is not well defined.

19.4.2 Coronary Sinus (CS)

If activity on a multi-electrode catheter in the CS precedes the P-wave during an ectopic beat, the origin of the ectopic beat can be from the CS musculature, LA myocardium at the inferior mitral annulus, or ligament of Marshall. Thus, mapping needs to be performed not only within the CS, but also

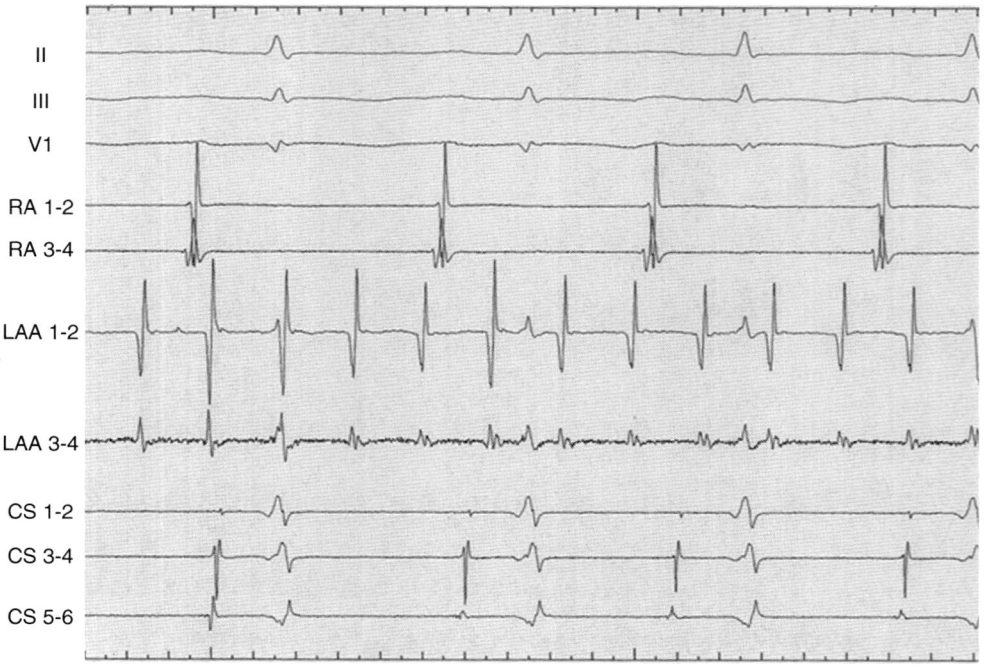

Fig. 19.3 A tachycardia confined inside the disconnected left atrial appendage (LAA). The intracardiac electrograms display a tachycardia in the LAA and sinus rhythm in the remaining atria. This demonstrates that the LAA was driving the atria before the isolation. *RAA* right atrium, *LAA* left atrial appendage, *CS* coronary sinus

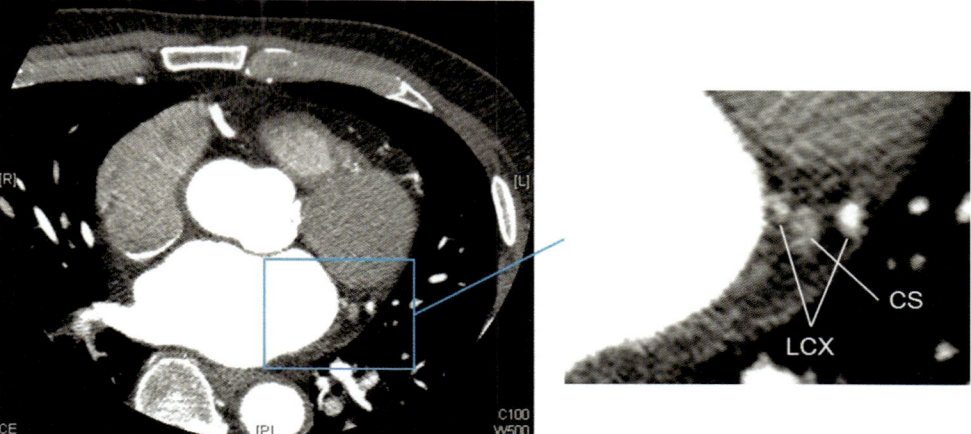

Fig. 19.4 Computed tomography image of the coronary sinus (CS) and left coronary circumflex artery (LCX). A small branch of the LCX is running between the LCX and left atrium. In this case, catheter ablation within the CS may cause thermal injury to the small branch of the LCX

on the endocardial surface of the inferior LA. To prove that the origin of the ectopic beat is the ligament of Marshall, a multi-electrode catheter should be deployed in the vein of Marshall. However, this is a complex procedure, which often requires retrograde angiography of the CS. Instead of the insertion of a multi-electrode catheter into the vein of Marshall, therefore, we usually perform mapping on the endocardial surface of the inferior LA to lateral LA along the possible location of the ligament of Marshall. If the earliest activation during an ectopic beat is located in the posterolateral LA, catheter ablation is performed at that site. However, ablation targeting the earliest activation site on the endocardium does not always eliminate the focus. Because the ligament of Marshall is an epicardial structure, catheter ablation from the endocardium occasionally modifies the electrical connections between the LA myocardium, and the abolition of the focus requires ablation at multiple sites including inside the CS.

For the elimination of CS triggers, isolation of the CS has previously been reported [19]. Because the CS musculature has multiple connections within the LA myocardium, extensive ablation both from the endocardium of the inferior LA and within the CS is required for isolation of the CS. A potential complication associated with ablation within the CS is coronary artery injury [20]. The relative anatomical relationship between the CS and coronary arteries is understood by computed tomography scanning before the ablation procedure (Fig. 19.4). In patients with coronary arteries running between the LA and CS, ablation within the CS should not be performed.

19.4.3 Persistent Left Superior Vena Cava (PLSVC)

A PLSVC is a common source of triggers, however, this anomaly is observed in less than 1% of the population. The muscular sleeve extends from the ostium of the CS to the

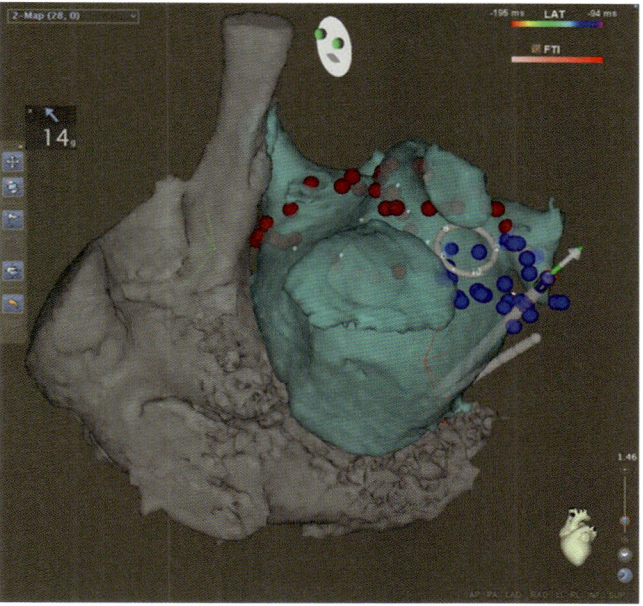

Fig. 19.5 Isolation of a persistent left superior vena cava (PLSVC). The left anterior oblique view of the CARTO image. The *red* and *blue tags* indicate the ablation lesions for the pulmonary veins and PLSVC, respectively. A circular multi-electrode catheter is deployed in the PLSVC

PLSVC up to 3–5 cm above the level of the left superior PV. Isolation of the PLSVC at the level of the left superior PV is feasible [21], while isolation at a lower level is challenging, because of the broad connections between the CS and LA myocardium. If PLSVC foci are suspected, it is important to identify whether the focus is distal to the level of the left superior PV. For mapping in the PLSVC, a circular multi-electrode catheter is deployed at the level of the left superior PV, and the activation timing of the ablation catheter distal to the circular catheter is determined. Use of a 3D mapping system is of great help for isolating the PLSVC (Fig. 19.5).

References

1. Haïssaguerre M, Jaïs P, Shah DC, Takahashi A, Hocini M, Quiniou G, et al. Spontaneous initiation of atrial fibrillation by ectopic beats originating in the pulmonary veins. N Engl J Med. 1998;339(10):659–66.
2. Hayashi K, An Y, Nagashima M, Hiroshima K, Ohe M, Makihara Y, et al. Importance of nonpulmonary vein foci in catheter ablation for paroxysmal atrial fibrillation. Heart Rhythm. 2015;12(9): 1918–24.
3. Takigawa M, Takahashi A, Kuwahara T, Okubo K, Takahashi Y, Watari Y, et al. Long-term outcome after catheter ablation of paroxysmal atrial fibrillation: Impact of different atrial fibrillation foci. Int J Cardiol. 2017;227:407–12.
4. Doshi RN, Wu TJ, Yashima M, Kim YH, Ong JJ, Cao JM, et al. Relation between ligament of Marshall and adrenergic atrial tachyarrhythmia. Circulation. 1999;100(8):876–83.
5. Lim PB, Malcolme-Lawes LC, Stuber T, Wright I, Francis DP, Davies DW, et al. Intrinsic cardiac autonomic stimulation induces pulmonary vein ectopy and triggers atrial fibrillation in humans. J Cardiovasc Electrophysiol. 2011;22(6):638–46. https://doi.org/10.1111/j.1540-8167.2010.01992.x.
6. Lu Z, Scherlag BJ, Niu G, Lin J, Fung KM, Zhao L, et al. Functional properties of the superior vena cava (SVC)-aorta ganglionated plexus: evidence suggesting an autonomic basis for rapid SVC firing. J Cardiovasc Electrophysiol. 2010;21(12):1392–9. https://doi.org/10.1111/j.1540-8167.2010.01787.x.
7. Hayashi K, Fukunaga M, Yamaji K, An Y, Nagashima M, Hiroshima K, et al. Impact of catheter ablation for paroxysmal atrial fibrillation in patients with sick sinus syndrome – important role of non-pulmonary vein foci. Circ J. 2016;80(4):887–94. https://doi.org/10.1253/circj.CJ-15-1384.
8. Akoum N, McGann C, Vergara G, Badger T, Ranjan R, Mahnkopf C, et al. Atrial fibrosis quantified using late gadolinium enhancement MRI is associated with sinus node dysfunction requiring pacemaker implant. J Cardiovasc Electrophysiol. 2012;23(1): 44–50. https://doi.org/10.1111/j.1540-8167.2011.02140.x.
9. Chang HY, Lin YJ, Lo LW, Chang SL, Hu YF, Li CH, et al. Sinus node dysfunction in atrial fibrillation patients: the evidence of regional atrial substrate remodelling. Europace. 2013;15(2): 205–11. https://doi.org/10.1093/europace/eus219.
10. Wongcharoen W, Lin YJ, Chang SL, Lo LW, Hu YF, Chung FP, et al. History of hyperthyroidism and long-term outcome of catheter ablation of drug-refractory atrial fibrillation. Heart Rhythm. 2015;12(9):1956–62. https://doi.org/10.1016/j.hrthm.2015.06.004.
11. Lo LW, Lin YJ, Tsao HM, Chang SL, Hu YF, Tsai WC, et al. Characteristics of complex fractionated electrograms in nonpulmonary vein ectopy initiating atrial fibrillation/atrial tachycardia. J Cardiovasc Electrophysiol. 2009;20(12):1305–12. https://doi.org/10.1111/j.1540-8167.2009.01617.x.
12. Elayi CS, Di Biase L, Bai R, Burkhardt JD, Mohanty P, Sanchez J, et al. Identifying the relationship between the non-PV triggers and the critical CFAE sites post-PVAI to curtail the extent of atrial ablation in longstanding persistent AF. J Cardiovasc Electrophysiol. 2011;22(11):1199–205. https://doi.org/10.1111/j.1540-8167.2011.02122.x.
13. Haissaguerre M, Hocini M, Denis A, Shah AJ, Komatsu Y, Yamashita S, et al. Driver domains in persistent atrial fibrillation. Circulation. 2014;130:530–8.
14. Lee S, Sahadevan J, Khrestian CM, Cakulev I, Markowitz A, Waldo AL. Simultaneous biatrial high-density (510–512 electrodes) epicardial mapping of persistent and long-standing persistent atrial fibrillation in patients: new insights into the mechanism of its maintenance. Circulation. 2015;132:2108–17.
15. Takahashi Y, Sanders P, Rotter M, Haïssaguerre M. Disconnection of the left atrial appendage for elimination of foci maintaining atrial fibrillation. J Cardiovasc Electrophysiol. 2005;16(8):917–9.
16. Di Biase L, Burkhardt JD, Mohanty P, Sanchez J, Mohanty S, Horton R, et al. Left atrial appendage: an underrecognized trigger site of atrial fibrillation. Circulation. 2010;122(2):109–18. https://doi.org/10.1161/CIRCULATIONAHA.109.928903.
17. Hocini M, Shah AJ, Nault I, Sanders P, Wright M, Narayan SM, et al. Localized reentry within the left atrial appendage: arrhythmogenic role in patients undergoing ablation of persistent atrial fibrillation. Heart Rhythm. 2011;8(12):1853–61. https://doi.org/10.1016/j.hrthm.2011.07.013.
18. Rillig A, Tilz RR, Lin T, Fink T, Heeger CH, Arya A, et al. Unexpectedly high incidence of stroke and left atrial appendage thrombus formation after electrical isolation of the left atrial appendage for the treatment of atrial tachyarrhythmias. Circ Arrhythm Electrophysiol. 2016;9(5):e003461. https://doi.org/10.1161/CIRCEP.115.003461.
19. Rotter M, Sanders P, Takahashi Y, Hsu LF, Sacher F, Hocini M, et al. Images in cardiovascular medicine. Coronary sinus tachycardia driving atrial fibrillation. Circulation. 2004;110(6):e59–60.
20. Takahashi Y, Jaïs P, Hocini M, Sanders P, Rotter M, Rostock T, et al. Acute occlusion of the left circumflex coronary artery during mitral isthmus linear ablation. J Cardiovasc Electrophysiol. 2005;16(10):1104–7.
21. Hsu LF, Jaïs P, Keane D, Wharton JM, Deisenhofer I, Hocini M, et al. Atrial fibrillation originating from persistent left superior vena cava. Circulation. 2004;109(7):828–32.

Stepwise Ablation for Persistent Atrial Fibrillation

Yoshihide Takahashi

Keywords

Stepwise ablation • Persistent atrial fibrillation • Pulmonary vein • Electrogram • Linear ablation

20.1 Introduction

Pulmonary vein (PV) isolation was developed in the late 1990s. Because of the impact of PV isolation on the management of patients with paroxysmal atrial fibrillation (AF), this ablation technique was also applied to persistent AF. However, its efficacy was not satisfying. In the early 2000s, various ablation techniques were developed particularly for persistent AF and were performed adjunctively to PV isolation. The ablation techniques commonly used in the 2000s were linear ablation and complex fractionated atrial electrogram (CFAE) ablation.

Thereafter, Haissaguerre hypothesized that AF is maintained by high-frequency electrical activities, the so-called drivers, and AF drivers are present dominantly in the PVs in paroxysmal AF, but ubiquitously present in the atria in persistent AF. It was considered that the elimination of AF drivers might be associated with better clinical outcomes. Based on this idea, he performed PV isolation, CFEA ablation, and linear ablation in a stepwise fashion until termination of AF [1]. This ablation strategy was named the "stepwise ablation."

20.2 Ablation Techniques Used in the Stepwise Ablation

20.2.1 Pulmonary Vein Isolation

It is unusual that PV isolation alone terminates AF in persistent AF. Before the stepwise ablation was started, the role of PV isolation in the ablative therapy for persistent AF was unclear. In fact, Nademanee does not perform PV isolation routinely when CFEA ablation has been performed. To clarify the role of PV isolation in persistent AF, the following ablation techniques were performed in a randomized order: (1) PV isolation, (2) isolation of the superior vena cava (SVC) and coronary sinus (CS), and (3) CFAE ablation [1]. Linear ablation was performed if all three of these steps failed to terminate AF. In this study, PV isolation increased AF cycle length. If PV isolation was performed after CFAE ablation, PV isolation often terminated AF. This result convinced us that PV isolation is also needed for persistent AF. After this study, PV isolation is performed as the initial step. In contrast, SVC isolation rarely increases AF cycle length and terminates AF in 2% of patients indicating a limited role of the SVC in perpetuation of AF. From this result, SVC isolation is performed, only if mapping demonstrates that consistent activation sequence from the SVC to the right atrium (RA).

20.2.2 Electrogram-Based Ablation

All of the atrial regions are targeted for an electrogram-based ablation, except for the sinus node region and vicinity of the atrioventricular node. The electrogram characteristics for this ablation technique are as follows: (1) continuous

Y. Takahashi, M.D.
Department of Cardiovascular Medicine, Tokyo Medical and Dental University, 1-5-45 Yushima, Bunkyo-ku, Tokyo 113-8510, Japan
e-mail: yoshihide_takahashi@oboe.ocn.ne.jp

electrical activity, (2) short cycle length activity, (3) centrifugal activation, and (4) activation gradient [1]. It is considered that all of these electrogram characteristics are associated with the presence of rapid activities which drive AF. The mechanism of such AF driver can be reentry or focal activity.

The duration of continuous electrical activity is associated with the impact of the ablation on the fibrillatory process, which is assessed by termination of AF or an increase in AF cycle length (Fig. 20.1) [2]. Ablation at a site displaying fractionated but not continuous electrograms with interruption with an isoelectric line has less impact. Recently, epicardial mapping of human AF has demonstrated that continuous activity is recorded in the center of a rotational propagation pattern [3]. Body surface mapping with phase map technique also has demonstrated that continuous electrical activity is recorded in the area where reentry is observed [4]. If there is a gradient in cycle length among atrial regions, the atrial region displaying activity with the shortest cycle length should play the role of a driver (Fig. 20.2). In case of the absence of cycle length gradient in the atria, activity propagates centrifugally from the AF drivers. However, identification of centrifugal activation patterns is infeasible when mapping is performed by conventional multi-electrode catheters. Exceptionally within the CS, centrifugal activation can be observed because of its unique structure (Fig. 20.3). The activation gradient between a distal and proximal bi-pole is considered to be associated with slow conduction. The repetitive appearance of this electrogram characteristic may represent the presence of a rotational wavefront in a localized area, which also contributes to the perpetuation of AF (Fig. 20.4). The activation gradient can be seen intermittently usually during several atrial cycles. Thus, careful observation is needed to identify this electrogram characteristics.

Fractionation is associated with shortening of cycle length [5]. Immediately after isolation of the PVs, cycle length is usually still short and fractionated continuous electrical activity is observed in wide areas. If electrograms are fractionated and continuous, neither local cycle length nor local propagation pattern is determined. Thus, continuous electrical activity must be targeted. The LA is the first

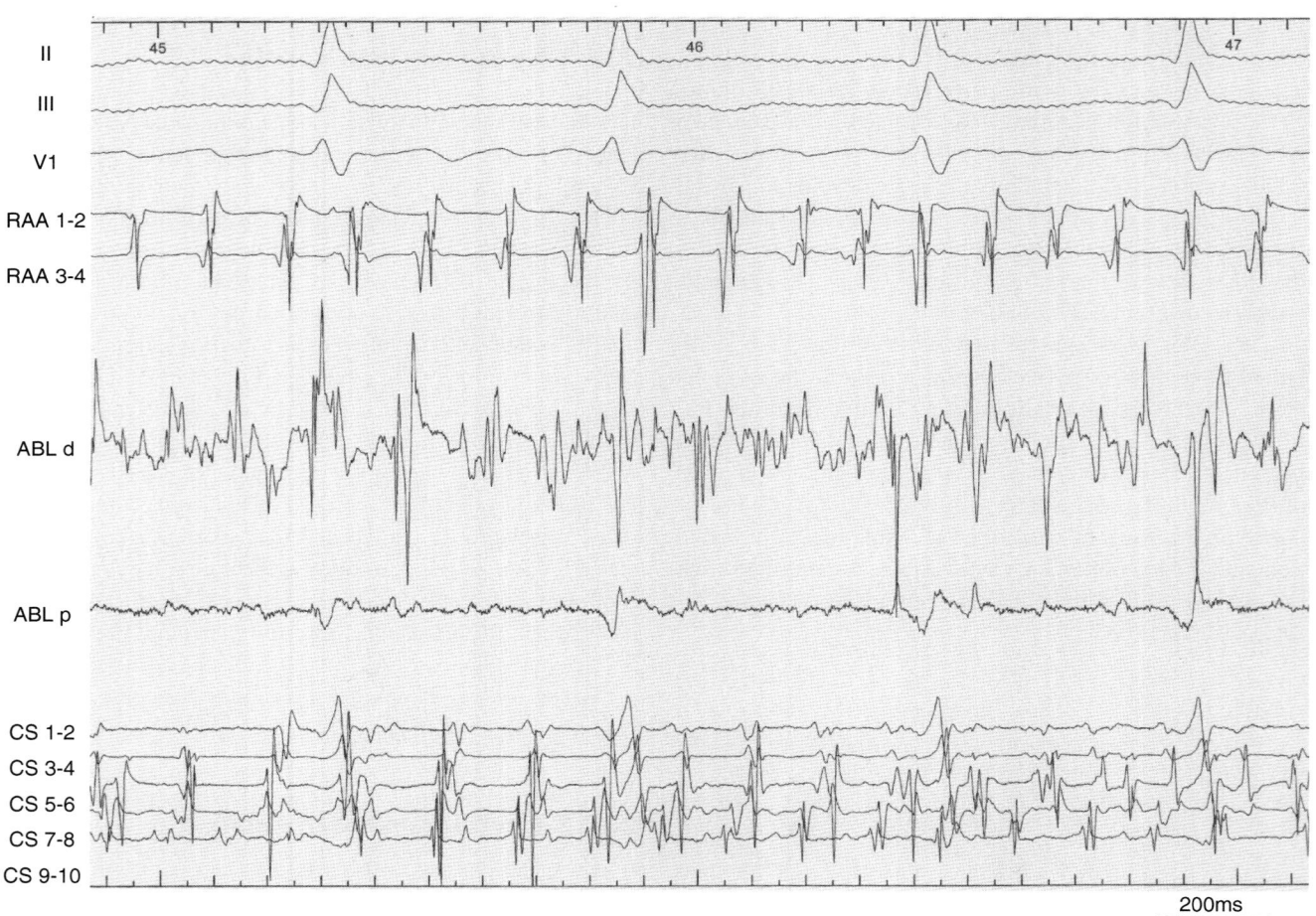

Fig. 20.1 Continuous electrical activity is recorded on distal bipolar electrograms on an ablation catheter. *RAA* right atrial appendage, *ABLd* distal bipolar electrogram on an ablation catheter, *ABLp* proximal bipolar electrograms on an ablation catheter, *CS* coronary sinus

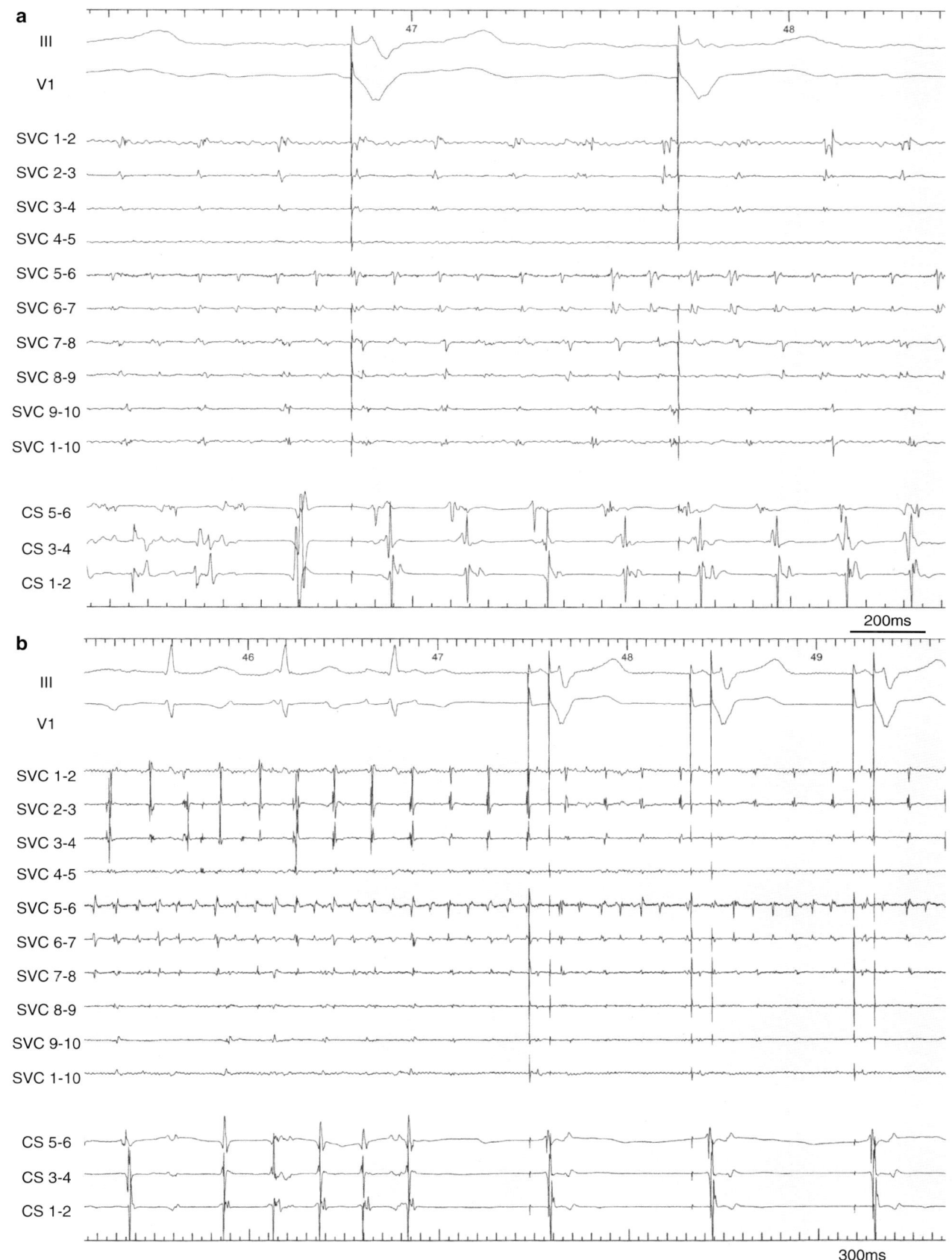

Fig. 20.2 Cycle length on SVC 5–6, 6–7, and 7–8 is shorter than that of the other electrograms in the SVC or CS. Cycle length gradient between the SVC and CS suggests that a driver is present in the SVC (**a**). Isolation of the SVC terminates atrial fibrillation, while arrhythmia continues within the SVC. This confirms a driving role of the SVC (**b**). *SVC* superior vena cava, *CS* coronary sinus

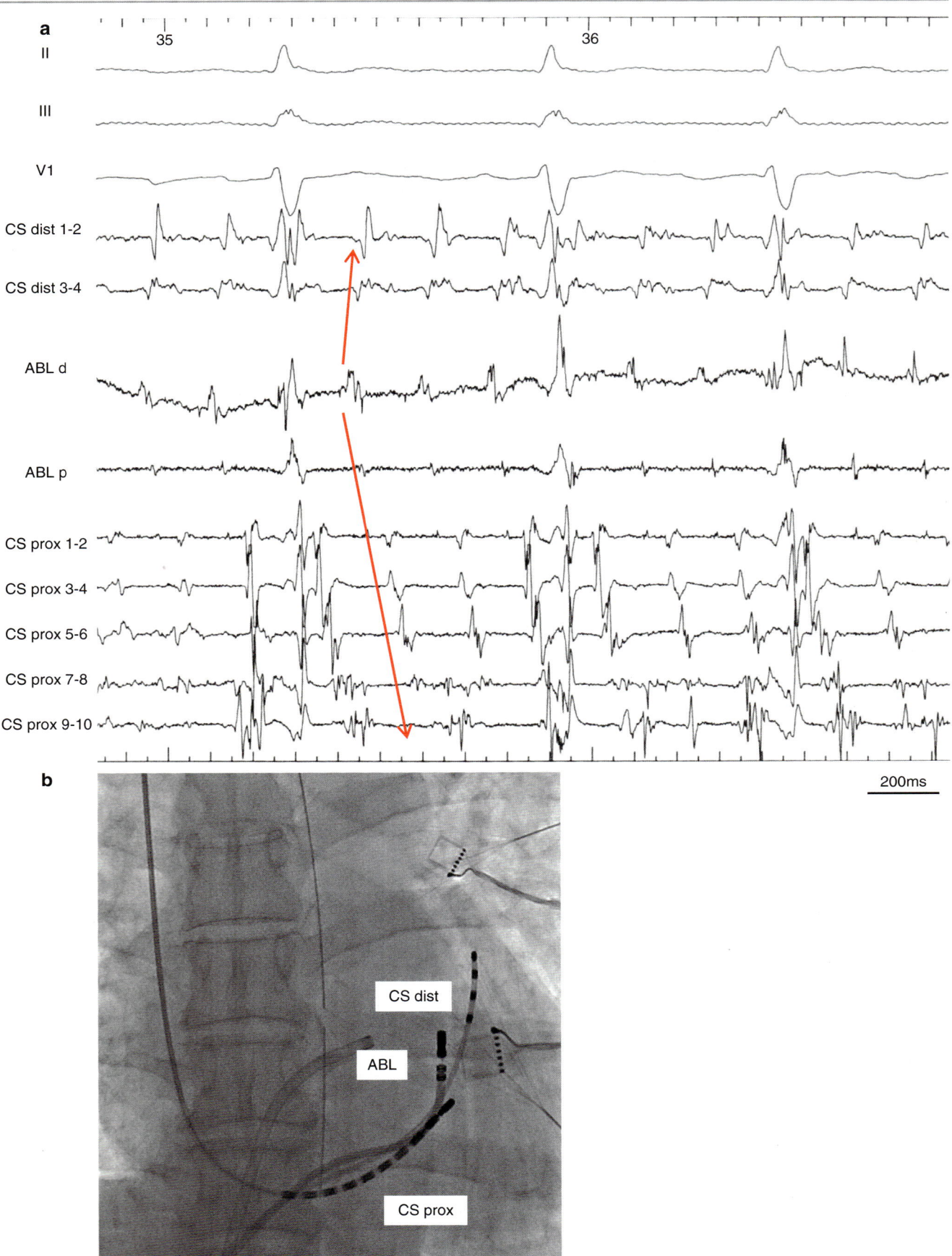

Fig. 20.3 Activation sequence is consistent during atrial fibrillation. Distal bipolar electrograms on an ablation catheter is the earliest activation site, and activity propagates to the surroundings (**a**). This activation sequence indicates centrifugal activation (**b**). Abbreviations as in Fig. 20.2

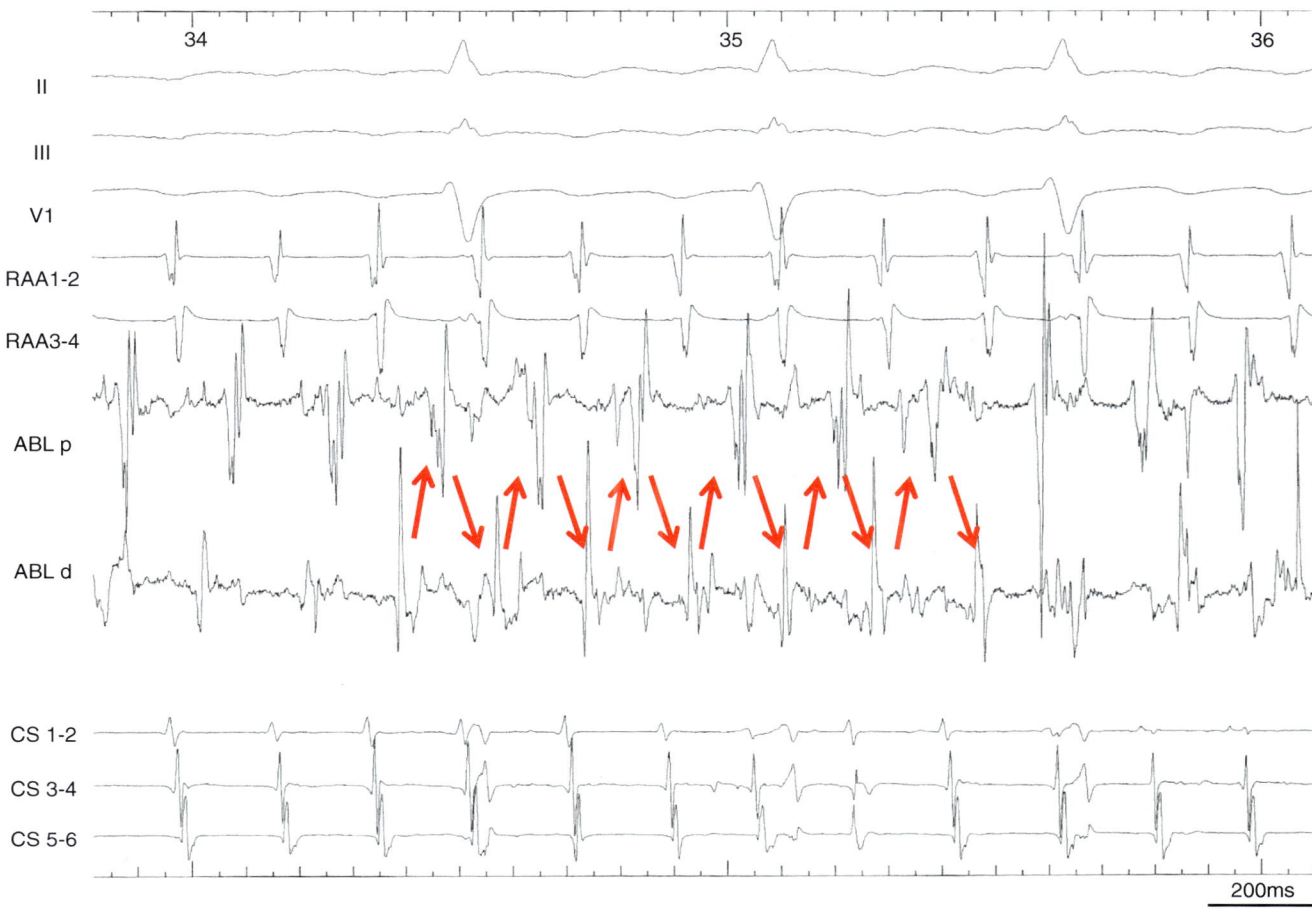

Fig. 20.4 Activation gradient between the proximal and distal bipolar electrograms is shown during six atrial cycles. Abbreviations as Fig. 20.1

chamber to be targeted because it was reported that AF is more often terminated by ablation of the LA compared to the RA [1]. However, if cycle length is shorter in the RA than the LA by >20 ms, this suggests that the RA is the driving chamber and the RA should be targeted. After ablation at continuous activity sites, local cycle length and propagation pattern can be determined due to an increase in AF cycle length and reduction in the fractionated electrograms. Then, short cycle length activity or centrifugal activation is targeted.

The efficacy of electrogram-based ablation is confirmed by an increase in AF cycle length because the elimination of AF drivers reduces the number of wavelets and increases AF cycle length. Eventually, AF is converted into atrial tachycardia (AT) or sinus rhythm is directly restored from AF. In 70% of cases, AF is converted into AT, the mechanism of which is focal or reentry. Occurrence of AT is explained by following hypothesis: (1) the mechanism of AT is masked by AF, or (2) prior ablation lesions are arrhythmogenic and responsible for occurrence of ATs. When the stepwise ablation was first reported by Haissaguerre et al. [1], electrogram-based ablation was performed without using a 3D-mapping system. Without using a 3D-mapping system, presumably there must have been conduction gaps between each ablation lesion, and those gaps served as a substrate for reentry. Before the use of a 3D-mapping system, we had recurrence of localized reentry in 10% of patients. Localized reentry involves a slow conduction area in its circuit, which may be a gap resulted from previous electrogram-based ablation and arises from the proximity of the ablation lesions for PV isolation [6]. Now, we use a 3D-mapping system for stepwise ablation. If we ablate within 1 cm from the PV isolation line, the ablation lesion is connected to the PV isolation line to eliminate conduction gaps (Fig. 20.5). After using a 3D-mapping system, the occurrence of localized reentry decreased to 1%.

One of the disadvantages of electrogram-based ablation is requirement of skill and experience of physicians, which enables mapping of all areas and immediate adjudication of chaotic electrograms in each site. An algorithm to quantify complex fractionated electrograms is equipped in 3D-mapping systems, but it appears to be insufficient. Thus, new mapping technologies to identify the AF drivers are being developed.

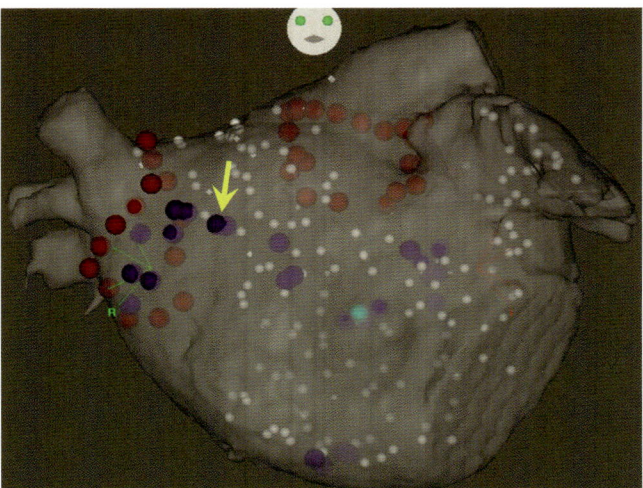

Fig. 20.5 Left atrial ablation lesions are displayed in an anterior-posterior view of a 3D-mapping system. *Red and purple dots* represent ablation lesions for pulmonary vein isolation and electrogram-based ablation, respectively. A *yellow arrow* indicates a site where continuous activity is recorded. Electrogram-based ablation starts from this site, and subsequent lesions are deployed between this site and pulmonary isolation line to eliminate a conduction gap

20.2.3 Linear Ablation

A common lesion set for LA linear ablation is a combination of roof line and mitral isthmus line. The roof line connects between both the left and right superior PVs, and the mitral isthmus line connects between the left inferior PV and postero-lateral mitral annulus. Although it is relatively less common, AF can be terminated during the linear ablation. This may suggest that macro-reentrant wavelets contribute to the perpetuation of AF. More importantly, linear lesions play a role in the prevention of macro-reentry occurring after the ablation procedure. However, a conduction gap in the linear lesions serves as a substrate critical for macro-reentry. If linear lesions are deployed, therefore, the line needs to be completely blocked. Formation of complete conduction block across the line often requires considerable procedural duration, and the acute success rate of the complete conduction block is <90%. Furthermore, conduction recovery of linear lesions is common. Thus, linear ablation, particularly mitral isthmus line, is performed at the last step in the stepwise ablation strategy. If sinus rhythm is restored before the mitral isthmus line, we do not have to deploy the line and save the procedural time. However, electrogram-based ablation often converts AF into macro-reentry during the ablation procedure. In such a case, linear ablation needs to be performed [7].

20.3 Predictors of Termination of AF During the Ablation Procedure

Termination of AF by ablation is predicted by the duration of the continuous AF and AF cycle length. It is reported that the specificity and sensitivity of continuous AF of <21 months is 93% and 62%, respectively, in predicting AF termination. AF cycle length of >142 ms is predictive of AF termination with a sensitivity and specificity of 93% and 70%, respectively [8]. The LA diameter is also associated with AF termination, but its predictive value is less than the duration of continuous AF and AF cycle length. AF cycle length is determined by averaging >30 consecutive atrial cycles. If atrial electrograms are fractionated and continuous, local cycle length cannot be evaluated. Thus, AF cycle length is often assessed in the LA appendage, where discrete potentials are commonly recorded. AF cycle length assessed by atrial electrograms is well correlated with cycle length of f waves on the 12-lead ECG, particularly lead V1. Thus, we can estimate AF cycle length from the 12-lead ECG before catheterization and predict whether ablation can terminate AF.

20.4 Atrial Tachycardia Occurring After Termination of AF During the Ablation Procedure

When AF is terminated by ablation, sinus rhythm is restored directly from AF in 10–20%. In the remaining patients, AF is converted into AT, and the type of the AT is macro-reentry, localized reentry, or focal tachycardia. Mapping of AT after termination of AF is often complex because local activation time cannot be annotated at the previous ablation sites. If double potentials are observed on a linear lesion, we need to consider complete conduction block or incomplete block with slow conduction. In the case of focal tachycardia, the conduction time from the earliest activation site to the latest is often greater than tachycardia cycle length due to intra-atrial conduction disturbances.

As mentioned in Sect. 20.2.2, localized reentry can be prevented by the elimination of a narrow isthmus with the use of a 3D-mapping system. Thus, currently macro-reentry more commonly occurs than localized reentry. Common reentry circuits are (1) around the mitral annulus (perimitral reentry), (2) around the ipsilateral PVs (LA roof dependent reentry), and (3) around the tricuspid annulus (common AFL). Upper or lower loop reentry may also occur although it is less common. Focal tachycardia can arise from any site in either atrium [7], but the LA origin is more common. Post-pacing interval is often used for mapping AT. Burst pacing should not be performed with cycle length less than 200 ms because pacing will degenerate AT into AF or change it into another AT.

20.5 Clinical Outcomes After the Stepwise Ablation

The arrhythmia-free rate at 1 year of follow-up after the stepwise ablation is 40% [9, 10]. Although arrhythmia recurrences commonly occur within 1 year after the ablation procedure, recurrences are not uncommon also beyond 1 year of follow-up. A gradual decrease in the arrhythmia-free rate during the long-term follow-up is not specific to the stepwise ablation, but also is observed after any ablation strategy for persistent AF [11]. Based on this evidence, the discontinuation of anticoagulants during the follow-up is not recommended after ablation of persistent AF.

Predictors of arrhythmia recurrences during follow-up are failure of AF termination, advanced age, female gender, larger LA diameters, greater duration of continuous AF, and structural heart disease [9, 10]. All of these predictors are associated with remodeling of the atria [12–14]. Progressive atrial remodeling is associated with a worse clinical outcome even after the aggressive ablation strategy. Thus, the management of risk factors such as hypertension, heart failure, obesity, or alcohol intake is important [15].

Termination of AF during the ablation procedure is associated with the type of recurrent arrhythmia during follow-up. In patients with AF termination, recurrence of AF is unusual, and most recurrent arrhythmias are AT. In contrast, if we fail to terminate AF, most patients have recurrence of AF. In general, AT is associated with a rapid ventricular response and being more symptomatic, compared to AF. However, the mechanism of AT can be determined with the use of a 3D-mapping system. Thus, AT can be eliminated in 90% of cases. As a result, the clinical outcome after a repeat ablation is favorable in patients with AF termination during the index ablation procedure, compared to that in those without AF termination. After a repeat ablation procedure, the arrhythmia-free rate is 70% at 1 year of follow-up.

Whether termination of AF is an appropriate procedural endpoint is controversial. In persistent AF, isolation of the PVs rarely terminates AF, but is effective in a fraction of patients. AF can be terminated by ablation in patients with less remodeled atria, such as small LA diameter, short duration of continuous AF, or no structural heart disease. It is often argued that patients who have AF termination may be treated successfully by PV isolation alone because of less remodeled atria. Additionally, extra-PV ablation lesions can be arrhythmogenic and attributable to recurrence of AT. If we draw two linear lesions, the opportunity of conduction recovery of at least one line would be doubled, compared to a single line. Extensive ablation is associated with the risk of iatrogenic arrhythmia recurrence. However, termination of AF suggests the elimination of atrial tissues critical for maintenance of AF. This idea is supported by the fact that recurrence of AF is uncommon in patients with AF termination. Therefore, a future direction of catheter ablation for persistent AF would be development of mapping techniques to precisely identify the atrial sites or areas critical for maintaining AF, which would facilitate AF termination by ablation and reduce the amount of ablation lesions.

20.6 Effects of the Stepwise Ablation on Left Atrial Electrical and Mechanical Properties

In patients with remodeled atria, extensively distributed arrhythmia substrate needs to be targeted for maintenance of sinus rhythm. However, extensive ablation lesions may adversely affect electrical and mechanical properties of the LA after the ablation procedure. Surface area of scar tissue was assessed by a 3D-mapping system ≥ 1 month after the stepwise ablation [16]. Scar area (bipolar voltage of <0.05 mV) and low-voltage area (bipolar voltage of <0.5 mV) accounted for $31 \pm 12\%$ and $32 \pm 17\%$ of the LA surface area, respectively. Scar area included the ablated PV regions, which accounted for $20 \pm 4\%$ of the LA surface area. Distribution of scar area was variable in each patient, depending on the location of previous ablation lesions or spontaneous scar or low-voltage area.

Spontaneous or iatrogenic scar affects intra-atrial conduction. In the previous report, the latest activation site in the LA was the appendage, posterior wall, or lateral wall. The latest activation of the LA was during or after the QRS complex in 22% of the patients [16]. Such intra-atrial conduction disturbances result in dyssynchronous contraction of the LA or simultaneous contraction of the LA and left ventricle, which adversely affect LA transport function. The activation delay in the LA is partly attributable to the tissue damage in the anterior LA, that is, the Bachmann bundle insertion region. Sixty percentage of patients with spontaneous low-voltage area in the LA have low-voltage tissue in this region [17]. Ablation at the low-voltage area readily results in conduction block. If conduction through the Bachmann bundle is blocked, activity propagates through the LA lateral wall to the LA appendage. Mitral isthmus line interrupts this pathway and causes isolation of the LA appendage, which is associated with thrombus formation in this structure and stroke during follow-up [18]. Thus, scarring in the anterior LA needs to be taken into consideration before mitral isthmus line ablation.

After the stepwise ablation, the healthy tissue is reduced and intra-atrial conduction is disturbed. Thus, LA contractile function should be depressed compared to that in normal population. In patients who underwent the stepwise ablation, however, echocardiograms confirm the presence of active LA contraction during sinus rhythm [16]. LA mechanical function is absent during AF, and AF would continue without ablation. Therefore, restoration of sinus rhythm after the stepwise ablation compensates for extensive atrial tissue damage by gain of LA mechanical function.

20.7 Recent Progress in the Ablation Strategy with an Endpoint of AF Termination

20.7.1 Body Surface Mapping

Recently, mapping techniques have been developed to identify AF drivers. Haissaguerre et al. used the body surface mapping technology, in which a 252-electrode vest is applied to the patient's torso and unipolar surface potentials are recorded from the electrodes on the vest [4]. From the unipolar surface potentials, 3D maps are created with the use of phase map technique. The major advantages of this technique are (1) mapping of the both atria is performed simultaneously, and (2) phase map technique reveals both focal and rotational activations. Rotational activation is often unclear when time-domain analysis is performed. Body surface mapping in the combined use of phase map demonstrates a median of four driver regions per patient, and 80% of them are reentry and the remaining 20% are focal activation. Reentrant drivers are commonly observed in the left and right PV regions, inferior LA, and upper RA, and focal drivers commonly arise from the PVs and LA and RA appendages.

Catheter ablation targeting such driver regions terminates AF in 63% of patients, and additional linear ablation terminates AF in another 17% of patients. The duration of radiofrequency energy deliveries is significantly shorter in driver ablation, compared to stepwise ablation, which confirms the accuracy of this new system. The extent of the lesions of driver ablation is less than that of stepwise ablation, but AT occurs during the ablation procedure after termination of AF in 66% of patients with AF termination. This fact may suggest that AT occurring after termination of AF is not always iatrogenic. Termination of AF by ablation is associated with a better clinical outcome, as is observed in the stepwise ablation. Even using this new mapping system, the AF termination rate and arrhythmia-free rate at 1-year follow-up are 45% and 50%, respectively, in long-standing persistent AF (continuous for >12 months). This is partly because body surface mapping is feasible only before the ablation procedure. In patients with a more advanced substrate, drivers may newly appear after elimination of drivers, which are not identified before the ablation procedure. Use of body surface mapping during the ablation procedure may improve the clinical outcomes in patients with a complex arrhythmia substrate.

20.7.2 High-Density Endocardial Mapping

A multi-electrode catheter with five radiating splines has been used to understand the wavefront propagation pattern during AF [19]. This catheter has four electrodes on each spline, for a total of 20 electrodes, and covers an area with a diameter of 35 mm. Using this high-density mapping catheter, focal activation pattern is demonstrated by displaying activity propagation from the proximal to distal electrodes on all five splines (Fig. 20.6). Focal activation is observed outside of the PVs in most patients with persistent AF, and appears repetitively for every 10–20 s at a discrete site. The duration of one episode is usually 0.5–2 s, but a persistent form of focal activation is also observed.

This catheter also enables the demonstration of rotational activation during AF, but rotational activation is infrequently observed. As mentioned above, body surface mapping has found reentry to be more common than focal drivers. The discrepancy between the findings using body surface mapping and high-density endocardial mapping may be explained by the following: (1) High-density mapping covers a small area of the atrium, thereby missing meandering reentries, and (2) body surface mapping uses phase map technique, which is often required for identification of reentry, but also generates false-positive reentry [20].

Epicardial mapping of human AF has also reported the presence of focal activation during AF [21]. However, the efficacy of catheter ablation targeting focal activation is unknown. We perform high-density mapping during AF after PV isolation, and subsequently perform electrogram-based ablation [22]. After the ablation procedure, high-density mapping data are analyzed and focal activation sites are determined. This study demonstrated that sites where ablation terminated AF were in the proximity of focal activation sites, suggesting a driving role of focal activation sites in AF.

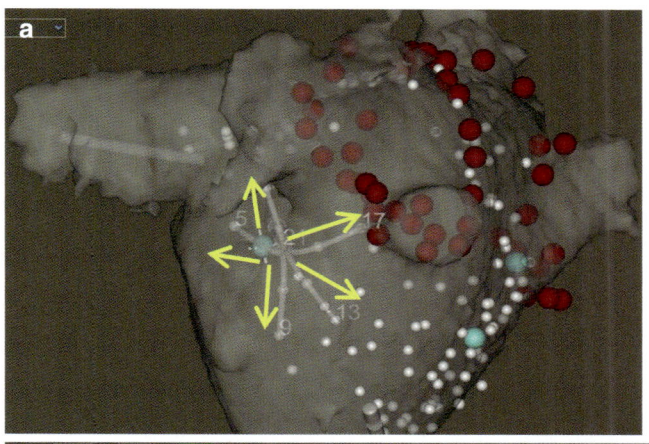
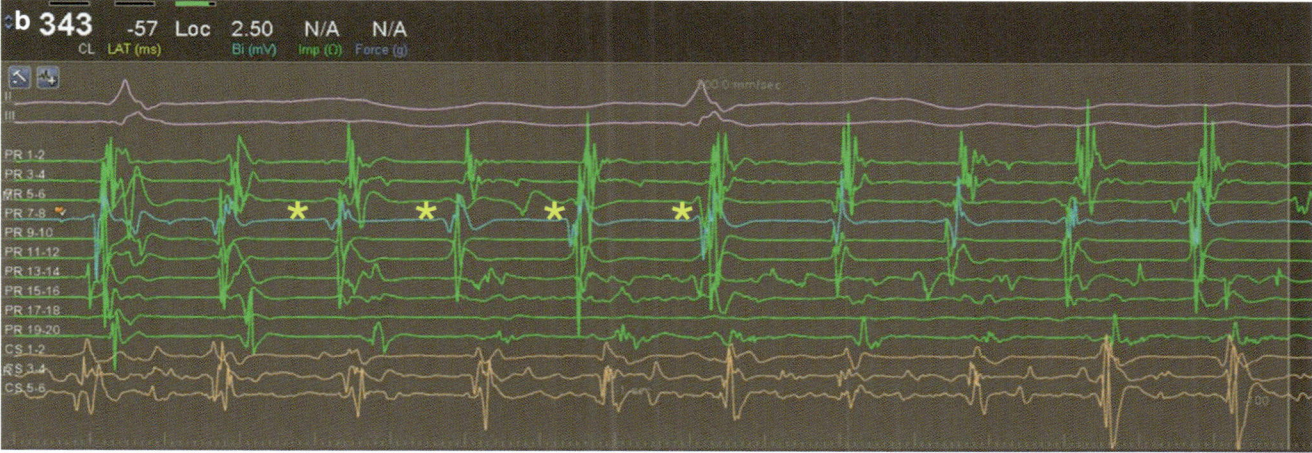

Fig. 20.6 A blue dot represents the focal activation site at the lateral wall of the left atrium in a left-posterior view of a 3D-mapping system (**a**). Electrograms from the high-density mapping catheter at this site shows the earliest activation on 7–8 on the high-density mapping catheter (*asterisk*) for four consecutive atrial cycles during atrial fibrillation. Red dots represent ablation lesions for pulmonary vein isolation

Conventional electrogram-based ablation enables the termination of AF, but the predictive value of the target electrogram characteristics for the presence of AF drivers is poor. This is associated with a prolonged procedural duration and occurrence of iatrogenic ATs. New mapping techniques to identify AF drivers will improve the clinical outcomes of the catheter ablation of persistent AF.

References

1. Haïssaguerre M, Hocini M, Sanders P, Sacher F, Rotter M, Takahashi Y, et al. Catheter ablation of long-lasting persistent atrial fibrillation: clinical outcome and mechanisms of subsequent arrhythmias. J Cardiovasc Electrophysiol. 2005;16:1138–47.
2. Takahashi Y, O'Neill MD, Hocini M, Dubois R, Matsuo S, Knecht S, et al. Characterization of electrograms associated with termination of chronic atrial fibrillation by catheter ablation. J Am Coll Cardiol. 2008;51(10):1003. https://doi.org/10.1016/j.jacc.2007.10.056.
3. Lee G, Kumar S, Teh A, Madry A, Spence S, Larobina M, et al. Epicardial wave mapping in human long-lasting persistent atrial fibrillation: transient rotational circuits, complex wavefronts, and disorganized activity. Eur Heart J. 2014;35:86–97. https://doi.org/10.1093/eurheartj/eht267.
4. Haissaguerre M, Hocini M, Denis A, Shah AJ, Komatsu Y, Yamashita S, et al. Driver domains in persistent atrial fibrillation. Circulation. 2014;130:530–8. https://doi.org/10.1161/circulationaha.113.005421.
5. Rostock T, Rotter M, Sanders P, Takahashi Y, Jaïs P, Hocini M, et al. High-density activation mapping of fractionated electrograms in the atria of patients with paroxysmal atrial fibrillation. Heart Rhythm. 2006;3:27–34.
6. Takahashi Y, Takahashi A, Miyazaki S, Kuwahara T, Takei A, Fujino T, et al. Electrophysiological characteristics of localized reentrant atrial tachycardia occurring after catheter ablation of long-lasting persistent atrial fibrillation. J Cardiovasc Electrophysiol. 2009;20:623–9. https://doi.org/10.1111/j.1540-8167.2008.01410.x.
7. Haïssaguerre M, Sanders P, Hocini M, Takahashi Y, Rotter M, Sacher F, et al. Catheter ablation of long-lasting persistent atrial fibrillation: critical structures for termination. J Cardiovasc Electrophysiol. 2005;16:1125–37.
8. Matsuo S, Lellouche N, Wright M, Bevilacqua M, Knecht S, Nault I, et al. Clinical predictors of termination and clinical outcome of

catheter ablation for persistent atrial fibrillation. J Am Coll Cardiol. 2009;54:788–95. https://doi.org/10.1016/j.jacc.2009.01.081.
9. Schreiber D, Rostock T, Fröhlich M, Sultan A, Servatius H, Hoffmann BA, et al. Five-year follow-up after catheter ablation of persistent atrial fibrillation using the stepwise approach and prognostic factors for success. Circ Arrhythm Electrophysiol. 2015;8:308–17. https://doi.org/10.1161/CIRCEP.114.001672.
10. Scherr D, Khairy P, Miyazaki S, Aurillac-Lavignolle V, Pascale P, Wilton SB, et al. Five-year outcome of catheter ablation of persistent atrial fibrillation using termination of atrial fibrillation as a procedural endpoint. Circ Arrhythm Electrophysiol. 2015;8:18–24. https://doi.org/10.1161/CIRCEP.114.001943.
11. Tilz RR, Rillig A, Thum AM, Arya A, Wohlmuth P, Metzner A, et al. Catheter ablation of long-standing persistent atrial fibrillation: 5-year outcomes of the Hamburg Sequential Ablation Strategy. J Am Coll Cardiol. 2012;60:1921–9. https://doi.org/10.1016/j.jacc.2012.04.060.
12. Kistler PM, Sanders P, Fynn SP, Stevenson IH, Spence SJ, Vohra JK, et al. Electrophysiologic and electroanatomic changes in the human atrium associated with age. J Am Coll Cardiol. 2004;44:109–16.
13. Sanders P, Morton JB, Davidson NC, Spence SJ, Vohra JK, Sparks PB, et al. Electrical remodeling of the atria in congestive heart failure: electrophysiological and electroanatomic mapping in humans. Circulation. 2003;108:1461–8.
14. John B, Stiles MK, Kuklik P, Chandy ST, Young GD, Mackenzie L, et al. Electrical remodelling of the left and right atria due to rheumatic mitral stenosis. Eur Heart J. 2008;29:2234–43. https://doi.org/10.1093/eurheartj/ehn329.
15. Abed HS, Wittert GA, Leong DP, Shirazi MG, Bahrami B, Middeldorp ME, et al. Effect of weight reduction and cardiometabolic risk factor management on symptom burden and severity in patients with atrial fibrillation: a randomized clinical trial. JAMA. 2013;310:2050–60. https://doi.org/10.1001/jama.2013.280521.
16. Takahashi Y, O'Neill MD, Hocini M, Reant P, Jonsson A, Jaïs P, et al. Effects of stepwise ablation of chronic atrial fibrillation on atrial electrical and mechanical properties. J Am Coll Cardiol. 2007;49:1306–14.
17. Rolf S, Kircher S, Arya A, Eitel C, Sommer P, Richter S, et al. Tailored atrial substrate modification based on low-voltage areas in catheter ablation of atrial fibrillation. Circ Arrhythm Electrophysiol. 2014;7:825–33. https://doi.org/10.1161/circep.113.001251.
18. Rillig A, Tilz RR, Lin T, Fink T, Heeger CH, Arya A, et al. Unexpectedly high incidence of stroke and left atrial appendage thrombus formation after electrical isolation of the left atrial appendage for the treatment of atrial tachyarrhythmias. Circ Arrhythm Electrophysiol. 2016;9:e003461. https://doi.org/10.1161/CIRCEP.115.003461.
19. Takahashi Y, Hocini M, O'Neill MD, Sanders P, Rotter M, Rostock T, et al. Sites of focal atrial activity characterized by endocardial mapping during atrial fibrillation. J Am Coll Cardiol. 2006;47:2005–12.
20. Vijayakumar R, Vasireddi SK, Cuculich PS, Faddis MN, Rudy Y. Methodology considerations in phase mapping of human cardiac arrhythmias. Circ Arrhythm Electrophysiol. 2016;9(11):pii:e004409.
21. Lee S, Sahadevan J, Khrestian CM, Cakulev I, Markowitz A, Waldo AL. Simultaneous biatrial high-density (510–512 electrodes) epicardial mapping of persistent and long-standing persistent atrial fibrillation in patients: new insights into the mechanism of its maintenance. Circulation. 2015;132:2108–17.
22. Takahashi Y, Iwai S, Yamashita S, Masumura M, Suzuki M, Yabe K, et al. Novel mapping technique for localization of focal and reentrant activation during atrial fibrillation. J Cardiovasc Electrophysiol. 2017;28(4):375–82.

Substrate Ablation of Persistent AF

Takeshi Tsuchiya, Takanori Yamaguchi, and Akira Fukui

Keywords

Ablation • Atrial fibrillation • Fibrosis • Low voltage zone • Voltage mapping

21.1 Current Situation of Substrate Ablations of Persistent and Long-Standing Persistent Atrial Fibrillation

Pulmonary vein antrum isolation (PVAI) is the cornerstone of atrial fibrillation (AF) ablation, which is an imperative first step in the ablation of any type of AF [1–3]. Although it seems adequate for eliminating paroxysmal AF, and when sometimes in conjunction with an appropriate addition of a non-PV foci or carvotricuspid isthmus ablation; however, it is insufficient to eliminate persistent or long-standing persistent AF in half of the cases. Many strategies have been attempted in order to destroy the remaining "substrate of AF outside the PVs" after the PVAI in those with persistent or long-standing persistent AF, including a complex fractionated atrial electrogram (CFAE) ablation and left atrial linear ablation. However, they have not been shown to have any benefit over the PVAI by a meta-analysis [2], and the STAR AF II trial [3], possibly because they are not a tailored ablation strategy for a patient-specific AF substrate. Further, the Cardiothoracic Surgical Trials Network (CSTN) investigators reported that they failed to find any significant difference in the rate of freedom from AF between patients who underwent a surgical PV isolation and those who underwent a bi-atrial maze procedure [4], indicating that an "empirical substrate ablation not based on a patient-specific background" is questionable.

Atrial fibrosis has attracted interest as a patient-specific AF substrate [5]. Fibrosis is well known to play an important role in ventricular tachyarrhythmias associated with structural heart disease. Atrial fibrosis seems to be a final common pathway, which results from a variety of comorbidities of AF including structural heart diseases, obesity, hypertension, sleep apnea, heart failure, and aging. Kottkamp et al. argued that atrial fibrosis can occur in an idiopathic fashion independent of these modulators of atrial fibrosis called fibrotic atrial cardiomyopathy (FACM) [6]. A body of evidence revealed that a more increased amount of atrial fibrosis has been observed in patients with AF compared to those with sinus rhythm [5–13]. The location of the fibrosis seems diverse and patient specific. It includes a collagen deposition produced by fibroblasts or the activated form of myofibroblasts mainly due to the reparative process for degenerating myocytes or due to the reactive process to local environmental changes in the tissue. It is also known that in fibrotic tissue, gap junction remodeling consisting of a decreased number and lateralization of gap junctions occurs, and both the fibroblasts and myofibroblasts proliferate [14–17]. These histological changes in the fibrotic tissue result in electrophysiological changes involving a conduction delay or block, generation of ectopy, and an abbreviation of the myocardial action potential duration, leading to arrhythmogenicity [17, 18].

21.2 Histological Changes in the Fibrotic Tissue

Fibrotic changes progress in different components of the atrial tissue in parallel over time. Along with AF sustaining, structural and pathological changes occur at the cellular level,

T. Tsuchiya (✉) • A. Fukui
EP Expert Doctors – Team Tsuchiya,
3-14-28, Koto, Higashi-ku, Kumamoto-shi 862-0909, Japan
e-mail: tsuchiya0210jupiter@yj8.so-net.ne.jp

T. Yamaguchi
Saga-ken Medical Center Koseikan,
Ooaza Nakahara 400, Kase-machi, Saga 840-8571, Japan

including myocyte hypertrophy, loss of myofibrils, changes in the mitochondrion size, disruption of the sarcoplasmic reticulum, and apoptotic or necrotic death of myocytes followed by interstitial fibrosis. Atrial fibrosis occurs in a patient-specific manner, mainly in the anterior, septal, and posterior LA where the number of myocytes decreases due to myocardial apoptosis and/or necrosis in association with collagen deposition, gap junction remodeling, and proliferation of fibroblasts and the activated form of myofibroblasts [14–23].

Gap junctions are formed by joining two hemichannels or connexins and are responsible for mediating the spread of cardiac excitation and direct intercellular metabolic communication between neighboring myocytes. Gap junctions in the human heart consist of connexins (CX) 31.9, 40, 43, and 45, among which CX 40 and 43 are said to mainly contribute to carrying myocardial excitation in the atrium. In patients with sinus rhythm, gap junctions are found at the intercalated disc and mediate the cell-to-cell electrical coupling and communication. However, in patients with atrial fibrillation the location changes to the lateral wall of the atrial myocytes called lateralization in most patients although there is controversy with regard to the reduction of the CX. The changes in the expression and distribution of the CX are well known as gap junction remodeling, which gives rise to a conduction delay and block, facilitating reentry. In fact, CX 43 gene therapy was reported to preserve the conduction velocity and prevent atrial fibrillation in a burst pacing induced AF model using experimental animals [18]. It is also noted that the magnitude of fibrosis is inversely correlated with the amount of CX 43 in patients with AF, suggesting that the expression of CX43 is reduced in fibrotic tissue [19]. Actually, in a rat experiment, AF became more inducible by atrial pacing after aortic banding in parallel with fibrosis and CX 43 remodeling.

Fibroblasts outnumber cardiomyocytes by two or threefold in the normal atrium, which interconnect with each other and produce extracellular structural proteins including collagen I and III, fibronectin, laminin, and elastic fibers to serve as a heart skeleton and provide the basic structure for cardiomyocytes to jointly contract as a pump [15, 16]. Fibrosis proliferation results from apoptotic or necrotic death of myocytes caused by a mechanical overload of the heart, infarction, aging, and so on while it can occur in response to mechanical and humoral stimulation. Along with fibrosis, the matrix proteins, mainly consisting of collagen, are disproportionally produced by fibroblasts or the activated form of myofibroblast. That results in a derangement of the muscle bundle architecture to form a collageneous septa and causes a separation between the bundles of myocytes, leading to a local conduction delay or block with a zig-zag conduction.

Myofibroblasts are not found in healthy hearts and are differentiated from fibroblasts in their response to myocardial damage or death, and humoral and mechanical stimulation [15]. They are characterized by their large size and multiple processes with the expression of α-smooth muscle actin. Myofibroblasts actively produce collagen, but are also known to secrete many cytokines, chemokines, extracellular matrix (ECM) proteins, proteases, and growth factors in a paracrine fashion, which facilitates fibroblasts to transform into myofibroblasts and causes further abbreviation of the action potential duration of the atrial myocytes. Fibroblasts and myofibroblasts are located next to myocytes and exert some electrophysiological effects on the myocytes. There is some evidence showing that there is an electrical coupling between fibroblasts/myofibroblasts and cardiomyocytes via gap junctions, suggesting an electrotonic cross-talk between the fibroblasts/myofibroblasts and cardiomyocytes. Both fibroblasts and myofibroblasts are electrically non-excitable, but have shallow membrane potentials ranging from −20 to −40 mV. The membrane potentials are less negative compared with the resting membrane potentials of atrial myocytes (during diastole) and much more negative than that during the depolarization and repolarization phases (during systole). Because of the electrical gap and cross-talk between the fibroblasts/myofibroblasts and atrial myocytes, for atrial myocytes, fibroblasts function as an electrical source during the polarization phase (diastole) leading to a shallowing of the resting membrane potential (partial depolarization during diastole), and as a sink during the depolarization and repolarization phases (systole) leading to a shortening of the action potential duration. This electrical cross-talk likely results in conduction slowing due to partially depolarized resting membrane potentials and a subsequent reduced availability of sodium channels. The abbreviation of the action potential duration indicates a shortened refractory period, facilitating reentry. Myofibroblasts are larger and more powerful than fibroblasts for exerting an electrical influence on neighboring atrial myocytes via an active collagen production, paracrine function, and electrical cross-talk.

During AF, fibroblast proliferation and differentiation into myofibroblasts seems more atrial selective even if the left ventricle is damaged. Some researches attempted to explain why and how this happens. It is noted that the morphology and contents of atrial fibroblasts are different from those of the ventricular ones and the fibrotic response in the left atrium was shown to be 20 times greater than that in the left ventricle in a canine AF model using ventricular tachypacing-induced heart failure [20]. Along with the advancement of heart failure, fibrosis progresses more prominently in the left atrium than in the left ventricle because of the atrium-selective fibroblast activation via the platelet-derived growth factor. This change occurs in parallel with a white cell infiltration, apoptosis, tissue angiotensin II increase, and MAP kinase and TGFβ1 activation. It is also known that transient receptor potential (TRP) receptors in atrial fibroblasts regulate the proliferation and phenotype switching into myofibroblasts during AF. TRP receptors mediate Ca^{2+} entry in excitable and unexcitable cells like fibroblasts, which activates the extracellular signal-related kinase signaling. TRP receptors are activated by various local environmental stimuli including receptor activation, oxidative stress, mechanical stretch, cellular metabolites, and thermal and sensory stimuli. TRP canonical-3 (TRPC3) and TRP melastatin-related 7 (TRPM7) are well known to increase during AF facilitating fibrosis, and it has been shown that the blockade of the TRP channel prevents fibrosis in an animal experimental model [21, 22]. These mechanisms seem to contribute to an atrium-selective fibrosis in spite of a lack of an obvious organic ventricular disease.

21.3 Electrophysiologic Changes Corresponding to the Histological Changes in Fibrotic Tissue

AF promotes electrical remodeling of atrial myocytes, including a reduction in the L-type calcium current (I_{ca-L}) along with an increase in the basal inward rectifier current (I_{k1}) and acetylcholine-dependent inward rectifier current ($I_{K, Ach}$), leading to a shortened action potential duration [23]. In addition to this electrical remodeling by AF, fibrotic tissue is characterized by some electrophysiological changes, including a low voltage, abbreviation of the effective refractory period, and conduction slowing/block. Each of those corresponds to three major histological changes in the fibrotic tissue, including collagen deposition, fibroblast/myofibroblast proliferation, and gap junction remodeling [24, 25] (Table 21.1). To begin with, fibrotic tissue exhibits low amplitude bipolar electrograms resulting from a decreased electromotive force due to the loss of myocytes and an increase in fibroblasts/myofibroblast and the extracellular matrix. Proliferation of fibroblasts and myofibroblasts causes a shallowing of the resting membrane potential of the atrial myocytes, leading to a reduced availability of sodium ion channels and a subsequent conduction slowing or block, and sometimes causes depolarization-induced ectopy. It also shortens the action potential duration of atrial myocytes, which means a shortening of the effective refractory period.

Table 21.1 Pathological changes and the corresponding electrophysiological changes

Pathological changes		Corresponding electrophysiological changes
Loss of myocytes and collagen deposition	→	Low voltage
Gap junction remodeling	→	Conduction delay or block
(Myo)fibroblast proliferation	→	APD abbreviation, conduction delay, or block

APD action potential duration

Gap junction remodeling, which is characterized by a reduced number and lateralization of the CX, causes conduction slowing and block.

McDowell et al. examined what factors play an important role in the initiation and maintenance of AF using a computer simulation model constructed based on a patient-specific atrial geometry and fibrotic distribution obtained from the cardiac MRI of AF patients [25]. They tested how a combination of a collagen deposition, fibroblast/myofibroblast proliferation, and gap junction remodeling would work to initiate and maintain AF, and found that the collagen deposition is not responsible for reentrant activation, but both the gap junction remodeling and proliferation of fibroblast/myofibroblast contribute to reentry formation. Further, the same group reported, using a computer simulation that reentrant drivers persist at intermingling sites with a high density of fibroblasts around the border of fibrotic tissue [26].

21.4 Reverse Remodeling of Fibrosis

If AF is associated with fibrosis, then, can fibrotic tissue be reversed after AF is restored to sinus rhythm? There are some papers that examined this issue. In a canine AF model created by mitral regurgitation and rapid atrial pacing for more than 8 weeks, AF was still easily induced by atrial pacing 7–14 days after restoration of sinus rhythm where structural changes remained unchanged, consisting of swollen myocytes, an increase in the extracellular matrix, an increased number or size of mitochondria, and destruction of the sarcoplasmic reticulum, but the number of ectopy and an abbreviation of the effective refractory period both recovered to the control level. In a goat model, burst atrial pacing was performed in order to sustain AF for 4 months, and what was occurring after sinus rhythm restoration was observed [27]. Of note, the extracellular matrix continued to increase even if 4 months had passed after restoration of sinus rhythm. Those findings suggested that the process of reverse remodeling of fibrosis is slow.

21.5 Clinical Aspects of Atrial Fibrosis

Atrial fibrosis is represented as a low voltage zone (LVZ) by voltage mapping during sinus rhythm using an electrode catheter, which has historically been defined as a site with a peak-to-peak bipolar voltage <0.5 mV. Recently, the amplitude cut-off value is in debate. Kottkamp et al. set the cut-off at 0.5 mV but they think 0.5–1.5 mV represents an "intermediate zone" for mild fibrosis [6]. Yang et al. defined the LVZ as 0.1–0.4 mV and a transitional zone as 0.4–1.3 mV, which were set based on findings taken from the voltage distribution of healthy controls and AF patients [12]. Jadidi et al. defined low

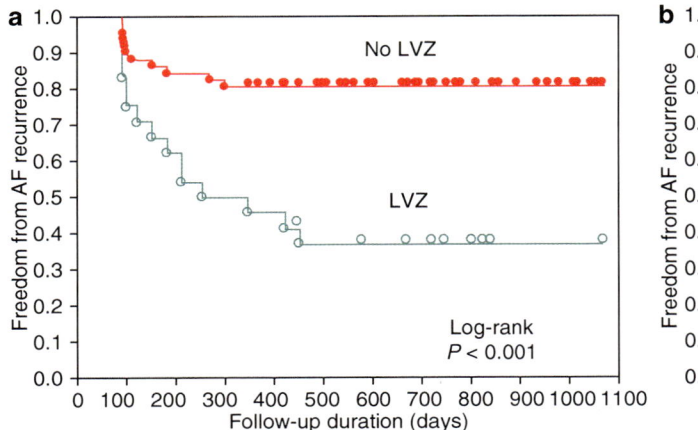
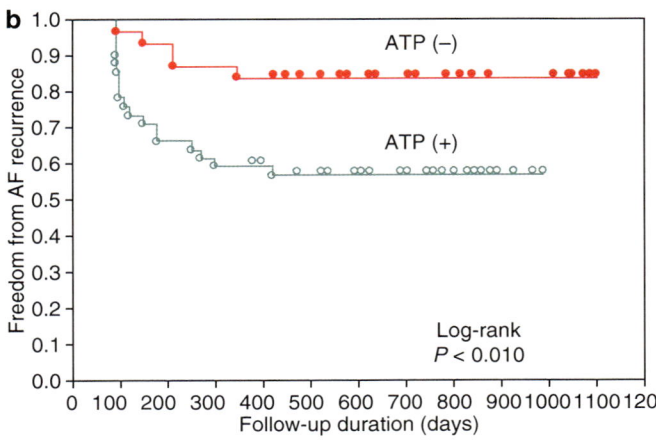

Fig. 21.1 Freedom from atrial fibrillation recurrence in patients undergoing pulmonary vein antrum isolation alone. Panel (**a**) shows the difference in the AF free ratio between those with a low voltage zone (LVZ) and those without. Panel (**b**) shows the difference in the AF free ratio between those with an ATP-induced acute PV reconnection and those without. Of note, ATP-induced acute PV reconnections were closed by a touch-up ablation during the same ablation procedure. *ATP* adenosine triphosphate (Permission from EP Europace, ref. [1]).

voltage areas as sites <0.5 mV during AF determined as the maximum bipolar voltage of two consecutive AF beats, and <1.0 mV during sinus rhythm [13]. In contrast, scar is defined as very low voltage ranging from <0.2 mV to no electrogram and no electric capture depending on the reports [6, 7, 10–13]. Fibrotic tissue and scar somewhat differ from each other because fibrotic tissue is arrhythmogenic by itself while scar represents a non-exciting tissue providing a conduction gap for reentry between scars and between scar and anatomical obstacles. Actually, we found that those with an LVZ have more frequent recurrences after pulmonary vein antrum isolation (PVAI) compared with those without an LVZ irrespective of the AF type, indicating that patients with an LVZ have more frequent recurrences even if they have paroxysmal AF while those without an LVZ have less frequent recurrences even though they have long-lasting persistent AF (Fig. 21.1) [7]. The clinical characteristics of the patients with an LVZ have an old age, greater female gender, LA enlargement, and structural heart disease [7, 10]. The LVZ is reported to have slow conduction, fractionated potentials during sinus rhythm and can be a source of AF [28].

Atrial fibrosis can also be expressed by delayed enhancement (DE) of cardiac MRI, the location and morphology of which are similar to the LVZ identified by voltage mapping using an electroanatomical mapping system and defined as <0.5 mV during sinus rhythm [8]. The tissue characterization of the LA wall by DE was correlated with that of fibrosis revealed by histology of specimens obtained from surgical biopsy in patients undergoing open heart surgery for diverse heart diseases with and without AF. The areas exhibiting some extent of DE matched with fibrosis in the surgical specimens while those without DE had normal tissue without any significant fibrosis. Sites with DE exhibit slow and more organized electrical activity rather than complex fractionated atrial electrograms during AF, but with a lower voltage than healthy atrial tissue. The amount of DE was strongly correlated with the outcome after the PV isolation followed by posterior wall and septal debulking. Recurrence after ablation was significantly higher in those with >30% fibrosis on the LA surface than in those without [9].

21.6 Tips and Tricks of Voltage Mapping

Accurate voltage mapping requires an accurate electrogram sampling with a stable catheter position and appropriate pressure application of the electrodes against the LA endocardium. We usually use a 20-pole spiral shaped ring electrode catheter for the voltage mapping with support of a long sheath in order to guarantee a pressure application of the electrodes. The amplitude and distinctive morphology of the electrograms are strongly related to the electrode length and interelectrode spacing. Anter et al. conducted a study comparing the amplitude and morphology of the LA electrograms between 3.5-mm tip ablation catheters and 1-mm multielectrode-mapping catheters in patients with structurally normal atria and with scar-related atrial arrhythmias, and they found that the bipolar electrograms recorded in the area with a low voltage using the 1-mm multielectrode-mapping catheter were significantly higher and more distinct than those recorded using the ablation catheter [29]. Further, the size of the low voltage area was reduced by 30% when it was identified using the 1-mm multielectrode-mapping catheter. Recognition of the morphology of the low amplitude electrograms is important because it sometimes exhibits fractionated electrograms, which suggest slow conduction or local conduction block.

21.7 Efficacy and Safety of Ablation of Fibrotic Areas (Table 21.2)

Rolf et al. firstly reported in 2014 the effects of substrate modification based on the LVZ in 47 patients with either paroxysmal ($n = 6$) or persistent AF ($n = 41$) [10]. They used a decapolar circular catheter to acquire sampling points, and the missing sites were complemented with a 4-mm tip ablation catheter. An LVZ was defined as ≥3 adjacent sites with a peak-to-peak bipolar electrogram of 0.2–0.5 mV during sinus rhythm. Electrograms of <0.2 mV were considered likely to represent scar. After a standard PVAI using their ablate and pace technique, they employed diverse approaches to ablate the LVZ, initially attempting to homogenize the diseased LA tissue with the endpoint of a significant reduction in the local electrograms, defractionation, and loss of capture while stimulating with the ablation catheter with a high output of 10 V and pulse width of 2 ms. When LVZ homogenization was difficult to achieve, strategic linear lesions were created to connect nonconducting tissues with other nonconducting anatomic structures traversing the target LVZ, or and encircling large LVZ ablation was performed to isolate them. After that, burst atrial pacing was performed to induce atrial tachycardia, and if any, it was ablated, and when AF was induced, no further substrate ablation was done. An LVZ was identified in 6 out of 62 patients (10%) with paroxysmal AF and 41 out of 116 patients (35%) with persistent AF, mainly at the LA roof, and anterior, septal, and posterior LA. According to a multivariate analysis, the age, sex, persistent AF, and low LA appendage flow velocity were found to be independent risk factors for predicting an LVZ. During a follow-up period of 15 ± 3 months, a single procedure success was achieved in 70% of patients undergoing an LVZ ablation after the PVAI while that was 27% in the patients with a sole PVAI despite having a similar size of the LVZ left untreated. Procedure-related complications were noted in 2 of 47 patients (4%), all of which were groin pseudoaneurysms.

Cutler et al. performed a retrospective analysis to examine whether using the presence or absence of regional low voltages in the posterior LA to guide the ablation beyond the PVAI improves the recurrence after AF ablation in 65 patients with persistent AF [11]. They performed voltage mapping in the posterior LA using an ablation catheter with the definition of an LVZ as areas >0.5 × 0.5 cm with electrogram amplitudes of <0.5 mV. They performed a voltage-guided posterior LA isolation, in which it was performed in addition to the PVAI when an LVZ was observed there, and it was not performed after the PVAI when no LVZ was present. The outcome of the voltage-guided posterior LA box isolation was compared with that of the standard ablation where additional lesions beyond the PVAI were performed at the discretion of the operator. Their voltage-guided ablation increased the 1-year atrial tachyarrhythmia-free survival compared to the standard ablation (80% vs. 57%, $P = 0.005$).

Kottkamp et al. also reported a similar effectiveness of the isolation of the LVZ, and what stood out in their strategy was that they performed a box isolation of the fibrotic areas (BIFA) anywhere in the LA, not only in the posterior LA, but also in the anterior and septal regions, and so forth [6]. They performed LA voltage mapping using a contact force-sensing ablation catheter with a contact force of 5–10 g. They defined an LVZ as a peak-to-peak bipolar voltage of <0.5 mV during sinus rhythm, but considered an area with an electrogram amplitude of 0.5–1.5 mV as an intermediate zone that did not mean substantial fibrosis, but was not normal atrial myocardium, and an area with no discrete electrograms and no local capture during pacing as scar. It was noted that the LVZ was unpredictably distributed with the individual location and extent, with no relationship to the cardiac risk factors and duration of sustained AF. They classified the patients into four categories according to the extent of the LVZ, in which an LA with no or a very limited LVZ was categorized as fibrotic atrial cardiomyopathy (FACM) 0–1, an LA with regional areas of low voltages as FACM 2, and atria with large confluent areas as FACM 3. The ablation strategy was a PVAI alone for patients with FACM 0–1, and PVAI followed by a BIFA for those with FACM 2–3. The BIFA was completed during sinus rhythm with confirmation of entrance block using a ring catheter, and the BIFA lines in the anterior/septal LVZs were typically extended to the right PV isolation line, and the BIFA

Table 21.2 Results of the LVZ ablation

Author	n	Age	LVZ location	Patients with LVZ, %	Follow-up (months)	Success rate, %	Complication rate, %
Rolf	178	61	Sept, ant, post, roof	26	15	70	4
Kottkamp	31	63	Ant, sept, post, inf	58	12.5	72	3.23
Yamaguchi	101	61	Ant, sept, roof, post	39	18	72	0
Yang	79	53	Ant, post, roof	70	30	66	3.5
Jadidi	85	63	Ant, sept, RA, CS	73	13	80	1.18
Cutler	65	62	Post	42	12	80	NA

Age indicates the mean age, n indicates the number of patients studied, % area of LVZ indicates the percent area of the LVZ over the left atrial surface. In the column labeled "LVZ location," *ant* anterior LA, *CS* coronary sinus, *LA post* = posterior LA, *LVZ* low voltage zone, *roof* LA roof, *RA* right atrium, *sept* septal LA. Dr. Cutler only assessed the electrogram voltage in the posterior LA

lines in the posterior/inferior/superior LA to the left and/or right PV isolation lines to prevent gap-related secondary atrial tachycardias. They conducted a study to test how the BIFA worked in ten patients with paroxysmal AF despite a durable PVI, and nine out of the ten patients remained in sinus rhythm during a mean follow-up of 20 ± 13 months. They further applied this strategy to 31 patients with persistent AF, and reported that a sole PVI was adequate in 13 patients (42%) with FACM 0–1 because outcomes 1 years after the single- and multiple-procedure were 69% and 85%, respectively. In the remaining 18 patients (58%) with FACM 2–3, the BIFA was successful with the outcome 1 year after a single- and multiple procedure of 72% and 83%, respectively. One patient had a global LA-LVZ and therefore, the concept of a BIFA could not be applied. It should be pointed out that their study included no control group in whom a PVI alone was performed despite an LVZ. There were no major complications but one groin hematoma occurred at the access site.

Our group examined the effectiveness and safety of the LVZ ablation in a prospective study, and the strength of our methodology was to perform an LVZ homogenization during ongoing AF [7]. We performed voltage mapping during sinus rhythm in 101 patients with persistent AF (persistent AF/long-lasting persistent AF = 68/33) using a 20-pole spiral shaped ring electrode in the LA. An LVZ was defined as an area with a bipolar peak-to-peak voltage amplitude of <0.5 mV during sinus rhythm and covering >5% of the LA body surface area, and scar as an area with that of <0.1 mV. An LVZ was found in 39 patients (39%) mainly in the anterior, septal, roof, and posterior LA with a mean area of 17.3 cm^2 occupying 20% of the LA surface area. An LVZ frequently exhibited fractionated potentials. Those with an LVZ were characterized by a female gender, high age, large LA volume, and long-lasting persistent AF. In patients who did not have an LVZ, the PVAI was performed without substrate modification, sometimes followed by isolation of the superior vena cava and a line creation at the carvotricuspid isthmus if necessary. When an LVZ was identified in the LA, the LVZ was ablated during re-induced AF in 35 of 39 patients (90%) with a procedural endpoint of an entire regional LVZ homogenization, attempting to clarify the acute effect of the LVZ ablation on AF. Of note, the ablation continued until the entire LVZ was ablated irrespective of acute AF slowing or termination (Fig. 21.2). The radiofrequency energy was delivered with the power set at 30 W, and the ablation catheter was moved point by point in a dragging fashion using a steerable sheath with a radiofrequency duration of 10 s at each point until a marked voltage reduction of <0.1 mV occurred. When the LVZ was large, strategic linear lines were created so as to connect the LVZ ablation area to anatomical obstacles including the PVI line, mitral annulus, and electrical scar areas to prevent any gap-related secondary atrial tachycardia. It should be emphasized that the LVZ ablation terminated AF in 14 out of 35 patients (40%) undergoing an LVZ ablation, in whom AF was terminated into sinus rhythm in five patients (36%) and transformed into atrial tachycardia in nine (64%). The outcome after the LVZ ablation was compared with that after the PVAI alone because of no LVZ ($n = 62$). An additional group of 16 consecutive patients with persistent AF and an LVZ did not undergo an LVZ ablation after the PVAI in spite of having a similar size of the LVZ to that in the patients undergoing the LVZ ablation, and they were used as a historical control group to compare the outcome with those undergoing an LVZ ablation. All patients were followed without any antiarrhythmic drugs. After a single session, no recurrence was observed in 28 out of 39 patients (72%) with an LVZ ablation and 49 out of 62 patients (79%) without an LVZ ablation because of no LVZ during 18 ± 7 months of follow-up (log-rank, $P = 0.400$). In the historical control group, no recurrence occurred in 1 out of 16 patients (6%) after a single session and in six patients (37%) after 1.8 sessions during 32 ± 7 months of follow-up (log-rank, $P < 0.001$ vs. LVZ ablation group) (Fig. 21.3). No major procedural complications were noted except for a vascular access complication in two patients.

Yang et al. advocated that substrate modification after the PVAI during sinus rhythm, consisting of homogenization of the LVZ, elimination of abnormal complex electrograms in the transitional areas, and dechanneling, is curative for AF and preventive for secondary atrial tachycardias [12]. They examined 79 patients with persistent AF (persistent/long-lasting persistent AF = 42/58). After the PVAI and carvotricuspid isthmus ablation, they performed bipolar voltage mapping in the LA during sinus rhythm using a 10-pole A-focus catheter to identify the LVZ and transitional zone. The LVZ was defined as 0.1–0.4 mV and the transitional zone as 0.4–1.3 mV, which were set according to their previous work. They also defined abnormal electrograms as any multiphasic electrogram with ≥3 positive or negative distinct peaks and an electrogram duration of ≥50 ms during sinus rhythm (AE-SR), and the AE-SRs in the transitional zone were included in a target for ablation because such electrograms may represent fibrotic tissue as well as a low voltage. Neither an LVZ nor AE-SR was found in 30% of the patients, and a PV isolation without any further ablation was performed, while 70% of the patients had an LVZ or AE-SR mainly at anterior wall (33%), posterior wall (25%), roof (30%), or septum (10%). It was noted that an LVZ and transitional zone were not found in the LA appendage in any patients. The entire LVZ and abnormal electrograms in the transitional zone were ablated in these patients with a maximal power of 35 W during sinus rhythm. They added an arbitral short line to traverse the potential conducting channel between the isolation lines or anatomical conduction barriers and LVZs (dechanneling), except for the areas exhibiting a

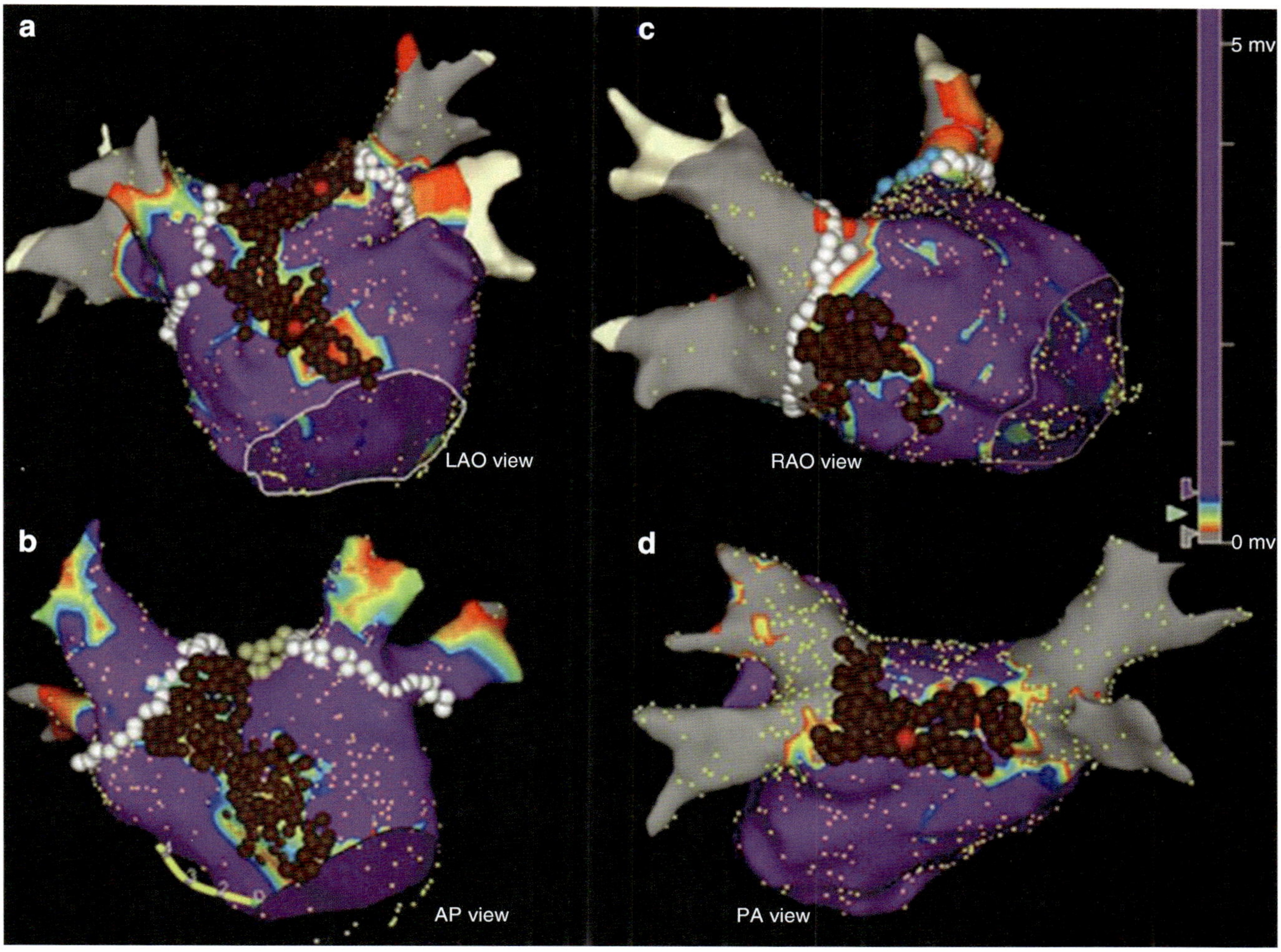

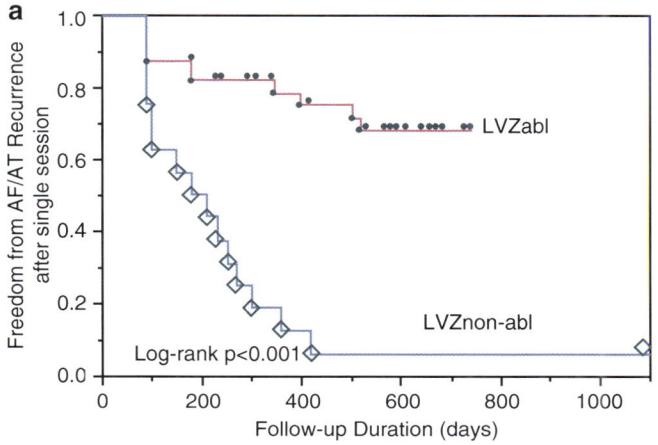

Fig. 21.2 Examples of an LVZ-guided ablation. Panels (**a–d**) show the entire LVZ ablation on the anterior wall and roof, anterior wall with an additional strategic roof line, on the septal wall, and on the posterior wall. The *red tags* indicate the termination sites of re-induced AF. *AF* atrial fibrillation, *AP* anterior-posterior, *AT* atrial tachycardia, *LVZ* low voltage zone, *PA* posterior-anterior, *PVAI* pulmonary vein antrum isolation, *RAO* right anterior oblique (Permission from Journal of Cardiovasc Electrophysiol, ref. [7])

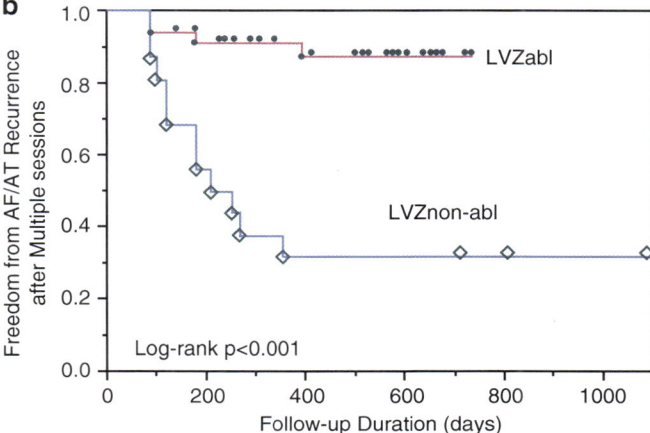

Fig. 21.3 Kaplan-Meier curve demonstrating the freedom from AF recurrence in patients undergoing an LVZ ablation and patients undergoing a PVI alone despite a similar size of the LVZs after a single session (panel **a**) and multiple sessions (panel **b**). *AF* atrial fibrillation, *LVZ* low voltage zone (Permission from Journal of Cardiovasc Electrophysiol, ref. [7])

width of >1.5 cm with local electrogram amplitudes of >1.3 mV. The outcome was compared with that of the historical cohort of the age- and sex-matched control group ($n = 78$), in which a stepwise approach consisting of a PVI, and linear ablation at the LA roof, posterior mitral, coronary sinus roof, and carvotricuspid isthmus followed by a CFAE ablation sequentially performed with the endpoint of AF termination. During a median follow-up period of 30 months, the freedom from AT/AF after a single session off antiarrhythmic agents was 66% (57/86) in all patients with and without an LVZ ablation while that of the historical control was 37% (29/78), which was translated into a SR maintenance of 69.8% versus 51.3% ($P = 0.011$) estimated from a Kaplan-Meier analysis at 24 months after the ablation. A subgroup analysis revealed that patients without LA substrates had a slightly higher success rate than the patients undergoing an LA substrate ablation. It was emphasized that AF recurred in 30% of patients receiving a voltage and AE-SR-guided ablation and atrial tachycardia in 3.5%. However, AF recurred in 32% of the patients receiving a stepwise approach, and the atrial tachycardia incidence was 30%, suggesting a voltage and AE-SR-guided ablation was similarly curative for AF and more preventive for secondary atrial tachycardia than the stepwise approach. Their procedure-related complications were femoral hematomas in two patients and a pseudoaneurysm in the groin in one.

Jadidi et al. performed a low voltage and specific electrogram-guided AF ablation in 85 patients with persistent AF sustaining from 7 days to 1 year. They gave all the patients DC shocks attempting to restore sinus rhythm 10 weeks before the ablation [13]. Sinus rhythm was maintained until the scheduled ablation date in 26 out of the 85 patients (31%). Interestingly, AF was not induced in 18 of the 26 patients in whom only a PVAI was performed in addition to the voltage mapping during sinus rhythm or CS pacing with a pacing cycle length of 800 ms with the definition of LVZ <1.0 mV. In the remaining 8 patients, AF was induced. A total of 67 patients with spontaneous AF despite a DC shock ($n = 59$) or induced AF ($n = 8$) underwent a PVAI during AF, which terminated the AF in five patients (7%). In the remaining 62 patients with AF after the PVAI, voltage mapping was performed during ongoing AF using an A-focus II and Lasso NaV with the definition of a low voltage as a maximal electrogram amplitude of <0.5 mV of consecutive two beats. When a low voltage was found, they used a contact force-sensing catheter at the site to confirm the low voltage area with the definition of an LVZ occupying >10% of the LA surface. They further defined the border zone as a 1 cm-tissue surrounding the LVZ. It was noted these patients with non-inducibility at the beginning of procedure had a low extent of the LVZ during a regular rhythm (sinus rhythm or CS pacing) and also those with AF termination by a PVAI alone had a limited extent of the LVZ during AF. An LVZ was frequently found in the 62 patients with persistent AF after the PVI, mainly in the anterior LA, septal right atrium (RA), and coronary sinus (CS). They applied radiofrequency energy to specific sites in the LVZ or at the border area, which were characterized by an electric activity of >70% of the AF cycle length on single or multiple electrodes of the ring catheter corresponding to a rotational activity or discrete rapid activity displaying a local cycle length of >10 ms shorter than the concomitant AF cycle length in the LA appendage or CS. Ablation at the electrically specific sites terminated AF in 45 out of the 62 patients (73%) it was attempted, and AF was directly restored to sinus rhythm in 14 patients (31%) and transformed into atrial tachycardia in 31 (69%). It should be emphasized that the AF termination sites were colocalized within the LVZ in 80% and at the border zone in 20%. The arrhythmia free outcome during a median of 13 months after a single session was achieved in 59 of 85 patients (69%), which was higher than that of the matched control group (53%, $n = 66$) in which only a conventional PVAI was performed. It was also noted that the outcome was similar between the patients who underwent a PVAI alone because of no or small amount of the LVZ and the patients who underwent the PVAI and ablation of the electrically specific sites in and around the LVZ. One patient developed a cardiac tamponade because of a steam pop during the carvotricuspid isthmus ablation and no other complications were noted.

The complication rate of the LVZ ablation was similar to that of the standard PVAI, which is about 1–4% depending on reports [6, 7, 10–13]. Those complications usually include vascular access complications, cardiac tamponade, embolization, and so on. Caution should be paid when an entire ablation of a broad LVZ in the anterior LA is performed because it may cause a bi-atrial atrial tachycardia, cut-off Backmann's bundle, damage the left-sided fast pathway, and cause secondary atrial tachycardias. A bi-atrial tachycardia is a huge macro-reentrant atrial tachycardia conducting through Backmann's bundle and the ablation of Backmann's bundle is necessary to eliminate it, which is a risk of a thrombus formation in the LA appendage and a stiff LA syndrome in addition to inadvertently cutting Backmann's bundle during the LVZ ablation. LVZ ablation-related secondary atrial tachycardias consist of a variation of a localized atrial tachycardia that rotates in relation to the damaged tissue, and macro-reentrant atrial tachycardias conducting through a gap between ablated areas of the LVZ, mitral annulus, or PVAI line. To avoid that, a strategical linear ablation is sometimes performed from the ablated LVZ to an anatomical obstacle or the PV isolation lines.

The types of recurrent atrial tachyarrhythmias are diverse depending on the researchers, possibly because of the different methodologies of the LVZ ablation. We and Cutler's group reported that the recurrence was due to atrial tachycardias in about half of the cases, while Yang et al. and Kottkamp et al. reported it was predominantly due to AF [6, 7, 11, 12]. This should be further examined in a large number of cases.

Acknowledgement We would like to acknowledge Mr. John Martin for his linguistic help in preparing this manuscript.

References

1. Yamaguchi T, Tsuchiya T, Nagamoto Y, Miyamoto K, Murotani K, Okishige K, et al. Long-term results of pulmonary vein antrum isolation in patients with atrial fibrillation: an analysis in regards to substrates and pulmonary vein reconnections. Europace. 2014;16:511–20.
2. Providência R, Lambiase PD, Srinivasan N, Ganesh Babu G, Bronis K, Ahsan S, et al. Is there still a role for complex fractionated atrial electrogram ablation in addition to pulmonary vein isolation in patients with paroxysmal and persistent atrial fibrillation? Meta-analysis of 1415 patients. Circ Arrhythm Electrophysiol. 2015;8(5):1017–29.
3. Verma A, Jiang CY, Betts TR, Chen J, Deisenhofer I, Mantovan R, et al. Approaches to catheter ablation for persistent atrial fibrillation. N Engl J Med. 2015;372:1812–22.
4. Gillinov AM, Gelijns AC, Parides MK, DeRose JJ Jr, Moskowitz AJ, Voisine P, et al.; CTSN Investigators. Surgical ablation of atrial fibrillation during mitral-valve surgery. N Engl J Med 2015;372(15):1399–1409.
5. Verma A, Wazni OM, Marrouche NF, Martin DO, Kilicaslan F, Minor S, et al. Pre-existent left atrial scarring in patients undergoing pulmonary vein antrum isolation: an independent predictor of procedural failure. J Am Coll Cardiol. 2005;45:285–92.
6. Kottkamp H, Berg J, Bender R, Rieger A, Schreiber D. Box isolation of fibrotic areas (BIFA): a patient-tailored substrate modification approach for ablation of atrial fibrillation. J Cardiovasc Electrophysiol. 2016;27(1):22–30.
7. Yamaguchi T, Tsuchiya T, Nakahara S, Fukui A, Nagamoto Y, Murotani K, et al. Efficacy of left atrial voltage-based catheter ablation of persistent atrial fibrillation. J Cardiovasc Electrophysiol. 2016;27(9):1055–63.
8. Oakes RS, Badger TJ, Kholmovski EG, et al. Detection and quantification of left atrial structural remodeling with delayed-enhancement magnetic resonance imaging in patients with atrial fibrillation. Circulation. 2009;119:1758–67.
9. McGann C, Akoum N, Patel A, Kholmovski E, Revelo P, Damal K, et al. Atrial fibrillation ablation outcome is predicted by left atrial remodeling on MRI. Circ Arrhythm Electrophysiol. 2014;7(1):23–30.
10. Rolf S, Kircher S, Arya A, Eitel C, Sommer P, Richter S, et al. Tailored atrial substrate modification based on low-voltage areas in catheter ablation of atrial fibrillation. Circ Arrhythm Electrophysiol. 2014;7:825–33.
11. Cutler MJ, Johnson J, Abozguia K, Rowan S, Lewis W, Costantini O, et al. Impact of voltage mapping to guide whether to perform ablation of the posterior wall in patients with persistent atrial fibrillation. J Cardiovasc Electrophysiol. 2016;27(1):13–21.
12. Yang G, Yang B, Wei Y, Zhang F, Ju W, Chen H, et al. Catheter ablation of nonparoxysmal atrial fibrillation using electrophysiologically guided substrate modification during sinus rhythm after pulmonary vein isolation. Circ Arrhythm Electrophysiol. 2016;9(2):e003382.
13. Jadidi AS, Lehrmann H, Keyl C, Sorrel J, Markstein V, Minners J, et al. Ablation of persistent atrial fibrillation targeting low-voltage areas with selective activation characteristics. Circ Arrhythm Electrophysiol. 2016;9(3):pii: e002962.
14. Kostin S, Klein G, Szalay Z, Hein S, Bauer EP, Schaper J. Structural correlate of atrial fibrillation in human patients. Cardiovasc Res. 2002;54:361–79.
15. Rohr S. Arrhythmogenic implications of fibroblast-myocyte interactions. Circ Arrhythm Electrophysiol. 2012;5(2):442–52.
16. Xu J, Cui G, Esmailian F, Plunkett M, Marelli D, Ardehali A, et al. Atrial extracellular matrix remodeling and the maintenance of atrial fibrillation. Circulation. 2004;109:363–8.
17. Chaldoupi SM, Loh P, Hauer RNW, Bakker JMT, van Rijen HVM. The role of connexin 40 in atrial fibrillation. Cardiovasc Res. 2009;84:15–23.
18. Igarashi T, Finet E, Takeuchi A, Fujino Y, Storm M, Greener IA, et al. Connexin gene transfer preserves conduction velocity and prevents atrial fibrillation. Circulation. 2012;125:216–25.
19. Luo M, Li YS, Yang KP. Fibrosis of collagen I and remodeling of connexin 43 in atrial myocardium of patients with atrial fibrillation. Cardiology. 2007;107:248–53.
20. Hanna N, Cardin S, Leung TK, Nattel S. Differences in atrial versus ventricular remodeling in dogs with ventricular tachypacing-induced congestive heart failure. Cardiovasc Res. 2004;63:236–44.
21. Du J, Xie J, Zhang Z, Tsujikawa H, Fusco D, Silverman D, et al. TRPM7-mediated Ca2+ signals confer fibrogenesis in human atrial fibrillation. Circ Res. 2010 Mar 19;106(5):992–1003.
22. Harada M, Luo X, Qi XY, Tadevosyan A, Maguy A, Ordog B, et al. Transient receptor potential canonical-3 channel-dependent fibroblast regulation in atrial fibrillation. Circulation. 2012;126(17):2051–64.
23. Wakili R, Voigt N, Kaab S, Dobrev D, Nattel S. Recent advances in the molecular pathophysiology of atrial fibrillation. J Clin Invest. 2016;121:2955–68.
24. Ashihara T, Haraguchi R, Nakazawa K, Namba T, Ikeda T, Nakazawa Y, Ozawa T, Ito M, Horie M, Trayanova NA. The role of fibroblasts in complex fractionated electrograms during persistent/permanent atrial fibrillation: implications for electrogram-based catheter ablation. Circ Res. 2012;110(2):275–84.
25. McDowell KS, Vadakkumpadan F, Blake R, Blauer J, Plank G, Macleod RS, et al. Mechanistic inquiry into the role of tissue remodeling in fibrotic lesions in human atrial fibrillation. Biophys J. 2013;104:2764–73.
26. Zahid S, Cochet H, Boyle PM, Schwarz EL, Whyte KN, Vigmond EJ, et al. Patient-derived models link re-entrant driver localization in atrial fibrillation to fibrosis spatial pattern. Cardiovasc Res. 2016;110(3):443–54.
27. Ausma J, van der Velden HM, Lenders MH, van Ankeren EP, Jongsma HJ, Ramaekers FC, et al. Reverse structural and gap-junctional remodeling after prolonged atrial fibrillation in the goat. Circulation. 2003;107(15):2051–8.
28. Miyamoto K, Tsuchiya T, Narita S, Yamaguchi T, Nagamoto Y, Ando S, et al. Bipolar electrogram amplitudes in the left atrium are related to local conduction velocity in patients with atrial fibrillation. Europace. 2009;11:1597–605.
29. Anter E, Tschabrunn CM, Josephson ME. High-resolution mapping of scar-related atrial arrhythmias using smaller electrodes with closer interelectrode spacing. Circ Arrhythm Electrophysiol. 2015;8:537–45.

Autonomic Ganglionated Plexi Ablation in Patients with Atrial Fibrillation

Hiroshi Nakagawa, Benjamin J. Scherlag, Deborah Lockwood, and Warren M. Jackman

Keywords

Catheter ablation • Atrial fibrillation • Autonomic nervous system • Ganglionated plexi

22.1 Introduction

Autonomic influences in the heart are generated by both the extrinsic (central) and intrinsic cardiac autonomic nervous systems. The extrinsic cardiac autonomic nervous system is formed by the vagosympathetic system from the brain and spinal cord to the heart. The intrinsic cardiac autonomic nervous system involves the automatic tissues on the heart, including clusters of autonomic ganglia located within epicardial fat pads of the left and right atria, known as ganglionated plexi (GP) [1–3]. The GP contain afferent neurons from the atrial myocardium to the extrinsic autonomic nervous system, efferent cholinergic and adrenergic neurons (with heavy innervation to the pulmonary vein [PV] myocardium and the atrial myocardium surrounding the GP), as well as an extensive array of interconnecting neurons. The interconnecting neurons create a communication network between the different GP and between the GP and the atrial and PV myocardium [1–3].

Recent studies in experimental models and in patients with atrial fibrillation (AF) have shown that activation of the GP plays a significant role in the initiation and maintenance of AF [4–17]. In this chapter, we will present the recent data on the role of the autonomic ganglia in the pathogenesis of AF and the impact of GP ablation in AF patients.

22.2 Basic Research on the Role of Intrinsic Cardiac Autonomic Nervous System in the Initiation and Maintenance of Atrial Fibrillation

Experimental studies have shown that AF induced by increased GP activity is caused by triggered firing resulting from early after depolarizations (EADs) [18, 19]. GP activation includes both parasympathetic and sympathetic stimulation of the atrium surrounding the GP and the closest PV. Parasympathetic stimulation markedly shortens action potential duration, with a much greater shortening in PV myocardium compared to the adjacent left atrial myocardium. Sympathetic stimulation increases calcium loading and calcium release from the sarcoplasmic reticulum (larger and longer calcium transient). The combination of short action potential duration, EADs, and longer calcium release results in high intracellular calcium concentrations during and immediately after repolarization. This, in turn, drives Na^+/Ca^{++} exchange with three Na^+ entering the cell for each Ca^{++} exiting the cell, resulting in a net inward current. The inward current produces EADs and triggered firing ("Calcium Transient Triggered Firing Hypothesis," Fig. 22.1) [18, 19]. Myocardial contractility, EADs, and triggered firing are enhanced by a pause, especially when the pause follows rapid rate. The rapid rate increases Ca^{++} loading in the cells (shorter diastolic periods prevent extrusion of all of the Ca^{++} entering the cell during systole), resulting in an increased Ca^{++} accumulation in the sarcoplasmic reticulum during the pause. Activation of the cell at the end of the pause results in an exaggerated release of Ca^{++} from the sarcoplasmic reticulum (increased calcium transient) with increased likelihood of triggered firing [19].

H. Nakagawa, M.D., Ph.D. (✉) • B.J. Scherlag, Ph.D.
D. Lockwood, B.M., B.Ch., M.A • W.M. Jackman, M.D.
Heart Rhythm Institute and Department of Medicine,
University of Oklahoma Health Sciences Center,
1200 Everett Drive (TUH-6E-103), Oklahoma City,
OK 73104, USA
e-mail: hiroshi-nakagawa@ouhsc.edu

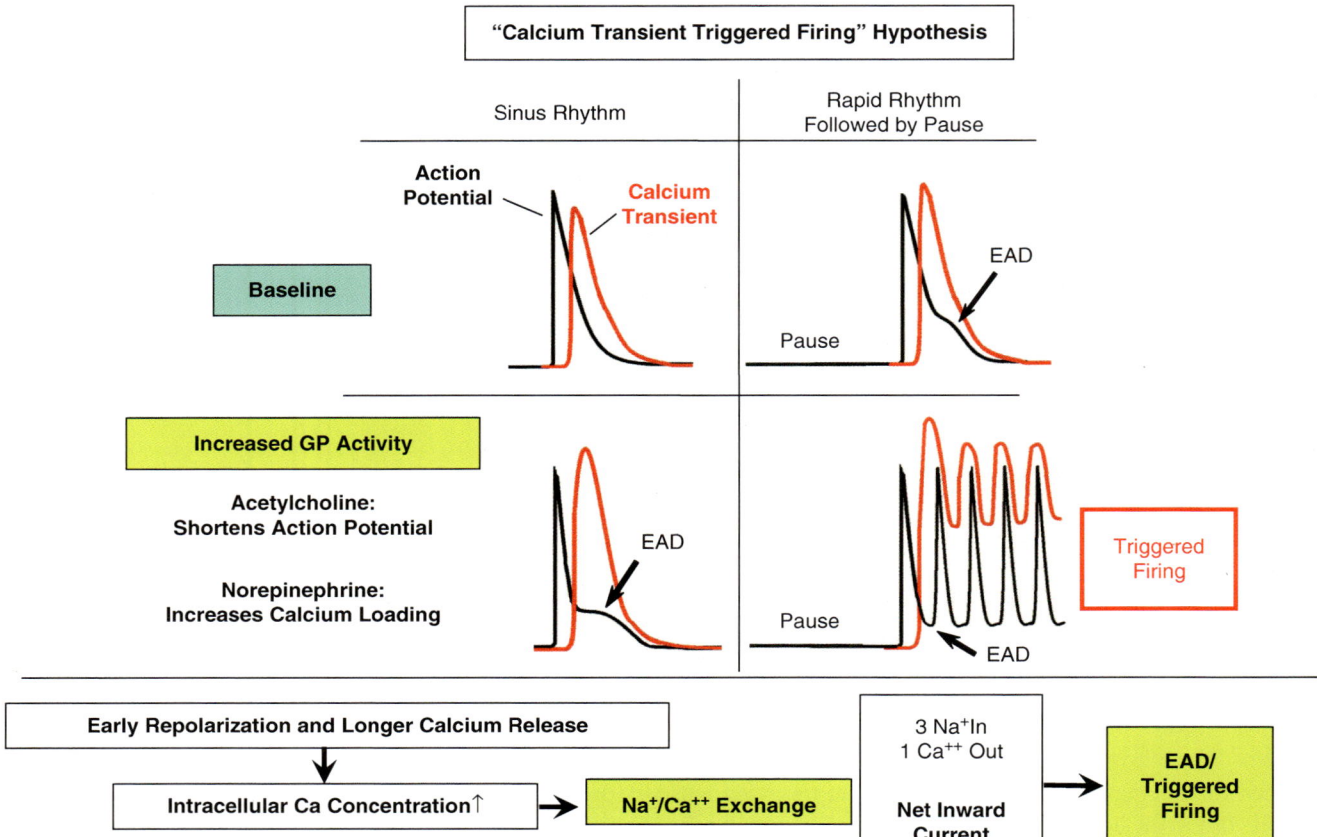

Fig. 22.1 Schematic representation of the "Calcium Transient Triggered Firing" hypothesis for the mechanism of short episodes (usually <1 s) of very rapid irregular firing in the pulmonary vein (PV) initiating atrial fibrillation (AF). Action potential is drawn in black and the calcium transient (intracellular calcium concentration) is drawn in *red*. Ganglionated plexi (GP) activation results in both sympathetic and parasympathetic stimulation. Acetylcholine shortens the action potential duration and norepinephrine enhances the calcium transient. The disparity between the short action potential duration and the enhanced and delayed calcium transient can produce an early afterdepolarization (EAD) due to the inward sodium–calcium exchange current. Further enhancement of the calcium transient is observed by a pause (flowing a rapid rhythm), initiating PV triggered firing. Modified with permission from ref. [19]

In a canine isolated left superior PV preparation (with a rim of adjacent left atrium), selective electrical stimulation (high-frequency stimulation [HFS] at a cycle length of 10 ms, 0.1 ms pulse width, train duration 300 ms) in the left atrial rim (stimulating axons from the GP to the PV) produced a striking shortening of action potential duration with EADs and triggered firing originating in the PV myocardium (Fig. 22.2) [18, 19]. The response to HFS was completely blocked by superfusion with tetrodotoxin in low concentration, which blocks neurons without affecting the action potential of the left atrial or PV myocardial cells. This confirmed that HFS exerts its effects by stimulating autonomic axons (mimicking GP activity), and not by direct electrical stimulation of the myocardial cells. In this model, atropine prevents the shortening of action potential duration by HFS and prevented triggered firing [18]. Atenolol allowed the shortening of action potential duration by HFS, but prevented the triggered firing. Ryanodine, which in high dose prevents the release of Ca^{++} from the sarcoplasmic reticulum, allowed some shortening of the action potential duration, but totally prevented EAD formation and triggered firing [19]. The response to ryanodine supports the role of the primary Ca^{++} release from the sarcoplasmic reticulum in the generation of EADs and triggered firing. The EADs and triggered firing in this preparation were increased by a pause following rapid pacing, similar to the pause-dependent pattern of PV firing seen clinically (Fig. 22.3) [15–17]. This pause-dependent PV firing is often manifested clinically as the immediate recurrence of AF (IRAF) after cardioversion or spontaneous termination of AF.

The magnitude of action potential shortening, EAD formation, and triggered firing produced by HFS (GP axon stimulation) was much greater in the PV myocardium than in the adjacent left atrial myocardium (Fig. 22.2) even though the left atrial myocardium was closer to the site of HFS [18]. These observations suggest that the PV myocardium is much more sensitive to autonomic stimulation than the adjacent left atrial myocardium. The increased sensitivity of the PV myocardium may help to explain the observation in patients with paroxysmal AF that the focal firing which triggers AF is usually located within the PV myocardial sleeves.

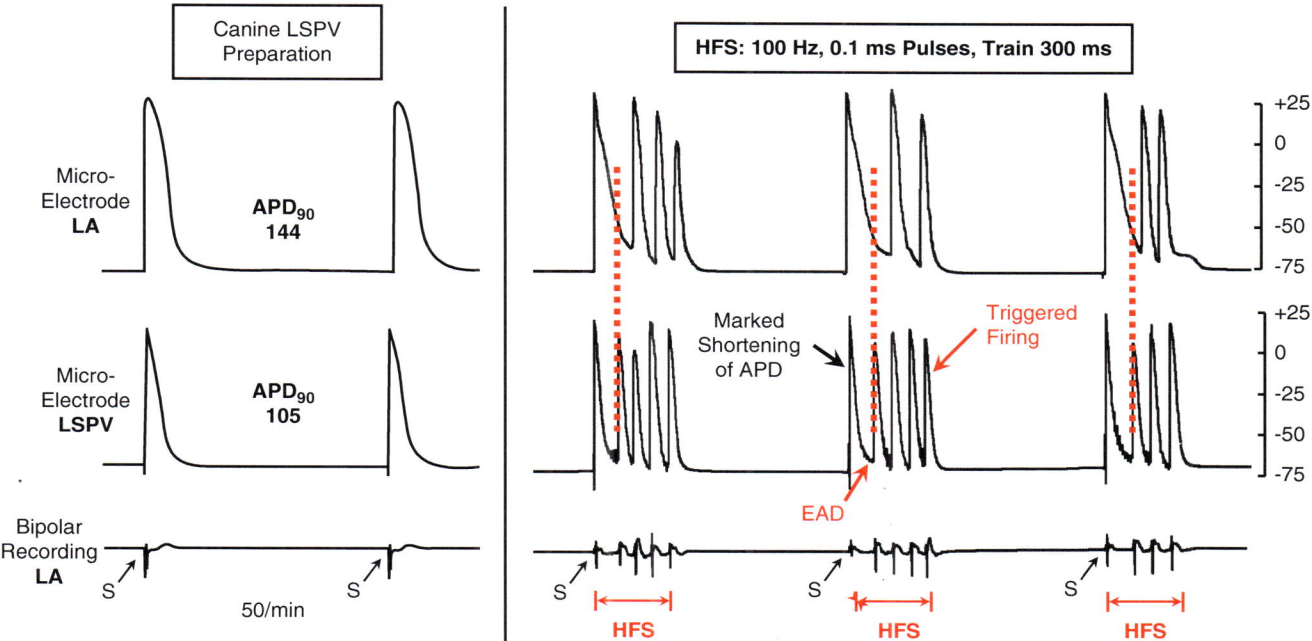

Fig. 22.2 Pulmonary vein triggered firing during high-frequency stimulation (HFS) of the axons extending from the ganglionated plexi (GP) to the left superior PV in a canine model. Tracings are microelectrode recordings from the left atrium (LA) and left superior pulmonary vein (LSPV) in the isolated canine preparation. *Left panel*: During LA pacing at 50/min without HFS, the action potential duration at 90% of repolarization (APD_{90}) is shorter in the PV myocyte (105 ms) than the LA myocyte (144 ms). *Right panel*: Short trains of HFS (cycle length 10 ms, 0.1 ms pulse width, train duration 300 ms, 100 V) are delivered to the LA pacing site, immediately after each pacing stimulus (without capture of the LA myocardium). HFS produces significant shortening of action potential duration in both the LA and LSPV myocytes, resulting in EADs and triggered firing. During the first beat of each episode of triggered firing, activation of the LSPV precedes LA activation, indicating that the triggered firing is occurring from the LSPV. The greater APD_{90} shortening and occurrence of triggered firing in the PV myocytes suggest the PV myocardium exhibits a greater response to GP stimulation than the LA myocardium. Modified with permission from ref. [18]

Experimental studies using an in vivo canine model have shown that HFS of the epicardial fat pad containing a GP produces: (1) a parasympathetic response (sinus bradycardia or AV block); (2) marked shortening of the atrial refractory period close to the stimulated GP; and (3) initiation of sustained AF either spontaneously or by a single atrial extrastimulus [5, 6, 13, 15–17]. Testing in the left atrium at a distance from the stimulated GP shows little or no decrease in atrial refractory period and sustained AF cannot be induced by a single atrial extrastimulus [5, 6]. During AF produced by HFS of a GP, rapid and fractionated atrial potentials (FAP) or complex fractionated atria electrograms (CFAE) [20] are consistently located in the adjacent PV and left atrium surrounding the stimulated GP (Fig. 22.4) [21–24]. The same pattern of FAP close to the GP occurs with pharmacological stimulation of the GP by injection of acetylcholine into the fat pad [21, 22]. Electrograms recorded at sites distant from the stimulated GP exhibit more organized atrial potentials and longer cycle lengths during AF. These data strongly suggest a relationship between FAP and autonomic activity arising from a GP. Other studies in canines showed that placing acetylcholine on the right (or left) atrial appendage induced AF. The AF often began nearly simultaneously in the right (or left) superior PV, then in the appendage. Blocking afferent and efferent neurons to the right atrial appendage prior to applying the acetylcholine prevented firing in both the appendage and PV, whereas blocking the neurons to the appendage after the onset of AF terminated firing in the appendage but not in the PV [21, 23]. These findings suggest that the effect of acetylcholine on the right (or left) atrial appendage was to produce afferent stimulation to activate the anterior right (or superior left) GP. Efferent stimulation from the GP resulted in firing in both the PV and the atrial appendage. In canines with AF induced by acetylcholine applied to the atrial appendage, serial ablation of four GP resulted in progressive slowing and then termination of AF. After serial ablation of four GP, sustained AF could not be induced by rapid pacing in the atrial appendage despite the continued application of acetylcholine [21–23]. The progressive organization of atrial activation with serial GP ablation suggests that communication between the GP (activation of one GP activates multiple other GP) facilitates the maintenance of AF [13, 21].

In the canine model, the GP can also be localized from the endocardium using HFS [15–17, 24]. When close to a GP, an endocardial application of HFS produces a parasympathetic response manifested by a marked lengthening of the R-R interval during AF (AV block). Endocardial RF ablation at those sites eliminated the parasympathetic response to repeat endocardial and even epicardial HFS. GP ablation often decreased or eliminated the FAP close to that GP [15–17, 22–24].

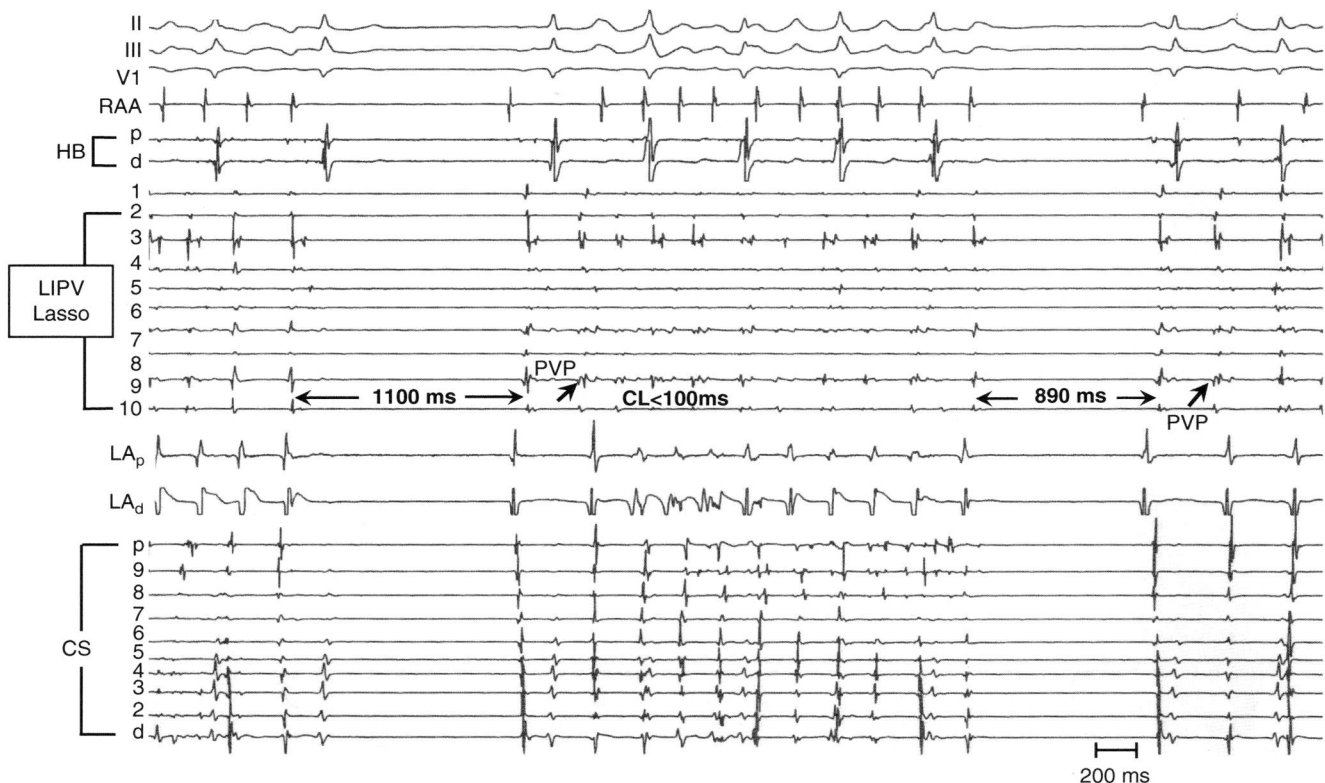

Fig. 22.3 Spontaneous pause-dependent PV firing from the left inferior pulmonary vein (LIPV) in a patient with paroxysmal AF. Tracings from the top are surface ECG leads II, III, V1, and intracardiac electrograms from the right atrial appendage (RAA), His bundle region (HB), the LIPV, the left atrium (LA), and the coronary sinus (CS). The spontaneous termination of a brief AF episode resulted in a sinus pause (1100 ms), followed by very rapid, irregular firing in the LIPV (*small arrow*, mean cycle length [CL] <100 ms), initiating AF. The second AF episode spontaneously terminated, resulting in another sinus pause (890 ms) and PV firing. *PVP* pulmonary vein potential, *d* distal bipolar electrode pair, *p* proximal bipolar electrodes pair. Modified with permission from ref. [17]

The above experimental studies suggest that the GP may play a significant role in clinical AF, especially in patients with paroxysmal AF, where PV focal firing is a dominant factor [15–17, 24].

22.3 Localization and Ablation of Left Atrial Ganglionated Plexi in Patients with Atrial Fibrillation

22.3.1 Localization of GP by Epicardial High-Frequency Stimulation in Patients Undergoing Thoracoscopic Surgical Ablation of Atrial Fibrillation

In patients undergoing thoracoscopic surgical ablation of AF, the left atrial epicardial fad pads can be visualized [15, 25–27]. A large epicardial fat pad is located anterior to the right superior and inferior to the right inferior PVs (Fig. 22.5a). Epicardial HFS (cycle length 50 ms, pulse width 1–5 ms) is performed over the fat pads, resulting in a positive response to HFS, defined as a ≥50% increase in mean R-R interval during AF (transient AV block and hypotension) [15, 26].

The GP exhibiting a positive response to HFS are located within the fat pad, shown in the red crossed-hatch areas in Fig 22.5a, corresponding to the Anterior Right GP and the Inferior Right GP, respectively. The Marshall tract GP is located within the fat pad anterior to the left superior PV and left inferior PV along the left atrial appendage ridge (Fig 22.5b), confirmed by a positive response to HFS. The Superior Left GP is located on the roof of the left atrium, medial to the LSPV, extending anteriorly towards the superior base of the left atrial appendage. The Inferior Left GP is located within the fat pad located infero-posteriorly to the LIPV (Fig 22.5b). Radiofrequency (RF) applications within the fat pads eliminate the positive response to HFS, confirming epicardial ablation of these five left atrial GP.

22.3.2 Localization of GP by Endocardial High-Frequency Stimulation in Patients Undergoing Catheter Ablation of Atrial Fibrillation

GP can also be identified and localized using endocardial HFS in patients undergoing catheter ablation of AF (Fig. 22.6)

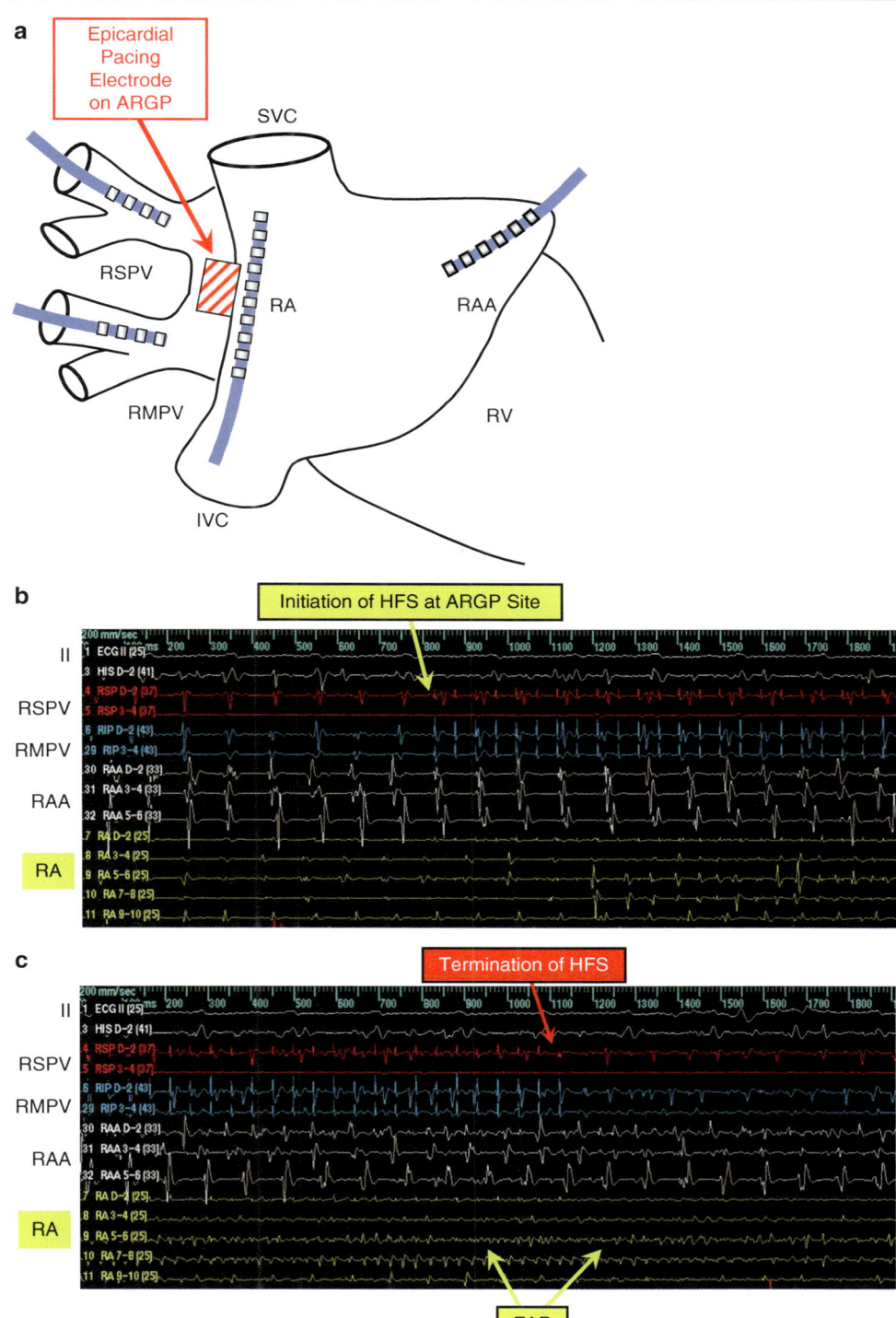

Fig. 22.4 Production of fractionated atrial potentials (FAP) during AF by high-frequency stimulation (HFS) at the anterior right ganglionated plexi (ARGP) in a canine model. (**a**) Schematic representation of the right atrium demonstrating the position of epicardial recording electrodes (blue electrode catheters) and epicardial pacing electrodes (red cross-hatched areas) over the fat pads containing the ARGP. The epicardial pacing electrode was used to deliver HFS to the ARGP. *RSPV* right superior pulmonary vein, *RMPV* right middle pulmonary vein, *RA* right atrium close to the ARGP, *RAA* right atrial appendage, *RV* right ventricle. (**b**) Rapid right atrial stimulation initiated only non-sustained episodes of relatively organized AF with long atrial cycle length (beginning of the tracing). HFS (without direct capture of the atrial myocardium) at the ARGP is initiated during AF (top *yellow arrow*). (**c**) With the continuation of selective ARGP stimulation (without direct atrial capture) for 30 s, AF became sustained and fractionated atrial potentials (FAP) with very short cycle lengths (<30–40 ms) appeared at sites close to the ARGP (RA D-2, 3–4, 5–6, and 7–8 electrograms). Notice that FAP continued even after the termination of HFS. Modified with permission from ref. [15]

[15–17, 24]. A high-density electroanatomical map (CARTO3, Biosense Webster, Inc) of the left atrium and each of the four PVs is obtained during AF to provide both an anatomical shell and the location of the areas of fractionated atrial potentials (FAP) in the left atrium and PVs. The left atrial FAP are located primarily in four areas: (1) LAA Ridge FAP area (between LAA and left PVs); (2) Superior Left FAP area; (3) Anterior Right FAP area; and (4) Infero-Posterior FAP area (Figs. 22.6 and 22.7). Endocardial HFS (cycle length 50 ms, 12 V actual output, 10 ms pulse width) is delivered through the distal pair of the electrodes on a mapping catheter to sites in the left atrium and proximal portions of the PVs [15–17, 23]. The sites with a positive HFS response (Fig. 22.6b) are localized in five major areas: (1) Marshall Tract GP; (2) the Superior Left GP; (3) Anterior Right GP; (4) Inferior Left GP; and (5) Inferior Right GP (Fig. 22.6a, Fig. 22.7). The sites of a positive HFS response are

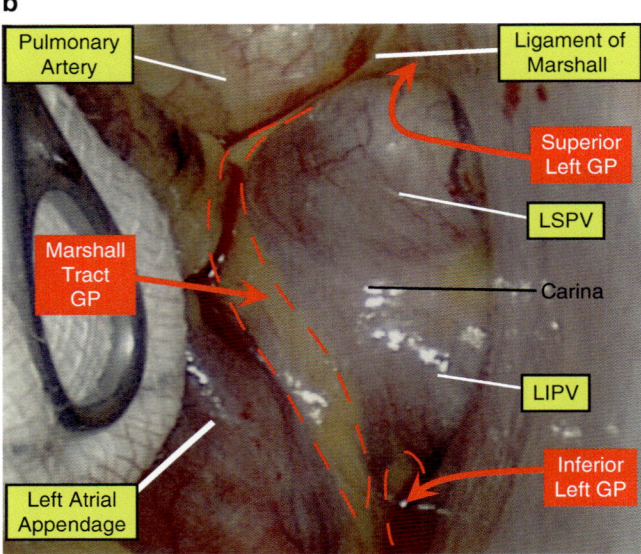

Fig. 22.5 Five major left atrial ganglionated plexi (GP) in patients undergoing thoracoscopic surgical ablation of AF. (**a**) A thoracoscopic photograph in the right side of the chest during surgical ablation in a patient with persistent AF. An epicardial left atrial fat pad (*black dashed line*) is located anterior to the right superior PV (RSPV) and another epicardial fat pad (*black dashed line*) is located infero-posterior to the right inferior PV (RIPV). HFS is delivered within the area of the fat pads. The sites exhibiting a parasympathetic response to HFS are limited to the *red crossed-hatch* areas, corresponding to the anterior right GP and the inferior right GP, respectively. (**b**) A thoracoscopic photograph in the left side of the chest in the same patient, demonstrating the left superior PV (LSPV), left inferior PV (LIPV), and the pulmonary artery. The left atrial appendage is retracted underneath the gauze. The fat pad is located between the left PVs and the left atrial appendage. HFS along this fat pad resulted in a transient AV block response, identifying the Marshall tract GP. The superior left GP is located deep within the pocket beneath the ligament of Marshall on the roof of the left atrium. The inferior left GP is located within the fat pad infero-posterior to the LIPV, confirmed by a positive HFS response. Modified with permission from ref. [15]

consistently located outside of the PVs, except for the Marshall Tract GP along the LAA ridge. The Superior Left GP, Anterior Right GP, Inferior Left GP, and Inferior Right GP are usually located more than 1 cm from the adjacent PV ostium. All five left atrial GP are located within large areas of FAP (Fig. 22.6, Fig. 22.7). HFS of a GP often produced increased fractionation in both the adjacent PV and PVs further away [6, 23, 24]. These observations suggest communication between GP (activation of one GP leads to activation of other GP) as well as a relationship between GP activation and the occurrence of FAP. Some FAP may represent the recording of "calcium transient triggered firing" in atrial myocardium initiated by GP activation [18, 19].

22.3.3 Catheter Ablation of Left Atrial GP

For endocardial catheter ablation of the GP, RF energy is applied to each site exhibiting a positive HFS response (usually 25–35 W for 30–60 s, but the RF power and/or time is reduced when close to the esophagus). If the positive HFS response is still present after ablation, RF energy is reapplied until the response is eliminated (generally only one or two RF applications are required). In our experience, ablation of each of the five GP areas requires 2–12 (median 5) RF applications [15–17, 24].

A positive HFS response may not identify cycle length the entire GP area. HFS-induced transient AV block is driven by activation of the Inferior Right GP. Therefore, activating the Marshall Tract GP, Superior Left GP, Anterior Right GP, or Inferior Left GP by HFS is followed by activation of other GP, including the Inferior Right GP, which innervates the AV node. The positive response to HFS (transient AV block) may not occur due to ablation of one of the intermediate GP connecting to the Inferior Right GP. Therefore, in order to minimize the loss of a positive HFS response, GP ablation in the left atrium should be performed in the following order: Marshall Tract GP, Superior Left GP, Anterior Right GP, Inferior Left GP, and finally Inferior Right GP [13, 15–17, 23]. Signs of activation of GPs other than the GP being stimulated directly (such as the onset of firing in a PV far from the stimulated GP) are occasionally observed during HFS which does not produce a transient AV block response, suggesting the limited sensitivity of AV block in identifying GP. Some reports describe targeting GP without HFS, delivering RF applications to the presumed anatomical locations of the GP [28].

The GP (identified by HFS) are consistently located within an area of fractionated atrial potentials (FAP), and the area of FAP is much larger than the area responsive to HFS. In 100 patients with paroxysmal AF, GP ablation alone (before PV antrum isolation) significantly decreased the occurrence of PV firing (74/100 patients before ablation vs. 14/100 patients after ablation, $p < 0.01$). GP ablation also decreased the inducibility of sustained AF (68/100 patients vs. 36/100 pts., $p < 0.01$) and markedly reduced or eliminated the left atrial FAP areas, despite GP ablation is covering only a small fraction of the overall FAP area (Fig 22.6a) [15–17, 24].

Katritsis et al. [29] performed a large clinical study, which randomized a total of 242 patients with paroxysmal AF to conventional PV isolation, PV isolation plus GP ablation, and GP ablation alone. Freedom from atrial

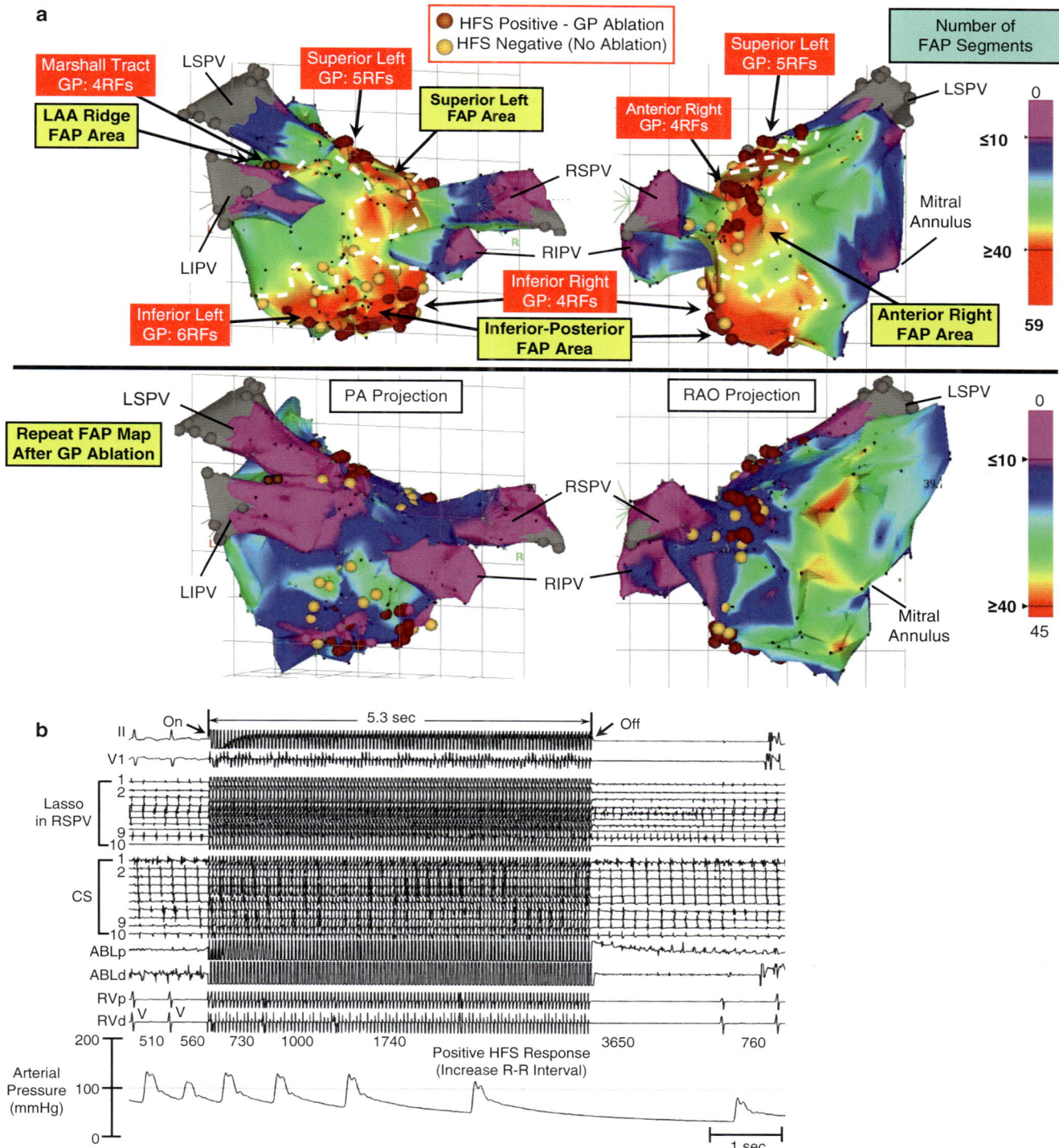

Fig. 22.6 Relationship between locations of fractionated atrial potentials (FAP) and ganglionated plexi (GP) in a 59-year-old man undergoing catheter ablation of paroxysmal AF. (**a**) FAP maps of the left atrium and all four PVs during AF before (*upper panel*) and after (*lower panel*) ablation of all five left atrial GP (*without PV isolation or other ablation*). An automated algorithm was used to identify segments between electrogram peaks of 15–80 ms duration. FAP was defined as an area with sites demonstrating more than 40 short intervals (15–80 ms) per 2.5 s (FAP regions are colored *red*). Areas with sites exhibiting large amplitude, discrete atrial potentials with average cycle length ≥180 ms are colored purple (FAP sites have ≤10 short intervals per 2.5 s). After ablation of all five GP in the left atrium, there is a marked decrease in the area of FAP represented by the red area, even though the areas of GP ablation are much smaller than the areas of FAP. *PA* posterior-anterior, *AP* anterior–posterior. Modified with permission from ref. [24]. (**b**) Identification of anterior right GP by endocardial HFS. The tracings from the top are ECG lead II, V1, and electrograms from the circular catheter in the right superior pulmonary vein (RSPV), coronary sinus (CS), right ventricle (RV), and arterial pressure. During AF, endocardial HFS (cycle length 50 ms, pulse width 10 ms, 5.3 s stimulation) delivered from the ablation catheter (ABL) positioned in the Anterior Right FAP Area resulted in transient AV block (R-R interval increased up to 3650 ms) and hypotension (positive HFS response), identifying the ARGP. Modified with permission from ref. [17]

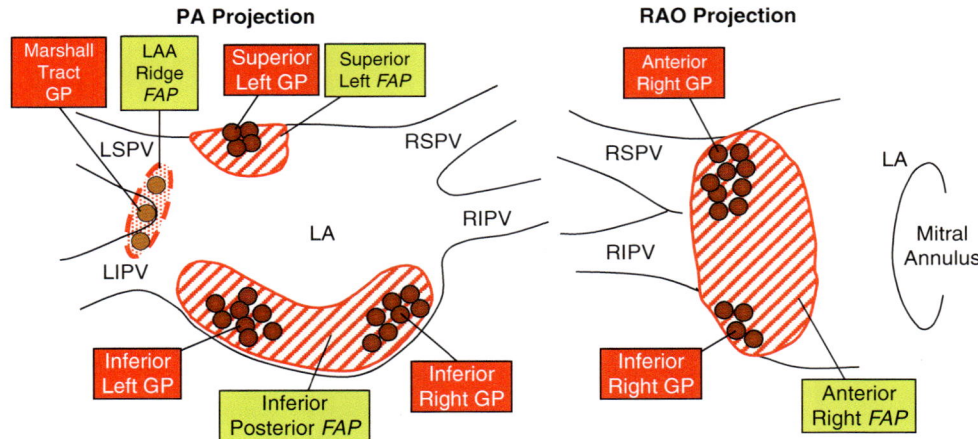

Fig. 22.7 Schematic representation of the relationship between the FAP areas and GP locations. *Brown tags* indicate sites with a positive HFS response (GP location). *Red crossed-hatch* areas indicate FAP areas. All five GP are located within one of the four FAP areas. *PA* posterior-anterior, *AP* anterior-posterior. Modified with permission from ref. [15]

tachyarrhythmias (over at least 2 years follow-up) was achieved in a similar number of patients in the conventional PV isolation group and the GP ablation alone groups (56% and 48%, respectively), and in a significantly greater number of patients in the PV isolation plus GP ablation group (74%; $p = 0.004$). In another randomized study including 264 patients with persistent or long-standing persistent AF, GP ablation as an adjunct to PV isolation resulted in higher rates of sinus rhythm maintenance at 3 years (49%) compared to PV isolation plus left atrial linear lesions (34%) [30]. In addition, left atrial tachycardias were less common with PV isolation plus GP ablation than with PV isolation plus linear lesions. GP ablation alone was also tested in patients with drug-refractory long-standing persistent AF, resulting in a lower but notable success rate (38% sinus rhythm maintenance at 2 years) [31].

22.4 Summary

Experimental and clinical studies suggest that GP activation plays a significant role in clinical AF in both: (1) the initiation of AF by producing PV firing ("Calcium Transient Triggered Firing"); and (2) the maintenance of AF with production of fractionated atrial potentials during AF. GP ablation should be additive to PV antrum isolation to prevent PV firing and eliminate (or decrease) FAP areas during AF.

Conflicts of Interest H. Nakagawa and W.M. Jackman are consultants for Biosense Webster, inc.

References

1. Armour JA, Hageman GR, Randall WC. Arrhythmias induced by local cardiac nerve stimulation. Am J Phys. 1972;223:1068–75.
2. Armour JA, Yuan BX, Macdonald S, et al. Gross and microscopic anatomy of the human intrinsic cardiac nervous system. Anat Rec. 1997;247:289–98.
3. Pauza DH, Skripka V, Pauziene N, et al. Morphology, distribution, and variability of the epicardiac neural ganglionated subplexuses in the human heart. Anat Rec. 2000;259:353–82.
4. Sharifov OF, Fedorov VV, Beloshajeko GG, et al. Roles of adrenergic and cholinergic stimulation in spontaneous atrial fibrillation in dogs. J Am Coll Cardiol. 2004;43:483–90.
5. Scherlag BJ, Yamanashi WS, Patel U, et al. Autonomically induced conversion of pulmonary vein focal firing into atrial fibrillation. J Am Coll Cardiol. 2005;45:1575–880.
6. Scherlag BJ, Nakagawa H, Jackman WM, et al. Electrical stimulation to identify neural elements on the heart: their role in atrial fibrillation. J Interv Electrophysiol. 2005;13:37.
7. Nishida K, Maguy A, Sakabe M, et al. The role of pulmonary veins vs. autonomic ganglia in different experimental substrates of canine atrial fibrillation. Cardiovasc Res. 2011;89:825–33.
8. Nishida K, Datino T, Macle L, Nattel S. Atrial fibrillation ablation: translating basic mechanistic insights to the patient. J Am Coll Cardiol. 2014;64:823–31.
9. Bettoni M, Zimmermann M. Autonomic tone variations before the onset of paroxysmal atrial fibrillation. Circulation. 2002;105:2753–9.
10. Choi EK, Shen MJ, Han S, et al. Intrinsic cardiac nerve activity and paroxysmal atrial tachyarrhythmia in ambulatory dogs. Circulation. 2010;121:2615–23.
11. Lemola K, Chartier D, Yeh YH, et al. Pulmonary vein region ablation in experimental vagal atrial fibrillation: role of pulmonary veins versus autonomic ganglia. Circulation. 2008;117:470–7.
12. Lin J, Scherlag BJ, Lu Z, et al. Inducibility of atrial and ventricular arrhythmias along the ligament of Marshall: role of autonomic factors. J Cardiovasc Electrophysiol. 2008;9:955–62.
13. Hou YL, Scherlag BJ, Lin J, et al. Interactive atrial neural network: determining the connection between ganglionated plexi. Heart Rhythm. 2007;4:56–63.
14. Yamazaki M, Vaquero LM, Hou L, et al. Mechanisms of stretch-induced atrial fibrillation in the presence and the absence of adrenocholinergic stimulation: interplay between rotors and focal discharges. Heart Rhythm. 2009;6:1009–17.
15. Nakagawa H, Scherlag BJ, Patterson E, et al. Pathophysiologic basis of autonomic ganglionated plexus ablation in patients with atrial fibrillation. Heart Rhythm. 2009;6:S26–34.
16. Nakagawa H, Yokoyama K, Scherlag BJ, et al. Ablation of autonomic ganglia. In: Calkins H, Jais P, Steinberg JS, editors. A practical approach to catheter ablation of atrial fibrillation. Philadelphia, PA: Wolters Kluwer/Lippincott Williams & Wilkins; 2008. p. 218–30.
17. Nakagawa H, Scherlag BJ, Jackman WM. Catheter ablation of autonomic ganglionated plexi in patients with atrial fibrillation. In: Hands-on ablation: the expert approach 2013. Eds: Al-Ahmad A, Callans D, Hsia H, Natale A, Oseroff O, Wang PJ. Cardiotext Publishing Minneapolis, MN 2013, pp 227–233.

18. Patterson E, Po SS, Scherlag BJ, et al. Triggered firing in pulmonary veins initiated by in vitro autonomic nerve stimulation. Heart Rhythm. 2005;2:624–31.
19. Patterson E, Lazzara R, Szabo B, et al. Sodium-calcium exchange initiated by the Ca2+ transient: an arrhythmia trigger within pulmonary veins. J Am Coll Cardiol. 2006;47:1196–206.
20. Nademanee K, McKenzie J, Kosar E, et al. A new approach for catheter ablation of atrial fibrillation: mapping of the electrophysiologic substrate. J Am Coll Cardiol. 2004;43:2044–53.
21. Scherlag BJ, Hou YL, Lin J, et al. An acute model of atrial fibrillation arising from a periferal atrial site: evidence for pulmonary and secondary triggers. J Cardiovasc Electrphysiol. 2008;19:19–27.
22. Po SS, Scherlag BJ, Yamanashi WS, et al. Experimental model for paroxysmal atrial fibrillation arising at the pulmonary vein-atrial junctions. Heart Rhythm. 2006;3:201–8.
23. Niu G, Scherlag BJ, Lu Z, et al. An acute experimental mode demonstrating 2 different forms of sustained atrial tachyarrhythmias. Circ Arrhythm Electrophysiol. 2009;2:384–92.
24. Stavrakis S, Nakagawa H, Po SS, et al. The role of the autonomic ganglia in atrial fibrillation. J Am Coll Cardiol. 2015;1-2:1–13.
25. Wolf RK, Schneeberger W, Osterday R, et al. Video-assisted bilateral pulmonary vein isolation and left atrial appendage exclusion for atrial fibrillation. J Thorac Cardiovasc Surg. 2005;130:797–802.
26. Edgerton JR, Jackman WM, Mack MJ. Minimally invasive pulmonary vein isolation and partial automatic denervation for surgical treatment of atrial fibrillation. J Interv Card Electrophysiol. 2007;20:89–93.
27. Yilmaz A, Van Putte BP, Van Boven WJ. Completely thoracoscopic bilateral pulmonary vein isolation and left atrial appendage exclusión for atrial fibrillation. J Thorac Cardiovasc Surg. 2008;136:521–2.
28. Pokushalov E, Romanov A, Artyomenko S, et al. Left atrial ablation at the anatomic areas of ganglionated plexi for paroxysmal atrial fibrillation. Pacing Clin Electrophysiol. 2010;33:1231–8.
29. Katritsis DG, Pokushalov E, Romanov A, et al. Autonomic denervation added to pulmonary vein isolation for paroxysmal atrial fibrillation: a randomized clinical trial. J Am Coll Cardiol. 2013;62:2318–25.
30. Pokushalov E, Romanov A, Katritsis DG, et al. Ganglionated plexus ablation vs linear ablation in patients undergoing pulmonary vein isolation for persistent/long-standing persistent atrial fibrillation: a randomized comparison. Heart Rhythm. 2013;10:1280–6.
31. Pokushalov E, Romanov A, Artyomenko S, et al. Ganglionated plexi ablation for longstanding persistent atrial fibrillation. Europace. 2010;12:342–6.

Part VI

Catheter Ablation of Atrio-ventricular Nodal Tachycardias

23. Slow Pathway Ablation for Atrioventricular Nodal Reentrant Tachycardia

Kenichiro Otomo

Keywords

Ablation · Slow pathway · Atrioventricular nodal reentrant tachycardia · Leftward posterior extension

23.1 Differentiation of Three Types of Atrioventricular Nodal Reentrant Tachycardia

Atrioventricular nodal reentrant tachycardia (AVNRT) is a reentry involving the atrioventricular node, a component of atrial myocardium, and two atrionodal connections (fast pathway and slow pathway) [1–7]. AVNRT is generally classified as three types, slow/fast type, fast/slow type, and slow/slow type, based on the antegrade and retrograde conductions of the reentrant circuit [8].

Slow/fast AVNRT, also referred to as "common type," is thought to use the slow pathway for antegrade conduction and the fast pathway for retrograde conduction (Fig. 23.1a). Antegrade slow pathway conduction is identified when tachycardia occurs with an abrupt (≥50 ms) increase in the A-H interval (A-H jump) and/or A-H interval during tachycardia is relatively long (usually ≥200 ms). Retrograde fast pathway conduction is identified by locating the site of earliest atrial activation at the anteroseptal right atrium near the His bundle region or superior to the tendon of Todaro [8]. H-A interval during tachycardia is relatively short (25–90 ms) (Fig. 23.1a). Antegrade slow pathway is the target for the ablation of this tachycardia.

Fast/slow AVNRT, also referred to as "uncommon type," is thought to use the fast pathway for the antegrade conduction and the slow pathway for the retrograde conduction (Fig. 23.1b). A-H interval during tachycardia is short (30–185 ms, median 80 ms [8]). Retrograde slow pathway conduction is identified by locating the site of earliest atrial activation at the posteroseptal right atrium between the tricuspid annulus and the coronary sinus ostium or inside the coronary sinus [8]. H-A interval during tachycardia is relatively long (135–435 ms, median 260 ms [8]) (Fig. 23.1b). Retrograde slow pathway is the target for the ablation of this tachycardia.

Slow/slow AVNRT, like slow/fast AVNRT, is thought to utilize the slow pathway for antegrade conduction, which is reflected by an initiation of the tachycardia with A-H jump and/or long A-H interval during tachycardia (≥200 msec, median 240 msec [8]) (Fig. 23.2). Same as fast/slow AVNRT, retrograde slow pathway conduction is identified by locating the site of earliest atrial activation at the posteroseptal right atrium between the tricuspid annulus and the coronary sinus ostium or inside the coronary sinus. H-A interval of slow/slow AVNRT shows a wide variety (−30 to 260 ms, median 120 ms [8]) (Fig. 23.2). This is because the H-A interval represents the difference in conduction time over the retrograde slow pathway and the lower common pathway. Lengthening of the conduction time over the lower common pathway results in a shortening of the H-A interval. The relatively short H-A interval (median 120 ms [8]) of this tachycardia often resulted in simultaneous atrial and ventricular activation, mimicking slow/fast AVNRT (Fig. 23.2b). In patients with simultaneous atrial and ventricular activation during tachycardia, identification of the retrograde atrial activation sequence to differentiate retrograde conduction over the slow pathway (slow/slow AVNRT) from the fast pathway (slow/fast AVNRT) by the use of late ventricular extrastimulus is important (Fig. 23.1a, Fig. 23.2b). Recurrence rate after slow pathway ablation in slow/slow AVNRT is much greater than slow/fast or fast/slow AVNRT.

K. Otomo
Department of Cardiology, Oume Municipal General Hospital, 4-16-5, Higashioume, Oume-shi, Tokyo 198-0042, Japan
e-mail: kenotomo-circ@umin.ac.jp

Fig. 23.1 (**a**) Slow/fast AVNRT. Antegrade slow pathway conduction was identified by the long A-H interval (435 ms). A single extrastimulus (S_2) delivered to the anterobasal right ventricular septum (para-Hisian region) advanced the timing of local ventricular activation (V_2). This revealed the retrograde atrial activation sequence with the earliest activation recorded at the anteroseptal right atrium in the HB electrogram (A), suggesting the retrograde conduction over the fast pathway. (**b**) Fast/slow AVNRT. Short A-H interval (130 ms) reflected the antegrade conduction over the fast pathway. Retrograde slow pathway conduction is identified by locating the site of earliest atrial activation in the coronary sinus, as well as the long H-A interval during the tachycardia (260 ms)

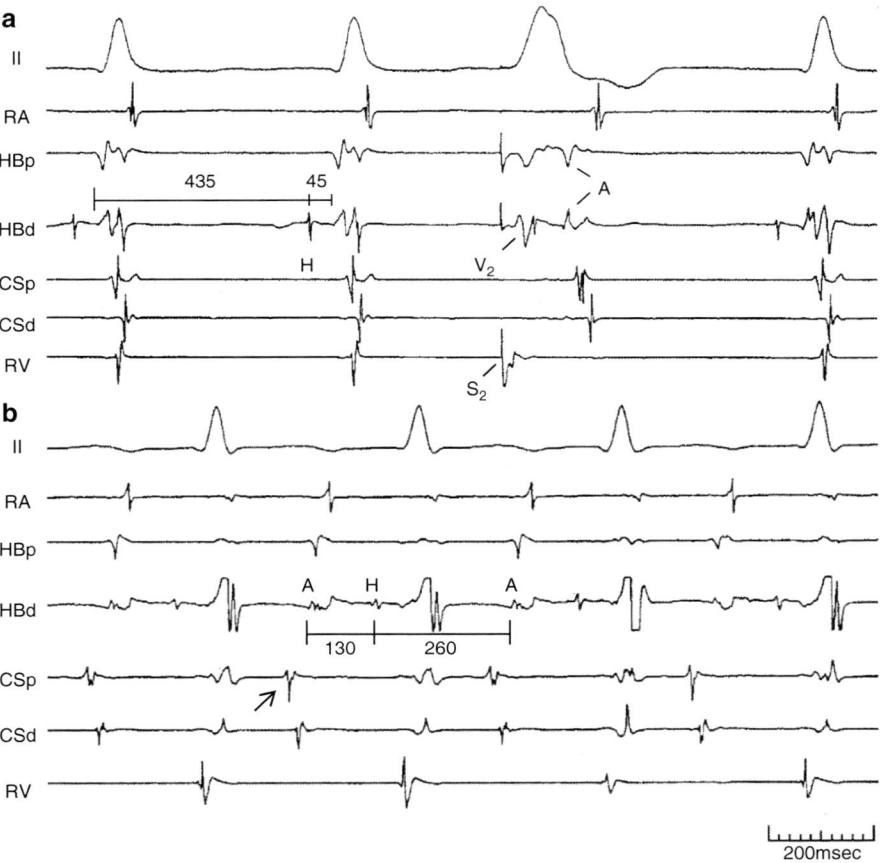

Fig. 23.2 Slow/slow AVNRT with various H-A interval. Antegrade slow pathway conduction was reflected by the long A-H interval in both panels (360 and 190 ms, respectively). In panel **a**, retrograde slow pathway conduction is easily identified by locating the site of earliest atrial activation in the posteroseptal right atrium (Asp) as well as the long H-A interval (235 ms). In the left part of panel b, a short H-A interval (70 ms) resulted in simultaneous atrial and ventricular activation which obscures retrograde atrial activation sequence and mimics slow/fast AVNRT. In the right part of panel **b**, a single extrastimulus (S_2) delivered to the anterobasal right ventricular septum advanced the timing of local ventricular activation (V_2), revealing the retrograde atrial activation sequence with the earliest activation recorded at the posteroseptal right atrium (Asp) followed by atrial activation within the proximal coronary sinus. This confirms the retrograde conduction over the slow pathway as well as the diagnosis as slow/slow AVNRT

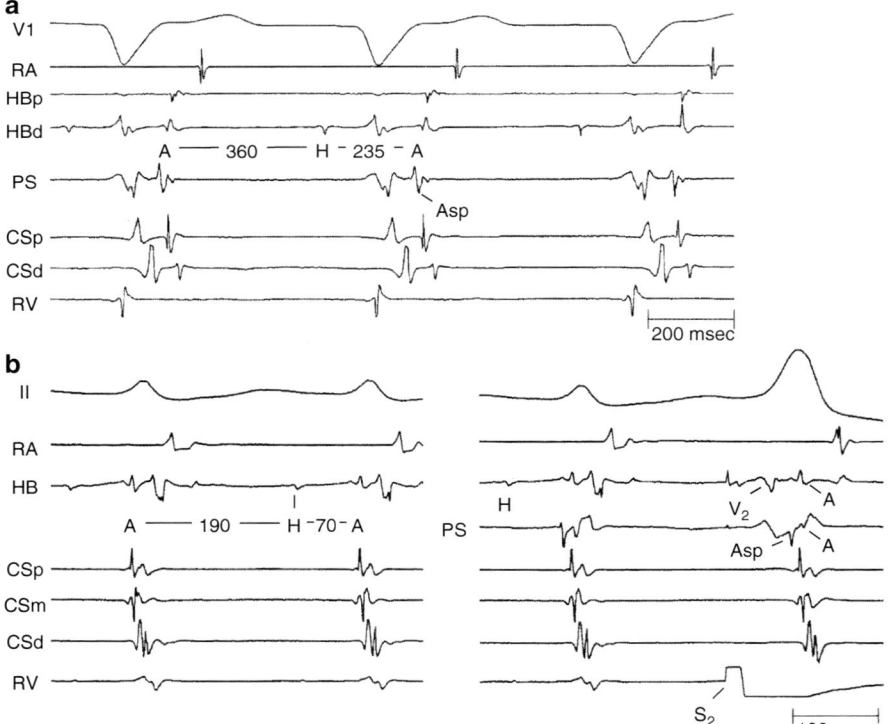

23.2 Slow Pathway Ablation for Atrioventricular Nodal Reentrant Tachycardia

23.2.1 Ablation of Antegrade Slow Pathway

Antegrade slow pathway is the target for ablation of slow/fast and slow/slow AVNRT. Ablation is generally performed with Asp potential as a successful electrogram marker [3]. Asp potential, referred to as representing the atrial connection to the slow pathway, is a high-amplitude high frequency potential which follows a small atrial potential during sinus rhythm and is recorded at posteroseptal right atrium between the tricuspid annulus and the coronary sinus ostium (Fig. 23.3). This potential is simultaneously recorded with a large ventricular potential since ventricular muscle lies underneath the right atrial muscle at this recording site (atrioventricular septum). The other electrogram marker for successful ablation of slow pathway is the slow potential, which is a low-amplitude activity with a slow rate of rise [6]. This potential is usually recorded at more anterior to the site recording Asp potential. Pure anatomical approach for slow pathway ablation is also reported [4, 5, 9]. The ablation is started at posteroseptal right atrium close to the tricuspid annulus at adjacent to the bottom half of the coronary sinus ostium. The only electrogram criterion used to select target sites is an atrial/ventricular electrogram ratio of ≤0.5. If the ablation attempt is unsuccessful, the site is moved slight anteriorly along the tricuspid annulus towards the His bundle recording site. Combination of both electrogram and anatomical approach is generally accepted nowadays. The ablation is initially attempted at posteroseptal right atrium adjacent to the coronary sinus ostium where Asp potential is recorded, then anatomically moved anteriorly along the tricuspid annulus. In order to avoid atrioventricular block, it is recommended that the ablation site be confined within lower two-thirds of the distance from the coronary sinus ostium to the proximal His bundle recording site [4, 5, 9]. Two posterior extensions of the human atrioventricular node which may represent the anatomical substrate for slow pathways are reported: the rightward extension along the tricuspid annulus and the leftward extension along the roof of the coronary sinus towards the mitral annulus [10] (Fig. 23.4a). Successful ablation of the slow pathway inside the coronary sinus is reported [3, 11, 12]. If the leftward extension serves as the slow pathway for AVNRT, successful ablation at inside the coronary sinus may be explained.

Radiofrequency current is generally applied at 20–30 W for 30–60 s. An appearance of an accelerated junctional rhythm is considered to be a marker of effective slow pathway ablation [13, 14]. Although the exact mechanism of accelerated junctional rhythm is unclear, automaticity due to a direct

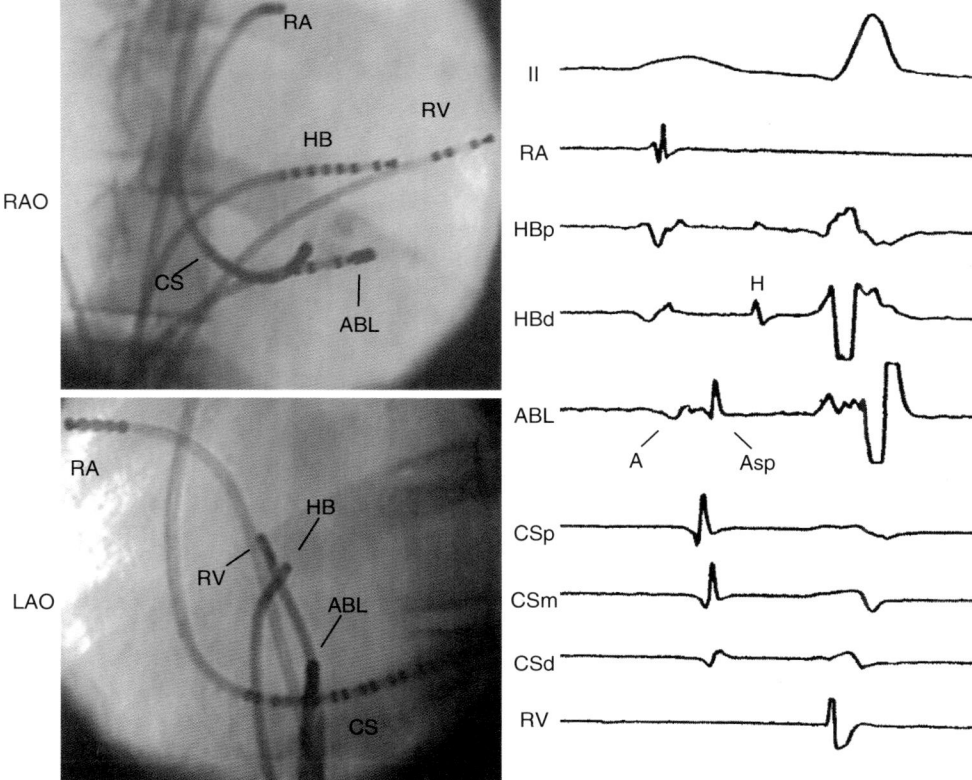

Fig. 23.3 Asp potential. *Left panel* shows radiograph taken in the right anterior oblique (RAO) and left anterior oblique (LAO) projections showing electrode catheters positioned in the right atrium (RA), His bundle region (HB), coronary sinus (CS), and right ventricle (RV). The ablation catheter (ABL) was positioned at posteroseptal right atrium between the tricuspid annulus and the coronary sinus ostium. *Right panel* shows the recording of a high-amplitude high frequency Asp potential which followed a small atrial potential in the ablation catheter. Note that the timing of Asp potential was after the timing of atrial activation in the proximal coronary sinus

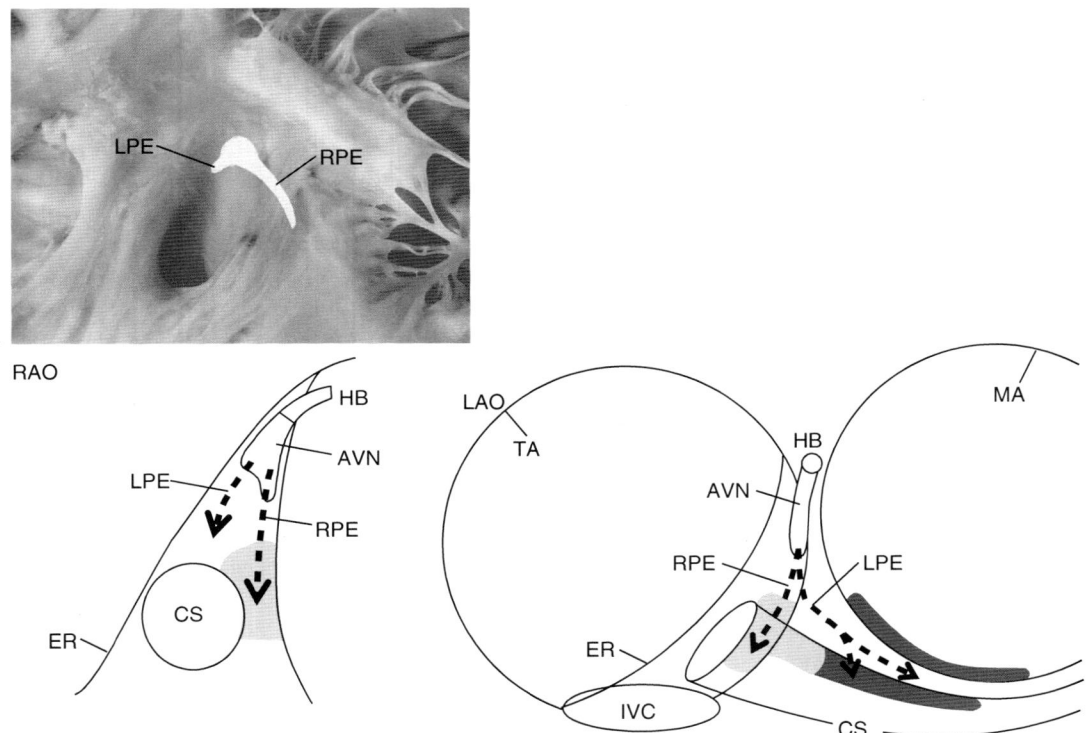

Fig. 23.4 (a) Rightward posterior extension (RPE) and leftward posterior extension (LPE) of the atrioventricular node. Reproduced and modified with permission from Circulation [10]. (b) Hypothetical route of the rightward posterior extension (RPE) and leftward posterior extension (LPE) of the atrioventricular node. Light and dark shaded area show the target site for the ablation of the RPE and LPE, respectively

heating of the tissue connected to the slow pathway is likely to be a mechanism and the radiofrequency current application should be continued at the same location until accelerated junction rhythm disappears. In order to avoid atrioventricular block caused by an injury of the atrioventricular node or the fast pathway, either confirming 1:1 retrograde conduction over the fast pathway to the atrium during accelerated junctional rhythm or overdrive atrial pacing to verify 1:1 antegrade fast pathway conduction is important [14].

Antegrade conduction over the slow pathway recognized by the A-H jump during atrial pacing often remains even after the effective slow pathway ablation because of the existence of multiple slow pathways. The endpoint of the slow pathway ablation is to achieve (1) inability to induce AVNRT, (2) no 1:1 antegrade slow pathway conduction during atrial pacing, and (3) one or less atrioventricular nodal echo during atrial and ventricular pacing with administration of isoproterenol (1–2 μg/min). Acute success rate and recurrence rate for slow pathway ablation for AVNRT have been reported as 90–95% and 1–5%, respectively [3–6].

23.2.2 Ablation of Retrograde Slow Pathway

Retrograde slow pathway is a target for ablation of fast/slow and slow/slow AVNRT. Ablation is generally performed at the site of retrograde Asp potential (Fig. 23.2) or the earliest atrial activation site during tachycardia or ventricular pacing (Fig. 23.1b).

The appearance of accelerated junctional rhythm depends on the existence of antegrade slow pathway conduction and is often not recognized during ablation for fast/slow AVNRT. The endpoint of the retrograde slow pathway ablation is the same as that of antegrade slow pathway ablation. In addition, no retrograde slow pathway conduction needs to be achieved especially for slow/slow AVNRT, since the recurrence rate after slow pathway ablation for slow/slow AVNRT is much greater than the other two types of AVNRT. Moreover, types of recurrence for slow/slow AVNRT is either slow/fast AVNRT or fast/slow AVNRT, not slow/slow AVNRT [8]. Therefore, more extensive ablation targeting both antegrade and

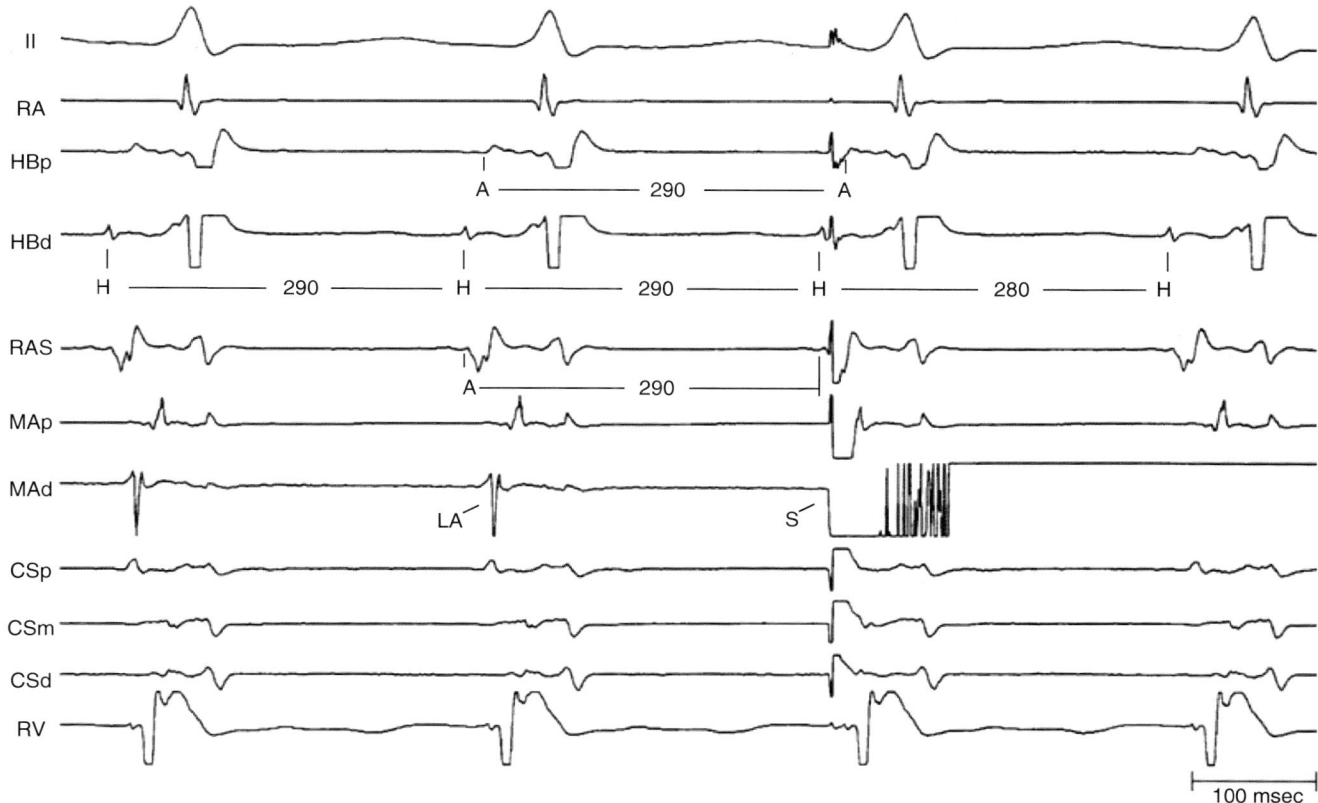

Fig. 23.5 Resetting of slow/fast AVNRT by a single atrial extrastimulus. A late atrial extrastimulus (S) was delivered at posterior mitral annulus (MAd) after the timing of the earliest atrial activation recorded at anteroseptal right atrium superior to the tendon of Todaro (RAS). This extrastimulus did not affect the timing of the retrograde atrial activation recorded in the His bundle region (HBp), advanced the subsequent His bundle electrogram (H-H = 280 ms, compared with 290 ms), and reset the tachycardia

retrograde slow pathway is necessary for ablation of slow/slow AVNRT.

23.2.3 Ablation at Deep Inside Coronary Sinus or Left Atrium

In rare cases, an endpoint for slow pathway ablation as mentioned above is not achieved in spite of an extensive ablation at sites posteroseptal right atrium between the tricuspid annulus and the coronary sinus ostium as well as inside the proximal coronary sinus. An alternative ablation site in these cases is either at site more anterior along the tricuspid annulus towards the His bundle region or deep inside the coronary sinus ≥3 cm from the ostium; however, the former ablation site may not be desirable from the perspective of avoiding atrioventricular block. Successful ablations of the slow pathway at sites deep inside the coronary sinus as well as the mitral annulus are reported [15–17]. One of the representative cases is shown in Figs. 23.5 and 23.6. A late atrial extrastimulus which delivered at posterior mitral annulus during slow/fast AVNRT advanced the subsequent His bundle electrogram without affecting the earliest atrial activation and reset the tachycardia, suggesting the close proximity of this pacing site to the tachycardia circuit (Fig. 23.5). A high-amplitude high frequency potential which followed a small atrial potential, mimicking the Asp potential, was recorded at the posterior mitral annulus (Fig. 23.6). Radiofrequency current application at this site provoked an accelerated junctional rhythm and successfully interrupted antegrade slow pathway conduction (not shown in the figure), resulted in an elimination of slow/fast AVNRT. If the atrial connection of the leftward posterior extension of the atrioventricular node which serves as the slow pathway for AVNRT locates deep inside the coronary sinus, ablation at deep inside the coronary sinus and/or the mitral annulus may be required (Fig. 23.4b).

Fig. 23.6 Successful ablation site of the slow pathway at the mitral annulus. An ablation catheter was positioned at the posterior mitral annulus (MA) in the *left panel*. A high-amplitude high frequency potential which followed a small atrial potential, mimicking the Asp potential, was recorded with the ablation catheter. Radiofrequency current application at this site provoked an accelerated junctional rhythm and successfully interrupted antegrade slow pathway conduction (not shown in the figure)

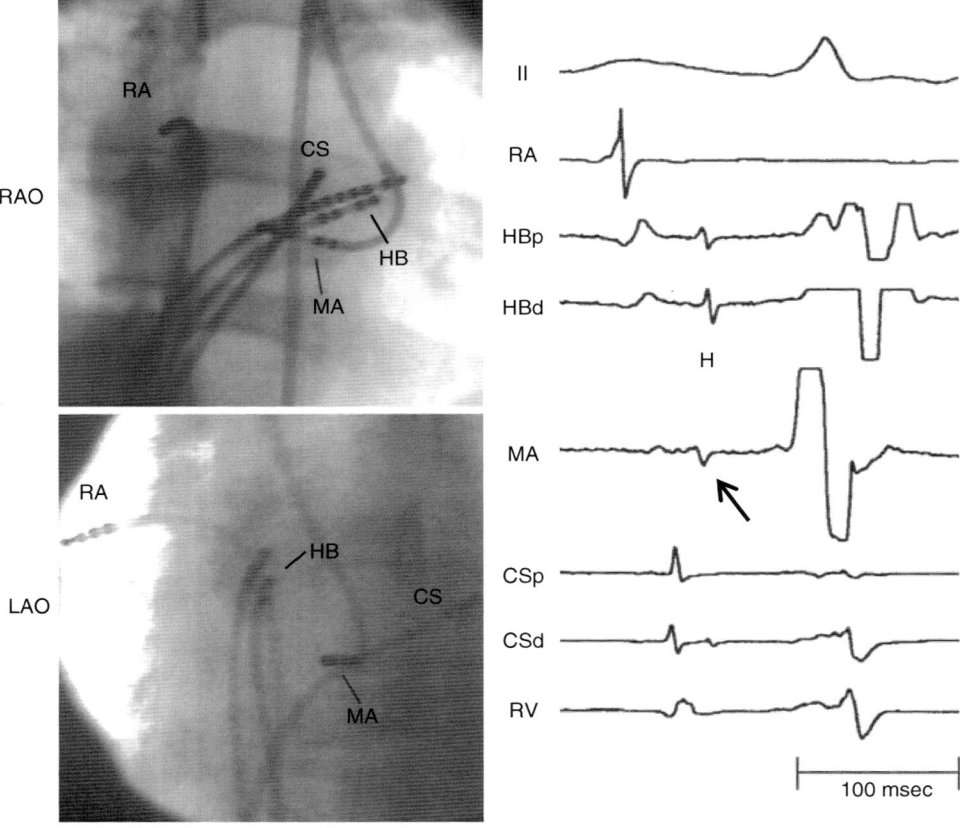

References

1. Sung RJ, Waxman HL, Saksena S, Juma Z. Sequence of retrograde atrial activation in patients with dual atrioventricular nodal pathways. Circulation. 1981;64:1059–67.
2. McGuire MA, Lau KC, Johnson DC, Richards DA, Uther JB, Ross DL. Patients with two types of atrioventricular junctional (AV nodal) reentrant tachycardia. Evidence that a common pathway of nodal tissue is not present above the reentrant circuit. Circulation. 1991;83:1232–46.
3. Jackman WM, Beckman KJ, McClelland JH, Wang X, Friday KJ, Roman CA, et al. Treatment of supraventricular tachycardia due to atrioventricular nodal reentry by radiofrequency catheter ablation of slow-pathway conduction. N Engl J Med. 1992;327:313–8.
4. Jazayeri MR, Hempe SL, Sra JS, Dhala AA, Blanck Z, Deshpande SS, et al. Selective transcatheter ablation of the fast and slow pathways using radiofrequency energy in patients with atrioventricular nodal reentrant tachycardia. Circulation. 1992;85:1318–28.
5. Kay GN, Epstein AE, Dailey SM, Plumb VJ. Selective radiofrequency ablation of the slow pathway for the treatment of atrioventricular nodal reentrant tachycardia. Evidence for involvement of perinodal myocardium within the reentrant circuit. Circulation. 1992;85:1675–88.
6. Haissaguerre M, Gaita F, Fischer B, Commenges D, Montserrat P, d'Ivernois C, et al. Elimination of atrioventricular nodal reentrant tachycardia using discrete slow potentials to guide application of radiofrequency energy. Circulation. 1992;85:2162–75.
7. McGuire M, Bourke J, Robotin M, Johnson D, Meldrum-Hanna W, Nunn G, et al. High resolution mapping of Koch's triangle using sixty electrodes in humans with atrioventricular junctional (AV nodal) reentrant tachycardia. Circulation. 1993;88:2315–28.
8. Otomo K, Wang Z, Lazzara R, Jackman WM. Atrioventricular nodal reentrant tachycardia: Electrophysiological characteristics of four forms and implication for the reentrant circuit. In: Zipes DP, Jalife J, editors. Caridac electrophysiology from cell to bedside. 3rd ed. Philadelphia, PA: WB Saunders; 2000. p. p504–21.
9. Kalbfleisch S, Strickberger SA, Williamson B, Vorperian VR, Man C, Hummel JD, et al. Randomized comparison of anatomic and electrogram mapping approach to ablation of the slow pathway of atrioventricular node reentrant tachycardia. J Am Coll Cardiol. 1994;23:716–23.
10. Inoue S, Becker AE. Posterior extensions of the human compact atrioventricular node: a neglected anatomical feature of potential clinical significance. Circulation. 1998;97:188–93.
11. Hwng C, Martin DJ, Goodman JS, Gang ES, Mandel WJ, Swerdlow CD, et al. Atypical atrioventricular node reciprocating tachycardia masquerading as tachycardia using a left-sided accessory pathway. J Am Coll Cardiol. 1997;30:218–25.
12. Nam GB, Rhee KR, Kim J, Choi K, Kim Y. Left atrionodal connections in typical and atypical atrioventricular nodal reentrant tachycardias: activation sequence in the coronary sinus and results of radiofrequency catheter ablation. J Cardiovasc Electrophysiol. 2006;17: 171–7.
13. Thakur RK, Klein GJ, Yee R, Stites W. Junctional tachycardia: a useful marker during radiofrequency ablation for atrioventricular node reentrant tachycardia. J Am Coll Cardiol. 1993;22:1706–10.
14. Jentzer JH, Goyal R, Williamson BD, Man KC, Niebauer MN, Daoud E, et al. Analysis of junctional ectopy during radiofrequency ablation of the slow pathway in patients with atrioventricular nodal reentrant tachycardia. Circulation. 1994;90:2820–6.
15. Jaïs P, Haïssaguerre M, Shah DC, Coste P, Takahashi A, Barold SS, et al. Successful radiofrequency ablation of a slow atrioven-

tricular nodal pathway on the left posterior atrial septum. PACE. 1999;22:525–7.

16. Altemose GT, Scott LR, Miller JM. Atrioventricular nodal reentrant tachycardia requiring ablation on the mitral annulus. J Cardiovasc Electrophysiol. 2000;11:1281–4.

17. Otomo K, Okamura H, Noda T, Satomi K, Shimizu W, Suyama K, et al. "Left-variant" atypical atrioventricular nodal reentrant tachycardia: electrophysiological characteristics and effect of slow pathway ablation within coronary sinus. J Cardiovasc Electrophysiol. 2006;17:1177–83.

Ablation of Superior Slow Pathway in Atypical Fast-Slow Atrioventricular Nodal Reentrant Tachycardia

24

Yoshiaki Kaneko

Keywords

Superior slow pathway · Atrioventricular nodal reentrant tachycardia · Ablation Electrophysiology

24.1 Introduction

Slow pathway (SP) ablation is a highly successful, curative therapy for atrioventricular (AV) nodal reentrant tachycardia (NRT), although some cases are refractory to the posterior delivery of therapy, behind the compact AV node [1–4]. The participation of a variant of the SP in the reentry circuit, behind the area that is usually treated, has been proposed as a cause of difficult ablation of AVNRT [5–12]. In patients presenting with atypical, fast-slow AVNRT, we recently reported a new type of SP located superiorly at the apex of Koch's triangle, serving as the retrograde limb of the reentry circuit, which we ablated successfully near the His bundle (HB) [7]. We named the tachycardia a superior type of fast-slow AVNRT (sup-F/S-AVNRT). In this chapter, we review the diagnosis and ablation therapy of this unique AVNRT.

24.2 History of Superior SP

Although the anatomic existence of a superior SP has never been confirmed in humans [13], several investigators have hypothesized its presence. Keim et al. first observed a single case of typical AVNRT in which the SP was identified anterior to the fast pathway (FP) by intraoperative ice mapping [8]. Nawata et al. reported three cases of atypical AVNRT in which the presence of the superior SP was hypothesized during an electrophysiologic study, but did not proceed with its ablation [12]. Jackman et al. referred to the presence of an "anterior superior SP" in his textbook, which can be successfully ablated in the noncoronary aortic cusp of Valsalva (NCC), but did not display any electrophysiological data [10].

In an anatomical and electrophysiological study using a canine preparation, Racker et al. reported the presence of an AV junctional pathway that originates posterior to the compact node and extends superiorly, i.e., superior atrionodal bundle [14, 15]. A recent anatomical and biochemical study of the specialized conduction system using a rat preparation demonstrated AV node-like tissue adjacent to the NCC, just above the central fibrous body, identified as the retroaortic node, but the presence of AV node-like tissue connecting the compact AV node and retroaortic node has not been confirmed [16, 17]. Recently, Inoue, the first author to describe the presence of rightward inferior extension, confirmed the presence of AV nodal tissue originating superiorly from the compact AV node, i.e., superior extension, in a pathological analysis of human hearts (unpublished).

24.3 Diagnosis of sup-F/S-AVNRT

In principle, the electrophysiological diagnosis of sup-F/S-AVNRT was based on (1) confirmation of the presence of superior SP, (2) long RP tachycardia with the earliest site of atrial activation at the HB region, and (3) exclusion of atrial tachycardia (AT) and AV reentrant tachycardia (AVRT).

24.3.1 Confirmation of the Presence of Superior SP

Initially, the presence of superior SP is suspected when retrograde conduction with the earliest site of atrial activation in

Y. Kaneko
Department of Cardiovascular Medicine, Gunma University Graduate School of Medicine, 3-39-22 Showa-machi, Maebashi, Gunma 371-8511, Japan
e-mail: kanekoy@gunma-u.ac.jp

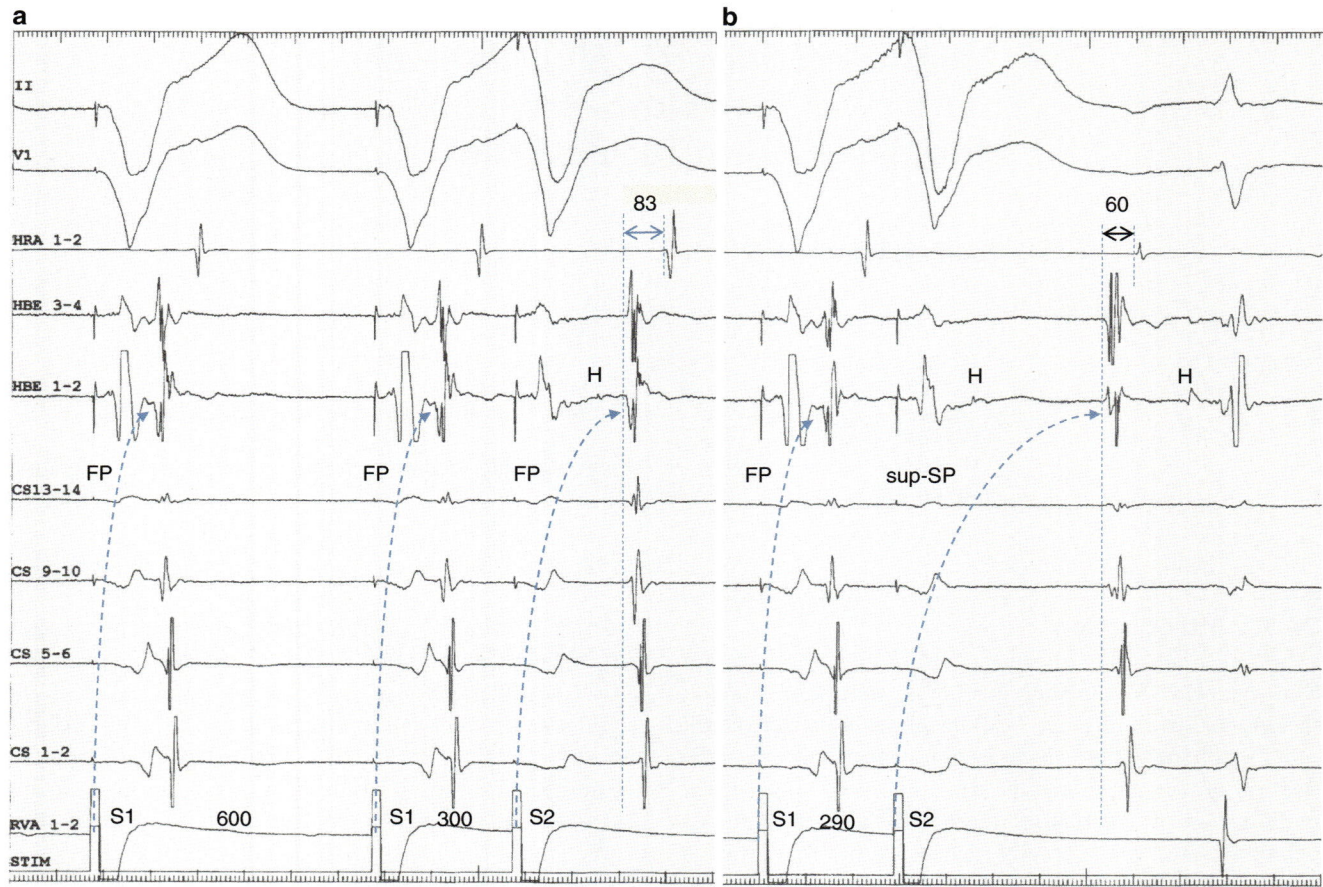

Fig. 24.1 A jump of His (H)-atrial (A) interval induced by right ventricular apical (RVA) extrastimulation, representing a switching of retrograde conduction (indicated by *curved dotted unidirectional arrows*) from fast pathway (FP) (**a**) to superior slow pathway (SP) (**b**) in a 70-year-old woman, whose successful ablation was in the anterolateral region along the tricuspid annulus. (**a**) During a burst stimulation of an S1–S1 cycle length of 600 ms, retrograde conduction via an FP is observed, characterized by the earliest site of atrial activation during His-bundle electrogram (HBE) recording and a short ventriculoatrial interval. Immediately after extrastimulation with an S1–S2 coupling interval of 300 ms, retrograde conduction via the FP also occurs, accompanied by a prolongation of ventricular-H interval. (**b**) Immediately after extrastimulation of an S1–S2 coupling interval of 290 ms, an H-A interval is abruptly prolonged with the earliest site of atrial activation during HBE recording, consistent with retrograde conduction via a superior SP. *Long* and *short vertical dotted lines* indicate the onset of atrial deflection in the HBE and high right atrium (HRA), respectively. Note that the interval between the onset of atrial deflection in the HBE and the HRA (indicated by *horizontal bidirectional arrows*) is shorter during retrograde conduction via a superior SP than via an FP. II and V1 = surface ECG, HBE1–2 to 3–4 = the distal to proximal HBE, CS1–2 to 13–14 = the distal to proximal coronary sinus

the HB region is observed immediately after ventricular stimulation (Fig. 24.1). Measurements of the ventriculoatrial (VA) interval are not always an absolute means of discrimination between FP and superior SP, since there may be some cases of superior SP with a short VA conduction time that mimics FP. Therefore, the presence of AV echo, i.e., antegrade conduction via an FP immediately following VA conduction after ventricular stimulation, is a landmark that can exclude the possibility of the FP as a retrograde pathway (Fig. 24.1). Similar to typical dual AV nodal physiology, a jump of His-atrial (H-A) interval is sometimes observed during ventricular extrastimulation (Fig. 24.1). Measurements of the interval between atrial deflection in HB recording and the subsequent atrial deflection in the high right atrium (RA) may be valid for discriminating between retrograde conduction via an FP and that via a superior SP, as the former is always longer than the latter (Fig. 24.1). Ultimately, the presence of a superior SP is confirmed by elimination or modification of the retrograde conduction via the superior SP after ablation near the HB region [7]. We believe that the confirmation of the presence of the superior SP is not necessarily a prerequisite for a diagnosis of sup-F/S-AVNRT, except when the tachycardia is terminated by ventricular stimulation without atrial capture.

24.3.2 Long RP Tachycardia

A 12-lead electrocardiogram (ECG) during tachycardia mostly represents long RP. The morphology of the P wave in inferior leads is characteristically biphasic in most patients,

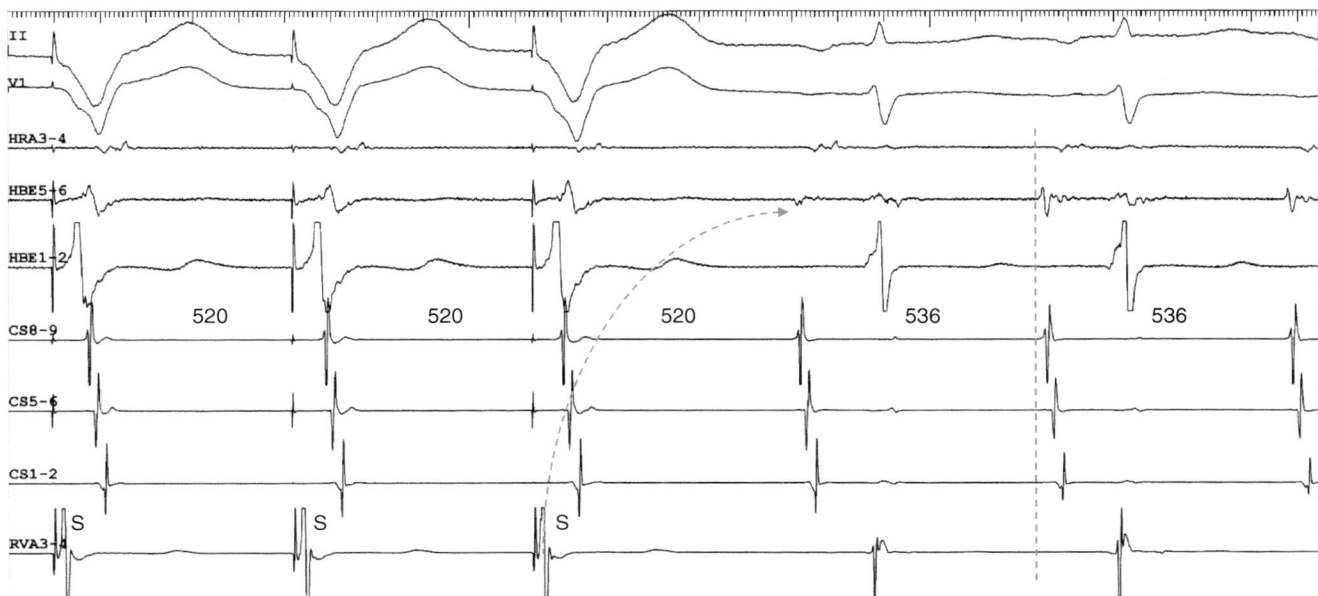

Fig. 24.2 Successful ventricular entrainment of the tachycardia with an initiating V-A-V activation sequence in a 73-year-old woman. Burst stimuli from the right ventricular apex (RVA) with an S–S cycle length of 520 ms capture the atria via a superior SP in a 1:1 ratio. The last stimulus captures the atria as indicated by a dashed arrow, followed by the reinitiation of the tachycardia, thereby representing a V-A-V activation sequence. *Vertical dotted line* indicates the onset of the earliest site of atrial deflection at the His region. II and V1 = surface ECG, HRA3–4 = the proximal high right atrium, HBE1–2 to 5–6 = the distal to proximal His-bundle recording, CS1–2 to 8–9 = the distal to proximal coronary sinus

but occasionally deeply negative. Intracardiac ECGs during tachycardia are characterized by (1) a longer H-A than atrio-His (A-H) interval and (2) an earliest site of atrial activation in the HB region during tachycardia, identical to the retrograde conduction observed over the superior SP during ventricular pacing. Therefore, for the diagnosis of sup-F/S-AVNRT, it is necessary to rule out AT originating near the HB and AVRT utilizing a slowly conducting AV accessory pathway as a retrograde limb located in the HB region.

24.3.3 Exclusion of AT

To exclude the diagnosis of AT, we always apply the following indicators that are observed during and/or after ventricular stimulation: (1) termination of the tachycardia by ventricular pacing without atrial capture and/or (2) V-A-V activation sequence after ventricular induction/reinitiation of the tachycardia, resulting from retrograde conduction over the superior SP, followed by anterograde conduction over the FP (Fig. 24.2), [7] including dual atrial responses (DARs) from simultaneous retrograde conduction over FP and superior SP after the last ventricular stimulus (Fig. 24.3). A DAR is diagnosed as a V-A-A-V activation sequence with an A-A interval shorter than the subsequent tachycardia cycle length and both earliest atrial activations in the HB region (Fig. 24.3) [7, 18–21]. However, the successful entrainment or termination of the sup-F/S-AVNRT by ventricular pacing is challenging, despite the confirmation of retrograde conduction over the superior SP before the onset of tachycardia, because a functional VA conduction block below the AV nodal reentrant circuit (the lower common pathway) during ongoing tachycardia frequently occurs due to an uncertain cause [7, 19, 21]. Moreover, particularly after ventricular induction, a DAR is frequently observed in patients with sup-F/S-AVNRT [7, 19]. Thus, to detect a V-A-V activation sequence or a DAR immediately after ventricular stimulation, irrespective of the presence or absence of retrograde conduction via a superior SP, we recommend repeatedly performing a ventricular burst or extra stimulation with/without preceding simultaneous AV-pacing drive, during control and/or during/after isoproterenol infusion [19]. We do not use any maneuvers of atrial pacing to discriminate between AT and AVNRT, because we believe that those are not absolute indicators for this purpose.

24.3.4 Exclusion of AVRT

To exclude orthodromic AVRT incorporating a slowly conducting AV or nodoventricular AP as the retrograde limb, we try to confirm one or all of the following observations: (1) inability to modify or entrain the tachycardia by ventricular overdrive pacing, i.e., presence of VA dissociation during ventricular overdrive pacing of the tachycardia (overdrive pacing criterion); (2) development of 2nd degree AV block

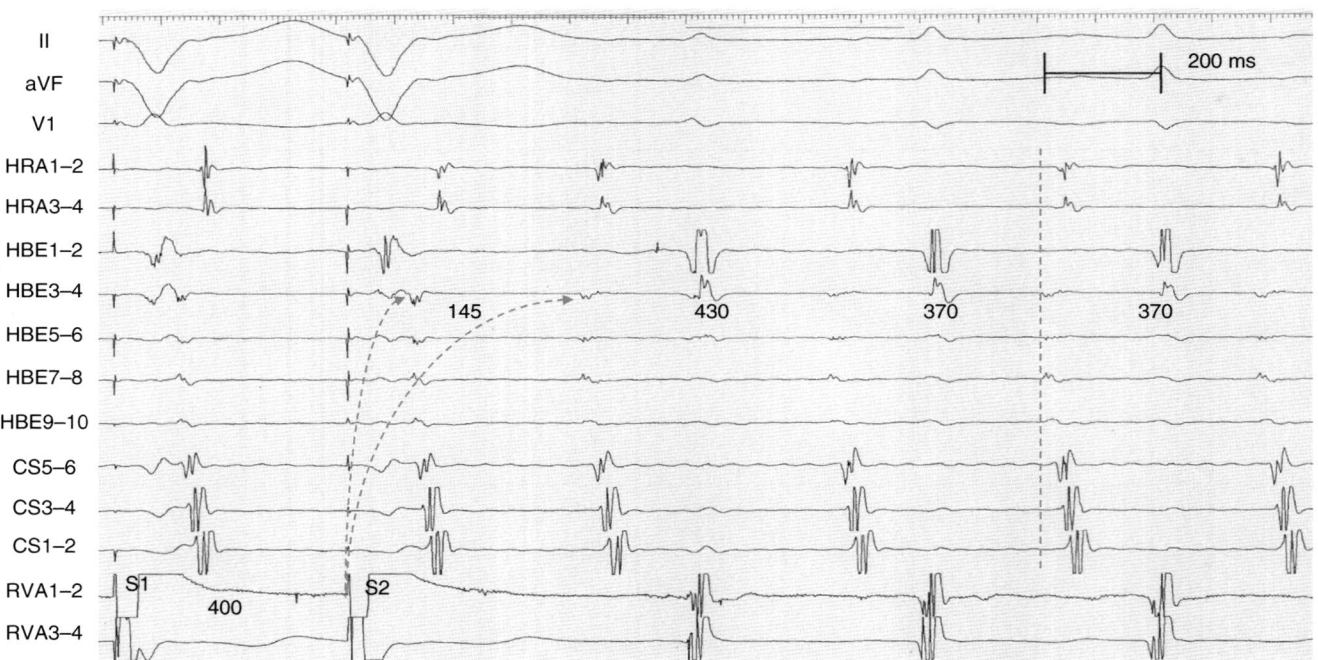

Fig. 24.3 Ventricular induction of tachycardia with an initiating double atrial response, representing V-A-A-V activation sequence in a 75-year-old woman, with successful ablation in the noncoronary aortic cusp of Valsalva. After the last burst stimulation from the right ventricular apex (RVA) at an S1–S1 cycle length of 600 ms, retrograde conduction over the fast pathway (FP) is visible, with the earliest site of atrial activation in the His-bundle region. The first and second atrial electrograms in response to ventricular extrastimuli (S2) at an S1–S2 coupling interval of 400 ms are activated in a retrograde manner (*dashed arrows*) via the FP and superior SP, respectively, followed by the reinitiation of tachycardia, thus representing a V-A-A-V activation sequence. *Numbers* indicate measurements of each atrial cycle. Note that the interval between first and second atrial electrograms of 145 ms is shorter than the tachycardia cycle length of 370 ms. I, II, and V1 = surface ECG, HRA1–2 to 3–4 = the distal to proximal bipoles of the high right atrium, HBE1–2 to 9–10 = the distal to proximal His-bundle recording, CS1–2 to 5–6 = the distal to proximal coronary sinus, RVA1–2 to 3–4 = the distal to proximal RVA

during ongoing tachycardia; and (3) a shorter stimulus-to-atrial-EGM interval during entrainment pacing from the RV apex than from the RV base (differential entrainment pacing) [7]. As described earlier, the inability to entrain the tachycardia with ventricular overdrive pacing is characteristic in most patients with the sup-F/S-AVNRT. In cases with the tachycardia which is successfully entrained with ventricular overdrive pacing (Fig. 24.2), differential entrainment pacing should be tried.

24.4 Ablation of sup-F/S-AVNRT

24.4.1 Mapping and Ablation Strategy

Our strategy of mapping and ablation is to search for and target the earliest site of atrial activation during the ongoing tachycardia in either the RA or NCC by using a contact electroanatomical mapping system. This strategy is based on the hypothetical concept that the reentry circuit is not confined within the AV node, i.e., it has no upper common pathway, and that the targeted site of the ablation corresponds to the putative atrial end of superior SP. When ablation at the earliest site of atrial activation is unsuccessful in either the RA or NCC, one could try to ablate from another side, thus obtaining successful ablation even at a less early site of atrial activation. The ratio of the amplitude of the atrial relative to the ventricular electrogram is always ≥1 (Fig. 24.4a). Moreover, an involvement of far-field components in the ventricular electrogram at the successful site may be characteristic, probably because the atrial end of the superior SP may be located away from the ventricular myocardium, due to the adjacent presence of the membranous septum, as described later (Fig. 24.5). To avoid an injury of the compact AV node, radiofrequency (RF) should not be delivered at the right-sided perihisian region based on a recording of an HB electrogram, or a higher and/or simply near-field ventricular electrogram. Moreover, excessive RF delivery should be avoided in the NCC for safety. We have not experienced the detection of delayed potentials during sinus rhythm that reflect antegrade activation over the superior SP. There may be a rare case in which successful ablation was obtained only by RF energy delivered at the left-sided interatrial septum, superior to the HB (personal communications).

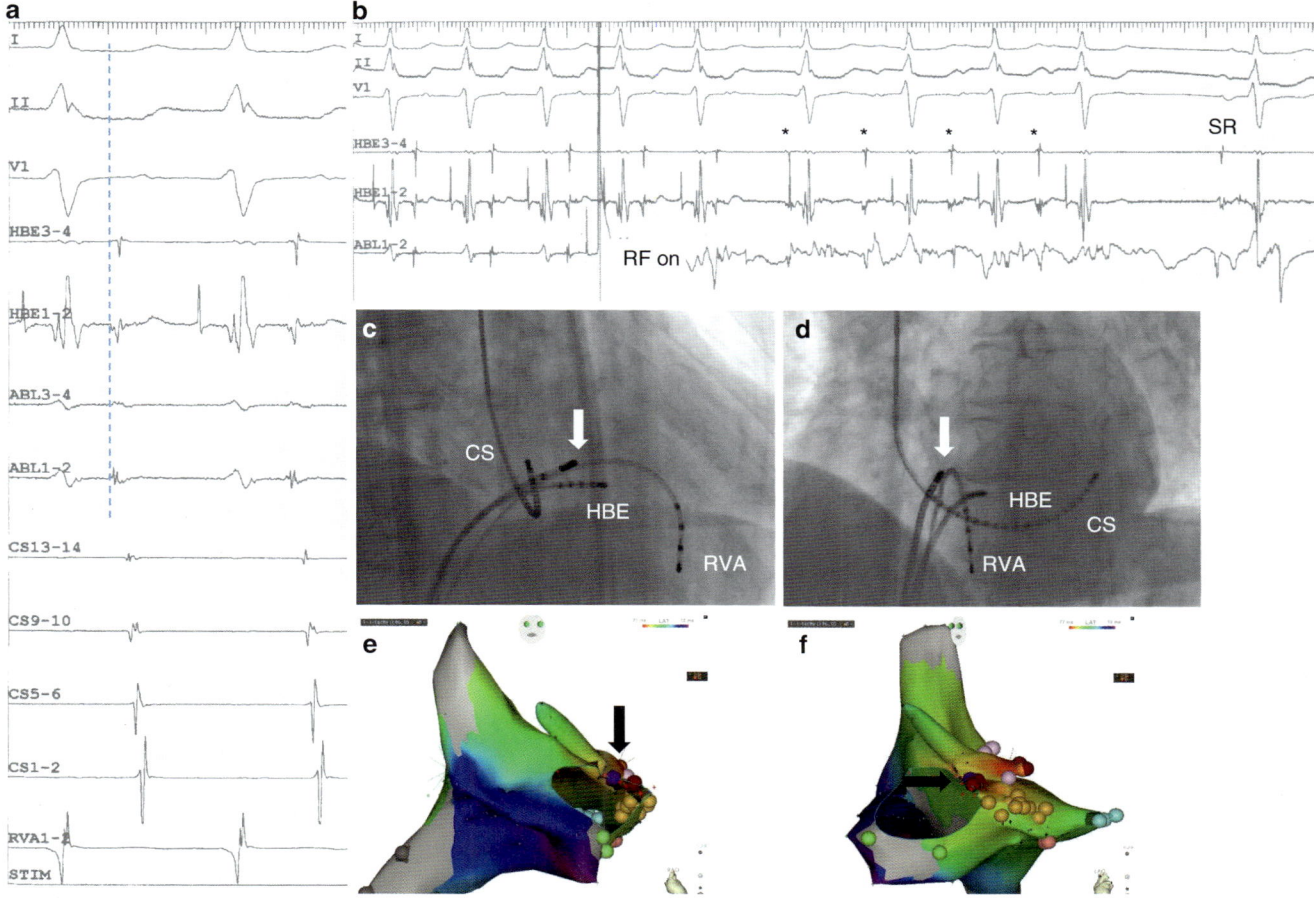

Fig. 24.4 Intracardiac recordings during tachycardia immediately before (**a**) and during (**b**) successful RF delivery, and fluoroscopic views showing the position of the catheters (**c, d**) and CARTO activation maps of the right atrium and noncoronary aortic cusp during tachycardia (**e, f**) in the right and left oblique projections, respectively, in an 81-year-old woman, with successful ablation in the right-sided perinodal region. (**a**) The atrial electrogram at the distal pole of the ablation catheter (ABL1–2) precedes the onset of the P wave by 45 ms. Note that the morphology of the ventricular electrogram is dull, consistent with a far-field activation. (**b**) The tachycardia ended 0.6 s after the RF delivery (RF on), followed by the development of several ectopic junctional cycles (*asterisks*) with the earliest activation in the HB region (HBE), before returning to sinus rhythm (SR). (**c, d**) The *white arrows point* to the tip of the ablation catheter at the site of successful ablation; *CS* coronary sinus catheter, *HBE* His-bundle electrogram, *RVA* right ventricular apical catheter. (**e, f**) The distance between the successful site (*purple tag* and *filled arrows*) and the nearest HB (*yellow tags*) measured 11.6 mm. I, II, and V1 = surface ECG, HRA3–4 = the proximal high right atrium, HBE1–2 = the distal His-bundle recording, CS1–2 to 13–14 = the distal to proximal coronary sinus

24.4.2 Hypothetical Location of Superior Slow Pathway

Considering the locational relationship between the successful ablation site and recording site of the HB electrogram, we hypothesize that the superior SP originates from the compact AV node and extends superiorly and just posterior to the membranous septum toward the NCC (Fig. 24.5). Importantly, the location of the atrial end of the superior SP seems to be individually variable. When the superior SP reaches to just underneath the NCC, it can be successfully ablated near the middle edge of the NCC. We believe that the anterior or posterior region in the NCC may be slightly separated from the superior SP coursing along the membranous septum. Notably, the NCC may be located closer to the HB than expected. In rare cases, the superior SP may extend anterolaterally along the tricuspid annulus (unpublished data).

Conclusions

The sup-F/S-AVNRT is a distinct clinical entity that involves a superior SP located above Koch's triangle as the retrograde limb, and that can be eliminated by RF ablation. In patients with confirmed fast-slow AVNRT, we recommend systematically mapping the retrograde activation of the SP before attempting its ablation.

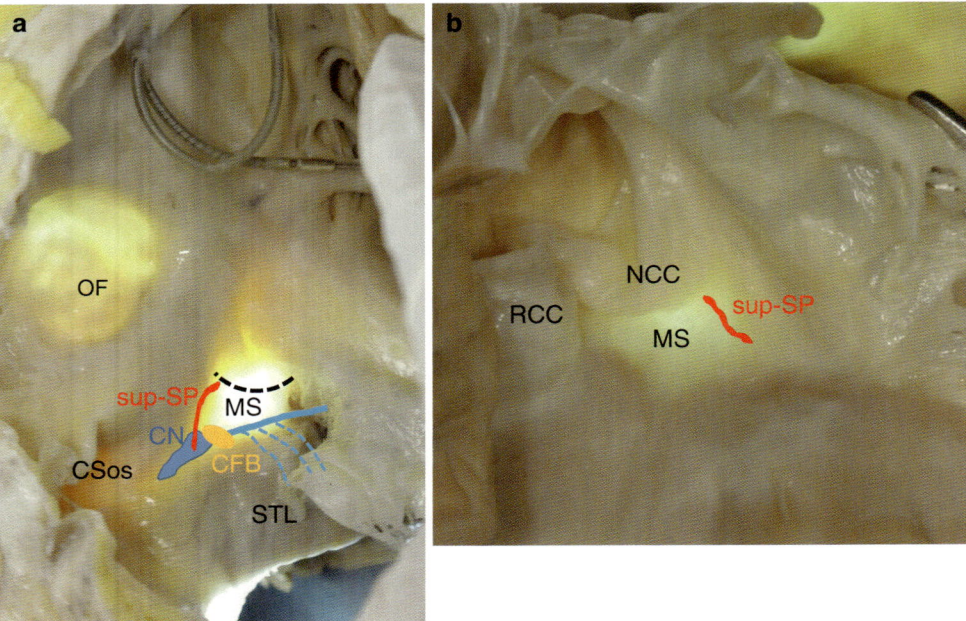

Fig. 24.5 The anatomical location of the superior SP (indicated by *bold red line*) hypothetically illustrated in the interval view of the right atrium (**a**) and left ventricle (**b**). Oval fossa (OF) and membranous septum (MS) are visualized by lighting effects from the left side. Specialized conduction system including compact node (CN), central fibrous body (CFB), and bundle branches (BB) are located just underneath the inferior margin of the MS. *Dashed line* indicates the presumed inferior margin of the noncoronary aortic cusp of Valsalva (NCC). See the text for details. *CSos* the ostium of coronary sinus, *RCC* right coronary aortic cusp. Courtesy of Prof Osamu Igawa, Nippon Medical School Tama-Nagayama Hospital, Tokyo, Japan

References

1. Clague JR, Dagres N, Kottkamp H, et al. Targeting the slow pathway for atrioventricular nodal reentrant tachycardia: initial results and long-term follow-up in 379 consecutive patients. Eur Heart J. 2001;22:82–8.
2. Estner HL, Ndrepepa G, Dong J, et al. Acute and long-term results of slow pathway ablation in patients with atrioventricular nodal reentrant tachycardia—an analysis of the predictive factors for arrhythmia recurrence. Pacing Clin Electrophysiol. 2005;28:102–10.
3. Hoffmann BA, Brachmann J, Andresen D, et al. Ablation of atrioventricular nodal reentrant tachycardia in the elderly: results from the German Ablation Registry. Heart Rhythm. 2011;8(7):981.
4. Feldman A, Voskoboinik A, Kumar S, et al. Predictors of acute and long-term success of slow pathway ablation for atrioventricular nodal reentrant tachycardia: a single center series of 1,419 consecutive patients. Pacing Clin Electrophysiol. 2011;34:927–33.
5. Otomo K, Okamura H, Noda T, et al. "Left-variant" atypical atrioventricular nodal reentrant tachycardia: electrophysiological characteristics and effect of slow pathway ablation within coronary sinus. J Cardiovasc Electrophysiol. 2006;17:1177–83.
6. Katritsis DG, Giazitzoglou E, Zografos T, et al. An approach to left septal slow pathway ablation. J Interv Card Electrophysiol. 2011;30:73–9.
7. Kaneko Y, Naito S, Okishige K, et al. Atypical fast-slow atrioventricular nodal reentrant tachycardia incorporating a "superior" slow pathway: a distinct supraventricular tachyarrhythmia. Circulation. 2016;133:114–23.
8. Keim S, Werner P, Jazayeri M, et al. Localization of the fast and slow pathways in atrioventricular nodal reentrant tachycardia by intraoperative ice mapping. Circulation. 1992;86:919–25.
9. Otomo K, Nagata Y, Taniguchi H, et al. Superior type of atypical AV nodal reentrant tachycardia: incidence, characteristics, and effect of slow pathway ablation. Pacing Clin Electrophysiol. 2008;31:998–1009.
10. Lockwood D, Nakagawa H, Dyer JW, Jackman WM. Electrophysiologic characteristics of atrioventricular nodal reentrant tachycardia: Implications for reentrant circuits. In: Zipes DP, Jalife J, editors. Cardiac electrophysiology: from cell to bedside. 6th ed. Philadelphia, PA: W.B. Saunders; 2014. p. 767–87.
11. Lin JF, Li YC, Yang PL, et al. Ablation of atrioventricular nodal reentrant tachycardia in a patient with reversal of slow and fast pathways inputs into the atrioventricular node. Pacing Clin Electrophysiol. 2012;35:e17–9.
12. Nawata H, Yamamoto N, Hirao K, et al. Heterogeneity of anterograde fast-pathway and retrograde slow-pathway conduction patterns in patients with the fast-slow form of atrioventricular nodal reentrant tachycardia: electrophysiologic and electrocardiographic considerations. J Am Coll Cardiol. 1998;32:1731–40.
13. Inoue S, Becker AE. Posterior extensions of the human compact atrioventricular node: a neglected anatomic feature of potential clinical significance. Circulation. 1998;97:188–93.
14. Racker DK. Sinoventricular transmission in 10 mM K+ by canine atrioventricular nodal inputs. Superior atrionodal bundle and proximal atrioventricular bundle. Circulation. 1991;83:1738–53.
15. Racker DK. Atrioventricular node and input pathways: a correlated gross anatomical and histological study of the canine atrioventricular junctional region. Anat Rec. 1989;224:336–54.
16. Atkinson AJ, Logantha SJ, Hao G, et al. Functional, anatomical, and molecular investigation of the cardiac conduction system and arrhythmogenic atrioventricular ring tissue in the rat heart. J Am Heart Assoc. 2013;2:e000246. https://doi.org/10.1161/JAHA.113.000246.

17. Yanni J, Boyett MR, Anderson RH, et al. The extent of the specialized atrioventricular ring tissues. Heart Rhythm. 2009;6:672–80.
18. Kaneko Y, Nakajima T, Irie T, et al. V-A-A-V activation sequence at the onset of a long RP tachycardia: what is the mechanism? J Cardiovasc Electrophysiol. 2015;26:101–3.
19. Kaneko Y, Nakajima T, Irie T, et al. Atrial and ventricular activation sequence after ventricular induction/entrainment pacing during fast-slow atrioventricular nodal reentrant tachycardia: new insight into the use of V-A-A-V for the differential diagnosis of supraventricular tachycardia. Heart Rhythm. 2017;pii:S1547-5271(17)30723-3.
20. Kaneko Y, Nakajima T, Irie T, et al. Successful ablation of atypical atrioventricular nodal reentrant tachycardia from a noncoronary sinus of Valsalva. Int Heart J. 2014;55:84–6.
21. Kaneko Y, Nakajima T, Irie T, et al. Differential diagnosis of supraventricular tachycardia with ventriculoatrial dissociation during ventricular overdrive pacing. Pacing Clin Electrophysiol. 2011;34:1028–30.

Retrograde Fast Pathway Ablation in Atrioventricular Nodal Reentrant Tachycardia

Yasuteru Yamauchi

Keywords

Retrograde fast pathway ablation • Prolonged PR interval • Dual AV nodal physiology • Cryoablation • AV block

25.1 Introduction

Atrioventricular nodal reentrant tachycardia (AVNRT) is a well known arrhythmia, and the initial experience of catheter ablation of slow-fast AVNRT targeted the fast pathway [1, 2]. However, the success rate of fast pathway ablation varied, and post-ablation PR interval prolongation was inevitable, and moreover, inadvertent second- or third-degree atrioventricular (AV) block sometimes occurred. Since the anatomic location of the slow pathway has been electrophysiologically elucidated, a slow pathway modification has been developed and produces a high successful rate, exceeding 98%. Therefore, slow pathway ablation has quickly become widespread as the first-line therapy for AVNRT, while fast pathway ablation has rarely been attempted, and is performed only when the slow pathway ablation fails. The antegrade fast pathway ablation has become completely obsolete. The most important complication of the slow pathway ablation is still AV block, and its incidence even now is 0.2–0.6%.

In the patients with a prolonged PR interval on the baseline ECG, slow pathway ablation may cause inadvertent AV block with a relatively high probability. Retrograde fast pathway ablation nowadays may be attempted in such AVNRT patients with a markedly prolonged PR interval, as an alternative approach to maintain the original AV conduction over the slow pathway.

25.2 Patient Selection for Those Suitable for Fast Pathway Ablation

In patients with AVNRT referred for catheter ablation, a prolonged PR interval on the baseline ECG is rarely encountered. In previous reports, the incidence of first-degree AV block at baseline was 2–3% in patients with AVNRT. There is great concern that slow pathway ablation in these patients may cause a subsequent higher AV block. The available clinical data concerning slow pathway ablation in patients with a prolonged PR interval are summarized in Table 25.1.

Even in such patients with a prolonged PR interval, there are some reports that careful slow pathway ablation is effective and well tolerated without any further AV conduction disturbance in most cases [3–5]. However, there are other reports that, in some patients with a prolonged PR interval, slow pathway ablation is associated not only with an intraoperative risk of higher degree AV block, but also with delayed advanced AV block during the follow-up period [6]. On the other hand, there are reports that the prolonged PR interval often shortens after successful slow pathway ablation [4, 7].

In previous reports showing that slow pathway ablation is effective and safe in AVNRT patients with a prolonged PR interval, an AH jump-up phenomenon during atrial extrastimuli suggesting the presence of dual AV nodal physiology is often observed. The prolonged PR interval appears to be caused by a long conduction time over a modestly impaired antegrade fast pathway, but not the complete absence of the antegrade fast pathway itself. In such patients, a prolonged PR interval is usually less than 300 ms. On the other hand, in patients with a markedly prolonged PR interval of more than 300 ms, the risk of complete AV block after slow pathway ablation may be significant. The optimal ablation approach in AVNRT patients with a markedly prolonged PR

Y. Yamauchi
Yokohama City Minato Red Cross Hospital,
3-12-1 Shinyamashita, Naka-ku, Yokohama, Kanagawa 231-8682, Japan
e-mail: yasuteru1020@gmail.com

Table 25.1 Slow pathway ablation in the patients with a prolonged PR interval

Author	Published year	n	Mean age (years)	PR interval (ms)	Dual AV nodal physiology (%)	Late AV block after SP ablation (%)	PM implantation after SP ablation (%)
Sra et al. [3]	1994	7	31	210-290	1 (14)	0	0
Rigden et al. [8]	1995	2	NA	300-400	NA	2 (100)	NA
Natale et al. [4]	1997	7	66	230-330	1 (14)	0	0
Lee et al. [10]	1997	8	57	210-300	8 (100)	1 (12)	1 (12)
Li et al. [6]	2001	18	62	235 ± 28	10 (55)	6 (33)	1 (5)
Pasquie et al. [5]	2006	10	69	200-240	6 (60)	0	0
Reithmann et al. [11]	2006	33	66	239 ± 31	33 (100)	4 (12)	4 (12)

AV atrioventricular, *SP* slow pathway, *PM* pacemaker, *NA* not available

interval, in order to avoid any further AV nodal dysfunction, has not well been defined.

Sra et al. described seven patients with a prolonged PR interval who underwent slow pathway ablation [3]. No patients had any AVNRT recurrence or developed any further AV block. However, the Wenckebach cycle length (WBCL) and AV nodal effective refractory period (ERP) were both significantly prolonged after the ablation. While dual AV nodal physiology was demonstrated in only one patient, the baseline PR interval in this series was from 210 to 290 ms (mean 237 ± 26 ms), and patients with a markedly prolonged PR interval of more than 300 ms were not included. Further, the mean age was as young as 31 ± 15 years.

Natale et al. also reported seven patients with a prolonged PR interval (230–330 ms) who underwent slow pathway ablation [4]. No patients had any AVNRT recurrence or AV block after a 3-month follow-up. The WBCL increased in all patients and the PR interval shortened in five patients. However, they did not evaluate the long-term follow-up data.

Pasquie et al. described the long-term outcome of slow pathway ablation in ten patients with a slightly prolonged PR interval (200–240 ms, mean 222 ± 15 ms) [5]. The mean age in the patients with a preexisting prolonged PR interval was 69 ± 15 years, which was older than that in the patients without a preexisting prolonged PR interval. Eight of ten patients had structural heart disease (80%). Dual AV nodal physiology was demonstrated in six patients (60%). After slow pathway ablation, six patients had complete slow pathway elimination, while four patients had transient or permanent AV conduction disturbances (blocked P waves in one, transient complete AV block in two, and a further prolonged PR interval in one patient). It was noteworthy that three of these four patients with transient or permanent AV nodal dysfunction had no evidence of dual AV nodal physiology. Although none had any AVNRT recurrence or developed any advanced AV block during the follow-up period, slow pathway ablation in patients without dual AV nodal physiology may be associated with a higher risk of AV block.

Rigden et al. reported two patients with a markedly prolonged PR interval (300 and 400 ms) in whom complete AV block inadvertently occurred after slow pathway ablation [8].

Li et al. compared 18 AVNRT patients with a prolonged PR interval to 328 AVNRT patients with a normal PR interval regarding the long-term safety and efficacy of slow pathway ablation [6]. In the baseline characteristics, the patients with a prolonged PR interval had a higher incidence of structural heart disease (6 of 18 vs. 19 of 328) and bundle branch block (7 of 18 vs. 19 of 328), and longer tachycardia cycle length (378 ± 72 vs. 320 ± 60 ms). In this study, 10 of 18 patients with a prolonged PR interval had dual AV nodal physiology. Although successful slow pathway modification was achieved in all patients in the acute phase, an intermittent higher degree AV block was observed in 6 of 18 (55%) patients with a prolonged PR interval compared to none in the 328 patients with a normal PR interval during the follow-up period. A predictor of a higher AV block was longer AV nodal ERP after ablation (492 ± 150 in the patients who developed AV block vs. 332 ± 101 ms in the patients who did not).

The available clinical data concerning retrograde fast pathway ablation in patients with a prolonged PR interval are summarized in Table 25.2. Verdino et al. reported three patients who underwent retrograde fast pathway ablation [9]. Of 490 consecutive patients undergoing catheter ablation of slow-fast AVNRT, 12 patients (2.4%) had a moderately prolonged PR interval (200–300 ms), and three patients (0.6%) had a markedly prolonged PR interval (more than 300 ms). Of particular note is that dual AV nodal physiology was present in 80%, 58%, and 0% of the patients with normal, moderately prolonged, and markedly prolonged PR intervals, respectively. All three patients with a markedly prolonged PR interval of more than 300 ms, all of whom had no dual AV nodal physiology, underwent retrograde fast pathway ablation and had successful elimination of AVNRT, and the post-ablation PR interval was unchanged. No patients had any AVNRT recurrence or advanced AV block the during long-term follow-up period.

Lee et al. reported 14 AVNRT patients with a prolonged PR interval (210–300 ms) [10]. Eight patients with dual AV nodal physiology received antegrade slow pathway ablation, and the remaining six patients without dual AV nodal physiology received retrograde fast pathway ablation. All patients

Table 25.2 Fast pathway ablation in the patients with a prolonged PR interval

Author	Published year	n	Mean age (years)	PR interval (ms)	Dual AV nodal physiology (%)	Late AV block after FP ablation (%)	PM implantation after FP ablation (%)
Original papers							
Lee et al. [10]	1997	6	54	210–300	0	0	0
Vendino et al. [9]	1999	3	71	310–458	0	0	0
Reithmann et al. [12]	1998	5	54	210–330	0	0	0
Reithmann et al. [11]	2006	10	66	289 ± 66	0	1 (10)	1 (10)
Case reports							
Varotto et al. [13]	1996	1	73	240	NA	0	0
Sato et al. [14]	2011	1	84	312	0	0	0
Linton et al. [15]	2012	1	53	418	0	0	0

AV atrioventricular, *FP* fast pathway, *PM* pacemaker, *NA* not available

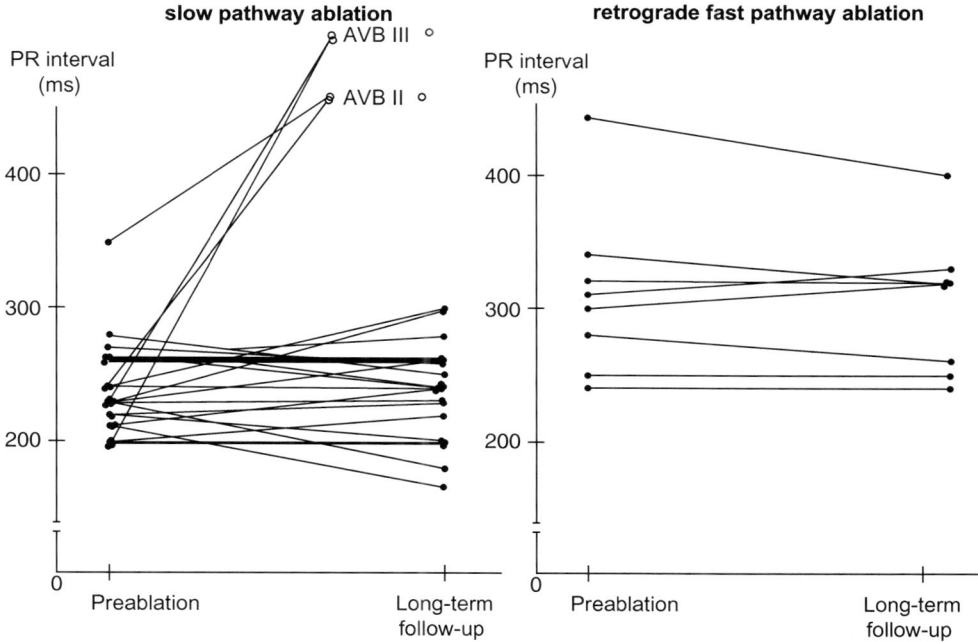

Fig. 25.1 The PR intervals immediately after ablation and during the long-term follow-up. Four patients developed delayed second- or third-degree AV block requiring pacemaker implantation after slow pathway ablation. The PR interval further increased during the follow-up after slow pathway ablation in six patients, remained the same in nine patients, and decreased in six patients. No delayed second- or third-degree AV block occurred in any of patients, and the PR interval remained unchanged after retrograde fast pathway ablation. The PR interval increased in two patients, remained the same in three patients, and decreased in three patients. *AVB* atrioventricular block

had successful elimination of AVNRT and the post-ablation AH interval remained unchanged in the acute phase. However, one patient who received slow pathway ablation developed 2:1 AV block with syncope during the follow-up period.

Similarly, Reithmann et al. reported on 43 AVNRT patients with a prolonged PR interval (200–430 ms) [11]. In 33 patients with demonstrable dual AV nodal physiology, slow pathway ablation was performed. Complete slow pathway elimination was obtained in 26 of 33 (79%) patients, and slow pathway modification was obtained in the remaining seven (21%) patients. Second-degree AV block occurred during the procedure in two patients, leading to pacemaker implantation in one patient. Notably, four (9.3%) patients required permanent pacemaker for advanced AV block, and six patients had a significant further prolongation of the PR interval (20–70 ms), and three patients suddenly died during the follow-up period (Fig. 25.1). In contrast, in ten patients without demonstrable dual AV nodal physiology, retrograde fast pathway ablation was performed. Although intraopera-

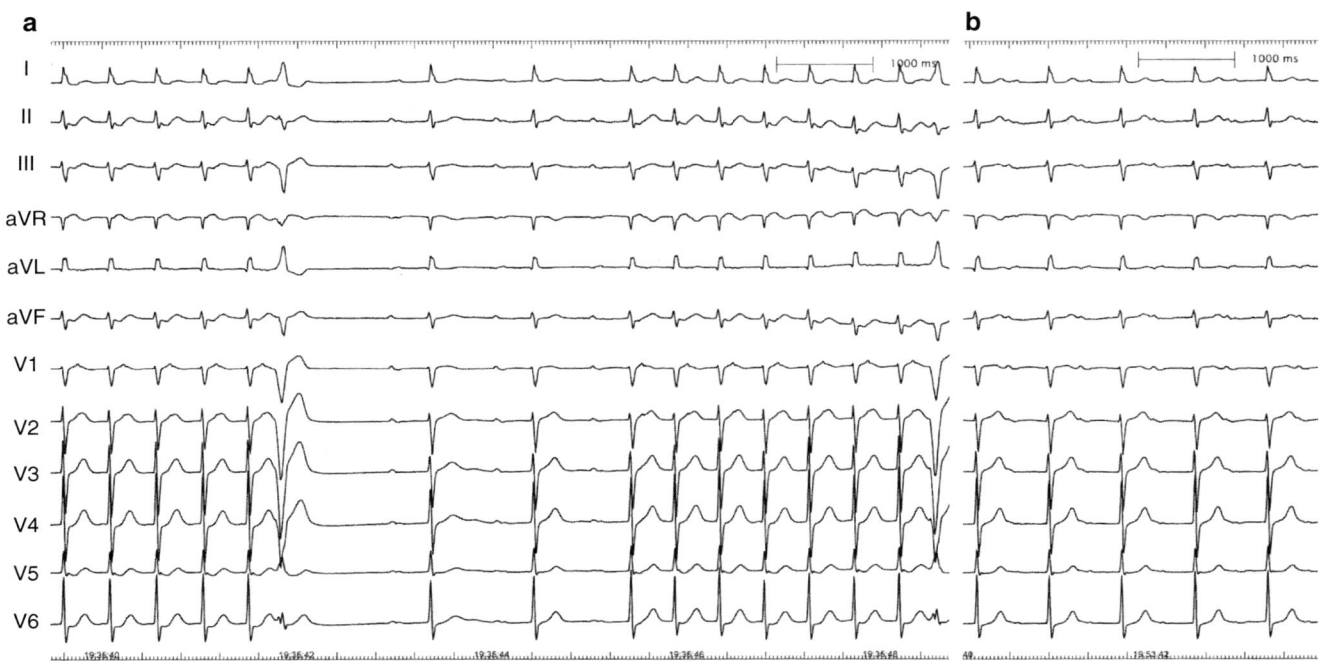

Fig. 25.2 The electrocardiograms (ECGs) during the tachycardia and sinus rhythm. (**a**) The ECG showed a regular supraventricular tachycardia of 122 beats/min, and the P wave was unclear. (**b**) The ECG during sinus rhythm exhibited a prolonged PR interval (370 ms)

tive complete AV block requiring permanent pacemaker implantation occurred in one patient, no delayed higher degree AV block occurred and the PR interval remained unchanged in the remaining nine patients during the long-term follow-up period (61 ± 39 months).

Based on these evidences, the indication for retrograde fast pathway ablation is the most suitable for patients in whom the antegrade fast pathway conduction is clearly absent without any demonstrable dual AV nodal physiology or a markedly prolonged PR interval of more than 300 ms before the ablation. Even if dual AV nodal physiology is demonstrated, slow pathway ablation may not be desirable in patients with severely impaired fast pathway conduction (for instance, a markedly prolonged PR interval or long ERP of the fast pathway conduction or documented second-degree AV block), and retrograde fast pathway ablation may rather be desirable in such a situation. These patients are usually elderly and tend to have structural heart disease. Further, slow-fast AVNRT is relatively slow, and is often incessant or easy to induce (Fig. 25.2). At any rate, when considering which pathway, antegrade slow or retrograde fast, should be ablated in patients with a prolonged PR interval, the most important thing is to electrophysiologically evaluate in minute detail whether dual AV nodal physiology is present or absent (Fig. 25.3) [12–14].

25.3 Retrograde Fast Pathway Ablation Procedure

The fast pathway is situated at the right atrial septal site posterior and superior to the apex of the triangle of Koch. A 7F deflectable quadripolar catheter with a 4 mm tip electrode is generally used for the fast pathway ablation. The ablation catheter is initially positioned along the His-bundle catheter to obtain the maximal amplitude of the His-bundle potential from the distal pair of the ablation catheter. The ablation catheter is then gradually withdrawn for several millimeters and slightly rotated anteriorly until the amplitude of the local atrial potential is at least 1–2 times as large as the local ventricular potential, and there is no His-bundle potential or it is definitely smaller than 0.1 mV (Fig. 25.4.). Clockwise torque is gently applied to the ablation catheter toward the right atrial septum to ensure better catheter contact. Then, the earliest atrial activation site via the retrograde fast pathway is precisely mapped using a 3D-mapping system during

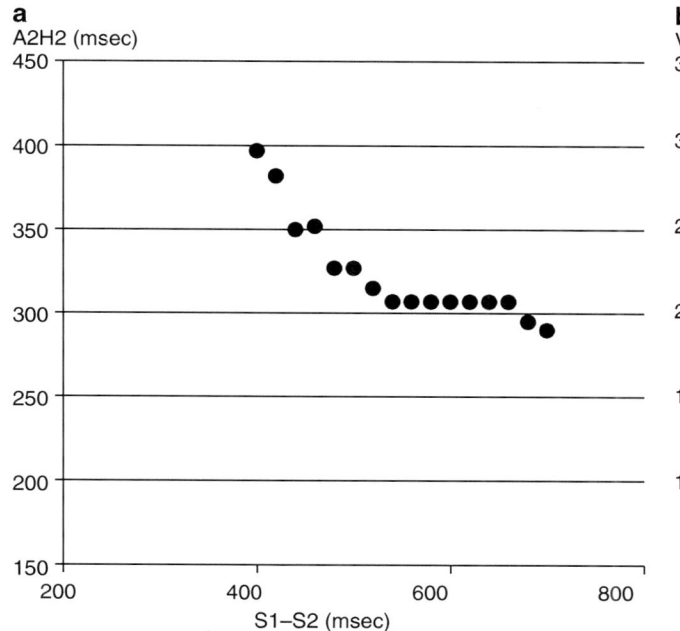 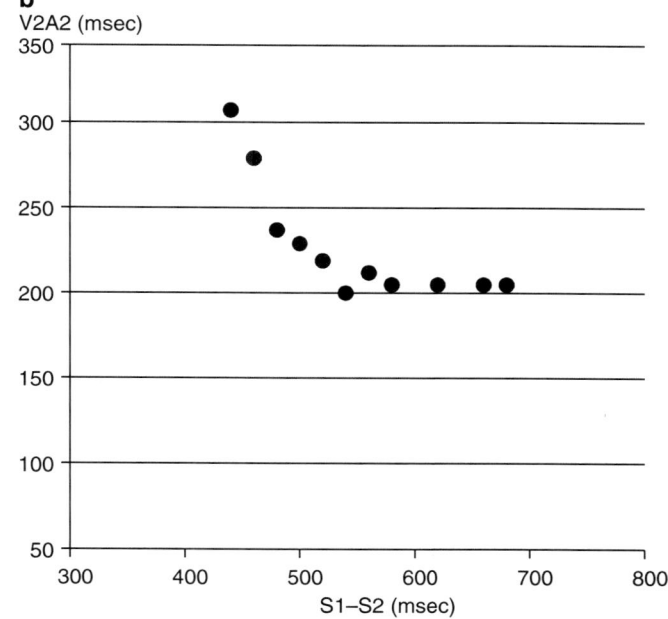

Fig. 25.3 The AH interval and VA interval conduction curves. (**a**) The A2H2 interval during atrial extrastimuli exhibits a decremental conduction property without a jump-up phenomenon. A markedly prolonged AH interval and the absence of a jump-up phenomenon suggest no antegrade fast pathway conduction. (**b**) The V2A2 interval during ventricular extrastimuli also exhibits a decremental conduction property without a jump-up phenomenon, suggesting retrograde AV nodal conduction without an accessory pathway

ventricular pacing or ongoing slow-fast AVNRT. Finally, it is necessary to confirm that the local atrial potential of the ablation catheter is earlier than or simultaneous with that of the His-bundle catheter. In the majority of patients, the optimal ablation site is 5–10 mm away from the largest His-bundle potential recording site. The LAO view is used to confirm that the tip of the ablation catheter is positioned on the anterior septum, and the RAO view is mainly used to carefully monitor that the ablation catheter dose not move.

Radiofrequency (RF) energy is initially delivered at 10 W and increased by 5 W every 10 s to a maximum of 25 W. In case of slow fast AVNRT without an antegrade fast pathway, an RF application targeting the retrograde fast pathway is usually applied during the tachycardia. If AVNRT terminates during ablation, the RF application is interrupted and it is necessary to confirm that the tachycardia termination is due to VA block, that is, retrograde fast pathway block. After confirmation of retrograde fast pathway block, the RF application at the same site is restarted. An RF application at an effective site invariably causes the emergence of an accelerated junctional rhythm. Whenever an accelerated junctional rhythm appears, it is advisable to pace the atrium at a faster rate (usually 100–120 beats/min) so as to meticulously monitor the AH interval over the antegrade slow pathway. If a much faster junctional rhythm than the pacing rate develops, the RF application should be stopped because a fast junctional rhythm often causes an impairment of the compact AV node leading to complete AV block. Thereafter, the RF application is restarted during a faster pacing rate. The initial RF power setting is always set at 10–15 W and is gradually titrated by 5 W until a total of 25 W for 30–60 s. During each RF application, the RF delivery is immediately terminated if a prolongation of the AH interval or fast junctional rhythm as well as complete AV block are noted.

After the RF energy delivery, ventricular pacing is performed to evaluate the retrograde conduction because the end-point of the procedure is to create complete retrograde fast pathway conduction block. If AVNRT remains inducible or retrograde fast pathway conduction still persists, the ablation catheter is slightly moved inferiorly toward the midseptum, and an RF application is attempted again. One of the technical difficulties in performing fast pathway ablation is getting good catheter stability in this small area close to the compact AV node. Because an RF application with catheter instability has a potentially high risk for complete AV block, the usage of a deflectable long sheath is recommended

25.4 Case Presentation: Retrograde Fast Pathway Ablation

The electrocardiogram during palpitation exhibits a narrow QRS tachycardia with a retrograde P wave just after QRS complex, while the PR interval is prolonged during sinus rhythm as in Fig. 25.2. From the electrophysiological study, the mechanism of tachycardia is a slow/fast type AV nodal reentrant tachycardia and the A-H interval during sinus rhythm is prolonged as in Fig 25.4a. The AV conduction curve and VA conduction curve, shown in Fig. 25.3, reveal that an antegrade fast pathway may not be present but retrograde fast pathway conduction exists. For retrograde fast pathway ablation, the ablation catheter is placed on the mid/anterior septum targeting the left-sided fast pathway as shown in Fig 25.4b. An RF energy application was effective in terminating the tachycardia, while it did not affect the PR interval during sinus rhythm (Fig 25.4c).

25.5 Cryoablation of the Retrograde Fast Pathway

Recently, cryoablation has become a widespread therapeutic approach for AVNRT with less risk of AV block [12]. Cryoablation has some advantages, especially with respect to fast pathway ablation, as compared to RF ablation. Ice mapping at −30 °C, of which any initial thermal injury is reversible, can be used to tentatively ascertain the unintentional risk of AV block as well as the effectiveness at the ablation site. Ice mapping does not cause permanent tissue damage if the ice mapping time is short and less than 60 s. Even if a prolongation of the AH interval or advanced AV block is observed during ice mapping, then immediate cessation of the ice mapping and rewarming can make it return back to the baseline AV conduction state.

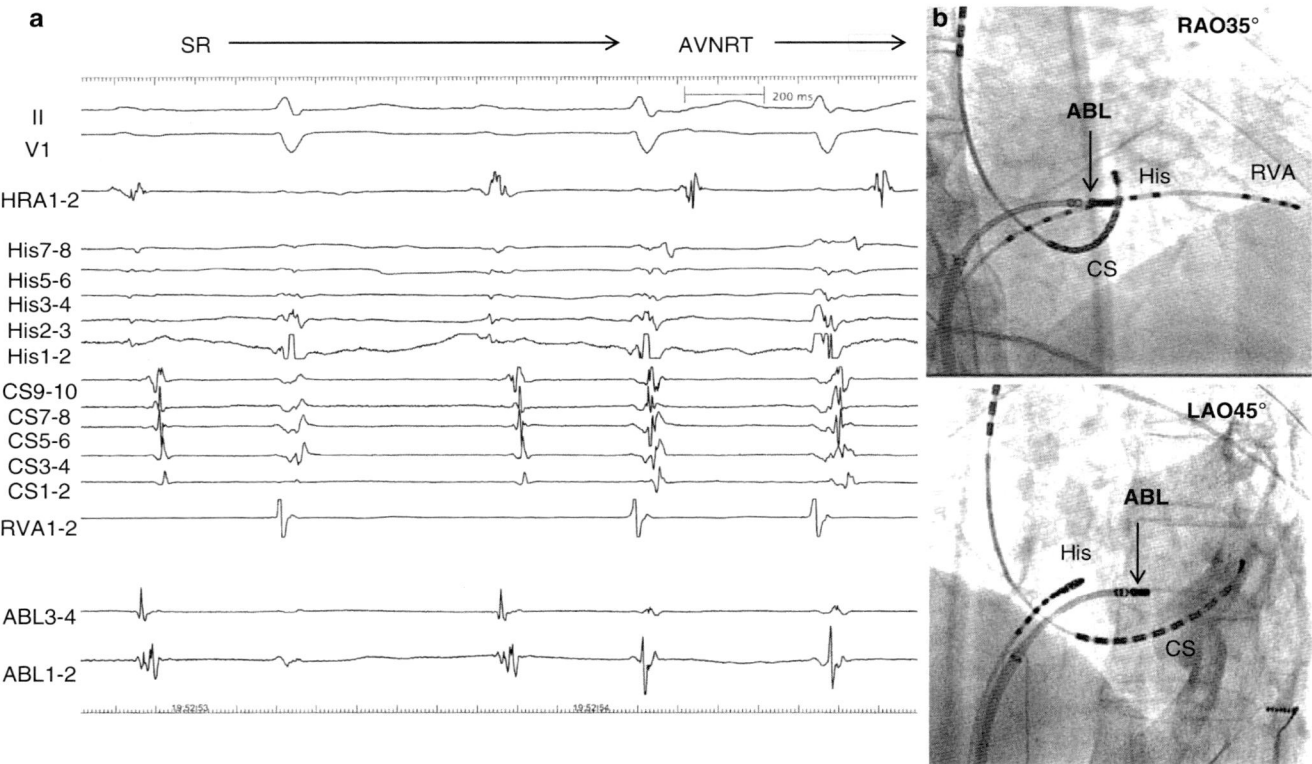

Fig. 25.4 The final successful retrograde fast pathway ablation site. We finally performed successful ablation of the retrograde fast pathway by a left-sided transseptal approach. (**a**) Recordings from surface ECG leads II and V1, and the intracardiac recordings from the distal pair of electrodes of the His-bundle (His), coronary sinus (CS), ablation (ABL), and right ventricular apex (RVA) catheters. AVNRT was initiated without an AH jump-up phenomenon. The AV electrogram amplitude ratio at the successful ablation site was more than 2, and no His-bundle potential was recorded. (**b**) The radiograms in the right anterior oblique 35 and left anterior oblique 45 projections presenting the location of the ablation catheter during the left-sided fast pathway ablation. (**c**) A radiofrequency application at that site terminated the tachycardia via VA block 2.7 s after the delivery of the radiofrequency current. The AH interval during sinus rhythm was unchanged after the ablation

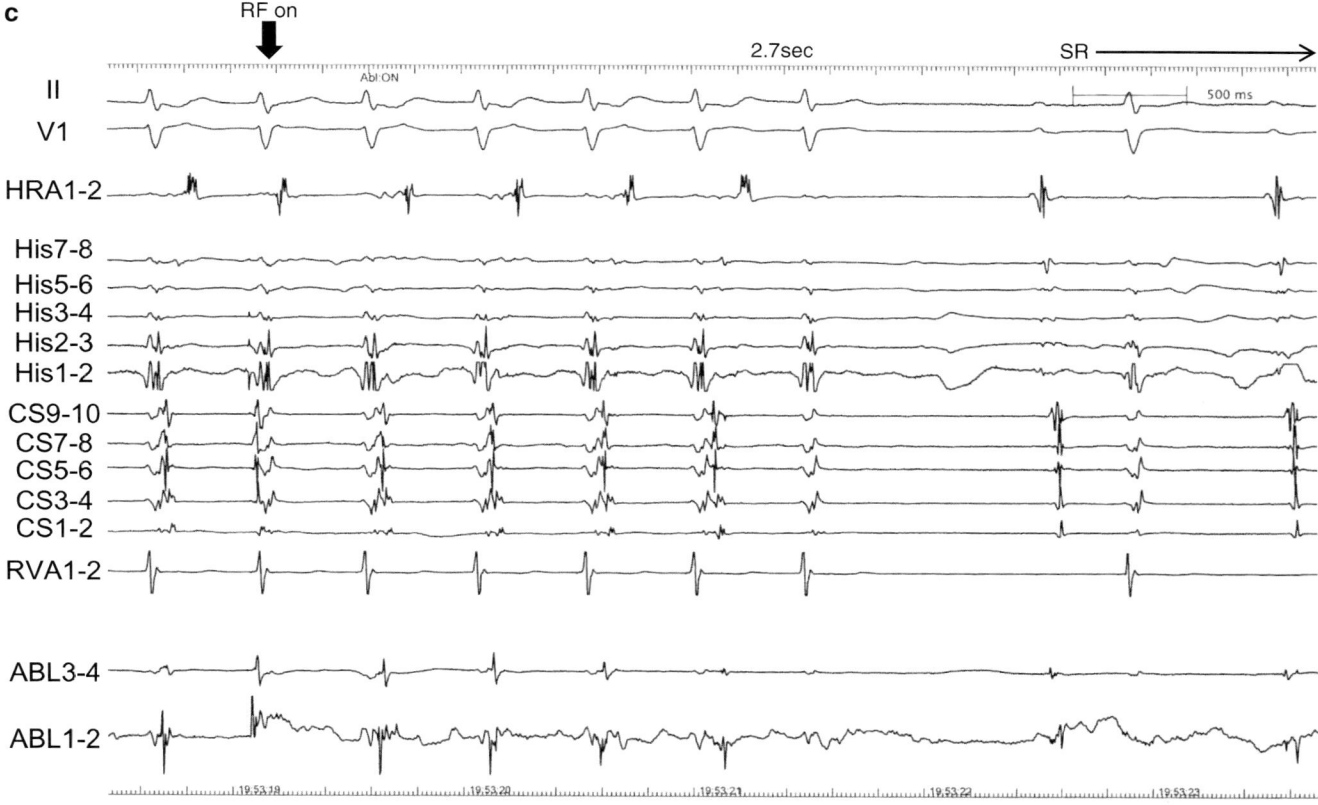

Fig. 25.4 (continued)

After a safe and effective ablation site is identified by ice mapping, cryoablation at −80 °C is executed at that same site. If AV nodal conduction disturbance is observed during the cryoablation, immediate cessation of cooling may restore it to the baseline AV nodal conduction status because a reversible damage zone always precedes any irreversible damage zone, and the lesion damage created by cryoablation progresses more slowly than RF ablation. The tip of the ablation catheter adheres to the ablative tissue firmly during cooling, which provides good catheter stability and can avoid any inadvertent catheter dislodgement. Unlike RF ablation, cryoablation usually does not provoke junctional rhythm. This enables stable continuous monitoring of the AH interval during ablation and contributes to a safer procedure. Cryoablation may be more suitable than RF ablation, especially for retrograde fast pathway ablation.

References

1. Haissaguerre M, Warin JF, Lemetayer P, et al. Closed-chest ablation of retrograde conduction in patients with atrioventricular nodal reentrant tachycardia. N Engl J Med. 1989;320:426–33.
2. Jazayeri MR, Hempe SL, Sra JS, et al. Selective transcatheter ablation of the fast and slow pathways using radiofrequency energy in patients with atrioventricular nodal reentrant tachycardia. Circulation. 1992;85:1318–28.
3. Sra JS, Jazayeri MR, Blanck Z, et al. Slow pathway ablation in patients with atrioventricular node reentrant tachycardia and a prolonged PR interval. J Am Coll Cardiol. 1994;24:1064–8.
4. Natale A, Greenfield RA, Geiger MJ, et al. Safety of slow pathway ablation in patients with long PR interval: further evidence of fast and slow pathway interaction. Pacing Clin Electrophysiol. 1997;20:1698–703.
5. Pasquie JL, Scalzi J, Macia JC, et al. Longterm safety and efficacy of slow pathway ablation in patients with atrioventricular nodal re-entrant tachycardia and pre-existing prolonged PR interval. Europace. 2006;8:129–33.
6. Li YG, Groenefeld G, Bender B, et al. Risk of development of delayed atrioventricular block after slow pathway modification in patients with atrioventricular nodal reentrant tachycardia and a pre-existing prolonged PR interval. Eur Heart J. 2001;22:89–95.
7. Hummel JP, DiMarco JP. Paroxysmal supraventricular tachycardia in a patient with a markedly prolonged PR interval. Heart Rhythm. 2004;1:519–20.
8. Rigden LB, Klein LS, Mitrani RD, Zipes DP, Miles WM. Increased risk of heart block following slow pathway ablation for AV nodal reentrant tachycardia in patients with marked PR interval prolongation during sinus rhythm. Pacing Clin Electrophysiol. 1995;18:II-918. (NASPE abstract)
9. Verdino RJ, Burke MC, Kall JG, et al. Retrograde fast pathway ablation for atrioventricular nodal reentry associated with markedly prolonged PR intervals. Am J Cardiol. 1999;83:455–8.
10. Lee SH, Chen SA, Tai CT, et al. Atrioventricular node reentrant tachycardia in patients with a long fast pathway effective refractory period: clinical features, electrophysiologic characteristics, and results of radiofrequency ablation. Am Heart J. 1997;134:387–94.
11. Reithmann C, Remp T, Oversohl N, et al. Ablation for atrioventricular nodal reentrant tachycardia with a prolonged PR interval dur-

ing sinus rhythm: the risk of delayed higher-degree atrioventricular block. J Cardiovasc Electrophysiol. 2006;17:973–9.
12. Reithmann C, Hoffmann E, Grünewald A, et al. Fast pathway ablation in patients with common atrioventricular nodal reentrant tachycardia and prolonged PR interval during sinus rhythm. Eur Heart J. 1998;19:929–35.
13. Varotto L, Storti C, Salerno-Uriarte JA. Fast pathway ablation in a patient with iterative atrioventricular nodal reentrant tachycardia and prolonged PR interval. Int J Cardiol. 1996;56:263–7.
14. Sato D, Otani H, Noda T, et al. Retrograde fast pathway ablation with the EnSite NavX mapping system for slow-fast atrioventricular node reentrant tachycardia and a prolonged PR interval during sinus rhythm. J Cardiol Cases. 2011;3:e143–8.
15. Linton NW, Davies DW, Mason A, Lefroy D. Fast pathway ablation using cryotherapy for a patient with a long PR interval in sinus rhythm and AVNRT. Pacing Clin Electrophysiol. 2012;35:e47–51.

Part VII
Catheter Ablation of Accessory Pathways

Free Wall Atrioventricular Accessory Pathways

Seiji Takatsuki

Keywords
Accessory pathway • Catheter ablation • Mapping

26.1 Outline

Atrioventricular (AV) accessory pathway is a myocardial fiber connecting the atrium and the ventricle. The accessory pathway can be a cause of the paroxysmal AV reciprocating tachycardia which affects patient's quality of life. Furthermore, the atrial fibrillation may develop in patients with an accessory pathway, which can be fatal if the effective refractory period of the accessory pathway is short [1]. Since the ventricular fibrillation can develop due to high ventricular rate during atrial fibrillation in such patients. The radiofrequency catheter ablation for the accessory pathway is an established and curative treatment for such symptomatic patients [2, 3].

The accessory pathway is able to conduct electrical excitation both from the atrium to the ventricle (anterograde) conduction and from the ventricle to the atrium (retrograde) conduction. Typically, 12 lead electrocardiography (ECG) shows a short PQ interval and a delta wave which is the slur at the onset of the QRS wave making QRS wave wider, reflecting the early ventricular activation is brought by an accessory pathway. The accessory pathway can have exclusively a retrograde conduction, which is called concealed pathway without exhibiting a delta wave on the surface ECG. The concealed accessory pathway accounts for 40% of the accessory pathway patients. Multiple accessory pathways account for 10% of the accessory pathways. The electrophysiological characteristics of the accessory pathway are considered to resemble with atrial myocardium. The conduction velocity is fast without showing a decremental property, whereas 10% of the accessory pathways have a slow and a decremental conduction property. In such cases, discrimination of the retrograde conduction between the accessory pathway and the AV node sometimes might be difficult.

26.2 Diagnosis of Accessory Pathway

26.2.1 Retrograde Conduction

Retrograde conduction of the accessory pathway must be discriminated from that of the AV node. The site of the earliest atrial activation and the decremental conduction property contribute to discriminate them. The earliest atrial activation site of the retrograde conduction of the fast pathway of the AV node is around His bundle electrogram recording site and that of the slow pathway is around the ostium of the coronary sinus (CS). In both of them, the retrograde atrial activation shows concentric propagation pattern. Although quite rate, it is reported that the earliest retrograde activation via the AV node can show eccentric pattern from the distal CS [4]. The earliest activation of the accessory pathway can be located at anywhere around the tricuspid and mitral annulus except for the fibrous trigone of the anteroseptal area of the mitral annulus where ventricular myocardium does not exist. The eccentric atrial activation pattern during ventricular pacing usually associates with the existence of the accessory pathway.

The change in the atrial activation sequence during ventricular programmed stimulation indicates multiple retrograde conduction pathways. With decreasing the pacing cycle length or the pacing interval of the extrastimuli of ventricular stimulation, retrograde conduction time via the AV

S. Takatsuki
Keio University School of Medicine,
35 Shinanomachi, Shinjukuku, Tokyo 160-8582, Japan
e-mail: seiji.takatsuki@gmail.com

node will increase and a Wenckebach block will be shown whereas that via the accessory pathway will not increase much.

Ventricular stimulation site will affect the ventriculoatrial conduction time. In the WPW syndrome, the accessory pathway connects the atrium and the ventricle at the annulus of the AV valves. So pacing from the base of the ventricle usually associates with the shortening of the retrograde conduction time in the accessory pathway. Whereas the pacing from the right ventricular apex close to the exit of the right bundle branch associates with shortening of the retrograde conduction time via the AV node.

The paraHisian pacing is a useful method to discriminate the retrograde conduction of the AV node and the accessory pathway [5] (which is detailed in the Chapter 4). During paraHisian pacing, the low output pacing exclusively captures the local ventricular myocardium accompanying wide QRS complex and the high output pacing captures both the local ventricular myocardium and the His bundle accompanying narrow QRS complex, which facilitates the earlier retrograde conduction via the AV node. Retrograde conduction pattern should be investigated comparing during wide QRS complex vs. narrow QRS complex. When the retrograde activation sequence changes, both retrograde conduction via the AV node and the accessory pathway exist. If narrow QRS complex associates with shortening of the ventriculoatrial conduction time about 40 ms, the retrograde pathway must be the AV node. For the free wall accessory pathway, it should be noted that the high output pacing can also shorten the ventriculoatrial conduction time by 10–15 ms due to His bundle capture can advance the local ventricular activation near the accessory pathway via His-Purkinje system conduction [6].

26.2.2 Anterograde Conduction

Anterograde conduction of the accessory pathway can be shown by ventricular preexcitation, so-called delta wave in 12 lead electrocardiography. The ventricular preexcitation might be obscured during sinus rhythm in patients with the left lateral accessory pathway since it is far from sinus node compared with the AV node. WPW syndrome can be classified into three types of QRS configuration of the lead V1. The type A is the right bundle branch block pattern or R pattern which indicates the left free wall accessory pathway. The type B is the rS pattern in lead V1 indicating the right free wall accessory pathway. The type C is qS pattern in lead V1 indicating the septal accessory pathway. Anterior accessory pathway has an inferior axis and the posterior accessory pathway has a superior QRS axis. More precise localization of the accessory pathway by delta wave was proposed [7].

To decrease pacing cycle length during constant atrial pacing or to decrease coupling interval during atrial extrastimulation might reveal ventricular preexcitation, which could slow the anterograde conduction of AV node. The atrial stimulation close to the accessory pathway can reveal ventricular preexcitation compared with sinus rhythm. In patients with WPW syndrome, 10% of the patients have multiple accessory pathways. In such patients, pacing applied from different atrial sites would reveal different delta waves [7].

26.2.3 Induction and Diagnosis of the Atrioventricular Reciprocating Tachycardia (AVRT)

In a patient with WPW syndrome, two types of atrioventricular reciprocating tachycardia (AVRT) can develop, which are orthodromic and antidromic AVRT. In the orthodromic AVRT, the activation comes down from the atrium to the ventricle via the AV node and goes up from the ventricle to the atrium via the accessory pathway. Hence, the orthodromic AVRT has a narrow QRS complex unless the bundle branch block does not develop. The antidromic AVRT uses the same tachycardia circuit with the orthodromic AVRT with a reversed direction which has wide QRS complex. The earliest ventricular activation is recorded at the accessory pathway connecting site and retrograde conduction, ventriculoatrial conduction passes via AV node or another accessory pathway.

The AVRT characteristically has one-to-one AV conduction, which is different from atrial tachycardia and AV nodal reentrant tachycardia. The diagnosis of AVRT is to prove that the accessory pathway is included in the tachycardia circuit. If a single ventricular extrastimulation at the timing of the His bundle refractoriness advances the tachycardia, the tachycardia must not be an AV nodal reentrant tachycardia or atrial tachycardia but an orthodromic AVRT (Fig. 26.1).

If the functional bundle branch block developing during tachycardia accompany the prolongation of the tachycardia cycle length, the tachycardia is assumed to be an AVRT having an accessory pathway at the same side with a blocked bundle branch [8] (Fig. 26.2). For example, if a left bundle branch block develops during narrow QRS tachycardia and the tachycardia cycle length prolongs, the tachycardia is AVRT with an accessory pathway at the left free wall. During narrow QRS tachycardia, the activation conducted from the AV node to the His bundle, the left bundle branch, the left ventricular myocardium and conducted to the accessory

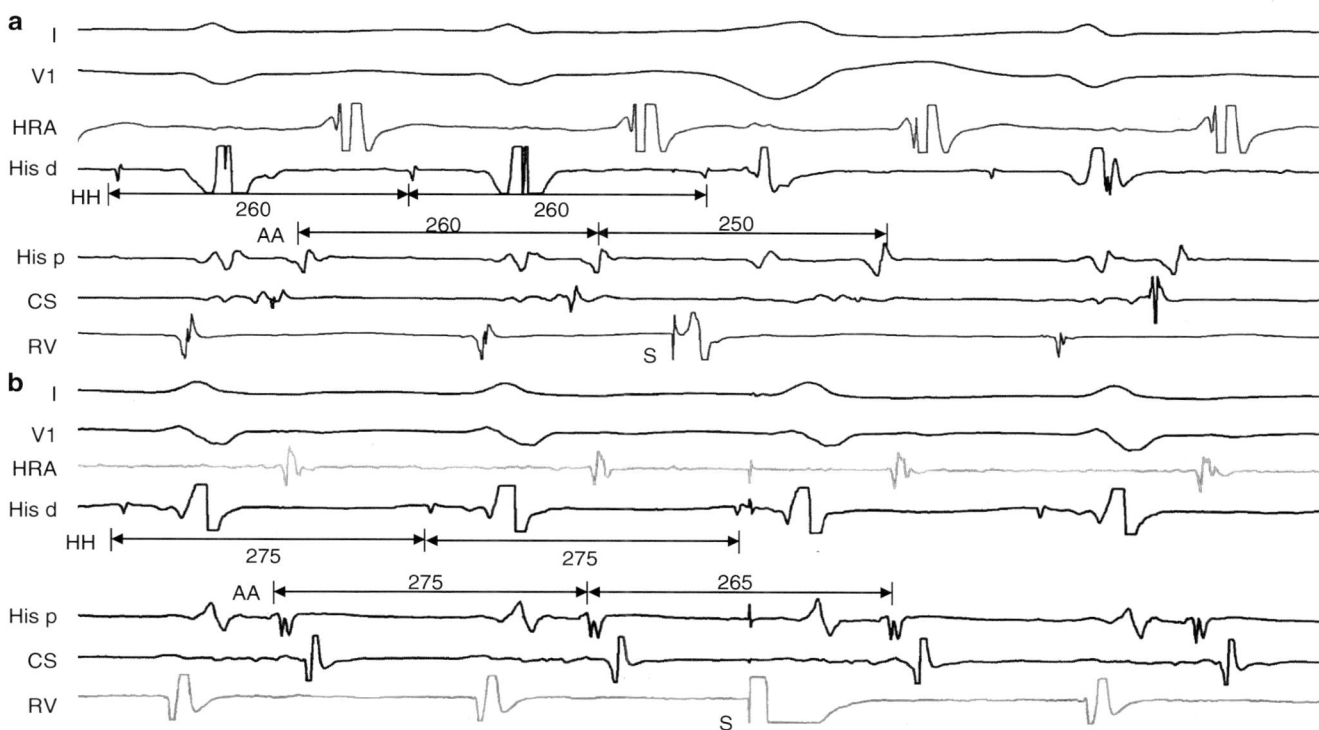

Fig. 26.1 Atrial early capture during orthodromic atrioventricular reciprocating tachycardia. (**a**) Atrial early capture in a patient with a left free wall accessory pathway. During orthodromic AVRT, an extrastimulus was applied from the right ventricular apex (RV), which advanced atrial activation by 10 ms (from 260 to 250 ms) without advancing His bundle activation. This finding confirmed ventriculoatrial conduction was via an accessory pathway, so the diagnosis of the orthodromic AVRT was defined. (**b**) Atrial early capture in a patient with a right free wall accessory pathway. During orthodromic AVRT, a ventricular extrastimulus advanced atrial activation by 10 ms. The timing of the extrastimulus was just after His bundle anterograde activation, that was refractory period of the His bundle activation. This confirmed the tachycardia was an orthodromic AVRT. Comparing (**a**) with (**b**), we could see that the atrial early capture was easily obtained in a patient with a right accessory pathway. The tachycardia circuit was far in a patient of the left free wall accessory pathway and was close in a patient of the right free wall accessory pathway from the pacing site of the right ventricle

pathway, but once the left bundle branch develops, activation from the AV node conducts to the His bundle, the right bundle branch, the ventricular septum, the left ventricle and finally to the accessory pathway. Hence, the tachycardia circuit is elongated and the tachycardia cycle length will increase.

Antidromic AVRT should be discriminated from the ventricular tachycardia with 1-to-1 retrograde conduction via AV node and the atrial tachycardia with bystander anterograde accessory pathway conduction. The surface electrocardiogram of the antidromic AVRT can mimic that of a ventricular tachycardia originated from the myocardium near the accessory pathway. To discriminate VT, an atrial extrastimulus should be applied near the accessory pathway. If an atrial extrastimulus can advance the next ventricular activation, it must not be a ventricular tachycardia. And if a ventricular extrastimulus advances the next atrial activation, the atrial tachycardia can be discriminated (Figs. 26.3 and 26.4).

The induction of the AVRT can be obtained by either atrial or ventricular programmed stimulation. For the initiation of the reentrant tachycardia, to provoke unidirectional conduction block is mandatory. The atrial burst stimulation or extrastimulation provokes conduction block of the accessory pathway and the activation conducts exclusively AV node, which propagates ventricular myocardium and turns up retrogradely to the atrium via the accessory pathway and the orthodromic AVRT initiates. Orthodromic AVRT induction by atrial programmed electrical stimulation sometimes can be accompanied by jump up of the AV nodal conduction, that is the switch from the fast pathway to the slow pathway of the AV nodal anterograde conduction.

The ventricular programmed stimulation can provoke retrograde conduction block of AV nodal conduction and the exclusive retrograde accessory pathway conduction can activate the atrial myocardium, which would lead to induction of orthodromic AVRT. The right ventricular programmed electrical

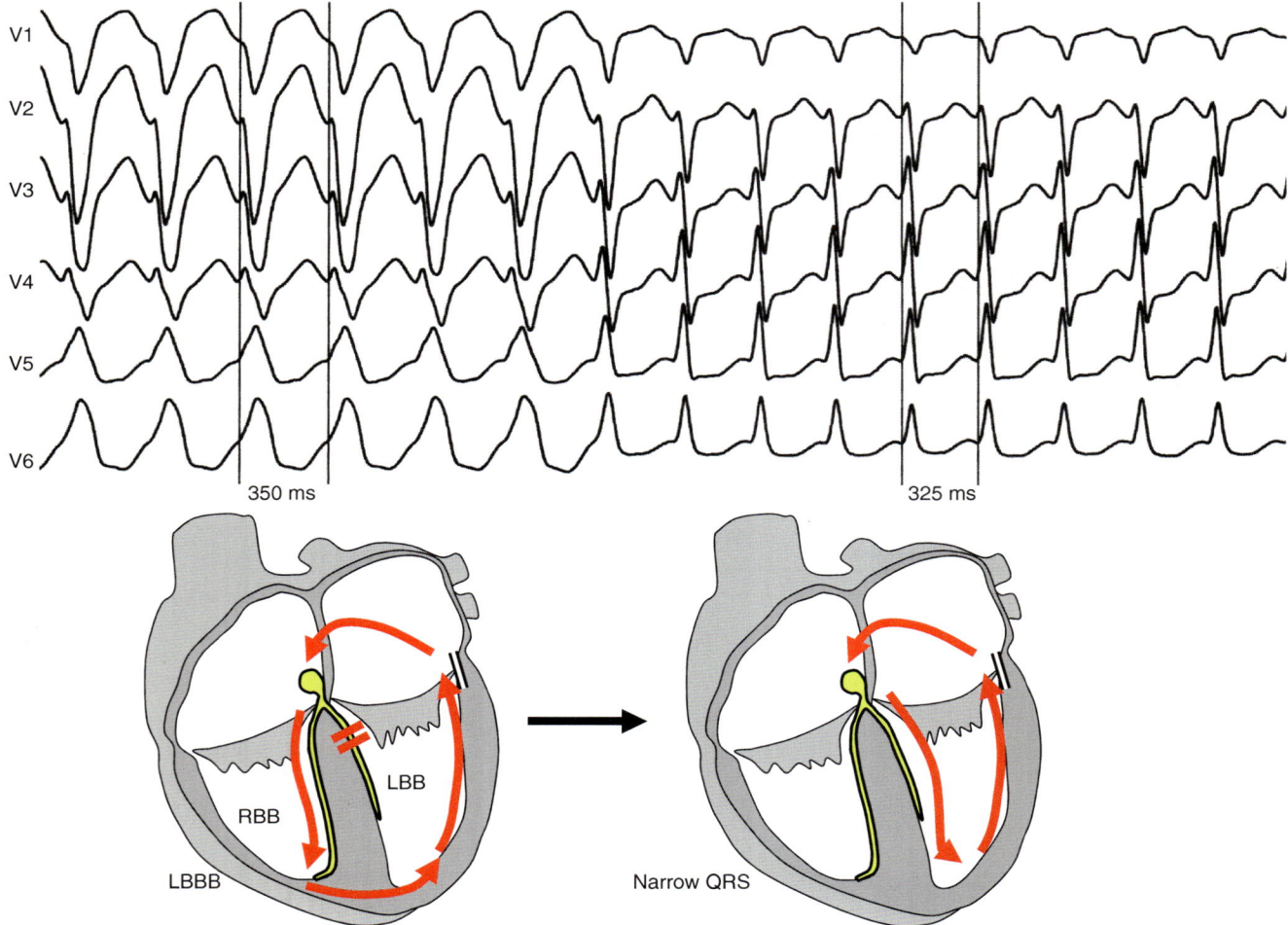

Fig. 26.2 The bundle branch block affecting tachycardia cycle length in a patient with WPW syndrome. In the upper panel, an AVRT with a left bundle branch block type aberrant conduction changed to narrow QRS complex with resolution of the left bundle branch block and the tachycardia cycle length shortened by 25 ms. In the lower panel, schemas showing the change of the tachycardia circuit was shown. With a left bundle branch block, the tachycardia circuit of an AVRT utilizing a left free wall accessory pathway detour to utilize the right bundle branch. In patients with AVRT, developing a functional right or left bundle branch block with elongation of the tachycardia cycle length associates with the existence of the ipsilateral accessory pathway

stimulation can induce one echo of the bundle branch reentry, which also can lead to the orthodromic AVRT induction caused by retrograde AV nodal conduction block.

26.3 Catheter Manipulation

26.3.1 Left Side Accessory Pathway

For the left side accessory pathway, both of the retrograde aortic approach and the transseptal approach can be taken. The retrograde approach needs puncture of the femoral artery and the ablation catheter goes through the aorta and passes through the aortic valve. Hence, if the patient has aortic sclerosis, aortic approach should be avoided. In patients with elongated and tortuous abdominal aorta, a long sheath which reaches below the aortic arch will help to manipulate the mapping catheter. By using the transaortic approach, the mapping catheter is easily going to the posterior mitral annulus in the left ventricle, whereas is difficult to reach the anterior annulus. To contact the anterior mitral annulus, using a large curve catheter would be successful. Just after passing through the aortic valve, to bend slightly the mapping catheter and the direction of the catheter should be determined. To ablate the left accessory pathway, the ablation catheter can be positioned either below the mitral

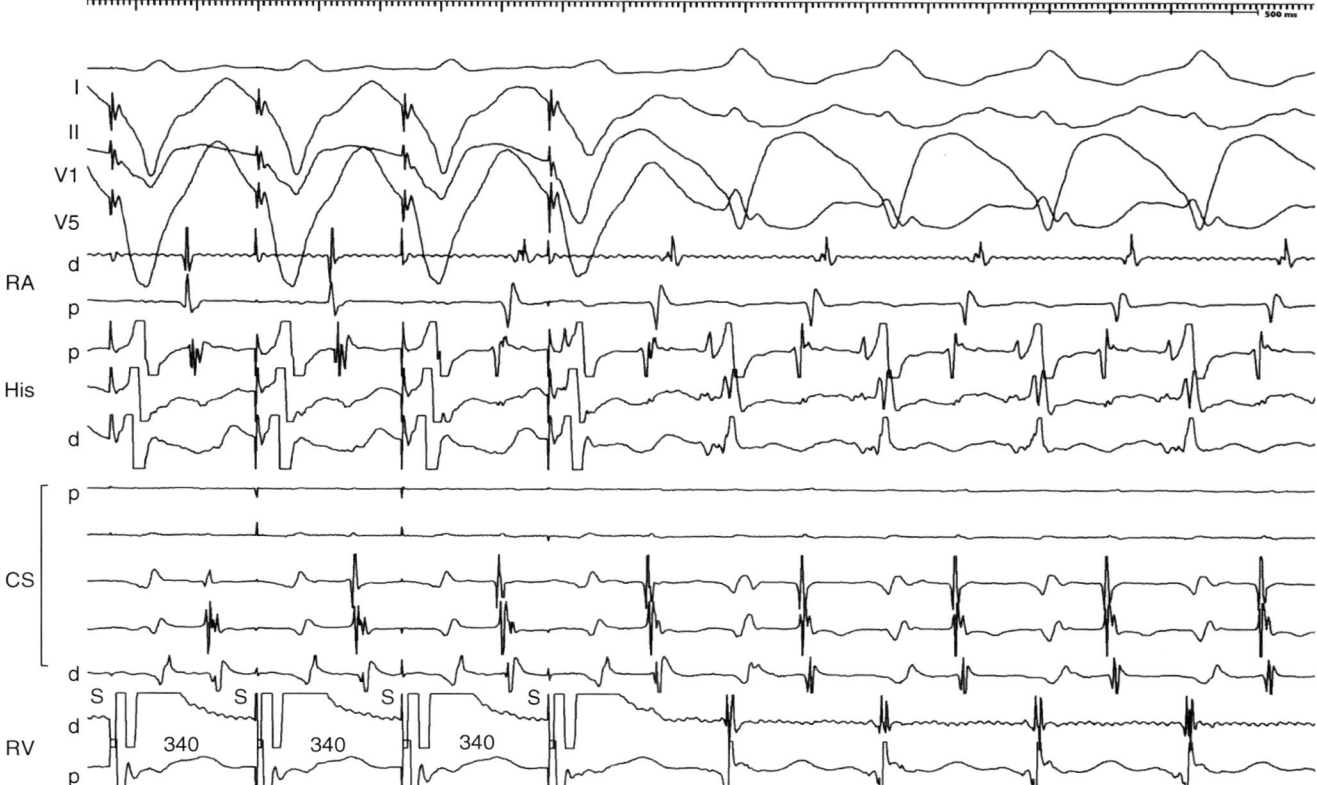

Fig. 26.3 Induction of the antidromic atrioventricular reciprocating tachycardia. Constant pacing (340 ms) from the right ventricle induced the antidromic atrioventricular reciprocating tachycardia. The ventriculoatrial conduction was via the right free wall accessory pathway during the first and second pacing stimulus and the retrograde conduction via an AP was blocked at the third stimulus which was shifted to the retrograde conduction via atrioventricular node and the tachycardia initiated. The tachycardia exhibited a left bundle branch block QRS morphology due to atrioventricular conduction via right free wall accessory pathway

valve (subvalvular approach) or over the valve (supravalvular approach). The subvalvular approach can obtain a good tissue contact of the ablation catheter, however, to map precisely or to move the ablation catheter subtly is difficult after the catheter reach below the valve. With the supravalvular approach, to take enough contact might be difficult, but catheter is easy to move. After mapping on the valve, the catheter should be pulled below the valve and then radiofrequency energy can be delivered. For the subvalvular approach, the catheter should be directed towards the location of the accessory pathway with advancing the catheter after passing the aortic valve.

With the supravalvular approach, after advancing the ablation catheter to the mitral annulus, the catheter tip must get across the mitral valve and go into the left atrium. Then pull the catheter slowly to where the tip of the ablation catheter locates the mitral annulus. To rotate the catheter counterclockwise with pulling back the catheter a little, the catheter goes posteriorly and to rotate the catheter clockwise with advancing the catheter, the catheter goes anteriorly.

Transseptal puncture can accompany some risk but physicians having many experience of atrial transseptal puncture would prefer the transseptal approach than the transaortic approach for the left free wall accessory pathway, in which the mapping catheter is easy to control. After transseptal puncture, to use a long sheath is mandatory to achieve an enough catheter contact. Using a steerable sheath makes the catheter manipulation easier especially for the larger left atrium. To change curve of the long sheath also might work according to the site of the accessory pathway.

26.3.2 Right Accessory Pathway

For the left accessory pathway, the CS can be an anatomical marker of the approximate position of the mitral annulus.

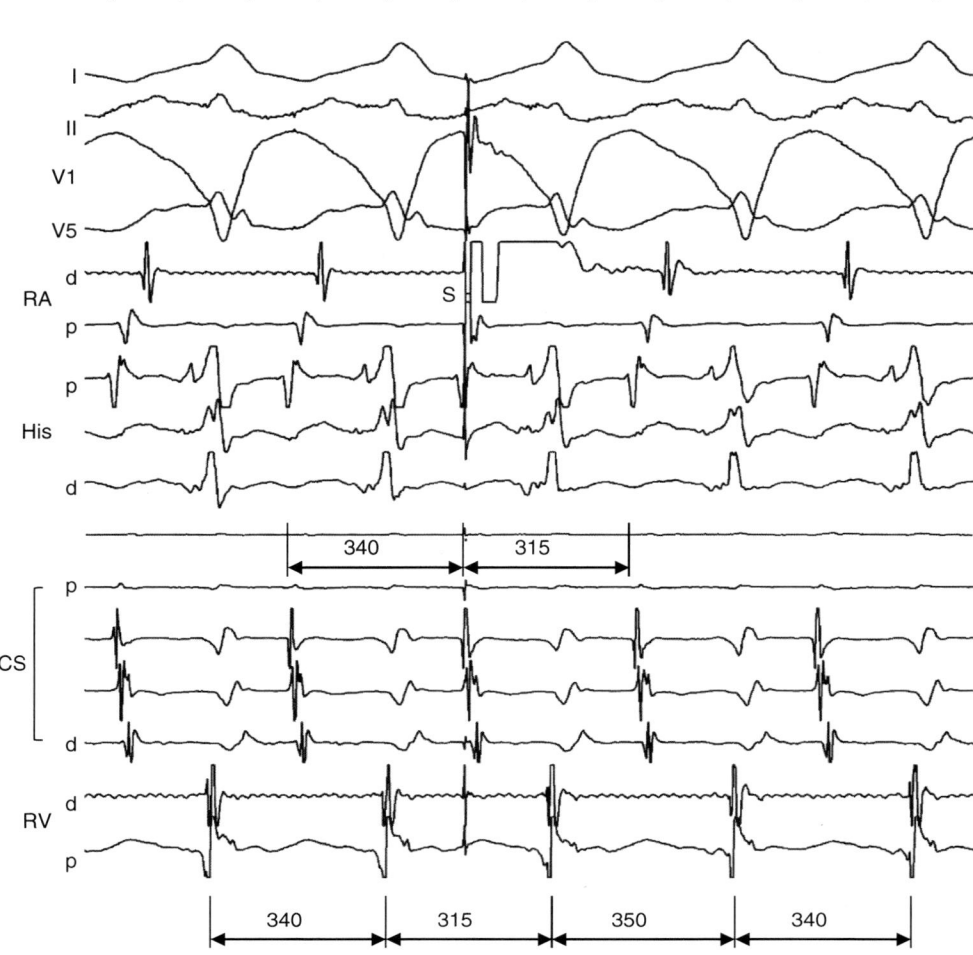

Fig. 26.4 Atrial extrastimulus during antidromic AVRT. During induced tachycardia in Fig. 26.4, an atrial extrastimulus was applied from the RA, which advanced the ventricular activation by 25 ms. Please note the timing of the atrial extrastimulus which applied just after the atrial activation of the His bundle area and also did not advance atrial activation of CS. These findings indicated the accessory pathway was located close to the RA and the ventricular activation was conducted via the right free wall accessory pathway during the tachycardia, which could deny the possibility of the ventricular tachycardia. And subsequently after the ventricular early capture, the atrial activation was also advanced from 340 to 315 ms. This finding indicated the atrial activation was conducted from the ventricle, which could exclude the diagnosis of atrial tachycardia

However, there is no anatomical marker for the tricuspid annulus where the accessory pathway can exist. The right atriography can reveal the anatomy of the right atrium and the ventricle, which can serve for the right free wall accessory pathway mapping. To use a steerable sheath is recommended for mapping the right free wall accessory pathway for good catheter contact, with which a better contact force can be obtained [9].

26.4 Mapping

26.4.1 Anatomical Consideration of Coronary Sinus

Accessory pathway is connecting the atrium and the ventricle and the target of the catheter ablation for the accessory pathway locates at the annulus of the AV valve. The left free wall accessory pathway accounts for 70% of the accessory pathways, and the rest is the right free wall accessory pathway and the septal accessory pathway.

The left free wall accessory pathway is located at the mitral annulus, where should be mapped. For mapping of the left free wall accessory pathway, a deca- or duodeca-polar electrodes catheter should be put into the CS, which tells us the activation sequence of the atrium during ventricular pacing and that of the ventricle during sinus rhythm or atrial pacing. The CS runs along the AV groove, however, which is shifted approximately 1 cm to atrial side from the true mitral annulus [10], so usually accessory pathway ablation site is a little bit ventricular side. The location of the CS can vary and if the CS runs close to the true mitral annulus, the mapping catheter can be very close to the CS catheter as a result. The important thing is to see the local electrocardiogram of the mapping catheter. The thickness of atrial myocardium is thinner than that of ventricular myocardium. The ratio of the amplitude of the atrial and the ventricular electrocardiogram to map the accessory pathway should be around 0.5–1. During mapping of the accessory pathway, if the amplitude of the atrial electrogram is higher than the ventricular electrocardiogram, the catheter is located at atrial side rather than the true mitral annulus.

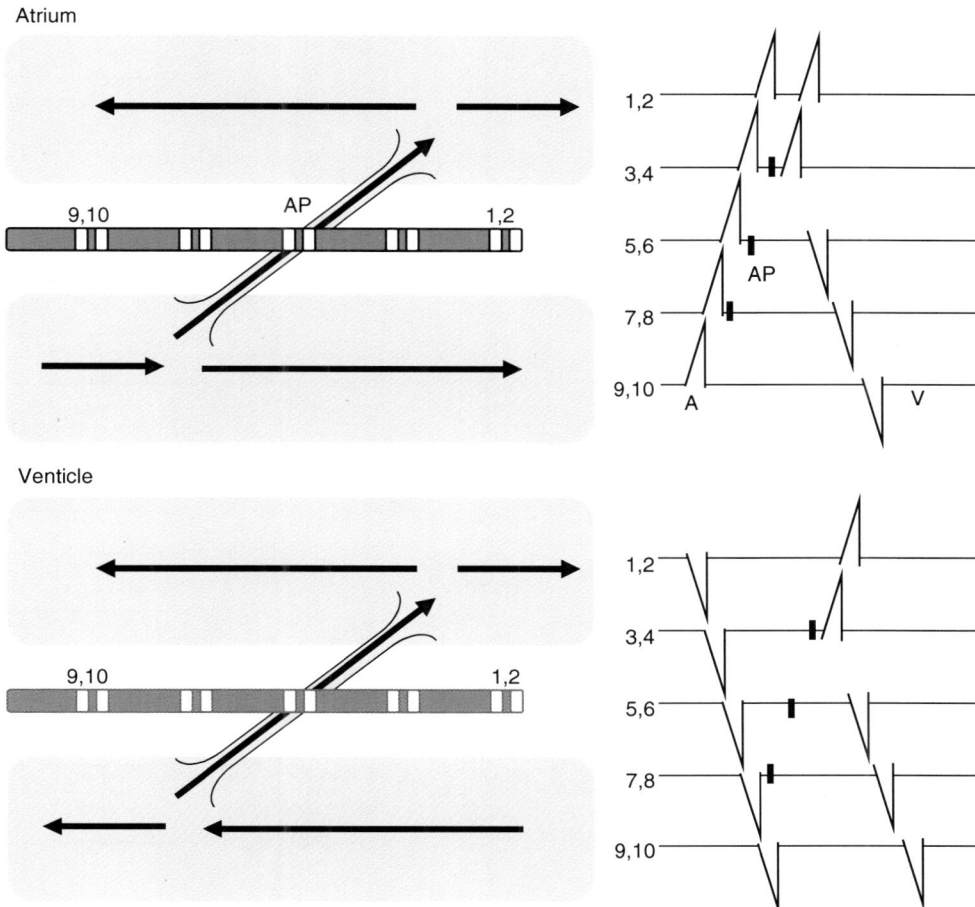

Fig. 26.5 Association of the direction of the oblique accessory pathway and the activation wave front. The *upper panel* illustrates activation sequence of the ventriculoatrial conduction during ventricular pacing via an oblique accessory pathway (AP). The ventricular activation wave front comes in the same direction with the AP, which does not lead to separate the atrial, AP, and the ventricular potentials. Please note the shortest AV interval is recorded both electrodes 1, 2 and 3, 4. In the lower panel, the ventricular activation wave front comes from opposite to the AP direction, which could separate the atrial, AP and the ventricular potentials. Most of the APs have such an oblique pathway. Pacing site should be determined to separate the potentials. In this figure, to apply ventricular pacing from the right side is preferable

26.4.2 Mapping During Sinus Rhythm, Pacing or Tachycardia?

For patients with manifest WPW syndrome who have delta wave on 12 lead ECG, mapping during sinus rhythm or atrial pacing is preferable since the timing of the earliest ventricular activation can be seen by the onset of delta wave. The recording speed of the EP lab system should be set at 200 mm/s or 400 mm/s and the intracardiac ECGs should be shown in sweep mode triggered on some atrial electrocardiogram. A vertical line should be put at the onset of the delta wave and the earliest ventricular activation site should be mapped by an ablation catheter and the accessory pathway potential should be soak and targeted as ablation therapy. To map the shortest AV interval recording site is misunderstanding. The shortest AV interval can be recorded at sites far from the accessory pathway opposite to the pacing site (Fig. 26.5).

For the concealed accessory pathway which exclusively has the retrograde conduction, mapping should be performed during the right ventricular pacing. The earliest atrial activation should be mapped and the accessory pathway potential should be explored. At the local intracardiac electrogram of the ablation catheter, sometimes to discriminate the atrial and ventricular electrograms is difficult. In such cases, to compare the electrograms of the ablation catheter during ventricular pacing and simultaneous ventricular and atrial pacing useful. The component of atrial electrogram is advanced during simultaneous ventricular and atrial pacing comparing during ventricular pacing.

If a patient has a fast retrograde conduction of the AV node, discrimination of retrograde conduction from the accessory pathway can be difficult especially when the accessory pathway is close to the AV node. To shorten the pacing cycle length for delaying the retrograde AV nodal conduction is the usual maneuver. But in case that method does not work, mapping should be done during the AVRT in which the retrograde conduction utilizes exclusively the accessory pathway.

26.4.3 Direction of the Pacing

The accessory pathway is a myocardial fiber connecting the atrial and ventricular myocardium, which is considered to take an oblique course at the AV annulus. In such case, the direction of the activation wavefront by the pacing stimulus

Fig. 26.6 Accessory pathway potential recorded at the successful ablation site. At the distal tip of the ablation catheter, an accessory pathway potential is recorded 15 ms prior to the onset of the delta wave. Accessory pathway potential is usually recorded as such a tiny and spiky potential. Unipolar electrogram of the distal tip shows QS pattern

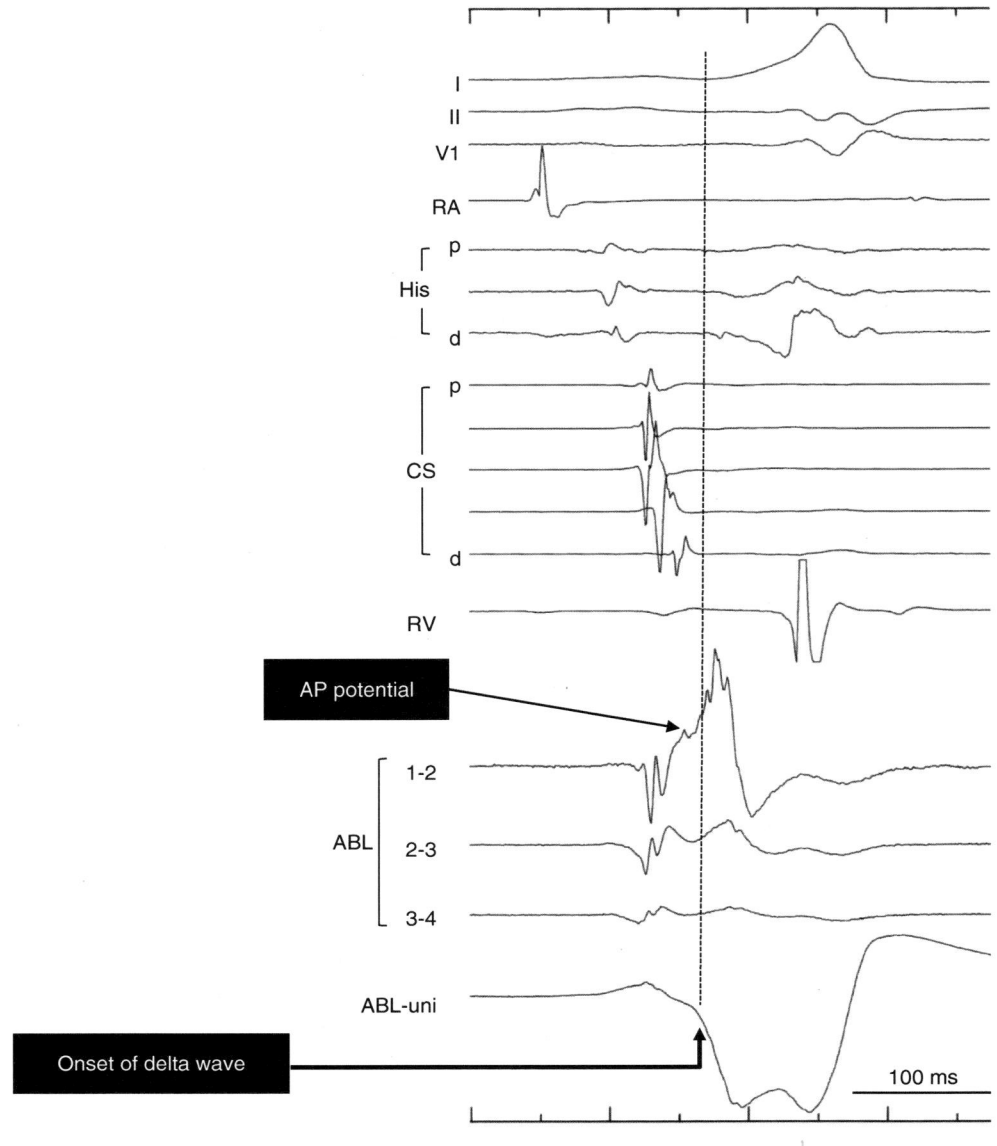

would affect the AV or ventriculoatrial conduction pattern, which can contribute to discriminate between atrial and ventricular electrograms (Fig. 26.5) [11]. In brief, considering the ventriculoatrial conduction, a ventricular activation wavefront propagated in the reverse direction to an accessory pathway can separate the ventricular and the atrial electrograms conducted through the accessory pathway. On the contrary, when the direction of the propagation of ventricular activation is same with that of the accessory pathway, the local ventriculoatrial interval will be shorter. During ventricular pacing, the earliest atrial activation or accessory pathway potential can more clearly be seen when the ventricular and atrial electrocardiograms are separated. If the accessory pathway is located at the lateral wall of the tricuspid annulus, to apply ventricular pacing from anterior or posterior to the accessory pathway site will serve to separate the ventricular and atrial potential. Of course, regarding the anterograde conduction, to apply atrial pacing from two different sites to the accessory pathway site can contribute to separate atrial and ventricular electrograms.

26.4.4 Accessory Pathway Potential

The accessory pathway potential can be seen between atrial and ventricular electrograms near the earliest ventricular activation recording site during sinus rhythm and between ventricular and atrial electrograms near the earliest atrial activation site during ventricular pacing (Fig. 26.6). The accessory pathway potential is usually a very tiny but spiky potential and can be seen as a part of atrial or ventricular electrogram. To prove a potential as an accessory pathway potential is usually difficult. In a case of concealed accessory pathway, if simultaneous pacing from both the atrium and the ventricle advanced the timing of a potential compared to that during ventricular pacing, we can conclude that potential is not a part of ventricular electrogram. It is important that such potential should be recorded largest at the distal bipoles. The ablation catheter has 4 electrodes and so three pairs of electrograms should always be shown, 1–2, 2–3, and 3–4 from distal to proximal. When we see an accessory pathway potential at the distal bipoles of 1–2, if we do not have the electrograms of 2–3 bipoles but just have 1–2 and 3–4, we cannot figure out whether the accessory pathway potential originates from the electrode 1 or 2. The distal tip of the ablation catheter, the electrode 1, should contact or be closest to the accessory pathway, so ideally, the accessory pathway potential should be recorded only at the 1–2 bipoles. Alternatively, unipolar recordings of the electrode 1 and 2 can show the origin of the accessory pathway potential if the noiseless and high quality unipolar signals can be recorded. But usually accessory pathway potential is too small to see in the unipolar electrogram and the QS pattern of the unipolar ventricular activation suffices.

26.4.5 Radiofrequency Application

Non irrigated tip ablation catheter is usually selected for the accessory pathway ablation. The duration of radiofrequency energy delivery is 30–60 s and the output of the radiofrequency energy and the maximum temperature is set at around 30 W and 50 °C. The conduction block of accessory pathway is usually obtained in a few seconds after radiofrequency energy delivery. So if conduction block is not obtained in 10 s, the radiofrequency energy application is usually terminated and the optimal position should be mapped again.

After radiofrequency application, adenosine or adenosine triphosphate can be administered for the induction of the dormant conduction of the accessory pathway. Spotnitz et al. reported dormant accessory pathway conduction was revealed by adenosine administration after ablation in 13 out of 109 accessory pathway patients [12]. Usually 30 min waiting time is considered to be enough to check the recurrence of the accessory pathway conduction.

If the patient has a retrograde conduction after ablation, paraHisian pacing should be applied to exclude an accessory pathway conduction. And also programmed electrical stimulation should be applied after catheter ablation since patients still might have a slow accessory pathway which is hidden by the retrograde conduction via the AV node. Rarely, an accessory pathway can have a supernormal conduction property, in which the accessory pathway conduction does not occur during the sinus rhythm or a longer pacing cycle length but occurs during a shorter cycle length [13]. In such instance, we can never see the accessory pathway conduction unless applying the rapid pacing.

For the patient with Ebstein anomaly, we should be more careful. Ebstein anomaly can be diagnosed by the echocardiography, who could have multiple accessory pathways especially in the right heart [14]. Patients having a venous anomaly such as persistent left superior vena cava, coronary sinus diverticulum, or coronary sinus atresia also might be associated with an accessory pathway [15, 16].

References

1. Montoya PT, Brugada P, Smeets J, Talajic M, Della Bella P, Lezaun R, et al. Ventricular fibrillation in the Wolff-Parkinson-White syndrome. Eur Heart J. 1991;12(2):144–50.
2. Jackman WM, Wang XZ, Friday KJ, Roman CA, Moulton KP, Beckman KJ, et al. Catheter ablation of accessory atrioventricular pathways (Wolff-Parkinson-White syndrome) by radiofrequency current. N Engl J Med. 1991;324(23):1605–11. https://doi.org/10.1056/NEJM199106063242301.
3. Chen SA, Tsang WP, Hsia CP, Wang DC, Chiang CE, Yeh HI, et al. Catheter ablation of free wall accessory atrioventricular pathways in 89 patients with Wolff-Parkinson-White syndrome—comparison of direct current and radiofrequency ablation. Eur Heart J. 1992;13(10):1329–38.
4. Otomo K, Nagata Y, Uno K, Fujiwara H, Iesaka Y. Atypical atrioventricular nodal reentrant tachycardia with eccentric coronary sinus activation: electrophysiological characteristics and essential effects of left-sided ablation inside the coronary sinus. Heart Rhythm. 2007;4(4):421–32. https://doi.org/10.1016/j.hrthm.2006.12.035.
5. Hirao K, Otomo K, Wang X, Beckman KJ, McClelland JH, Widman L, et al. Para-Hisian pacing. A new method for differentiating retrograde conduction over an accessory AV pathway from conduction over the AV node. Circulation. 1996;94(5):1027–35.
6. Takatsuki S, Mitamura H, Tanimoto K, Fukuda Y, Ieda M, Miyoshi S, et al. Clinical implications of "pure" Hisian pacing in addition to para-Hisian pacing for the diagnosis of supraventricular tachycardia. Heart Rhythm. 2006;3(12):1412–8. https://doi.org/10.1016/j.hrthm.2006.08.028.
7. Arruda MS, McClelland JH, Wang X, Beckman KJ, Widman LE, Gonzalez MD, et al. Development and validation of an ECG algorithm for identifying accessory pathway ablation site in Wolff-Parkinson-White syndrome. J Cardiovasc Electrophysiol. 1998;9(1):2–12.
8. Coumel P, Attuel P. Reciprocating tachycardia in overt and latent preexcitation. Influence of functional bundle branch block on the rate of the tachycardia. Eur J Cardiol. 1974;1(4):423–36.
9. Kimura T, Takatsuki S, Oishi A, Negishi M, Kashimura S, Katsumata Y, et al. Operator-blinded contact force monitoring during pulmonary vein isolation using conventional and steerable sheaths. Int J Cardiol. 2014;177(3):970–6. https://doi.org/10.1016/j.ijcard.2014.09.189.
10. Takatsuki S, Yamada M, Fukumoto K, Tanimoto K, Jinzaki M, Kuribayashi S, et al. Extracardiac structures are frequently present within close proximity to the left atrium: Relevance to catheter ablation. Heart Rhythm. 2009;6(11):1559–64. https://doi.org/10.1016/j.hrthm.2009.07.049.
11. Otomo K, Gonzalez MD, Beckman KJ, Nakagawa H, Becker AE, Shah N, et al. Reversing the direction of paced ventricular and atrial wavefronts reveals an oblique course in accessory AV pathways and improves localization for catheter ablation. Circulation. 2001;104(5):550–6.

12. Spotnitz MD, Markowitz SM, Liu CF, Thomas G, Ip JE, Liez J, et al. Mechanisms and clinical significance of adenosine-induced dormant accessory pathway conduction after catheter ablation. Circ Arrhythm Electrophysiol. 2014;7(6):1136–43. https://doi.org/10.1161/CIRCEP.114.002140.
13. Przybylski J, Chiale PA, Sanchez RA, Pastori JD, Francos HG, Elizari MV, et al. Supernormal conduction in the accessory pathway of patients with overt or concealed ventricular pre-excitation. J Am Coll Cardiol. 1987;9(6):1269–78.
14. Iturralde P, Nava S, Salica G, Medeiros A, Marquez MF, Colin L, et al. Electrocardiographic characteristics of patients with Ebstein's anomaly before and after ablation of an accessory atrioventricular pathway. J Cardiovasc Electrophysiol. 2006;17(12):1332–6. https://doi.org/10.1111/j.1540-8167.2006.00617.x.
15. Lesh MD, Van Hare G, Kao AK, Scheinman MM. Radiofrequency catheter ablation for Wolff-Parkinson-White syndrome associated with a coronary sinus diverticulum. Pacing Clin Electrophysiol. 1991;14(10):1479–84.
16. Takatsuki S, Mitamura H, Ieda M, Ogawa S. Accessory pathway associated with an anomalous coronary vein in a patient with Wolff-Parkinson-White syndrome. J Cardiovasc Electrophysiol. 2001;12(9):1080–2.

Posteroseptal Atrioventricular Accessory Pathways

27

Junichi Nitta

Keywords
Posteroseptal accessory pathway • Coronary sinus • Middle cardiac vein

27.1 Characteristics of Posteroseptal Accessory Pathways

27.1.1 Prevalence

Approximately 20% of accessory atrioventricular connections are posteroseptal in location [1–3]. Wen et al. reported that out of the 652 patients with Wolff–Parkinson–White (WPW) syndrome who underwent radiofrequency ablation in their laboratory, 139 patients (21%) were found to have a total of 146 posteroseptal APs [2]. Of these, 94 instances were successfully ablated in the left posteroseptal region and 45 in the right posteroseptal region. In three instances, successful ablation of the APs required delivery of current to the proximal coronary sinus, and in one instance, to the atrial and ventricular aspects of the tricuspid valve in the right posteroseptum. Thus, APs were successfully ablated in 143 (98%) of 146 instances, or in 136 (98%) patients. In three patients, however, ablation was unsuccessful despite delivery of current to the left posteroseptum, the right posteroseptum, the proximal coronary sinus, and the middle cardiac vein.

27.1.2 12-Lead Electrocardiogram

Predicting the location of APs in WPW syndrome is important for the proper planning of ablation and to minimize catheter-related injuries. Several algorithms, each with varying degrees of complexity and accuracy, have attempted to localize APs based on the morphologies of QRS and delta waves on a 12-lead electrocardiogram (ECG) [4–10]. Maden et al. compared the accuracy of three such algorithms in predicting the location of APs among adult patients with Wolff–Parkinson–White syndrome [11]. They found that the algorithm designed by Arruda et al. [5] demonstrated better predictability than the other two and using it while planning an ablation may be advantageous. This algorithm, shown in Fig. 27.1, is particularly useful in accurately localizing anteroseptal (sensitivity 75%, specificity 99%) and mid-septal (sensitivity 100%, specificity 98%) APs, as well as pathways that require ablation from within the ventricular venous branches or anomalies of the coronary sinus (sensitivity 100%, specificity 100%). In the algorithm, posteroseptal region is divided into the following three subregions: (1) posteroseptal tricuspid annulus (PSTA), including APs located near the coronary sinus ostium (CSO), (2) posteroseptal mitral annulus (PSMA), and (3) subepicardial posteroseptal APs, that require ablation from within the subepicardial venous system (occasionally at the left posterior region), including the middle cardiac vein and other coronary veins; or in anomalies of the coronary sinus, such as a diverticulum (subepicardial). The algorithm begins with identification of a septal or right free-wall accessory AV pathway if either the delta wave in lead I is not negative or isoelectric, or the amplitude of R wave is greater than that of S wave in lead V1 (Step 1). Once this is done, a negative delta wave in lead II helps in identifying subepicardial posteroseptal AP (Step 2). However, if the delta wave in lead II is isoelectric or positive, a negative or isoelectric delta wave in lead V1 indicates a septal AP. After the septal AP has been identified, a negative delta wave in lead aVF indicates that the AP is in the posteroseptal tricuspid annulus or at the coronary sinus ostium and surrounding region (PSTA/CSO);

J. Nitta, M.D., Ph.D.
Department of Cardiology, Japanese Red Cross Saitama Hospital, 1-5 Shintoshin, Chuo-ku, Saitama 338-8553, Japan
e-mail: jnitta-ind@umin.net

Fig. 27.1 ECG algorithm for determining the location of accessory pathway. *RA* right anterior, *RAL* right anterolateral, *RL* right lateral, *RPL* right posterolateral, *RP* right posterior, *PSTA* posteroseptal tricuspid annulus, *CSO* coronary sinus ostium, *MSTA* mid-septal tricuspid annulus, *AS* anteroseptal, *RAPS* right anterior paraseptal, *MCV* middle cardiac vein (coronary vein), *CS* coronary sinus, venous anomaly (coronary sinus diverticulum), *PSMA* posteroseptal mitral annulus, *LP* left posterior, *LPL* left posterolateral, *LL* left lateral, *LAL* left anterolateral, *HB* His bundle [5]

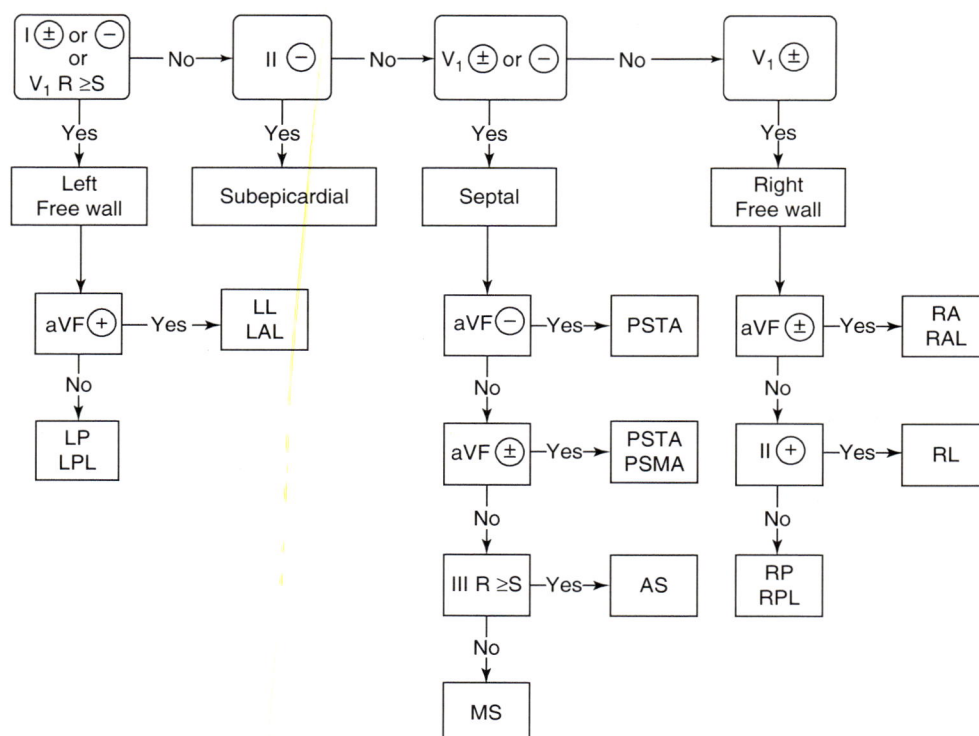

if it is isoelectric, then the AP may be located close to the posteroseptal tricuspid annulus (PSTA) or the posteroseptal mitral annulus (PSMA). Takahashi et al. also reported that posteroseptal APs ablated within the coronary venous system have highly specific features such as the combination of a steep positive delta wave in lead aVR and a deep S wave in lead V6 (R wave < S wave) during maximal preexcitation. The highest sensitivity, however, is with the identifying of a negative delta wave in lead II [12].

27.2 Identification of the Pathways by Electrophysiological Study

Mapping of manifest posteroseptal APs usually identifies the site of the earliest ventricular activation to be around the coronary sinus ostium. Haissaguerre et al. reported that the so-called "PQS pattern" obtained by unipolar recording at the ablation site is an independent predictor of successful RF ablation and it can help to determine the appropriate ablation site of accessory pathways with manifest antegrade conduction [13]. This unipolar pattern is characterized by upward P waves followed immediately by downward QS complexes without an intervening isoelectric interval (Figs. 27.2c, 27.3c, and 27.4c). Jackmann et al. demonstrated that catheter delivery of radiofrequency current guided by direct recordings of accessory pathway activation is highly effective in ablating APs [1, 14].

Mapping of retrograde atrial activation, best performed during orthodromic reciprocating tachycardia to avoid the confounding effects of retrograde atrioventricular (AV) nodal conduction, demonstrates earliest atrial activation in the same areas. In ventricular pacing, pacing cycle length and pacing site are very important for the differentiation of retrograde AV nodal conduction and retrograde AP conduction. If the pacing cycle length is shorter, then the retrograde atrial activation by AP is clearer because of the decremental property of AV node. Right ventricular outflow tract pacing is preferred to right ventricular apex pacing because the apex is closer to the peripheral inputs of the His-Purkinje system [15].

In order to precisely differentiate from AV nodal reentrant tachycardia, the presence or absence of retrograde AP conduction can be determined by delivering a late ventricular extrastimulus during supraventricular tachycardia to initiate atrial activation while the His bundle is refractory [16–23], or by an early ventricular extrastimulus during programmed ventricular stimulation to determine the presence or absence of significant delay in the timing of retrograde atrial activation while the His bundle activation is delayed. Sometimes, it may be difficult to differentiate retrograde AP conduction from retrograde AV nodal conduction when sustained supraventricular tachycardia cannot be induced, especially when retrograde conduction is present only at long pacing cycle lengths. One solution is to move the right ventricular pacing catheter from the apex towards the site of the earliest retrograde atrial activation [15, 24, 25]. Hirao et al. provided another solution—Para-Hisian Pacing, in which right ventricular pacing is performed close to the His bundle or proximal right bundle branch [26].

In some patients with a posteroseptal AP, extensive endocardial mapping of antegrade and retrograde activation, with right as well as left sided approaches, fails to reveal a specific site that activates earlier than its neighboring sites. This may indicate that the AP is epicardial, such as within the coronary sinus, middle cardiac vein, its branches, or diverticulum [27–29].

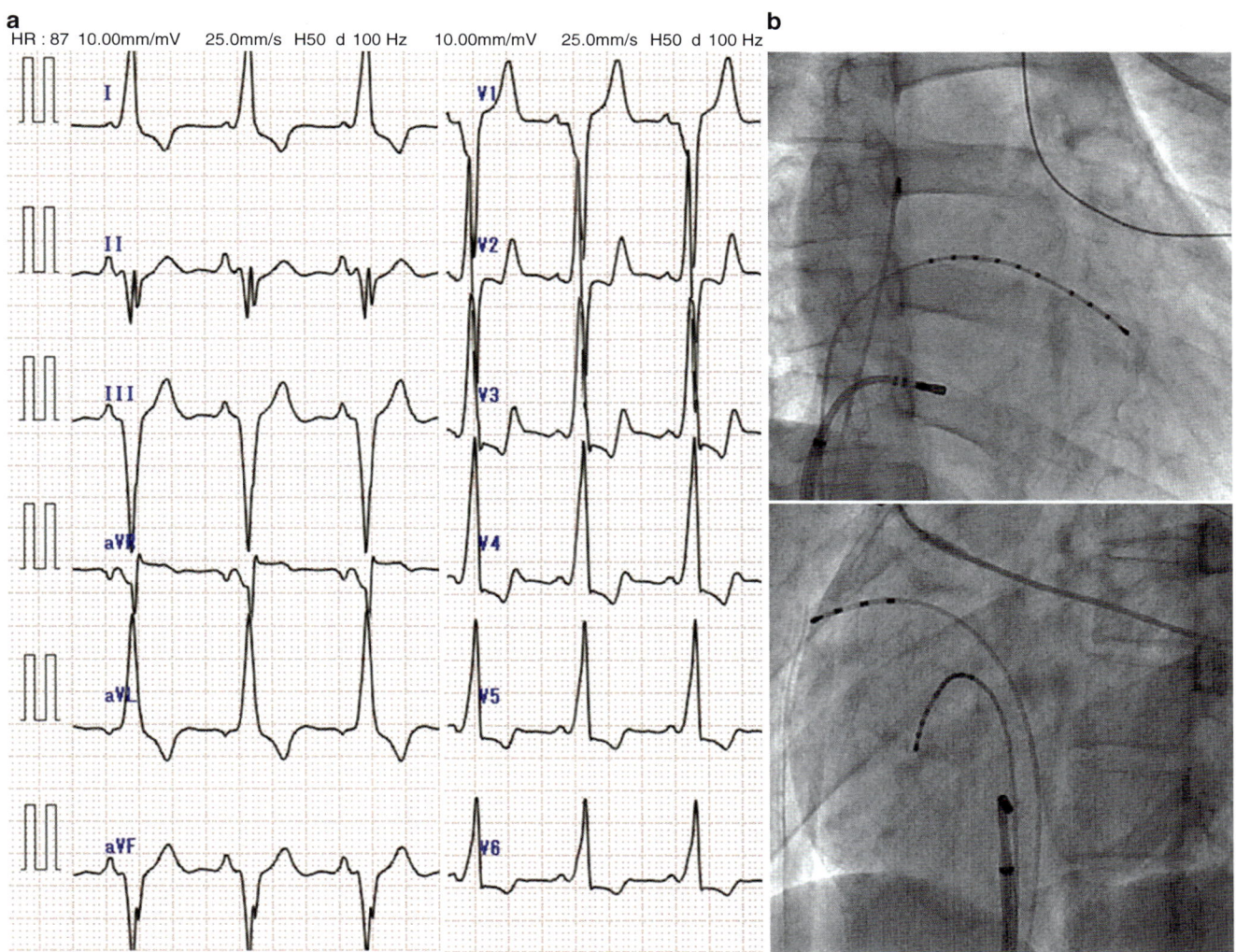

Fig. 27.2 A case of right posteroseptal pathway. (**a**) 12-Lead electrocardiogram in a patient with right posteroseptal AP. (**b**) Catheter position at the successful ablation site. (**c**) Intracardiac electrocardiogram at the successful ablation site. (**d**) Intracardiac electrocardiogram during RF delivery at the successful ablation site

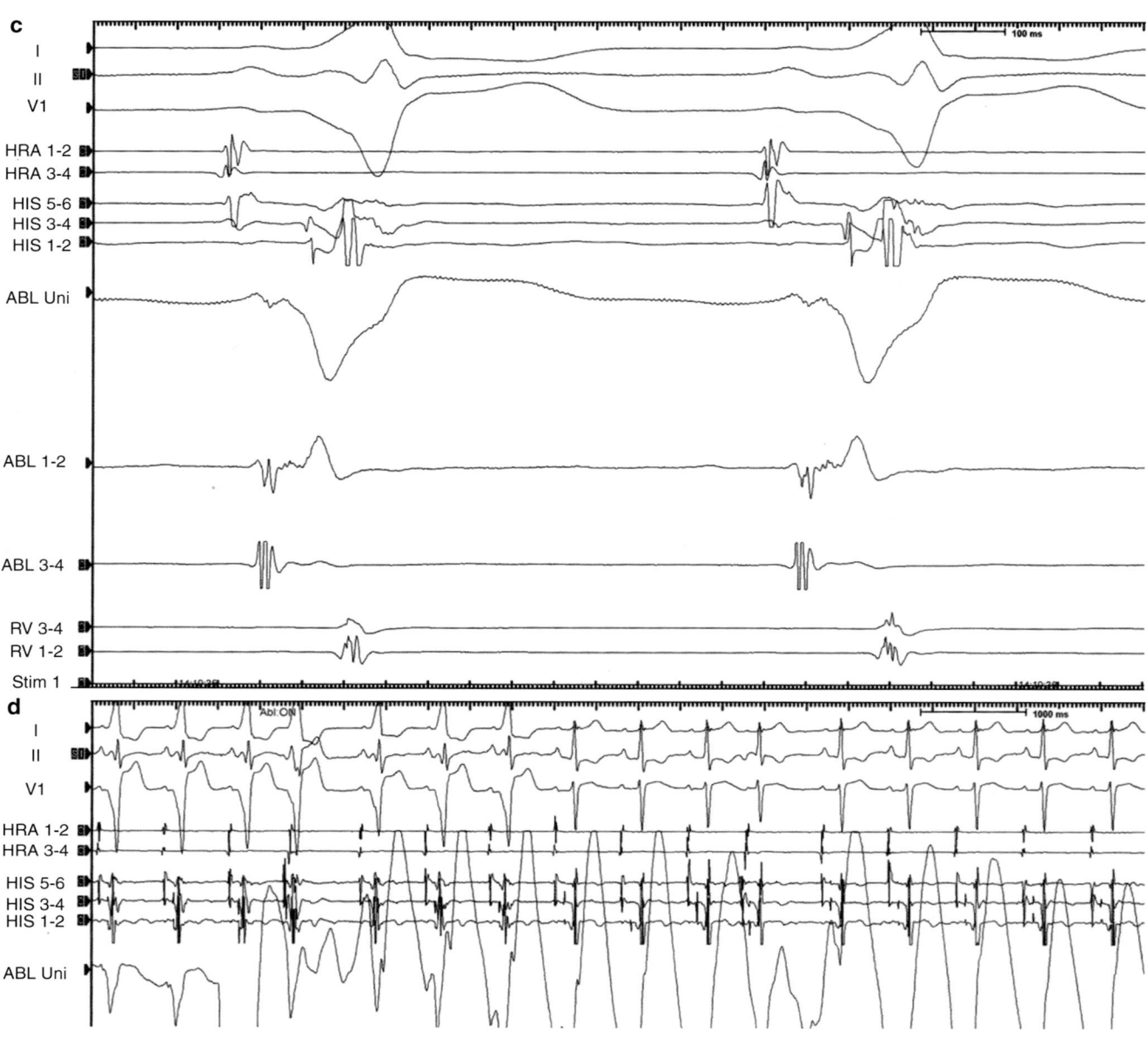

Fig. 27.2 (continued)

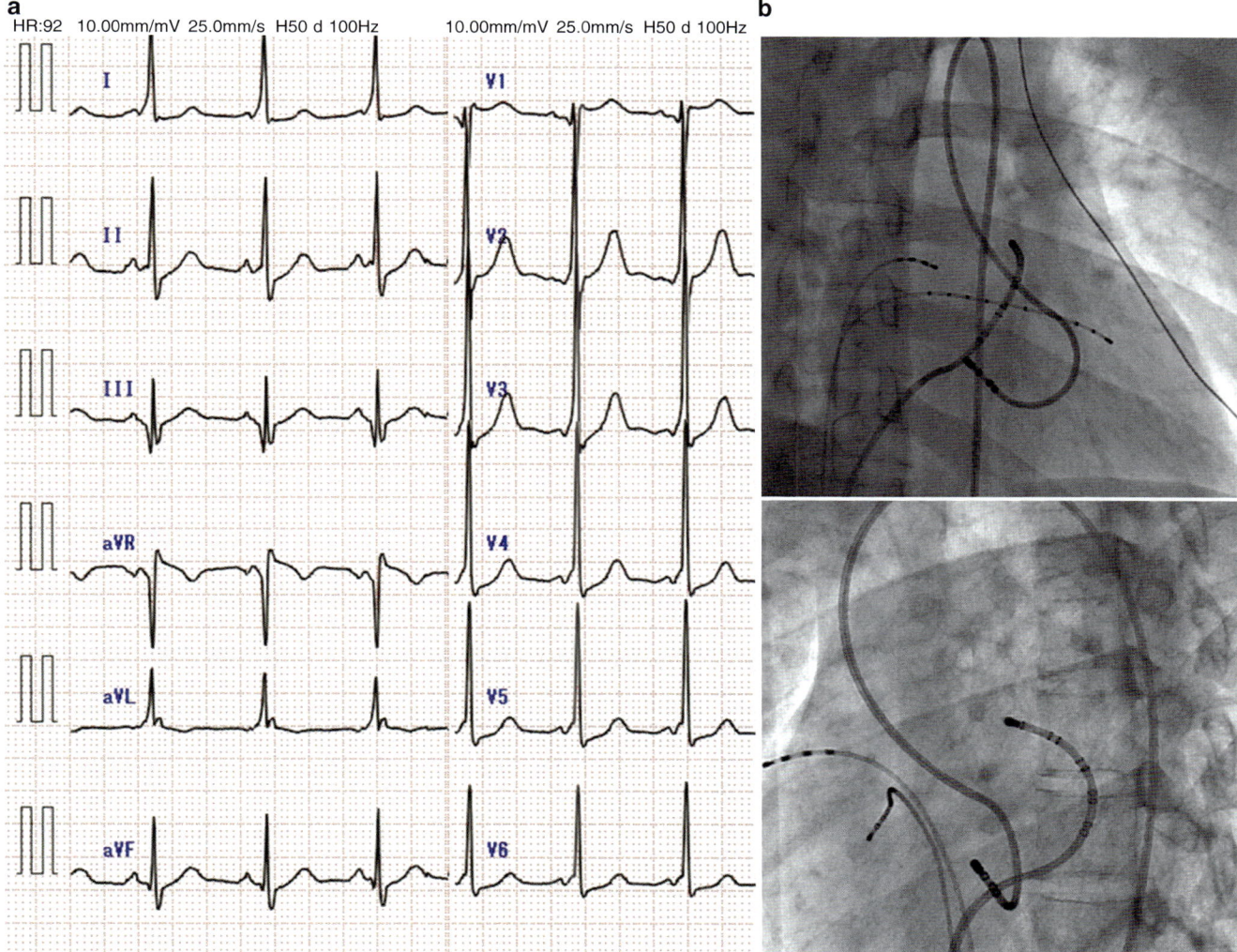

Fig. 27.3 A case of left posteroseptal pathway. (**a**) 12-Lead electrocardiogram in a patient with left posteroseptal AP. (**b**) Catheter position at the successful ablation site. (**c**) Intracardiac electrocardiogram at the successful ablation site. (**d**) Intracardiac electrocardiogram during RF delivery at the successful ablation site

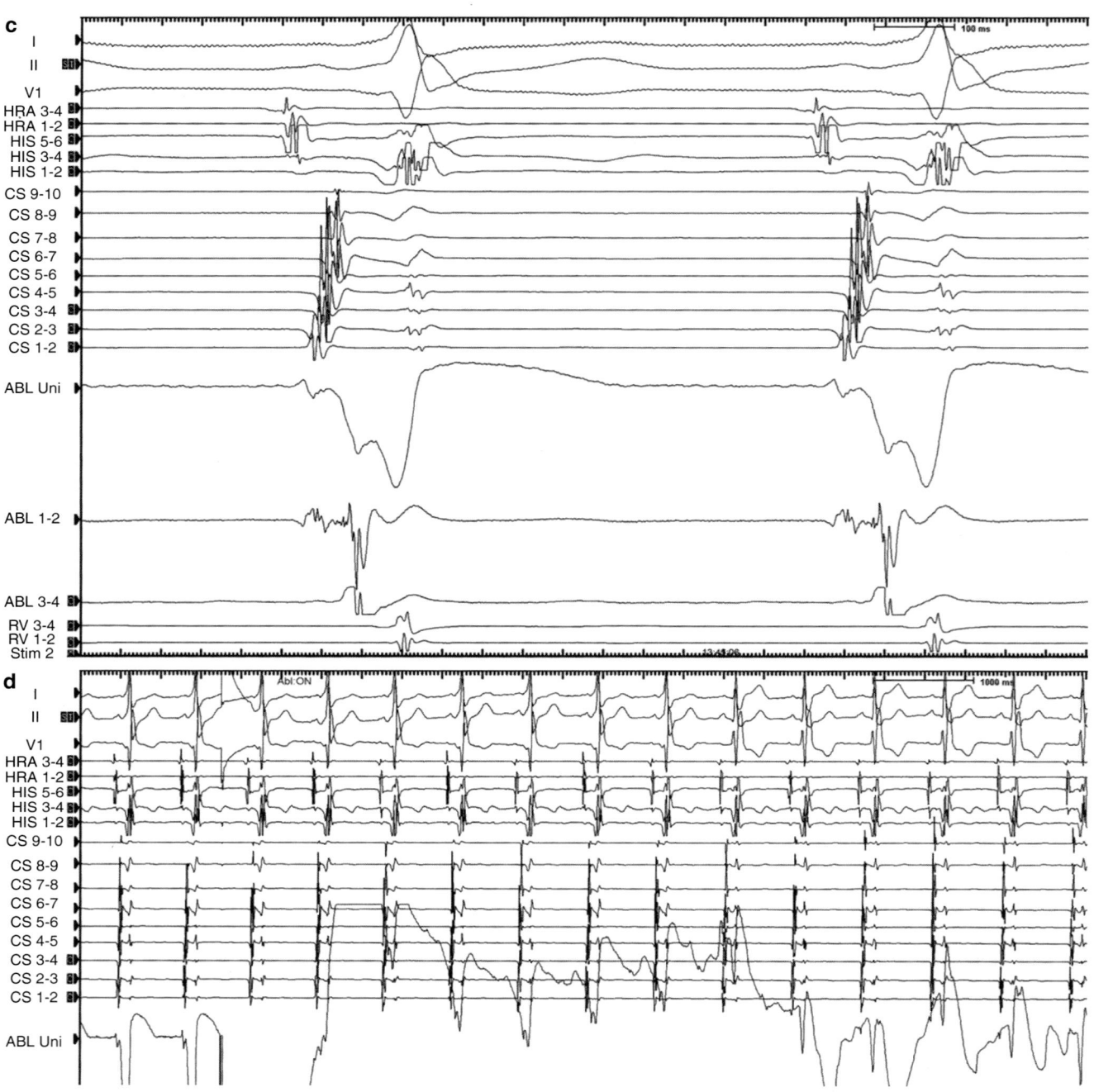

Fig. 27.3 (continued)

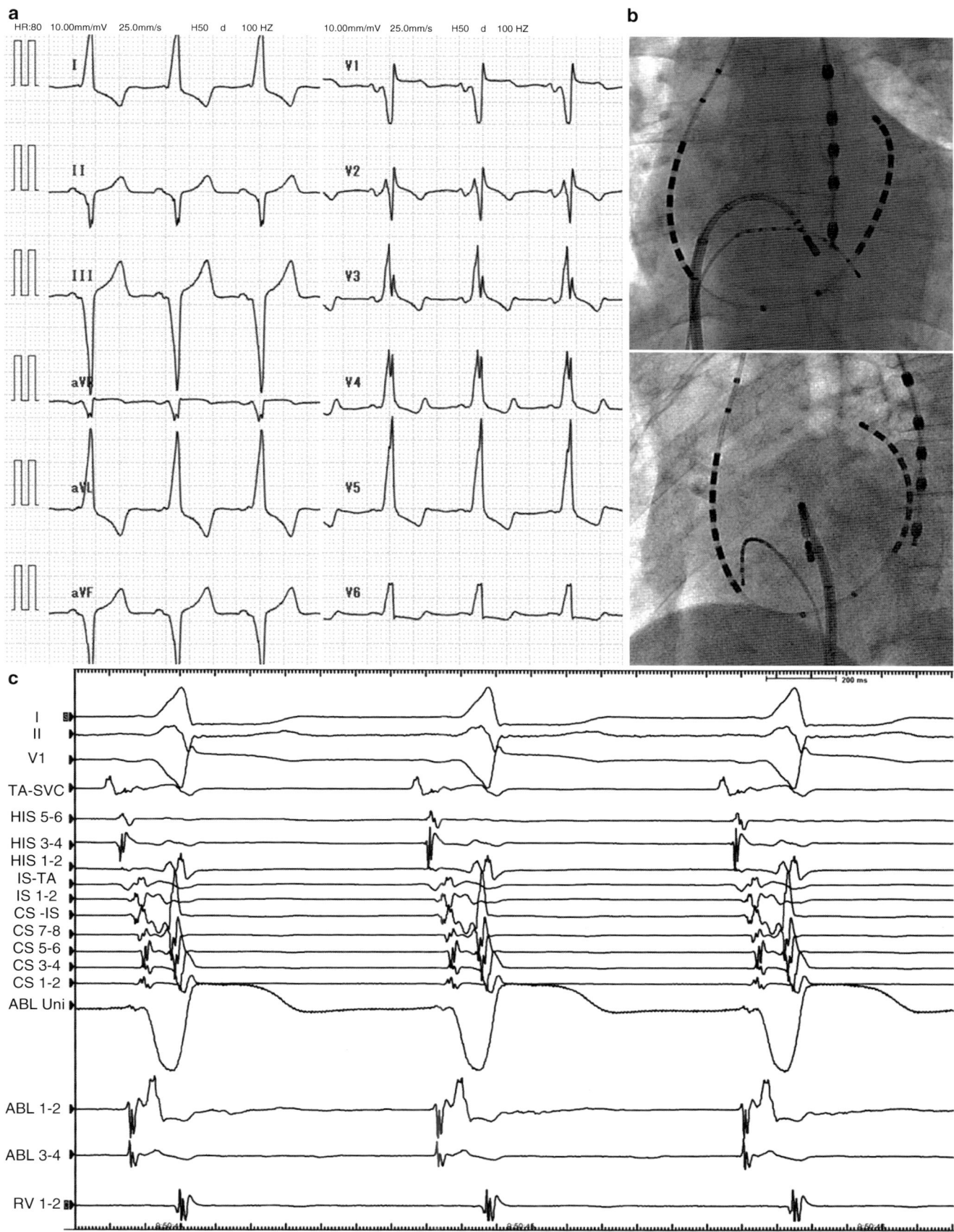

Fig. 27.4 Another case of left posteroseptal pathway. (**a**) 12-Lead electrocardiogram in another patient with left posteroseptal AP. (**b**) Catheter position at the successful ablation site. (**c**) Intracardiac electrocardiogram at the successful ablation site. (**d**) Intracardiac electrocardiogram during RF delivery at the successful ablation site

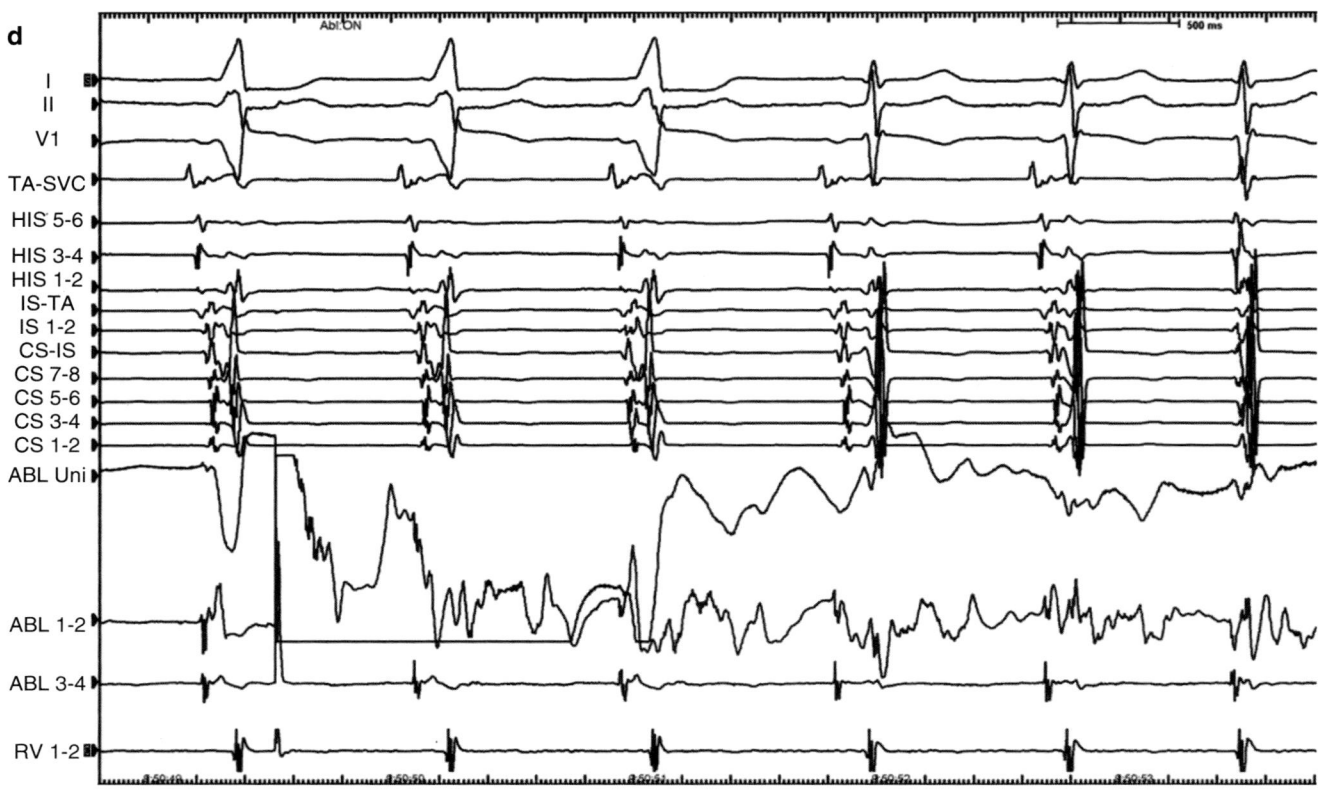

Fig. 27.4 (continued)

27.3 Case Presentation of Ablation of Posteroseptal Accessory Pathways

27.3.1 Endocardial Ablation

27.3.1.1 Right-Sided Pathway

Figure 27.2a shows 12-lead ECG of a patient with right posteroseptal pathway. The successful ablation site and the endocardial intracardiac ECG at the site are shown in Fig. 27.2b, c. The ablation catheter was positioned on the tricuspid valve and the unipolar recording by ablation catheter shows the "PQS pattern," while bipolar recording demonstrates direct recording of accessory pathway activation. The AP conduction ceased 3.2 s after the initiation of radiofrequency current (Fig. 27.2d).

27.3.1.2 Left-Sided Pathway

Figure 27.3a shows 12-lead ECG of a patient with left posteroseptal pathway. The successful ablation site and the endocardial intracardiac electrogram at the site are shown in Fig. 27.3b, c. The ablation catheter was introduced into the left ventricle by trans-aortic approach and positioned below the mitral valve. In this case, we were able to confirm the PQS pattern, but without a direct recording of AP activation. The AP conduction ceased 4.9 s after the initiation of radiofrequency current (Fig. 27.3d).

Figure 27.4 demonstrates the 12-lead ECG of a patient with episodes of pseudo-ventricular tachycardia with paroxysmal atrial fibrillation. Pre-procedural electrocardiogram showed negative delta waves in lead II, but not in the catheter laboratory because of a slight change of limb lead position. Initially, we sought the earliest ventricular activation site around the ostium of coronary sinus and middle cardiac vein but later we found that the earliest site was the endocardial left posteroseptal region (Fig. 27.4b, c). AP was ablated by the trans-septal approach before pulmonary vein isolation (Fig. 27.4d).

27.3.2 Epicardial Ablation

Figure 27.5a shows the 12-lead ECG of a patient with AP located in the ostium of the middle cardiac vein with a diverticulum (Fig. 27.5b). It was the earliest ventricular activation site, although AP activation was not directly recorded (Fig. 27.5c). In this case, AP conduction ceased 4.2 s after the initiation of radiofrequency current (Fig. 27.5d).

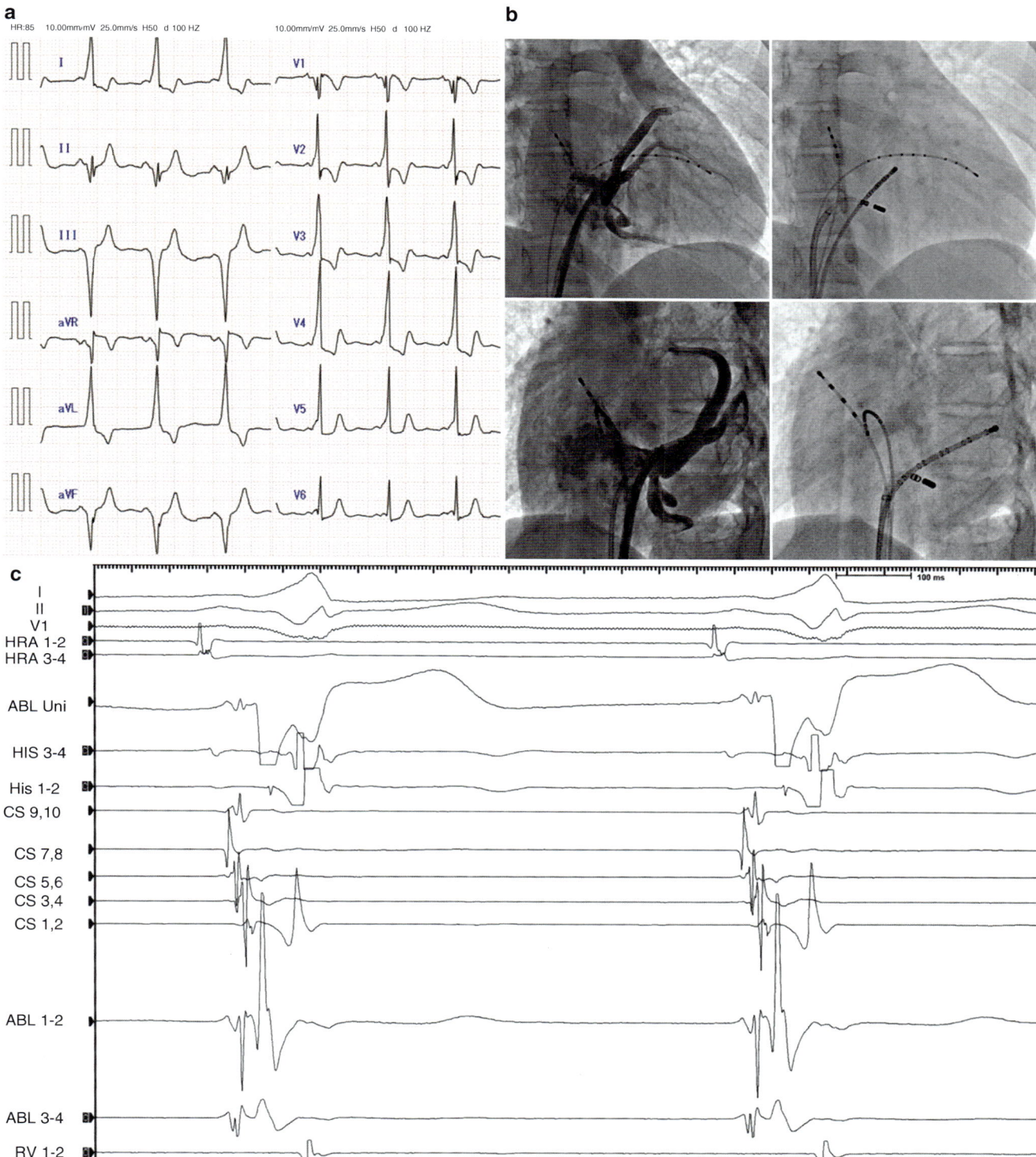

Fig. 27.5 A case of epicardial posteroseptal pathway. (**a**) 12-Lead electrocardiogram in a patient with epicardial posteroseptal AP. (**b**) Coronary sinus venography and catheter position at the successful ablation site. (**c**) Intracardiac electrocardiogram at the successful ablation site. (**d**) Intracardiac electrocardiogram during the RF delivery at the successful ablation site

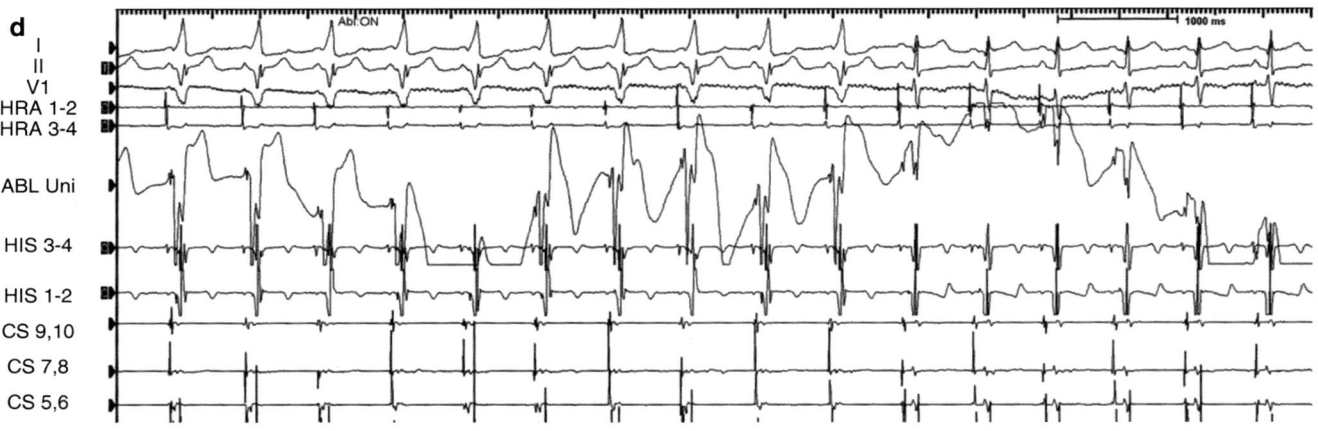

Fig. 27.5 (continued)

27.3.3 Drawbacks of Evaluating Retrograde Ventriculoatrial (VA) Conduction Through the AP

The location of AP is identified only by the evaluation of VA conduction in a patient with concealed WPW syndrome. Figure 27.6, demonstrating intracardiac electrocardiogram in a case of concealed WPW syndrome, reveals that it is difficult to differentiate between retrograde AP conduction and retrograde AV nodal conduction at the ventricular pacing cycle length of 600 ms (Fig. 27.6a) because of their fusion; however, it becomes easier at 300 ms (Fig. 27.6b). The earliest site of atrial activation, in this case, was in a superficial part of the middle coronary sinus (CS 6–7). We initially attempted to ablate this area. The ablation catheter was introduced into the left ventricle by the trans-aortic approach and positioned below the mitral valve in this area. However, the AP was not ablated. Finally, the AP was ablated at the posteroseptal region (Fig. 27.6c, d). CS 9–10 was not reflecting the endocardial activation of posteroseptal region. The atrial activation recorded by the ablation catheter was earlier at the posteroseptal site than the atrial activation recorded by any coronary sinus electrodes (Fig. 27.6c) because proximal coronary sinus (CS9–10) reflects activation of epicardial or CS musculature, but not endocardial activation.

27.4 Complication of Posteroseptal Accessory Pathway Ablation

Distinctive complications associated with posteroseptal AP ablation have been reported. These include high-degree AV block [1, 30, 31], cardiac tamponade [1], coronary sinus stenosis [32], coronary artery spasm [33], and coronary artery injury [34]. Therefore, care must be taken to avoid high-degree AV block if the patient has a baseline abnormality in AV nodal conduction. Other complications were associated with ablation of posteroseptal APs from within the coronary sinus, or one of its branches, including the middle cardiac vein. The risk of these complications can be minimized by avoiding high-energy delivery to high-impedance regions such as small branches of the coronary sinus.

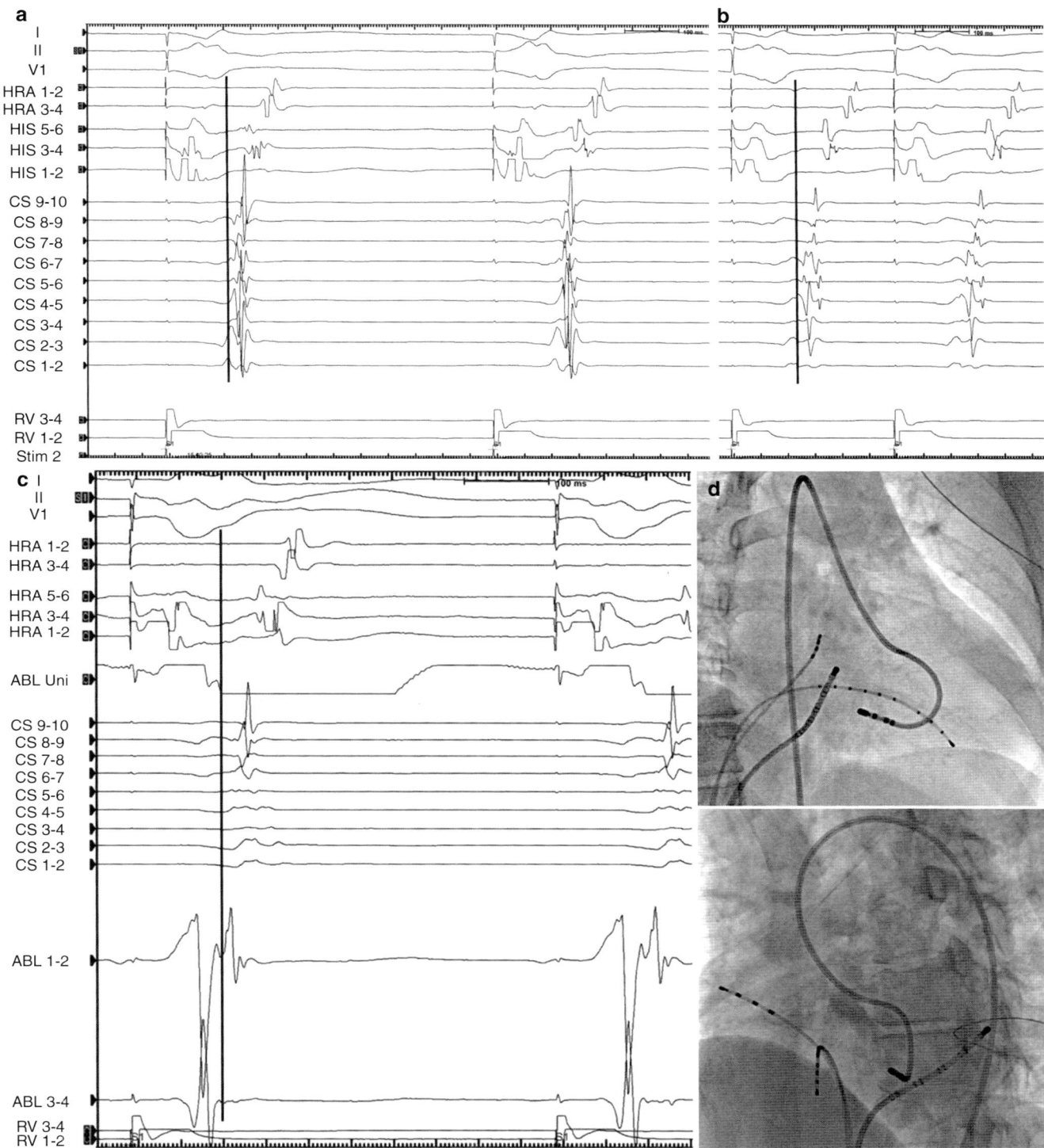

Fig. 27.6 Drawback of evaluating retrograde VA conduction. (**a**) Intracardiac electrocardiogram during ventricular pacing at cycle length of 600 ms in a case of concealed WPW syndrome. (**b**) Intracardiac electrocardiogram during ventricular pacing at cycle length of 300 ms. (**c**) Intracardiac electrocardiogram at the successful ablation site. (**d**) Catheter position at the successful ablation site. Position at the successful ablation site

References

1. Jackman WM, Wang XZ, Friday KJ, et al. Catheter ablation of accessory atrioventricular pathways (Wolff-Parkinson-White syndrome) by radiofrequency current. N Engl J Med. 1991;324:1605–11.
2. Wen MS, Yeh SJ, Wang CC, et al. Radiofrequency ablation therapy of the posteroseptal accessory pathway. Am Heart J. 1996;132:612–20.
3. Calkins H, Yong P, Miller JM, et al. Catheter ablation of accessory pathways, atrioventricular nodal reentrant tachycardia, and the atrioventricular junction. Circulation. 1999;99:262–70.
4. Chiang CE, Chen SA, Teo WS, et al. An accurate stepwise electrocardiographic algorithm for localization of accessory pathways in patients with Wolff-Parkinson-White syndrome from a comprehensive analysis of delta waves and R/S ratio during sinus rhythm. Am J Cardiol. 1995;76:40–6.
5. Arruda MS, McClelland JH, Wang X, et al. Development and validation of an ECG algorithm for identifying accessory pathway ablation site in Wolff-Parkinson-White syndrome. J Cardiovasc Electrophysiol. 1998;9:2–12.
6. d'Avila A, Brugada J, Skeberis V, et al. A fast and reliable algorithm to localize accessory pathways based on the polarity of the QRS complex on the surface ECG during sinus rhythm. Pacing Clin Electrophysiol. 1995;18:1615–27.
7. Boersma L, García-Moran E, Mont L, Brugada J. Accessory pathway localization by QRS polarity in children with Wolff-Parkinson-White syndrome. J Cardiovasc Electrophysiol. 2002;13:1222–6.
8. Fitzpatrick AP, Gonzales RP, Lesh MD, et al. New algorithm for the localization of accessory atrioventricular connections using a baseline electrocardiogram. J Am Coll Cardiol. 1994;23:107–16.
9. Iturralde P, Araya-Gomez V, Colin L, et al. A new ECG algorithm for the localization of accessory pathways using only the polarity of the QRS complex. J Electrocardiol. 1996;29:289–99.
10. Xie B, Heald SC, Bashir Y, et al. Localization of accessory pathways from the 12-lead electrocardiogram using a new algorithm. Am J Cardiol. 1994;74:161–5.
11. Maden O, Balci KG, Selcuk MT, et al. Comparison of the accuracy of three algorithms in predicting accessory pathways among adult Wolff-Parkinson-White syndrome patients. J Interv Card Electrophysiol. 2015;44:213–9.
12. Takahashi A, Shah DC, Jaïs P, et al. Specific electrocardiographic features of manifest coronary vein posteroseptal accessory pathways. J Cardiovasc Electrophysiol. 1998;9:1015–25.
13. Haissaguerre M, Dartigues JF, Warin JF, et al. Electrogram patterns predictive of successful catheter ablation of accessory pathways. Value of unipolar recording mode. Circulation. 1991;84:188–202.
14. Jackman WM, Friday KJ, Fitzgerald DM, et al. Localization of left free-wall and posteroseptal accessory atrioventricular pathways by direct recording of accessory pathway activation. Pacing Clin Electrophysiol. 1989;12:204–14.
15. Singh A, Beckman K, McClelland J, et al. Selection of optimal RV pacing site for mapping retrograde accessory pathway conduction. Pacing Clin Electrophysiol. 1994;17:741.
16. Coumel P, Attuel P. Reciprocating tachycardia in overt and latent preexcitation: influence of functional bundle branch block on the rate of the tachycardia. Eur J Cardiol. 1974;1:423–36.
17. Spurrell RAJ, Krikler DM, Sowton E. Retrograde invasion of the bundle branches producing aberration of the QRS complex during supraventricular tachycardia studied by programmed electrical stimulation. Circulation. 1974;50:487–95.
18. Zipes DP, DeJoseph RL, Rothbaum DA. Unusual properties of accessory pathways. Circulation. 1974;49:1200–11.
19. Neuss H, Schlepper M, Thormann J. Analysis of re-entry mechanisms in three patients with concealed Wolff-Parkinson-White syndrome. Circulation. 1975;51:75–81.
20. Wellens HJJ, Durrer D. The role of an accessory atrioventricular pathway in reciprocal tachycardia: observations in patients with and without the Wolff-Parkinson-White syndrome. Circulation. 1975;52:58–72.
21. Tonkin AM, Gallagher JJ, Svenson RH, et al. Antegrade block in accessory pathways with retrograde conduction in reciprocating tachycardia. Eur J Cardiol. 1975;3:143–52.
22. Gallagher JJ, Gilbert M, Svenson RH, Sealy WC, Kasell J, Wallace AG. Wolff-Parkinson-White syndrome: the problem, evaluation and surgical correction. Circulation. 1975;51:767–85.
23. Sellers TD Jr, Gallagher JJ, Cope GD, Tonkin AM, Wallace AG. Retrograde atrial preexcitation following premature ventricular beats during reciprocating tachycardia in the Wolff-Parkinson-White syndrome. Eur J Cardiol. 1976;4:283–94.
24. Benditt DG, Benson DW Jr, Dunnigan A, et al. Role of extrastimulus site and tachycardia cycle length in inducibility of atrial preexcitation by premature ventricular stimulation during reciprocating tachycardia. Am J Cardiol. 1987;60:811–9.
25. JD M'n-A, Almendral J, Arenal A, et al. Identification of concealed posteroseptal Kent pathways by comparison of ventriculoatrial intervals from apical and posterobasal right ventricular sites. Circulation. 1994;89:1060–7.
26. Hirao K, Otomo K, Wang X, et al. Para-Hisian pacing. A new method for differentiating retrograde conduction over an accessory AV pathway from conduction over the AV node. Circulation. 1996;94:1027–35.
27. Pedersen AK, Benetis R, Thomsen PE. A posteroseptal accessory pathway located in a coronary sinus aneurysm: diagnosis and radiofrequency catheter ablation. Br Heart J. 1992;68:414–6.
28. Tebbenjohanns J, Pfeiffer D, Jung W, et al. Radiofrequency catheter ablation of a posteroseptal accessory pathway within a coronary sinus diverticulum. Am Heart J. 1993;126:1216–9.
29. Sun Y, Arruda M, Otomo K, et al. Coronary sinus-ventricular accessory connections producing posteroseptal and left posterior accessory pathways: incidence and electrophysiological identification. Circulation. 2002;106:1362–7.
30. Calkins H, Kim YN, Schmaltz S, et al. Electrogram criteria for identification of appropriate target sites for radiofrequency catheter ablation of accessory atrioventricular connections. Circulation. 1992;85:565–73.
31. Liu J, Dole LR. Late complete atrioventricular block complicating radiofrequency catheter ablation of a left posteroseptal accessory pathway. Pacing Clin Electrophysiol. 1998;21:2136–8.
32. Wang SY, Yeh SJ, Lin FC, Wu D. Coronary sinus stenosis as a late complication of catheter ablation in Wolff-Parkinson-White syndrome. Catheter Cardiovasc Diagn. 1997;42(1):70–2.
33. Swartz JF, Tracy CM, Fletcher RD, et al. Radiofrequency endocardial catheter ablation of accessory atrioventricular pathway atrial insertion sites. Circulation. 1993;87:487–99.
34. Stavrakis S, Jackman WM, Nakagawa H, et al. Risk of coronary artery injury with radiofrequency ablation and cryoablation of epicardial posteroseptal accessory pathways within the coronary venous system. Circ Arrhythm Electrophysiol. 2014;7:113–9.

28

Catheter Ablation of Antero-septal (Supero-paraseptal) and Mid-septal (True Septal) Accessory Pathways

Takashi Kurita and Ryobun Yasuoka

> **Keywords**
> Supero-paraseptal accessory pathways · Mid-septal accessory pathways · Reset of tachycardia at His refractoriness · Para-Hisian pacing (Hirao's method) · Entrainment phenomenon

28.1 Introduction

Since the 1980s when the standard technique of catheter ablation was established, catheter ablation targeting accessory pathways (APs) has become the usual treatment used by all electrophysiologists. However, procedures for septal APs that are very close to His bundle are still challenging even for skilled operators because they may cause injury to the normal conduction system. Because relatively young patients are prone to be candidates for catheter ablation of APs, the occurrence of severe atrioventricular (AV) block imposes permanent artificial pacing on patients for more than 30–40 years. In this chapter, we will discuss the safe and reliable techniques for detecting the precise location of the AP and how to eliminate the AP conduction based on a correct recognition of the anatomical relationship between the cardiac septum and APs.

28.2 Anatomy and Definition of Supero-paraseptal (Antero-septal) and Mid-septal Accessory Pathways

The nomenclature "antero-septal" AP has been used traditionally to indicate a pathway with a connection between the atrial and ventricular septum at or above the apex of Koch's triangle (at the anterior region of the His bundle). However, as shown in Fig. 28.1, the anterior site of the His bundle no longer belongs to the "atrial septum" because the aortic root separates the right and left atrial walls. Therefore, this site theoretically should be considered the "supero-paraseptal" right free wall [1, 2]. Similarly, a so-called "postero-septal AP," which is located in the region of the coronary sinus ostium, should be defined as a "postero-paraseptal AP," since there is no atrial septum in that region (Fig. 28.1). A "mid-septal" AP, which is located between the two boundaries consisting of the His bundle and coronary sinus ostium, can be defined as a true "septal" AP [1, 2]. According to the above considerations we will use the terminology "supero-paraseptal AP" instead of "antero-septal AP," which represents the site at or above the apex of Koch's triangle (electrophysiologically, the His potential recording site), and will use "mid-septal AP" as the pathway that represents the floor of Koch's triangle (electrophysiologically between the His potential recording site and ostium of the coronary sinus as marked by the vortex of the curvature of the catheter in the coronary sinus on fluoroscopy) (Fig. 28.2) [1, 2].

28.3 ECG Manifestations

28.3.1 Supero-paraseptal APs

Supero-paraseptal APs are relatively rare (6–7% among all types of APs) and 80% of these are manifest (positive delta waves). In cases with a manifest AP, the morphology of the delta wave on the surface ECG is positive in all the inferior leads (II, III, and aVF) and lateral leads (V3–6), and negative

T. Kurita, M.D., Ph.D. (✉) · R. Yasuoka, M.D., Ph.D.
Faculty of Medicine, Division of Cardiology,
Department of Medicine, Kindai University,
377-2 Onohigashi, Osaka-Sayama, Osaka 589-8511, Japan
e-mail: kuritat@med.kindai.ac.jp

© Springer Nature Singapore Pte Ltd. 2018
K. Hirao (ed.), *Catheter Ablation*, https://doi.org/10.1007/978-981-10-4463-2_28

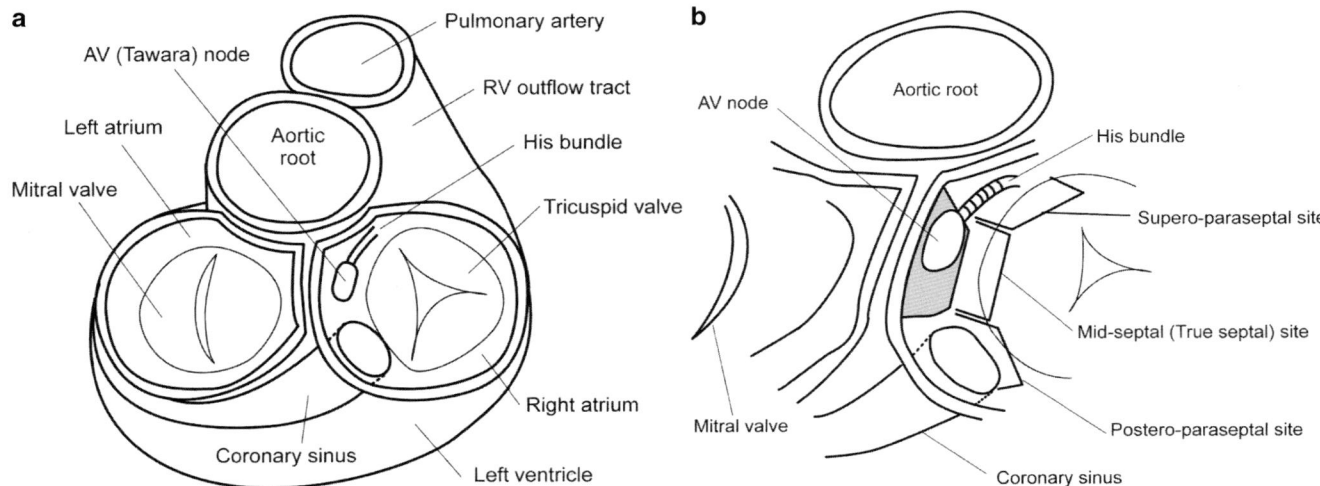

Fig. 28.1 Panel (**a**) shows the global cranial view of the atrioventricular groove by removing most of the atrial muscle. The location of the tricuspid and mitral annuli, and roots of the aortic and pulmonary arteries are illustrated. Note the anatomical relationship among the atrioventricular (AV) node, His bundle, and coronary sinus. Panel (**b**) is a magnified view focusing on the so-called "atrial septum." The anterior site of the His bundle no longer belongs to the "atrial septum" because the aortic root separates the right and left atrial walls. Therefore, theoretically this site should be considered as the "supero-paraseptal" right free wall (panel **b**). Similarly, the so-called "postero-septal AP," which is located in the region of the coronary sinus ostium, should be defined as "postero-paraseptal," since there is no atrial septum in that region (panel **b**). A "mid-septal" AP, which is located between the two boundaries of the His bundle and coronary sinus ostium, can be defined as a true "septal" AP (*shaded area* in panels **a** and **b**)

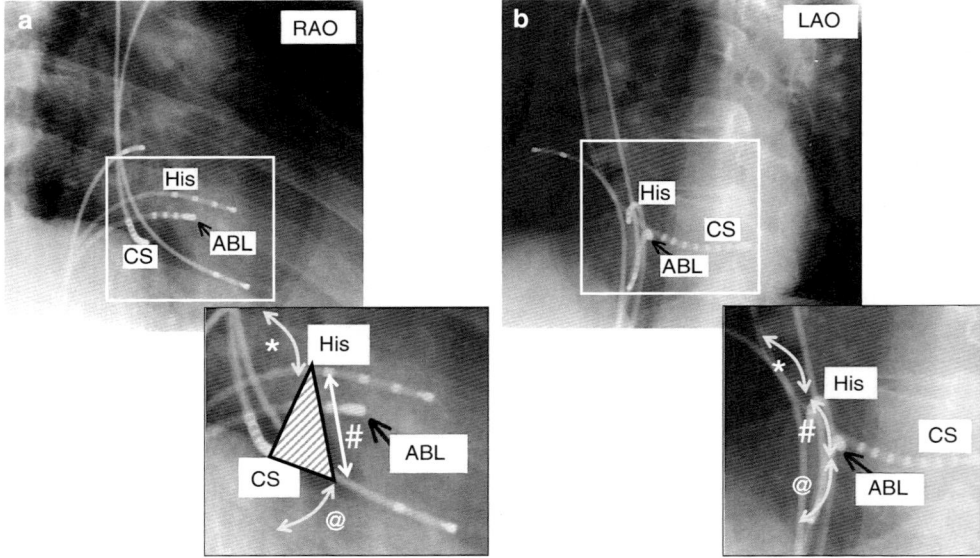

Fig. 28.2 Identification of supero-paraseptal (*asterisk*), mid-septal (*hash*), and postero-paraseptal (symbol "*commercial at*") sites using fluoroscopic images. In this case, the ablation catheter (ABL) is placed in a mid-septal position. The precise recognition of the catheter position around Koch's triangle is possible by placing diagnostic catheters at the His bundle and into the coronary sinus (CS). The *shaded triangle* in panel (**a**) indicates Koch's triangle

in V1 (and occasionally in V2) (Fig 28.3a). Retrograde P waves during orthodromic AV reciprocating tachycardia (AVRT) can been seen after the QRS wave, and are positive in the inferior leads, concordant with the vector of the delta wave (Fig 28.3b) [3].

Mid-septal APs are also relatively rare (5–6% among all types of APs) and 85% of those are manifest (positive delta waves). In the case of manifest APs, the delta waves on the ECG are positive in leads I, II, aVL, and V3 (2)-6 with negative or isoelectric waves in leads III, aVF, and V1 (Fig 28.4a) [3]. During orthodromic AVRT, the retrograde P waves following the QRS are isoelectric or negative in the inferior leads because of their more posterior location (Fig 28.4b).

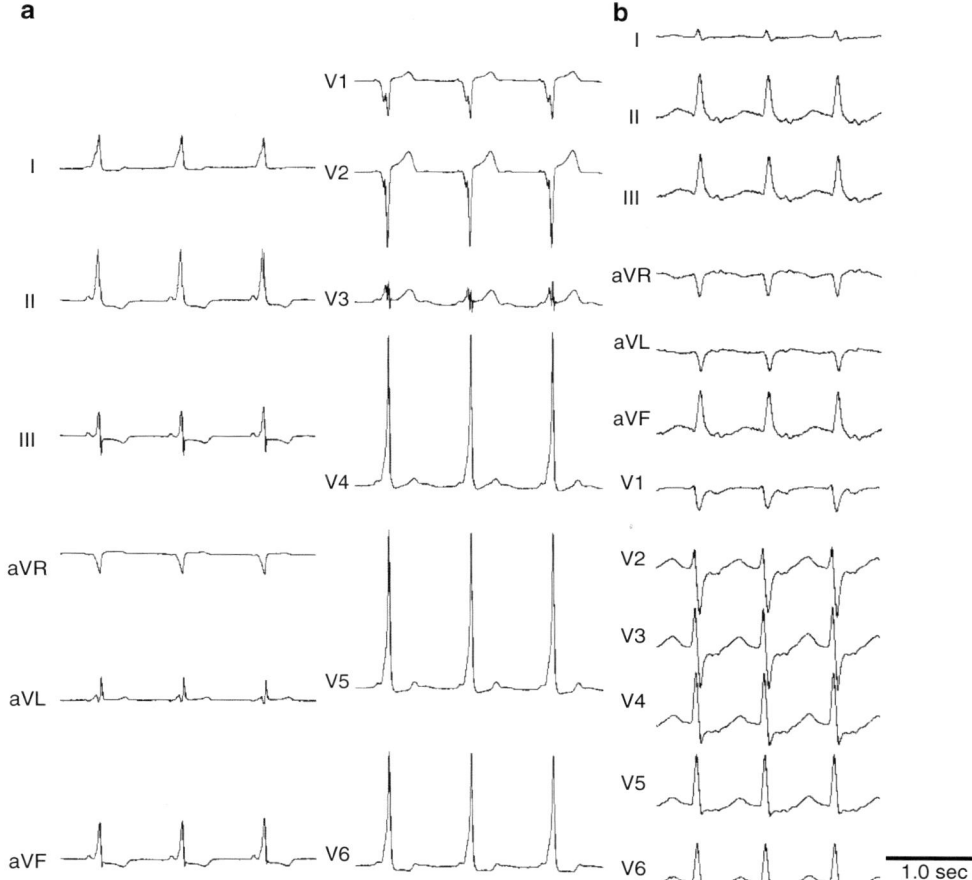

Fig. 28.3 A standard 12 lead electrocardiogram during sinus rhythm (panel **a**) and during atrioventricular reentrant tachycardia (panel **b**) in a patient with a supero-paraseptal accessory pathway. The delta waves during sinus rhythm are positive in leads II, III, and aVF, and negative in leads V1 and V2. Retrograde P waves during the atrioventricular reentrant tachycardia are positive in leads II, III, and aVF, and negative in leads V1 and V2

28.4 Diagnosis of AVRT [Differential Diagnosis of AV Nodal Reciprocating Tachycardia (AVNRT)]

In the case of concealed APs (AP with only retrograde conduction), the correct diagnosis completely depends on the electrophysiologic properties during retrograde conduction via the AP (by provocation of AVRT or ventricular pacing). Because the sequence of the retrograde conduction of a septal AP is similar to that of the AV node, proper techniques are required to differentiate between AVRT and AVNRT. During the tachycardia, a single extra-stimulus from the right ventricle (RV) at a timing when the His is refractory can produce a "reset" of the tachycardia, i.e., earlier capture of the atrial activity (Fig. 28.5). This phenomenon suggests that the RV is included in the reentrant circuit. Among the paroxysmal supraventricular tachycardias (PSVT), AVRT is the only tachyarrhythmia that utilizes the ventricles as part of the critical reentrant pathway. To promote this phenomenon, the operator should place an RV stimulation catheter at an RV septum basal site (as close to the reentrant circuit as possible). Constant pacing at a site close to the His bundle (para-Hisian pacing, so-called Hirao's method) is another effective procedure to distinguish retrograde conduction over an AP from that over the AV node [4]. Para-Hisian pacing should be started from the highest output, and then gradually decrease the output. At the high output, both the His bundle and ventricle can be captured simultaneously, which produces a relatively narrow QRS, and thereafter, with the low output, it loses His capture and captures only the ventricle, which can be recognized by a sudden widening of the QRS morphology (Fig. 28.6). When retrograde conduction is only via a septal AP, the interval from the stimulus to the atrial activity (St-A interval) and the sequence of the atrial activity are constant (same propagation process to the atrium, Fig. 28.6a). In the case of only retrograde conduction over the AV node, the St-A interval prolongs suddenly during RV pacing accompanied by a wide QRS while keeping the same

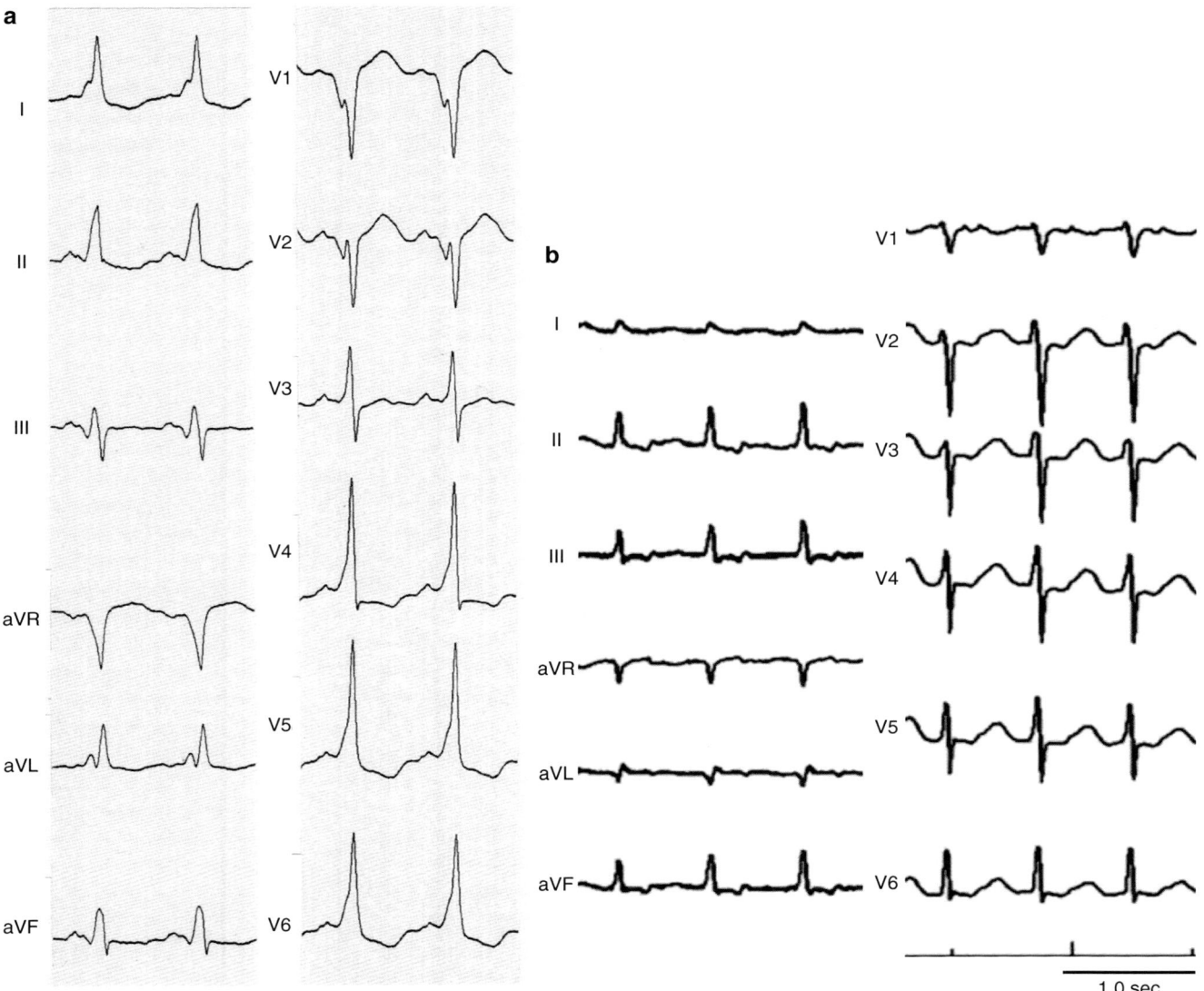

Fig. 28.4 A standard 12 lead electrocardiogram during sinus rhythm (panel **a**) and during atrioventricular reentrant tachycardia (panel **b**) in a patient with a mid-paraseptal accessory pathway. The delta waves during sinus rhythm are positive in lead II, isoelectric or slightly negative in leads III and aVF, and negative in leads V1 and V2. The retrograde P waves during the atrioventricular reentrant tachycardia are flat or slightly negative in leads II, III, and aVF, and negative in leads V1 and V2

sequence of the atrial activity (the excitation wavefront first travels to an apical site and then enters the His-Purkinje system, Fig. 28.6b). Although the case of retrograde conduction over both the AP and AV node is relatively complex, a change in the retrograde atrial excitation during para-Hisian pacing enables us to recognize the dual exits. During a narrow QRS (simultaneous AP and AVN conduction, Fig. 28.7), the excitation sequence around the atrial septum is more identical than that for a wide QRS (only AP conduction).

A comparison of the retrograde conduction time (St-A intervals) at two different RV pacing sites (RV basal septum and apical septum) can provide another option. Since a septal AP connects directly to the RV basal septum, the St-A interval from that site is much shorter than that from the RV apex. On the other hand, in the case of only retrograde AV node conduction, the St-A interval from the basal site becomes longer than that from the RV apex because the basal site is the most distant from the AV node electrophysiologically.

Fig. 28.5 Single extra-stimulus from the right ventricle at a timing when the His is refractory creates an early atrial activation (atrial capture). (**a**) The pacing artifact (*filled inverted triangle*) can be seen slightly after the His deflection (*up-arrow*). The A-A interval is shortened from 340 ms to 335 ms after the stimulus. (**b**) The pacing artifact can be seen just at the His deflection (*filled-inverted triangle*). The A-A interval is shortened from 340 to 325 ms after the stimulus. (**c**) Although the pacing artifact (*filled inverted triangle*) can be seen slightly before the His deflection (*up-arrow*), it still fulfills the condition of His refractoriness. The constant His to His intervals mean that the His bundle excites antegradely (*dotted arrows*). On the contrary, the A-A interval is shortened from 340 to 315 ms after the stimulus (*solid arrows*). *HRA* high right atrium, *His d* His distal, *His p* His paroxysmal, *CS d* coronary sinus distal, *CS p* coronary sinus proximal

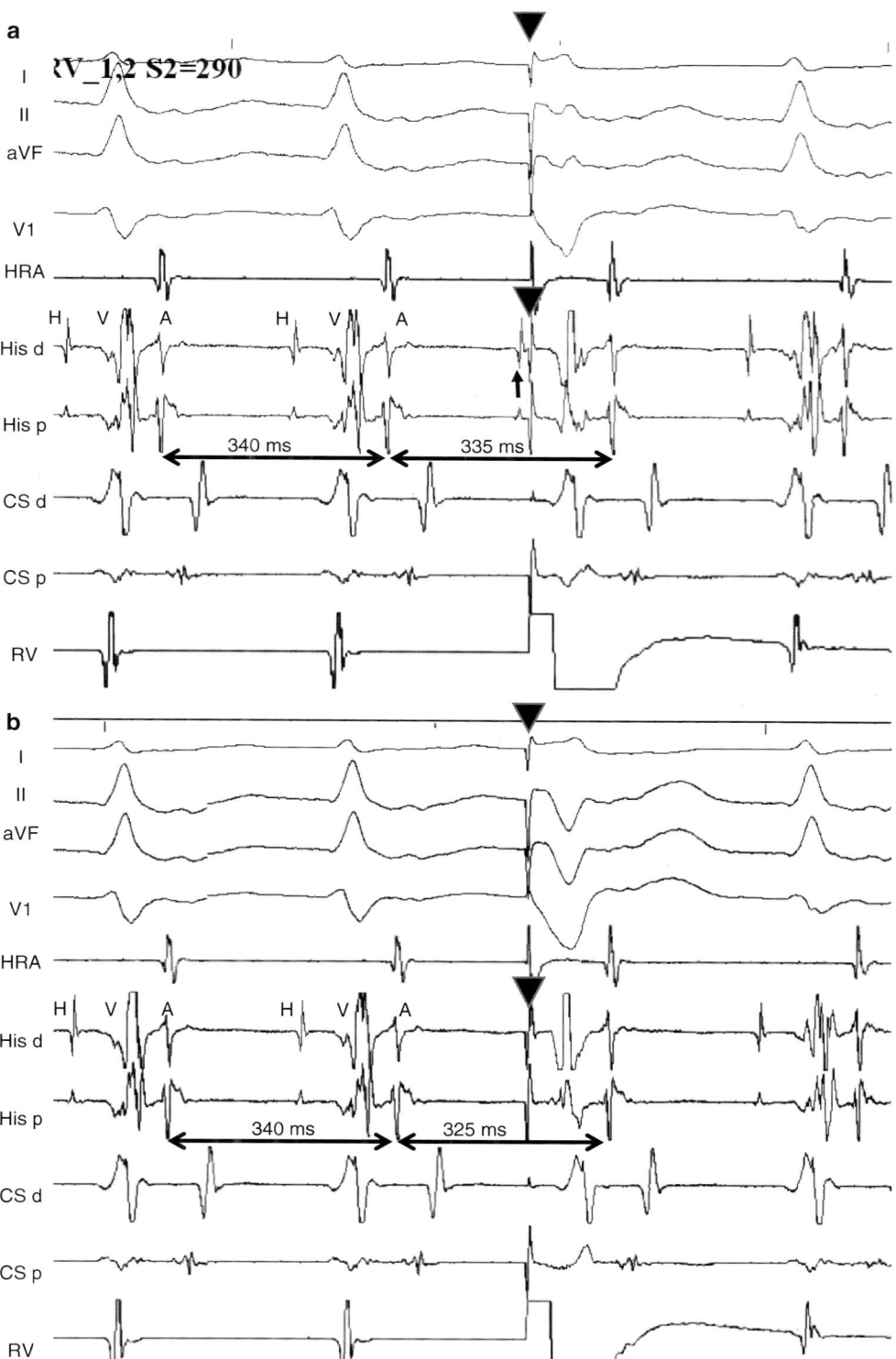

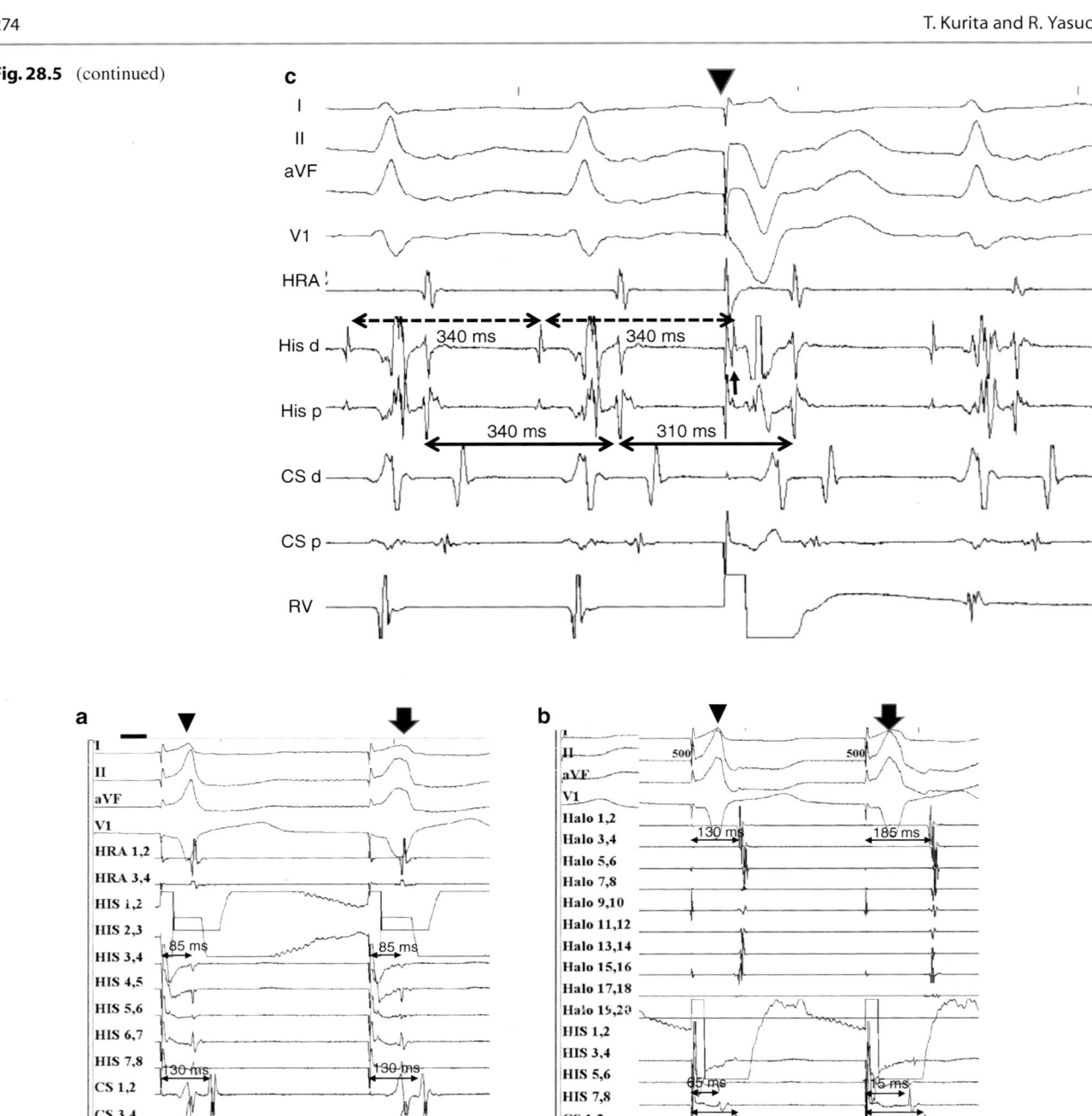

Fig. 28.6 Para-Hisian pacing (Hirao's method) in a patient with a supero-paraseptal accessory pathway (AP) before and after a successful catheter ablation (panels **a** and **b**). Pacing impulses are delivered to the distal portion of the His bundle (a significant pacing artifact can be seen). A relatively narrow QRS with high output pacing (*filled inverted triangle*) indicates that the pacing spike captures the ventricle including the His bundle. With a decreasing pacing output, the QRS width suddenly increases indicating the loss of the His bundle capture (*down arrow*). (**a**) Para-Hisian pacing in patient with supero-paraseptal accessory pathway (AP) before ablation. The stimulus to A interval and sequence of the atrial potentials are constant during either a wide or narrow paced QRS, which demonstrates that the retrograde conduction is utilizing only the AP, which is completely independent of the conduction of the His bundle. (**b**) Para-Hisian pacing in the same patient after successful ablation. A significant prolongation of the stimulus to A interval can be seen after a widening of the paced QRS without any sequential change in the atrial activity. This means that a retrograde conduction pathway is connected to the His bundle, namely, there is only retrograde conduction over the AV node. *HRA* high right atrium, *CS* coronary sinus, *RV* right ventricle, *STIM* stimulus

Fig. 28.7 Para-Hisian pacing in patient with retrograde conduction over both the mid-septal accessory pathway (AP) and atrioventricular (AV) node. During the narrow QRS (*filled inverted triangle*; when retrograde excitation is utilizing both pathways), the stimulus to A (St-A) interval at the His and coronary sinus ostium (CS OS) are similar (St-A interval of 105 and 120 ms, respectively). However, during the wide QRS (*down arrow*; when retrograde excitation is utilizing only the AP), the St-A interval at the His potential suddenly prolongs (from 105 to 160 ms), but that at the CS OS is kept almost constant (120 and 125 ms). *His d* His distal, *His p* His paroxysmal, *CS d* coronary sinus distal, *CS p* coronary sinus proximal

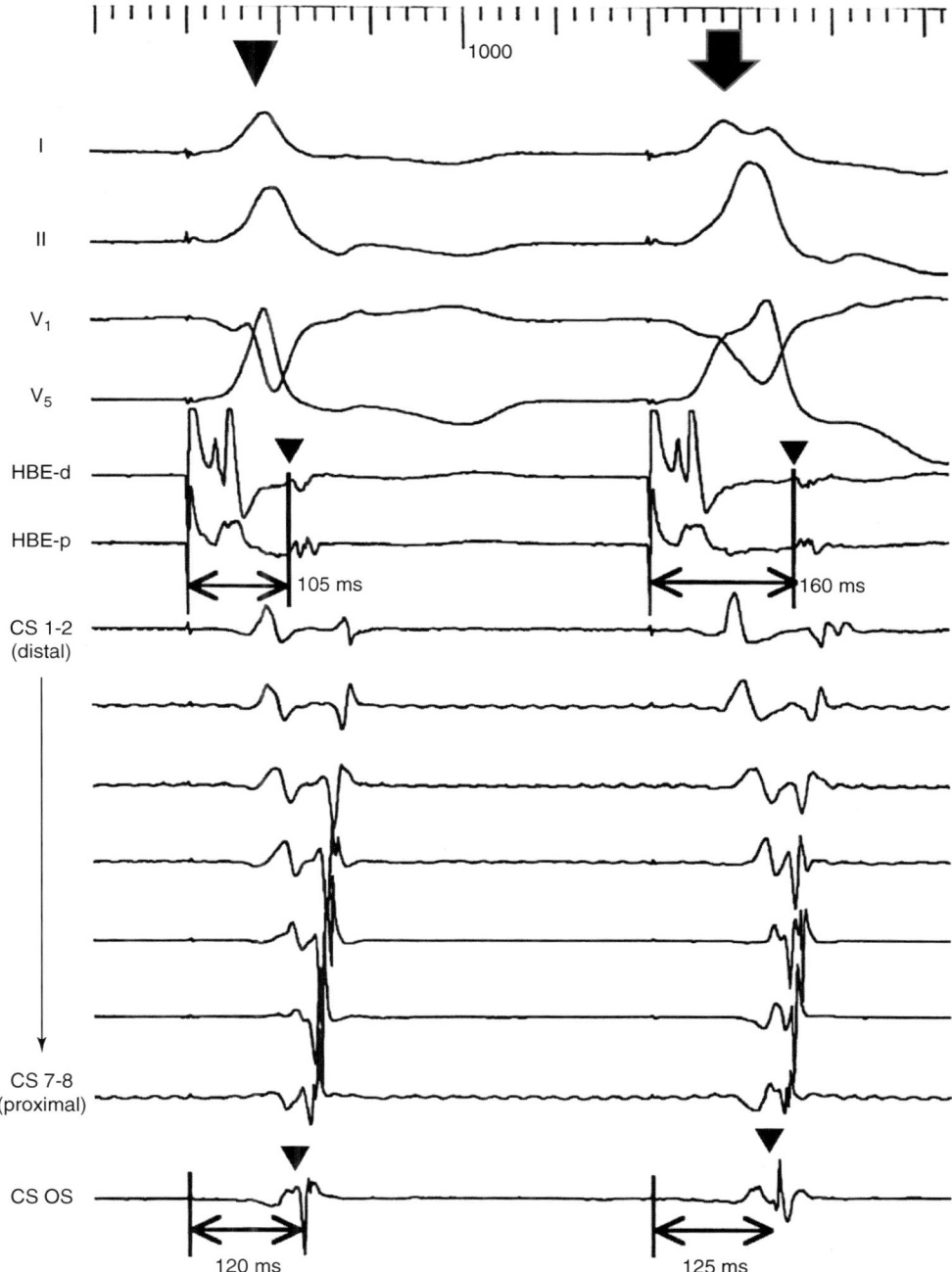

Manifest entrainment (constant and progressive fusion of the QRS morphologies) during RV pacing helps us to confirm that an AVRT utilizing a right AP is the mechanism of the PSVT (Fig. 28.8) [6]. To elucidate this phenomenon, the initial pacing cycle length should be set at 5–10 ms shorter than that of the tachycardia with a relatively long coupling interval, and repeated by decrementing the cycle length by 5–10 ms every step until the tachycardia terminates. In the case of AVNRT, RV pacing during the tachycardia produces an exclusive paced QRS morphology (not a fused QRS). Decremental conduction properties (rate-dependent conduction delay) are commonly observed in the AV node. However, this trend is sometimes observed with septal APs (especially mid-septal APs). Therefore, a differential diagnosis based on this electrophysiologic feature is probably misleading.

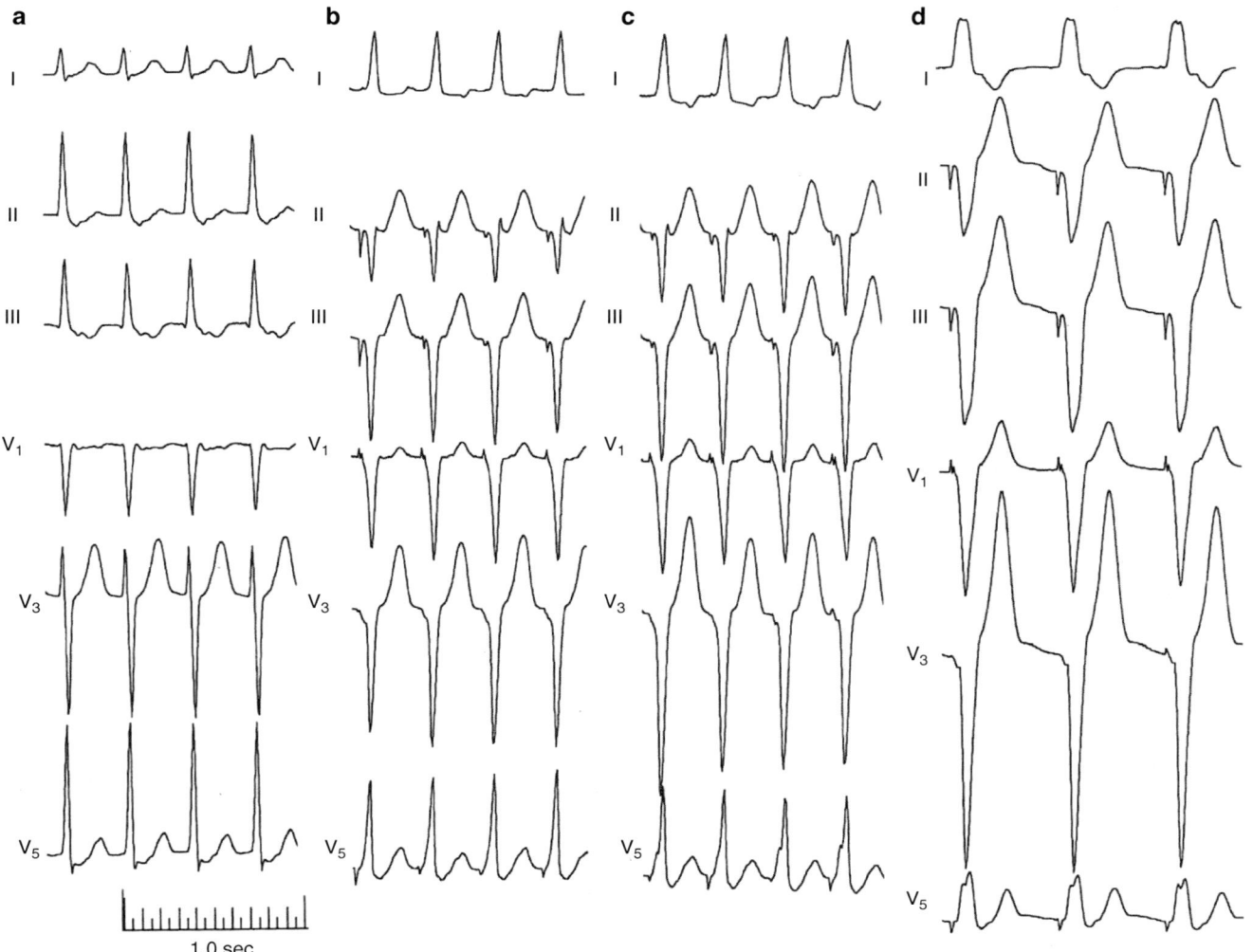

Fig. 28.8 Entrainment phenomena on the surface ECG produced by right ventricular (RV) pacing during an atrioventricular reciprocating tachycardia (AVRT) utilizing a right accessory pathway (AP). Panel (**a**) shows a narrow QRS tachycardia (AVRT) with a cycle length of 390 ms. The retrograde P waves can be seen following the QRS. RV pacing was performed during AVRT with cycle lengths of 380 ms (panel **b**) and 370 ms (panel **c**). Panel (**d**) demonstrates RV pacing during sinus rhythm (exclusively a paced QRS). By comparing the QRS morphologies in panels **a–d**, a constant and progressive fusion (first and second criteria of entrainment) is clearly demonstrated, which means that the reentrant circuit involves the RV. AVRT is the only tachycardia that utilizes the ventricles as the reentrant critical circuit among the so-called paroxysmal supraventricular tachycardias (PSVTs). Note a gradual QRS widening with a decreasing RV pacing cycle length

28.5 Localization of APs During Electrophysiologic Testing (EPS) and the Technical Aspects of the Catheter Ablation

The exact localization of septal APs is especially important in order to avoid any damage to the AV node (Tawara's node) or His bundle during the catheter ablation. A conventional ablation using radio-frequency (RF) energy at Koch's triangle has been reported to create AV block with an incidence of 5–10% [1, 2, 5]. Ordinarily, a trans-inferior vena cava approach is selected as the initial strategy by using a long vascular sheath that reaches into the right atrium to stabilize the ablation catheter at the target site [1, 2, 5]. In the case of a supero-paraseptal AP, some investigators recommend manipulating the ablation catheter via the superior vena cava or via the non-coronary cusp [1, 2, 7–10]. By utilizing the various techniques as described in this chapter, elimination of the AP conduction can be achieved with a success rate of more than 95%. On the other hand, the recurrence rate of antero-paraseptal and mid-septal AP conduction after a successful catheter ablation has been reported in up to 15% [1]. This relatively high recurrence rate may be due to the poor contact of the ablation catheter with the tissue or an unavoidable lack of courage of the operator to provide an adequate amount of energy or number of applications.

28.5.1 How to Localize and Ablate APs

28.5.1.1 Manifest Supero-paraseptal APs

As with other types of manifest APs, the earliest excitation of the potential generated by the AP or ventricle should be searched for by manipulating an ablation catheter at the apex of Koch's triangle [1, 2, 5]. In many cases, clearly distinguishing between the AP potential and that of the ventricle is difficult, but fractionated activity observed between the atrial and ventricular signals (continuous activity) may represent the AP-potential (Fig. 28.9a). It is recommended that the operator manipulates the ablation catheter back and forth, little by little, while careful watching for a change in the electrograms recorded both from the distal and proximal pairs of electrodes (the atrial potential becomes bigger and ventricular potential smaller at the proximal position of the electrodes), which may allow the recognition of several different components among the complex potentials. In the case of a relatively long refractory period of the AP, atrial extra-stimulus or burst pacing may be useful to distinguish between the atrial or non-atrial (AP or ventricular) potentials of the continuous potentials by creating atrio-AP block (Fig. 28.9a, b) [1, 2].

The onset of the ventricular (or AP) potential should precede the delta wave on the surface ECG by more than 15 ms (ideally more than 30 ms) (Fig. 28.9a). When mapping during sinus rhythm, the His potential cannot be recorded in the Koch's triangle region in many cases because an early non-atrial potential overrides it. To avoid the worst case scenario, which is the creation of conduction block of the AV node or His bundle without any effect on the AP, the exact recognition of the His potential recording site is essential. Induction of orthodromic AVRT is the simplest method to identify whether the His potential can be seen at the target site with the earliest atrial signal (Fig. 28.10), and "tagging" the His recording sites during the AVRT under the guidance of a 3D mapping system promotes a relatively safe procedure.

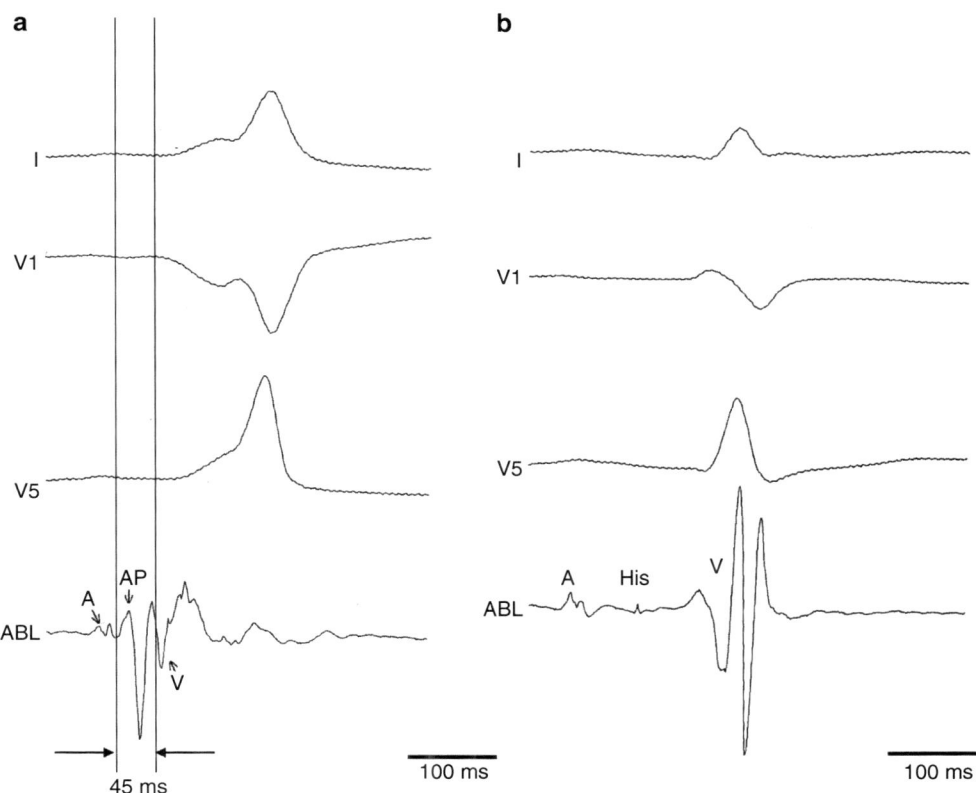

Fig. 28.9 Surface electrocardiogram (I, V1, and V5) and electrocardiograms at the site of a manifest supero-paraseptal accessory pathway before (panel **a**) and after (panel **b**) a successful catheter ablation. (**a**) Note the spiky and continuous activity between the atrial (A) and ventricular (V) potentials suggestive of an accessory pathway (AP) potential, which precedes the onset of the delta wave by 45 ms. (**b**) The elimination of the antegrade conduction of the AP reveals an apparent His potential at the ablation site. The amplitude of the His potential is less than 0.1 mV, and we could avoid any injury to the atrioventricular node and His bundle. A comparison of the local electrograms between that before and after the catheter ablation allowed us to distinguish between the atrial activity and subsequent "non-atrial" potentials (probable AP and ventricular potentials). *ABL* ablation catheter, *A* atrial activity, *AP* accessory pathway activity, *V* ventricular activity

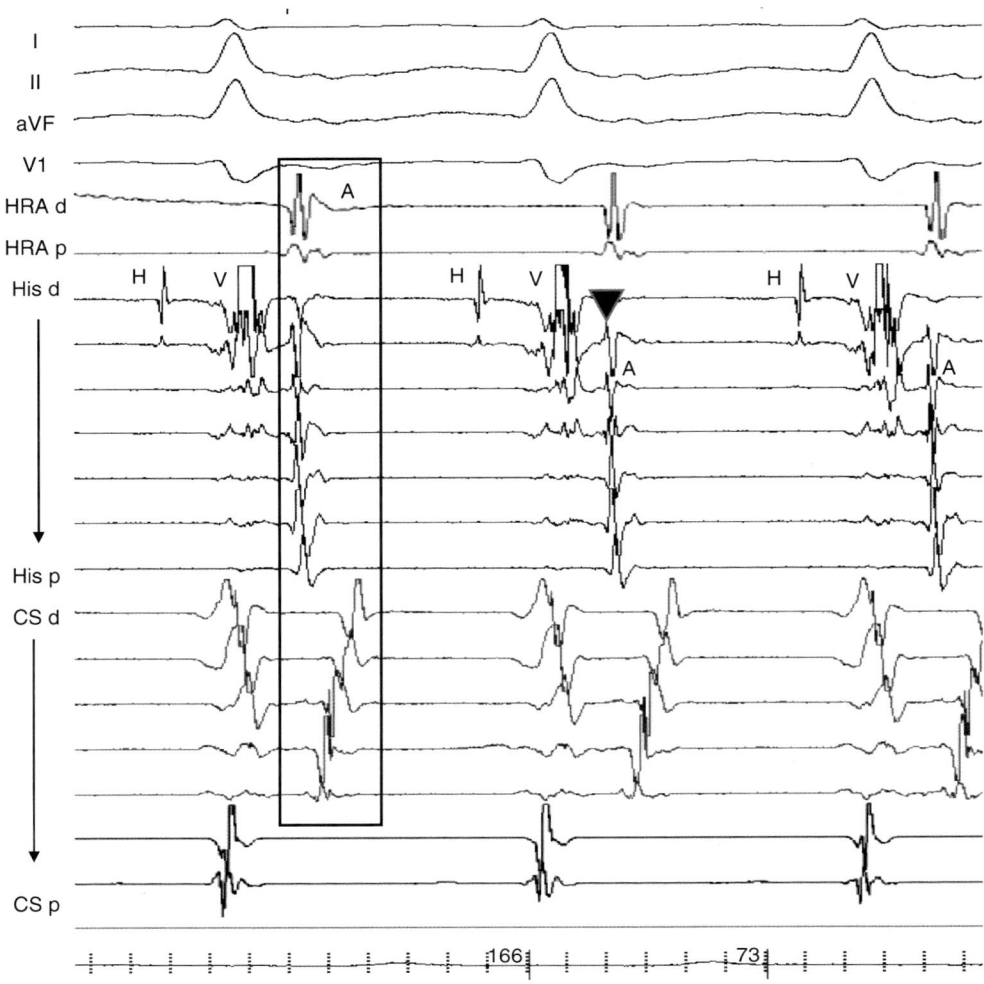

Fig. 28.10 Surface electrocardiogram (I, II, aVF, and V1) and electrocardiograms during atrioventricular reentrant tachycardia. The retrograde atrial potential (A, within the enclosed square) is the earliest at the His recording site (*filled inverted triangle*). *H* His potential, *V* ventricular potential, *HRA d* high right atrium distal, *HRA p* high right atrium proximal, *His d* His distal, *His p* His proximal, *CS d* coronary sinus distal, *CS p* coronary sinus proximal

The AP conduction can be safely eliminated at a site with a His potential of less than 0.1 mV (Fig. 28.9b). RF current should be started at the site with the earliest ventricular potential or biggest AP-potential based on the utmost detailed mapping within Koch's triangle (Fig. 28.2a, b). It is recommended to start the RF application at a relatively low energy (20–30 W) and with a low temperature (40–50°). When a relatively large His potential (>0.1 mV) is recorded at the most optimal site for ablation of the AP (true para-Hisian AP), titration of the RF current should be used by starting from 5 W and increasing it with 5 W steps every 10 s up to 40 W.

During the delivery of the RF current, careful attention to the QRS morphology is required. Since widening of the QRS (an exclusive QRS conducting AP) may indicate a conduction disturbance of the AV node or His-Purkinje system. If there is no effect on the antegrade conduction of the AP after 10–15 s into the RF delivery, it should be terminated to avoid any severe myocardial damage around the area of AP, which may result in distortion of the electrical activity and the formation of a tough physiological barrier (edematous tissue) for subsequent procedures [1]. The occurrence of junctional rhythm during the RF current may cause one to misunderstand it for the elimination of the delta wave because of the appearance of a narrow QRS complex [2]. In that situation, overdrive atrial pacing is useful to determine the efficacy of the ablation. However, termination of the RF current may be relatively safe especially in the case of a rapid junctional rhythm (>150 min^{-1}). When several applications are ineffective, the physician should evaluate the preserved AV node and His-Purkinje function, and consider an alternative strategy to improve the catheter contact with the tissue or to obtain a closer approach toward the site of the AP (e.g., cranial or trans-aortic approach) [7–11]. Some investigators prefer to advance the ablation catheter from the jugular vein by inserting the tip of the catheter beneath the tricuspid valve, because the His bundle is likely to be protected by central fibrous tissue [11].

The trans-aortic approach to antero-paraseptal APs was first reported by Tada et al. [7], and it has been widely known as a novel and alternative approach [8–11]. Since the non-coronary sinus of Valsalva is bound by the apex of Koch's triangle, RF current from this lesion may directly effect the antero-paraseptal AP. It has been reported that RF applications from all three coronary cusps of Valsalva are safe when targeting particular focal ventricular tachycardias or atrial tachycardias [12–14]. The results from the previous case reports suggest the presence of variant types of antero-paraseptal APs. Some investigators used a trans-aortic approach just to avoid any injury to the AV conduction system (a trans-atrial approach can be partially effective or effective); however, others used that approach only after recognizing either insufficient electrophysiologic features (such as a far-field nature of the local electrograms) or an unsuccessful RF delivery. The latter indicates that some antero-paraseptal APs may be located toward the left side of the heart. When detailed mapping around Koch's triangle does not demonstrate any local electrograms with earliest and spiky (near-field) characteristics, including a possible "AP potential" (Fig 28.8a), switching to a trans-aortic approach without any RF delivery around the tricuspid annulus may be relatively effective and safe. Some previous reports have demonstrated that the non-coronary cusp of Valsalva is the only site where a possible AP potential can be recorded [8, 11]. However, thrombo-embolic complications and injury to the coronary arteries can be a concern, especially in older patients. Confirmation by aortography or coronary arteriography of a distance between the ablation point and orifices of the left and right coronary arteries of at least 10 mm is required before any delivery of RF current. When one can create an exact merge of the CT image of the anatomy of the coronary cusp and artery to coordinate the axis of the patient's body, arteriography is not always necessary.

28.5.1.2 Concealed Antero-paraseptal APs

In the case of a concealed AP (AP with only retrograde conduction), the correct localization completely depends on the electrophysiologic properties during retrograde conduction over the AP (induction of AVRT or ventricular pacing, Figs. 28.10 and 28.11). The optimal target is the earliest excitation of the retrograde atrial potential especially accompanied by a fractionated and continuous potential (AP potential, Fig. 28.11). In the case of a relatively long refractory period, RV paired or burst pacing to produce retrograde conduction block over the AP is useful to recognize the origin of the complex potentials [1, 2]. When patient has both

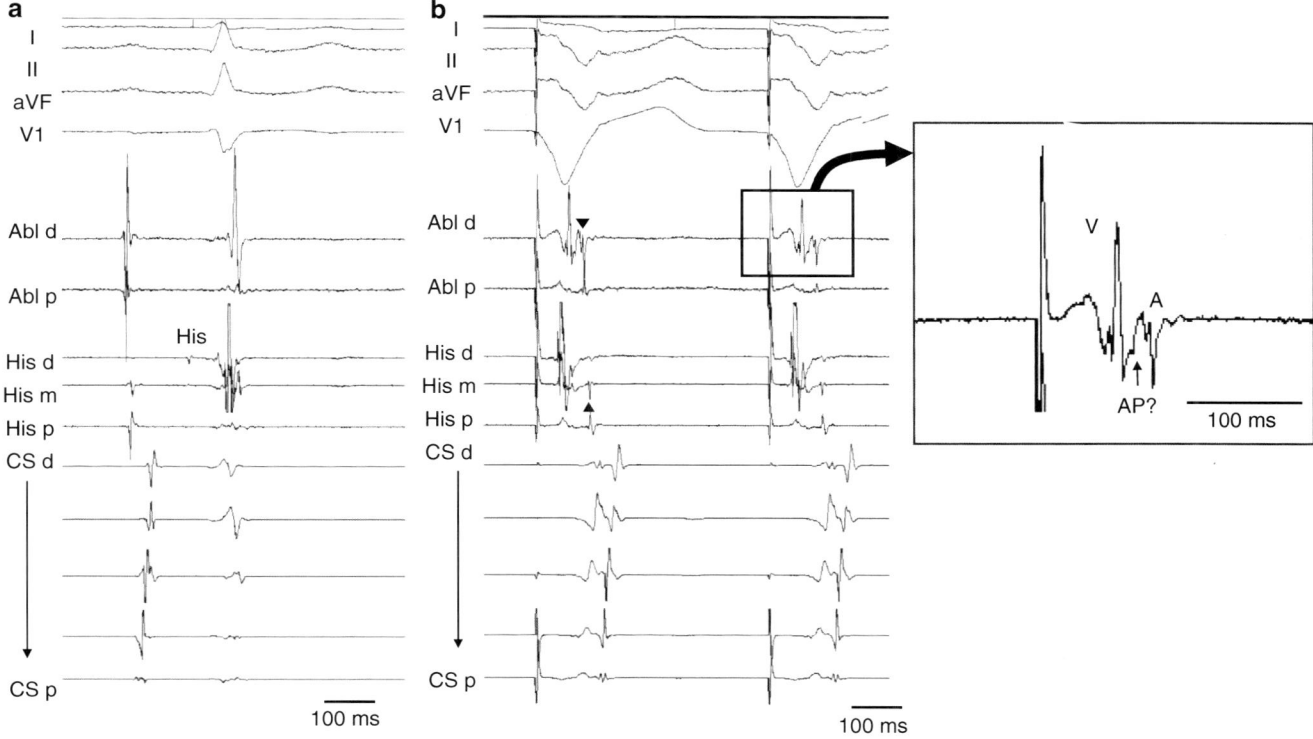

Fig. 28.11 Surface electrocardiogram (I, II, aVF, and V1) and electrocardiograms during sinus rhythm (panel **a**) and right ventricular (RV) pacing (panel **b**) in a patient with a concealed supero-paraseptal accessory pathway (AP). The ablation catheter is positioned at a superior site of the His recording catheter. No His potential is observed at that site (panel **a**). During RV pacing (panel **b**), the retrograde atrial conduction at the ablation catheter is earlier (*filled inverted triangle*) than that at the His recording site (*filled triangle*). Note that the continuous potential between the atrial and ventricular activation suggests the activity of the AP (*up-arrow* in the magnified electrogram). The sequence of the retrograde atrial conduction during RV pacing is identical to that during the atrioventricular reentrant tachycardia (refer to Fig. 28.9). *Abl d* ablation distal, *Abl p* ablation proximal, *His d* His distal, *His m* His middle, *His p* His proximal, *CS d* coronary sinus distal, *CS p* coronary sinus proximal

retrograde conduction over the AP and AV node, ventricular pacing from the RV basal septum (near the AP site) or induction of AVRT is helpful to create a clear sequential difference in the atrial signals.

Catheter ablation during RV pacing while observing the responses of the retrograde conduction is the easiest way to evaluate the efficacy of the ablation of the AP, but this method does not allow us to see any preserved function of the AV node and His bundle until cessation of the RV pacing. On the other hand, catheter ablation during sinus rhythm is the best way to determine any injury to the AV node and His bundle by monitoring the PR prolongation and appearance of any junctional rhythm. However, the simultaneous or instantaneous evaluation of the retrograde AP conduction during the RF delivery is impossible.

To resolve these issues, several alternative methods have been proposed. Catheter ablation during AVRT helps us understand both retrograde conduction block over the AP by termination of the tachycardia and the maintenance of normal AV conduction after the restoration of sinus rhythm [11]. If the tachycardia terminates due to AV block, the RF delivery should be terminated immediately. Sudden changes in the rate and chronologic A-V relationship after termination of the tachycardia may induce dislodgement of the ablation catheter that could increase the risk of injury to the AV conduction system and result in an inadequate lesion at the AP. Approaches from the non-coronary sinus of Valsalva or underneath the tricuspid valve may provide appropriately firm contact with the tissue even after exposure to a sudden hemodynamic change [8, 11, 12]. Another way is to deliver the RF current during atrial entrainment of the AVRT [1, 2]. Atrial pacing with a cycle length 5–10 ms shorter than that of the AVRT may induce entrainment with fusion of the orthodromic conduction and antidromic conduction in the atrium. Therefore, the earliest excitation of the retrograde atrial signal over the AP can still be seen on the ablation catheter during the entrainment (before RF delivery). Further, any apparent sequential change in the atrial activation (sudden prolongation of the V-A interval observed on the ablation or His recording catheters) tells us we have created successful AP conduction block while maintaining a similar hemodynamic condition. Using this method, the stabilization of the ablation catheter can be maintained even after termination of the AVRT because the heart rate is kept constant.

28.5.1.3 Mid-septal (True Septal) APs

Techniques to localize the exact site of a mid-septal AP (with either manifest or concealed properties) and preserve the function of the AV node and His bundle are almost the same as those for a super-paraseptal AP. Many mid-septal APs can be treated by RF applications on the tricuspid annulus (Fig. 28.2). To avoid any AV node or His bundle injury, the usage of a long vascular sheath that reaches into the right atrium to stabilize the ablation catheter, and to target relatively ventricular sites of the tricuspid annulus are recommended to protect the His bundle. During the RF delivery, the operators are recommended to anticipate a much higher incidence of junctional rhythm (tachycardia) compared with that during catheter ablation of supero-paraseptal APs, and it is observed approximately 50% of the time [1]. When one observes a relatively high rate of junctional tachycardia (>150 beats/min), discontinuation of the RF current may be a safe choice [2]. However, in the case of junctional rhythm or a tachycardia of less than 100 beats/min, atrial pacing helps to recognize the disappearance of the antegrade AP conduction and/or a preserved AV conduction. The achievement of a successful ablation of mid-septal APs has been reported to be relatively higher (approximately 98%) than that of supra-paraseptal APs, with a lower risk of AV block (about 1%) [1].

If several RF applications are unsuccessful or no satisfactory electrophysiologic features (e.g., a local potential preceding the onset of the delta wave by less than 10 ms or the absence of a possible AP potential) are identified around the tricuspid annulus, an alternative approach from the left atrium (trans-aortic or trans-septal approach) can be another option [1].

28.5.1.4 Cryo-mapping and Cryo-ablation
[1, 2, 15, 16]

Cryo-mapping and cryo-ablation provide some advantages, especially to avoid any permanent injury to the AV node and His bundle compared to RF ablation. The cryo-mapping method (approximately 0 to −30 °C for up to a 60 s cooling of the myocardial tissue) produces reversible conduction block, which allows us to confirm the efficacy of the AP ablation while allowing the observation of a preserved normal A-V conduction system. When cryo-mapping is not effective in eliminating the AP conduction within 30 s or an AV node or His bundle conduction disturbance is observed, the cryo-mapping can be discontinued. After confirmation of the AP conduction block during the cryo-mapping (test shot), the temperature of catheter tip should be decreased to −75 to −80 °C (cryo-ablation) to create permanent tissue damage around the AP. A rapid decrease in the temperature demonstrates firm contact of the catheter tip with the endocardial tissue. However, if there is slow decline in the temperature, some repositioning of the catheter to obtain a firm contact is necessary. Another advantage of cryo-ablation is that the likelihood of a catheter dislodgement is less possible owing to the adhesion of the catheter tip to the tissue due to an ice ball formation (cryo-adherence), particularly for ablation during AVRT. The overall successful rate has been reported to be less than 80%. However, we should be aware that this number is mainly based on cases with failure of a previous RF ablation. The disadvantages of cryo-ablation are thought to be as follows: (1) disappearance of the local electrogram (mixing of significant noise) during the cooling procedure due to an ice ball formation, (2) relatively high recurrence rate (approximately 20%) of the AP conduction during the remote phase, and (3) the less flexible feature of the cryo-ablation catheter [2].

References

1. Miller JM, Das MK, Yadav AV, Bhakta D. Catheter ablation of superoseptal ("anteroseptal") and midseptal accessory pathways. In: Shoei K, Huang S, Wood MA, editors. Catheter ablation of cardiac arrhythmias. Philadelphia, PA: Elsevier Sounders; 2006. p. 413–25.
2. Issa ZF, Miller JM, Zipes DP. Ablation of supraparaseptal and midseptal bypass tracts. In: Issa ZF, Miller JM, Zipes DP, editors. Clinical arrhythmology and electrophysiology. 2nd ed. Philadelphia, PA: Elsevier Sounders; 2012. p. 462–7.
3. Arruda MS, McClelland JH, Wang X, et al. Development and validation of an ECG algorithm for identifying accessory pathway ablation site in Wolff-Parkinson-White syndrome. J Cardiovasc Electrophysiol. 1998;9:2–12.
4. Hirao K, Otomo K, Aang X, et al. Para-Hisian pacing: a new method for differentiating retrograde conduction over an accessory AV pathway from conduction over the AV node. Circulation. 1996;94:1027–35.
5. Schlüter M, Kuck KH. Catheter ablation from right atrium of anteroseptal accessory pathways using radiofrequency current. JACC. 1992;19:663–70.
6. Suyama K, Ohe T, Kurita T, et al. Significance of ventricular pacing site in manifest entrainment during orthodromic atrioventricular reentrant tachycardia with left-sided accessory pathway. Pacing Clin Electrophysiol. 1992;15:1114–21.
7. Tada H, Naito S, Nogami A, et al. Successful catheter ablation of atrial tachycardia originating near the atrioventricular node from the noncoronary sinus of valsalva. J Cardiovasc Electrophysiol. 2003;14:544–6.
8. Huang H, Wang X, Ouyang F, Antz M. Catheter ablation of anteroseptal accessory pathway in the non-coronary aortic sinus. Europace. 2006;8:1041–4.
9. Suleiman M, Brady PA, Asirvatham SJ, et al. The noncoronary cusp as a site for successful ablation of accessory pathways: electrogram characteristics in three cases. J Cardiovasc Electrophysiol. 2011;22:203–9.
10. Miyauchi Y, Kobayashi Y, Morita N, et al. Successful radiofrequency catheter ablation of an anteroseptal (superoparaseptal) atrioventricular accessory pathway from the left ventricular outflow tract. PACE. 2004;27:668–70.
11. Tao S, Ihara K, Shirai Y, et al. Electrophysiological characteristics of successful ablation of supraparaseptal Kent from noncoronary cusp. Clin Cardiac Electrophysiol 2015;38:123–132 (in Japanese).
12. Hachiya H, Aonuma K, Yamauchi Y, et al. How to diagonose, locate, and ablate coronary cusp ventricular tachycardia. J Cardiovasc Electrophysiol. 2002;13:551–6.
13. Ouyang F, Fotuhi P, Ho SY, et al. Repetitive monomorphic ventricular tachycardia originating from the aortic sinus cusp: electrocardiographic characterization for guiding catheter ablation. J Am Coll Cardiol. 2002;39:500–8.
14. Ouyang F, Ma J, Ho SY, et al. Focal atrial tachycardia originating from the non-coronary aortic sinus: electrophysiological characteristics and catheter ablation. J Am Coll Cardiol. 2006;48:122–31.
15. Miyazaki A, Blaufox AD, Fairbrother DL, Saul P. Cryo-ablation for septal tachycardia substrates in pediatric patients: mid-term results. JACC. 2005;45:581–8.
16. Lemola K, Dubuc M, Khairy P. Transcatheter cryoablation part II: clinical utility. PACE. 2008;31:235–44.

Atriofascicular Accessory Pathways

29

Yukio Sekiguchi

Keywords
Atriofascicular pathway • Mahaim fiber • Paroxysmal supraventricular tachycardia

29.1 Introduction

Around 1940, Mahaim firstly reported the existence of Mahaim fibers which connected His bundle or the atrioventricular node to the ventricle anatomically [1–3]. Although some reports were published about these fibers after his report, no one knew the electrophysiological characteristics of them at that time. In 1975, Lev et al. described that Mahaim fibers histologically passed from the atrioventricular node to the left and to the right side of the posterior ventricular septum [4], and these pathways might play a role in the genesis of the preexcitation [5, 6]. In same year, Anderson proposed that Mahaim fibers might be classified into two anatomical types [7]. One was nodoventricular (NV) fibers connecting between the atrioventricular node and the ventricle, and the other was fasciculoventricular (FV) fibers connecting between the His bundle or the bundle branches and ventricle. However, there were rare cases having NV fibers or FV fibers, and the demonstration of reentrant circuit during reciprocating tachycardias might be difficult [6, 8]. In 1988, Tchou proposed that an accessory pathway which behaved a typical NV fiber actually arose directly from the right atrium and inserted into the right bundle branch, named as atriofascicular accessory pathway [9]. Many data have supported this proposal [10–12], and most accessory pathways with anterograde decremental conduction properties referred to as Mahaim fibers have been recognized as originating from the right lateral atrium in these days.

Y. Sekiguchi, M.D.
Cardiovascular Division, Faculty of Medicine,
University of Tsukuba, 1-1-1 Tennodai,
Tsukuba, Ibaraki 305-8575, Japan
e-mail: yseki@md.tsukuba.ac.jp

29.2 Classification of Mahaim Fibers in Cardiac Arrhythmias

Uncommon accessory pathways presenting decremental properties and inserting into the right ventricle have been frequently described as Mahaim pathways, and these fibers are distinct form of preexcitation. Recently, these anomalous pathways are subdivided into three types (Fig. 29.1), and it is said that most of those pathways in fact originate from the right atrial free wall near the tricuspid annulus and terminate in the distal right bundle branch, which is called as atriofascicular pathways. The most important feature in Fig. 29.1 is that the circuit of atriofascicular pathway includes right atrial muscle, in contradistinction to other circuit of Mahaim pathways. By using this feature, atriofascicular pathways can be ruled out of other Mahaim pathways. The differential diagnosis between atriofascicular pathway and other Mahaim pathways are noted in the following section. This Fig. 29.1 also indicates that Mahaim fibers including atriofascicular pathways can play a role of only anterograde pathway when macro reentrant reciprocating tachycardia occurs. These pathways typically conduct only in the anterograde direction.

29.3 Electrocardiographic Characteristics of Atriofascicular Pathway

The electrocardiogram during preexcited tachycardia using atriofascicular pathway is usually recorded as left bundle branch block pattern and left axis deviation, since the distal part of atriofascicular pathway connects to right ventricle or right bundle branch. On the other hand, although the detailed electrocardiogram depends on the transmission velocity or insertion site of these fibers, typical electrocardiogram

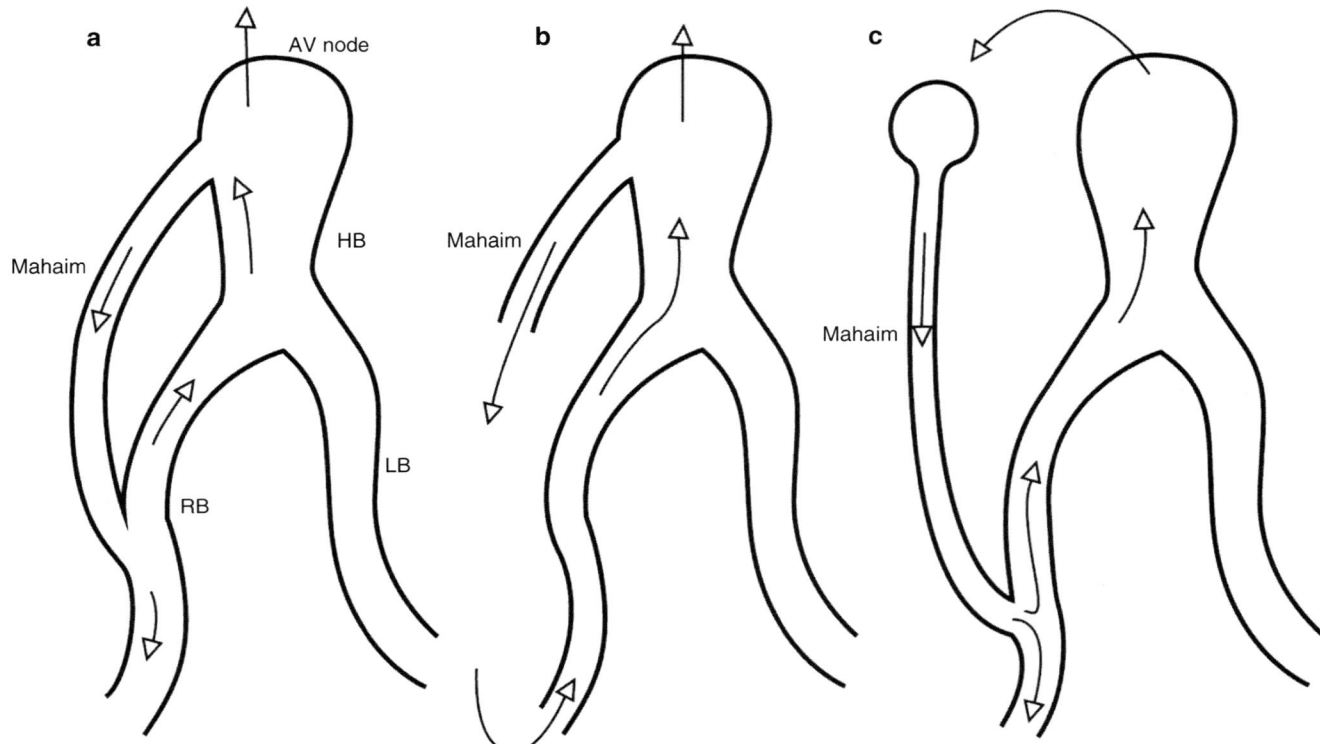

Fig. 29.1 Three types of schematic representations of antidromic reciprocating tachycardia containing Mahaim fibers. (**a**) Nodofascicular fibers connecting between the atrioventricular node and the right bundle. (**b**) Nodoventricular fibers connecting between the atrioventricular node and the right ventricle. (**c**) Atriofascicular fibers connecting between the right atrium and the right bundle. *AV node*; atrioventricular node, *LB* left bundle, *RB* right bundle

of the patients with atriofascicular pathway shows little or no preexcitation during sinus rhythm. Häissaguerre also reported that ten patients with atriofascicular pathways had narrower QRS complexes than seven patients with atrioventricular accessory pathways (133 ± 10 versus 165 ± 26 milliseconds, $p = 0.02$) [13], and narrower initial r wave in leads V_2 through V_4 during maximal preexcitation. As those pathways have the characteristics of decremental property, PR duration is normal in most cases.

29.4 Electrophysiological Characteristics of Atriofascicular Pathway

29.4.1 Differentiation Between Atriofascicular Pathway and Atrioventricular Pathway

Atriofascicular pathways electrophysiologically differ from typical atrioventricular pathways in some respects. First, these atriofascicular pathways are found to conduct only in the anterograde direction with a long conduction time, and these pathways can only form antidromic tachycardia or as bystanders during atrioventricular nodal reentrant tachycardia or atrial fibrillation. Therefore, the antidromic reentrant tachycardia using atriofascicular pathway has characteristic features which demonstrate a relatively short ventriculoatrial interval and a long atrioventricular interval. Second, these pathways characterize decremental conduction property as like atrioventricular node. Needless to say, typical atrioventricular accessory pathways have no decremental conduction property. Third, these pathways are vulnerable to atrioventricular block by administering adenosine, which also seem to be acted as like atrioventricular node. Moreover, the timing of the right ventricular apical electrocardiogram may be helpful in distinguishing an atriofascicular pathway from a slowly conducting, right free-wall atrioventricular pathway [14]. The right ventricular apical electrocardiogram is relatively early in the former and late in the latter, compared to the delta wave on the surface electrocardiogram.

29.4.2 Differentiation Between Atriofascicular Pathway and Other Mahaim Pathways

There are also several differences of electrophysiological characteristics between atriofascicular and other Mahaim pathways. However, it is very difficult to distinguish and identify those three types of Mahaim fibers by checking the earliest atrial activation site during ventricular pacing, or by using para-Hisian pacing method, as these pathways conduct only in the anterograde direction. To diagnose and elucidate the circuit with atriofascicular pathways, recordings of both right bundle branch and His electrocardiogram are firstly needed.

Especially, it is important to confirm the relationship between the activation sequence of His and right bundle potential. During sinus rhythm, surface electrocardiogram shows little or no preexcitation, and activation of His potential precedes right bundle potential since that the stimulus from sinus node goes through atrioventricular node pathway. However, His bundle to right bundle activation sequence reverses during right atrial rapid pacing at cycle lengths of associated with maximal preexcitation (Fig. 29.2). This reversed sequence demonstrated that the right bundle branch and His bundle were activated in a retrograde direction when electrocardiogram showed maximal preexcitation of the QRS configuration.

Seconds, insertion of a single late atrial pacing can make reset the tachycardia in the cases with atriofascicular pathways. An atriofascicular pathway mostly plays a role of antidromic reciprocating tachycardia, in which the anterograde circuit is the accessory pathway and the retrograde route is atrioventricular node. During tachycardia, ventricular activation was advanced by the atrial pacing delivered at the time of refractoriness of the atrial septum, while the morphology of the QRS configuration was exactly same as that during tachycardia [9]. It suggested that the origination of the accessory pathway directly from the right atrium rather than from the atrioventricular node. However, it should be taken care that the advanced ventricular electrocardiogram could not be obtained by atrial pacing at random location. This lack of advancement was due to the distance from the pacing site to the reentrant circuit of tachycardia. As might be expected, the advanced ventricular electrocardiogram resets the tachycardia by atrial pacing located near the pathway of accessory fibers.

Third, the intra-electrocardiograms of the patients who have nodoventricular fibers occasionally represent ventriculoatrial dissociation during tachycardias. The tachycardia shows wide QRS configuration and each ventricular response is preceded by a His deflection. It clarifies that an atrial tissue is not involved in the circuit of reciprocating tachycardia. Gallagher reported that ventriculoatrial dissociation occurred during tachycardia in three of the six patients with having nodoventricular fibers, and the mechanism of this tachycardia circuit is a macroreentry using the nodoventricular fiber for the anterograde limb and the His-Purkinje system with a portion of the atrioventricular node for the retrograde limb [6].

With regard to fasciculoventricular pathway, no reciprocating tachycardia using this pathway could be observed [6].

29.5 Catheter Ablation

About thirty years ago, surgical operation of Mahaim fibers has been reported by several institutions for drug-refractory antidromic reciprocating tachycardia [11, 12]. In that era, some therapeutic approaches to patients with Mahaim fibers were also carried out including pharmacological therapy [15] and His bundle ablation [16]. Next, Häissaguerre described that three patients whose Mahaim fibers were successfully ablated by endocardial DC shocks applied at the ventricular insertion of the pathway in 1990 [17]. All three patients were free from tachycardia during 12–16 months of follow-up. Since then, a lot of cases of successful catheter ablation for Mahaim fibers were reported [13, 18–24], and the utility of radiofrequency catheter ablation for those fibers has been established. Especially, catheter ablation for atriofascicular pathway targeting Mahaim potential at tricuspid

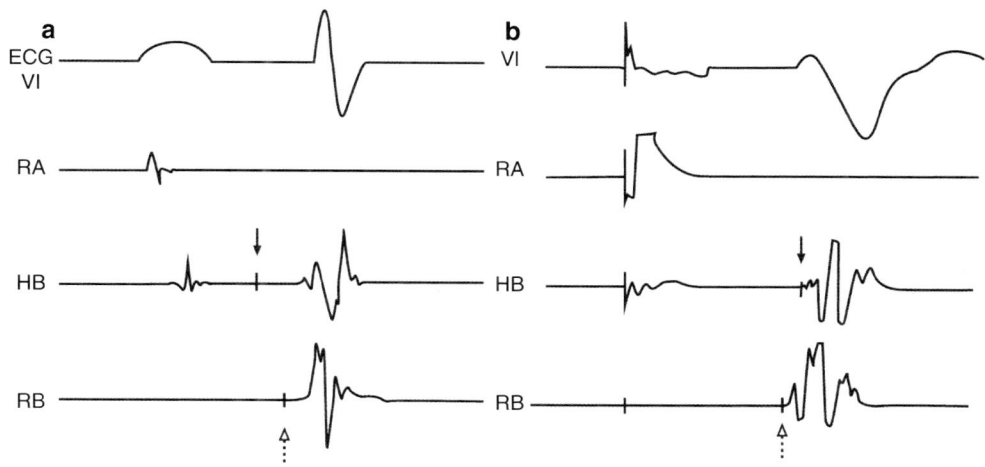

Fig. 29.2 Intra-electrocardiagraphic findings of the relationship between His bundle activation and right bundle activation. (**a**) His bundle activation (*solid arrow*) precedes right bundle branch activation (*dot arrow*) during sinus rhythm. (**b**) Right bundle branch activation precedes His bundle activation during right atrial pacing with preexcited QRS morphology. *ECG* electrocardiogram, *HB* His bundle, *RA* right atrium, *RB* right bundle

annulus is useful and widely recognized. In this chapter, several methods of catheter ablation for atriofascicular pathway are noted.

29.5.1 Catheter Ablation of Ventricular Insertion of Atriofascicular Pathway (Fig. 29.3)

As already described, Häissaguerre reported successful catheter ablation of Mahaim fibers in three patients [17]. Their ablation target sites of those fibers were ventricular insertion of the pathway found by using the criteria of concordance between paced and spontaneous QRS morphologies during pace mapping and the earliest onset of local electrocardiogram relative to surface preexcited QRS morphology. The complication related to the procedure in this paper was the creation of a permanent right bundle branch block in two of the three patients, but anomalous conduction in right bundle branch was present before the procedure in one of these two patients. Five years later, they also described the characteristics of the ventricular insertion sites of Mahaim fibers in ten patients with atriofascicular pathway and in eleven with atrioventricular accessory pathway [13]. In the first eleven patients, radiofrequency energy was delivered to the distal ventricular insertion sites of accessory pathway with a mean of 8 ± 5 applications. Although electrocardiographic preexcitation patterns have been changed either progressively in three patients or suddenly in one patient and right bundle branch block occurred in one patient by catheter ablation, successful catheter ablation at this site was obtained in only two patients. The procedure outcome in those cases might indicate that those pathways have a broad distal ventricular insertion supporting by the fact that spike potentials fusing with the earliest bipolar ventricular potentials could be recognized over the wide areas. Ventricular insertion of

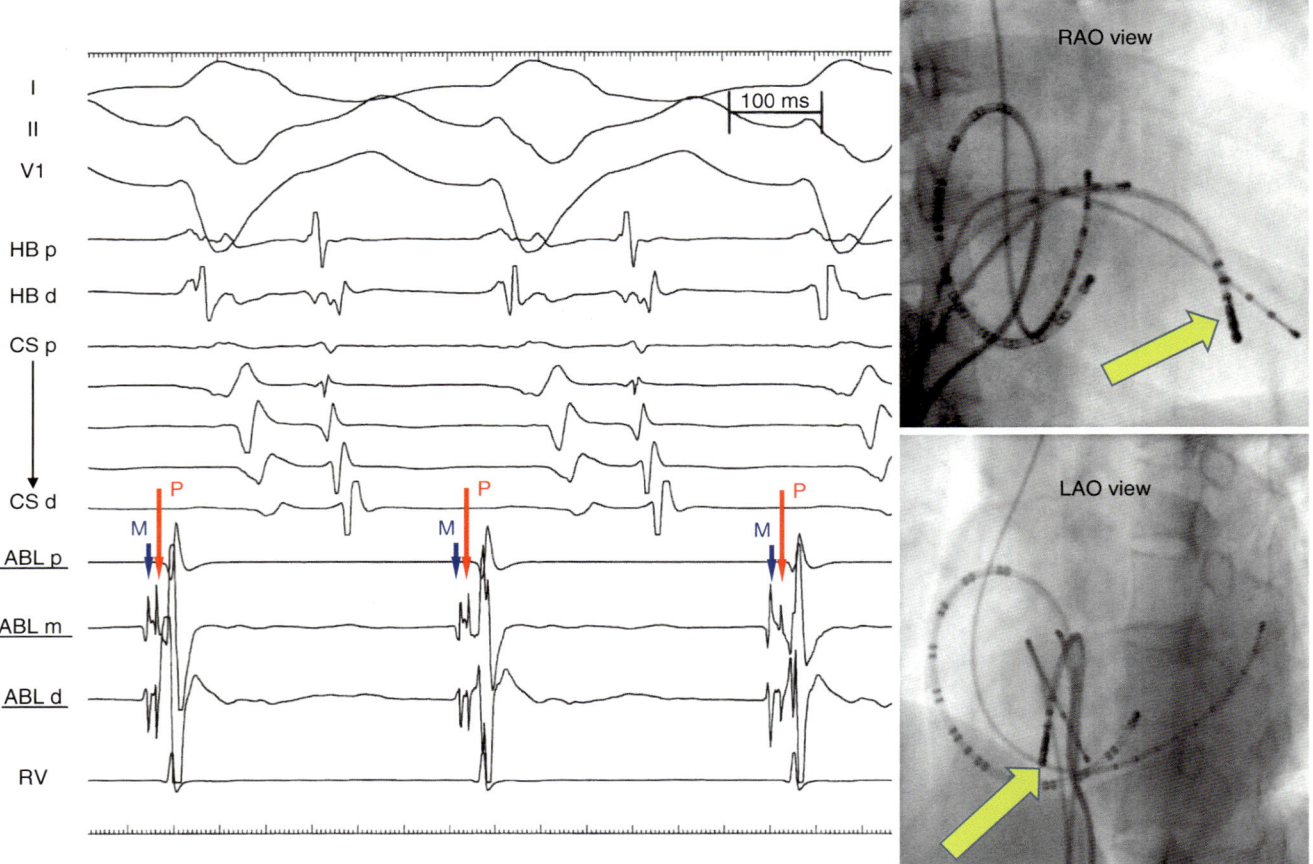

Fig. 29.3 The electrocardiogram recorded by ablation catheter located at the ventricular insertion site of atriofascicular pathway during antidromic reciprocating tachycardia (*yellow arrow*). ABLd, ABLm, ABLp; distal, mid, and proximal electrodes of ablation catheter, P (*red arrow*); Purkinje potential, M (*blue arrow*); Mahaim potential, LAO; left anterior oblique, RAO; right anterior oblique

atriofascicular fibers usually occur near the right ventricular apex. It might be difficult that the distal insertion of those pathways can be separated from the right bundle branch by a few applications of catheter ablation.

29.5.2 Catheter Ablation of Atrial Insertion of Atriofascicular Pathway

Due to the distal arborization of atriofascicular pathway fibers, radiofrequency catheter ablation of the atrial insertion of those fibers was performed [18, 25]. The atrial insertion site of this pathway is identified by introducing premature atrial stimulations at the tricuspid annulus during tachycardia to determine the site from which the latest atrial pacing beat preexcited right ventricle without advancing the atrium. This "reset phenomenon" clarified that the pacing site might be located on the circuit of antidromic reciprocating tachycardia, that is, on the atrial insertion site of atriofascicular pathway. The other approach is stimulus-to-delta wave mapping [18, 25]. Pace mapping in the right atrium during sinus rhythm can lead an atrial origin of accessory pathway, and the atrial insertion site was predicted by seeking the shortest stimulus-to-delta wave interval around the tricuspid annulus. However, those two techniques have a big same problem which each atrial pacing site at the tricuspid annulus should be severely limited. Moreover, the catheter is likely to be moved during tachycardia, and reliable stimulus-to-delta wave measurements might be difficult to obtain during the mapping procedure by changing heart rate or autonomic tone.

29.5.3 Catheter Ablation Targeting to the Tricuspid Annulus

Although atriofascicular pathways do not insert at the tricuspid annulus, the fact that they always pass through the annulus gave an important clue to separate those pathways [18, 19, 26, 27]. When the atriofascicular pathway mapping is performed during sinus rhythm, it is useful to be targeted to look for a single, discrete, high-frequency accessory pathway potential recorded between atrial and ventricular electrocardiogram. The catheter position and the timing of the accessory pathway potential serve to distinguish it from His potential. McClelland reported that those potential was recorded at the lateral, anterolateral, or posterolateral tricuspid annulus in 22 of the 23 patients 63 ± 12 ms after the local atrial potential and 83 ± 23 ms before the local ventricular potential during sinus rhythm [26]. Although the pathway potential can be identified from the mapping catheter only at a limited space at the tricuspid annulus, accessory pathway potentials were recognized at multiple sites along the right ventricular free wall, between the tricuspid annulus and the distal insertion near the right ventricular apex in many cases. As approaching right ventricular free wall close to the apex, this potential was recorded later. This suggests that an atriofascicular fiber runs through between the tricuspid annulus and the distal right bundle branch. From the previous paper, the right atriofascicular pathway was successfully ablated in a single session in all 23 patients [26]. The successful application of radiofrequency catheter ablation was performed close to the tricuspid annulus in 20 patients and at the right ventricular free wall in three patients [26].

Catheter ablation should be performed during right atrial pacing or antidromic reciprocating tachycardia to confirm the separation of accessory pathway in real-time. During radiofrequency energy, accessory pathway automaticity sometimes occurs, and presence of Mahaim automatic rhythm and its abolition during ablation is associated with long-term success of the procedure [28]. Besides, catheter trauma occasionally eliminates accessory pathway conduction, which clarifies that the atriofascicular pathways run through superficial right ventricular endocardium. Transient block of anterograde conduction induced by catheter manipulation at the subannular level proved to be reliable for precise mapping of atrial insertion of the accessory pathway [19].

Electroanatomical mapping is also useful for successful ablation of atriofascicular accessory pathway, as well as other various arrhythmias. Conventional mapping has a risk of prolonged traumatic loss of accessory pathway conduction. On the other hand, electroanatomical mapping can decrease such risk and make easy to perform the earliest ventricular activation mapping during preexcitation [21].

29.5.4 Catheter Ablation in the Patients Who Have No Mahaim Potential

Now that, a large, high-frequency Mahaim accessory pathway potential is helpful to identify an alternative site for catheter ablation. However, this potential could not be found along the tricuspid annulus in 14 of 29 study patients (48%) who had an atriofascicular pathway [23]. Catheter ablation targeting at the ventricular insertion is an option for such cases [24]. And, Mahaim potential mapping using electroanatomical mapping system during tachycardia seems to be another therapeutic option. We experienced a patient who had an antidromic reciprocating tachycardia related to an atriofascicular pathway. In this case, although a discrete accessory pathway potential could be recognized at free wall of right ventricle during tachycardia, we failed to identify this potential around the tricuspid annulus. Since right bundle branch block occurred by the catheter ablation targeting at ventricular insertion (Fig. 29.4), we speculate the atrial insertion site of the accessory pathway at the tricuspid annulus by using Mahaim potential mapping using electroanatomical mapping system, which could clearly visualize the course of this pathway (Fig. 29.5). When the ablation catheter was shifted to the presumed atrial insertion site during right atrial pacing, the delta wave was suddenly disappeared, which suggested atriofascicular pathway was transiently eliminated by catheter trauma. Radiofrequency energy was delivered at this site in order to achieve complete ablation lesion, which led to favorable long-term outcome.

29.5.5 The Outcome of Catheter Ablation

The acute success rate of catheter ablation of atriofascicular accessory pathway is more than 95%, and the recurrence rate is not so high [13, 18, 23, 26].

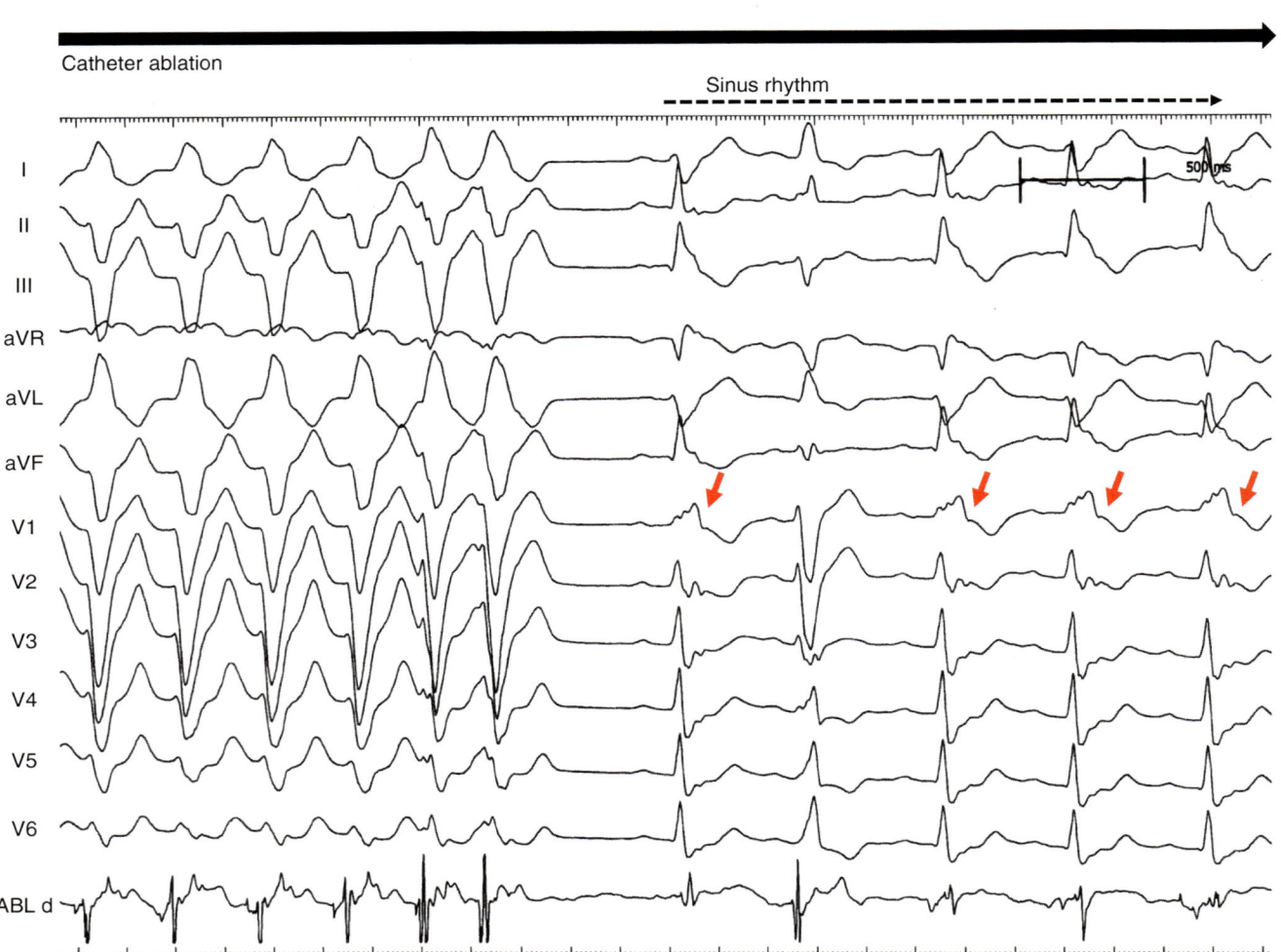

Fig. 29.4 Radiofrequency catheter ablation during antidromic reciprocating tachycardia. Tachycardia was terminated and transient right bundle branch block occurred (*red arrow*) by catheter ablation. Ablation catheter was placed at the ventricular insertion site of atriofascicular pathway

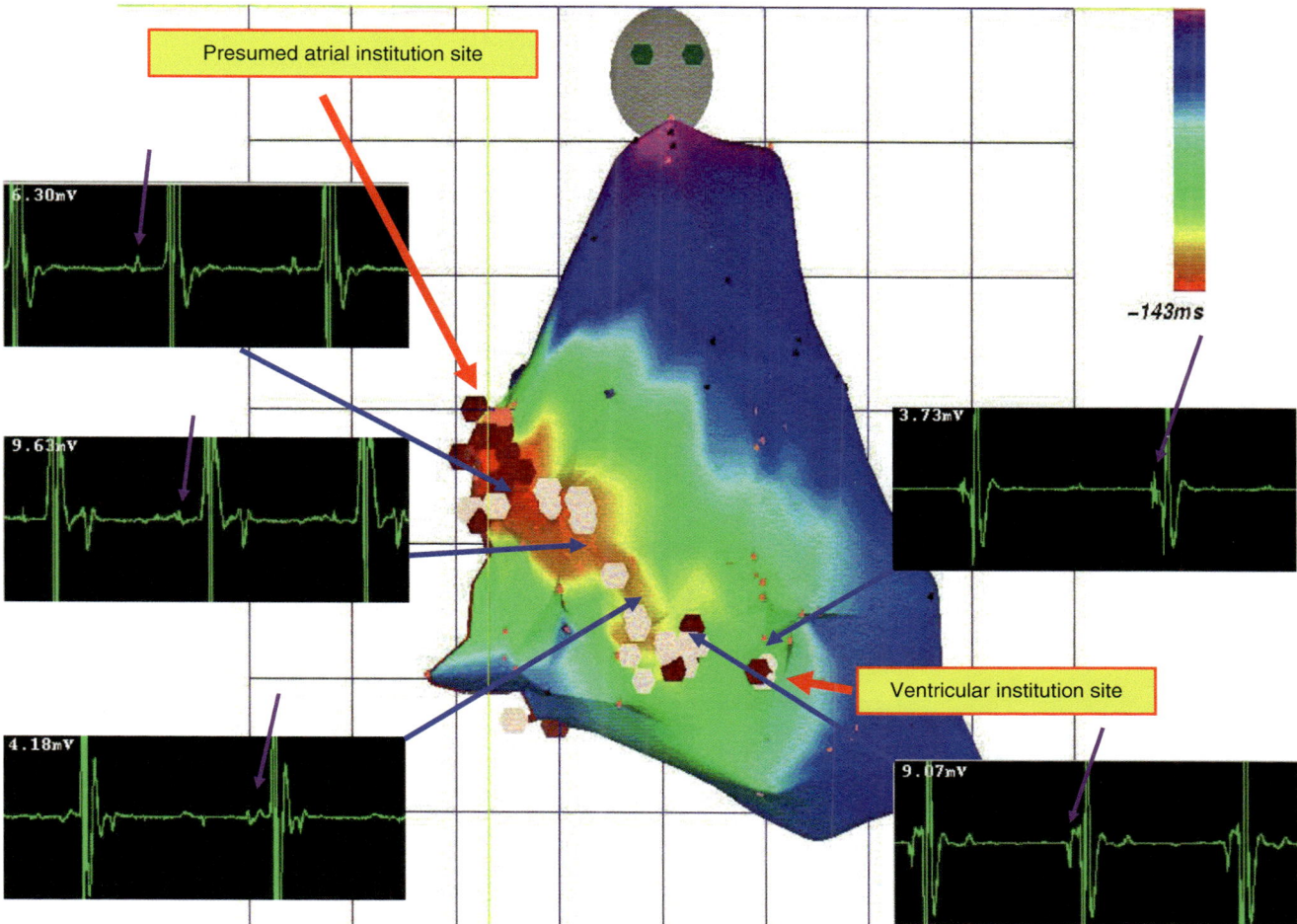

Fig. 29.5 Mahaim potential mapping during antidromic reciprocating tachycardia. *Purple arrow* shows Mahaim potential. Electroanatomical mapping system (CARTO; Biosense Webster, Inc., Diamond Bar, California, USA) can clearly visualize the course of the atriofascicular pathway during tachycardia

Conflicts of Interests None declared.

References

1. Mahaim IBA. Nouvelles recherches sur les connexions superieures de la branche gauche du faisceau de His-Tawara avec cloison interventriculaire. Cardiologia. 1938;1:61–73.
2. Mahaim I. Kent's fibers and the A-V paraspecific conduction through the upper connections of the bundle of His-Tawara. Am Heart J. 1947;33(5):651–3.
3. Mahaim IWM. Recherches d' anatomie compar6e et de pathologie experimentale sur les connexions hautes du faisceau de His-Tawara. Cardiologia. 1941;5:189.
4. Lev M, Fox SM III, Bharati S, Greenfield JC Jr, Rosen KM, Pick A. Mahaim and James fibers as a basis for a unique variety of ventricular preexcitation. Am J Cardiol. 1975;36(7):880–8.
5. Tonkin AM, Dugan FA, Svenson RH, Sealy WC, Wallace AG, Gallagher JJ. Coexistence of functional Kent and Mahaim-type tracts in the pre-excitation syndrome. Demonstration by catheter techniques and epicardial mapping. Circulation. 1975;52(2):193–200.

6. Gallagher JJ, Smith WM, Kasell JH, Benson DW Jr, Sterba R, Grant AO. Role of Mahaim fibers in cardiac arrhythmias in man. Circulation. 1981;64(1):176–89.
7. Anderson RH, Becker AE, Brechenmacher C, Davies MJ, Rossi L. Ventricular preexcitation. A proposed nomenclature for its substrates. Eur J Cardiol. 1975;3(1):27–36.
8. Bardy GH, German LD, Packer DL, Coltorti F, Gallagher JJ. Mechanism of tachycardia using a nodofascicular Mahaim fiber. Am J Cardiol. 1984;54(8):1140–1.
9. Tchou P, Lehmann MH, Jazayeri M, Akhtar M. Atriofascicular connection or a nodoventricular Mahaim fiber? Electrophysiologic elucidation of the pathway and associated reentrant circuit. Circulation. 1988;77(4):837–48.
10. Inoue H, Matsuo H, Takayanagi K, Ishimitsu T, Murao S. Antidromic reciprocating tachycardia via a slow Kent bundle in Ebstein's anomaly. Am Heart J. 1983;106(1 Pt 1):147–9.
11. Klein GJ, Guiraudon GM, Kerr CR, Sharma AD, Yee R, Szabo T, et al. "Nodoventricular" accessory pathway: evidence for a distinct accessory atrioventricular pathway with atrioventricular node-like properties. J Am Coll Cardiol. 1988;11(5):1035–40.
12. Gillette PC, Garson A Jr, Cooley DA, McNamara DG. Prolonged and decremental antegrade conduction properties in right anterior accessory connections: wide QRS antidromic tachycardia of left bundle branch block pattern without Wolff-Parkinson-White configuration in sinus rhythm. Am Heart J. 1982;103(1):66–74.
13. Haissaguerre M, Cauchemez B, Marcus F, Le Metayer P, Lauribe P, Poquet F, et al. Characteristics of the ventricular insertion sites of accessory pathways with anterograde decremental conduction properties. Circulation. 1995;91(4):1077–85.
14. Chugh ABF, Morady F. Cather ablation of cardiac arrhythmias. catheter ablation of accessory pathways. Carlton, VIC: Blackwell Futura; 2008.
15. Strasberg B, Coelho A, Palileo E, Bauernfeind R, Swiryn S, Scagliotti D, et al. Pharmacological observations in patients with nodoventricular pathways. Br Heart J. 1984;51(1):84–90.
16. Bhandari A, Morady F, Shen EN, Schwartz AB, Botvinick E, Scheinman MM. Catheter-induced His bundle ablation in a patient with reentrant tachycardia associated with a nodoventricular tract. J Am Coll Cardiol. 1984;4(3):611–6.
17. Haissaguerre M, Warin JF, Le Metayer P, Maraud L, De Roy L, Montserrat P, et al. Catheter ablation of Mahaim fibers with preservation of atrioventricular nodal conduction. Circulation. 1990;82(2):418–27.
18. Klein LS, Hackett FK, Zipes DP, Miles WM. Radiofrequency catheter ablation of Mahaim fibers at the tricuspid annulus. Circulation. 1993;87(3):738–47.
19. Cappato R, Schluter M, Weiss C, Siebels J, Hebe J, Duckeck W, et al. Catheter-induced mechanical conduction block of right-sided accessory fibers with Mahaim-type preexcitation to guide radiofrequency ablation. Circulation. 1994;90(1):282–90.
20. Okishige K, Goseki Y, Itoh A, Tsuboi N, Sasano T, Azegami K, et al. New electrophysiologic features and catheter ablation of atrioventricular and atriofascicular accessory pathways: evidence of decremental conduction and the anatomic structure of the Mahaim pathway. J Cardiovasc Electrophysiol. 1998;9(1):22–33.
21. Paydak H, Piros P, Scheinman MM, Dorostkar PC. Localization and radiofrequency ablation of atriofascicular pathways using electroanatomic mapping. J Electrocardiol. 2003;36(2):105–10.
22. Silva MA, Berardi G, Kraemer A, Nadalin E, Jorge JC. Catheter ablation of atriofascicular Mahaim fibers guided by the activation potential. Arq Bras Cardiol. 2003;80(1):66–70.
23. Kothari S, Gupta AK, Lokhandwala YY, Vora AM, Kerkar PG, Thakur RK. Atriofascicular pathways: where to ablate? Pacing Clin Electrophysiol. 2006;29(11):1226–33.
24. Ducceschi V, Vitale R, Ottaviano L, Sokola EA, Sangiuolo R, Gregorio G. Ablating the ventricular insertion of atrio-fascicular Mahaim fiber: what selection criteria should we use? J Interv Card Electrophysiol. 2009;25(3):207–11.
25. Okishige KSS, Walsh EP, Saul JP, Friedman PL. Catheter ablation of the atrial origin of a detrimentally conducting atriofascicular accessory pathway by radiofrequency current. J Cardiovasc Electrophysiol. 1991;2:465–75.
26. McClelland JH, Wang X, Beckman KJ, Hazlitt HA, Prior MI, Nakagawa H, et al. Radiofrequency catheter ablation of right atriofascicular (Mahaim) accessory pathways guided by accessory pathway activation potentials. Circulation. 1994;89(6):2655–66.
27. Heald SC, Davies DW, Ward DE, Garratt CJ, Rowland E. Radiofrequency catheter ablation of Mahaim tachycardia by targeting Mahaim potentials at the tricuspid annulus. Br Heart J. 1995;73(3):250–7.
28. Singh B, Gupta RK, Dhall A, Ghose T, Trehan R, Kaul U. Mahaim automatic accelerated rhythm: a marker of successful radiofrequency ablation. Indian Heart J. 2004;56(3):215–9.

30. Nodofascicular/Nodoventricular Accessory Pathway

Nitish Badhwar and Melvin M. Scheinman

Keywords
Nodofascicular tachycardia • Nodoventricular tachycardia

30.1 Introduction

Mahaim was the first to describe accessory pathways arising from AV node inserting in fascicles or ventricular myocardium [1]. This has to be differentiated from typical AV accessory pathway (Kent fiber seen in WPW syndrome) and fasciculo-ventricular fibers that never participate in tachycardia (Fig. 30.1) [2–6]. The term "Mahaim tachycardia" is often inappropriately used for atriofascicular tachycardia that is antidromic tachycardia with left bundle branch left axis morphology on 12 lead ECG. The antegrade limb is a decremental AV node like fiber that courses over the lateral tricuspid annulus and inserts into or near the right bundle branch and the retrograde limb is the AV node (Fig 30.2a). The atrium is an integral part of this circuit and successful ablation is usually performed in lateral tricuspid annulus at the proximal insertion site of the atriofascicular fiber. True Mahaim tachycardia is manifest or concealed NF/NV tachycardia using the Mahaim fiber as an antegrade or retrograde limb and AV node as the other limb (Fig 30.2b). The atrium is not an integral part of the circuit in this form of SVT. Recent studies have shown this to be an important differential diagnosis in SVT that presents with VA dissociation.

30.2 Clinical Presentation

Patients with NFT/NVT present with paroxysmal SVT similar to other mechanisms of SVT (AVNRT, AVRT, and atrial tachycardia). Symptoms include sudden onset palpitations, shortness of breath, dizziness, and rarely syncope if the rates are too fast. Rarely these patients can present with incessant SVT that can lead to tachycardia induced cardiomyopathy. The 12 lead ECG usually shows narrow complex SVT (concealed NFT/NVT), while wide complex tachycardia is inscribed in antidromic NFT/NVT (Fig. 30.3) and has to be differentiated from ventricular tachycardia. SVT with aberrancy in patients with rapid concealed NFT/NVT can also present as wide complex tachycardia. Incessant NVT has been reported in a patient with AV block who was s/p pacemaker implantation [7]. Presence of AV dissociation during narrow complex SVT on 12 lead ECG is a clue to the diagnosis of NFT/NVT. This form of SVT terminates with Valsalva, carotid sinus massage and adenosine as the circuit involves the AV node. These patients may respond to AV nodal blocking drugs (beta-blockers or Ca channel blockers).

30.3 Manifest NFT/NVT

Antidromic conduction down the NF/NV fiber will lead to a wide preexcited QRS complex. This can manifest as

1. Double fire (one atrial complex leading to narrow QRS due to ventricular activation via His bundle and wide QRS due to ventricular activation via NF/NV fiber).
2. Bystander preexcited tachycardia (SVT with ventricular activation via NF/NV fiber).

N. Badhwar, M.D. (✉) • M.M. Scheinman, M.D.
Section of Cardiac Electrophysiology, Division of Cardiology, University of California San Francisco,
500 Parnassus Avenue, MUE- 431, Box 1354,
San Francisco, CA 94143, USA
e-mail: nitish.badhwar@ucsf.edu

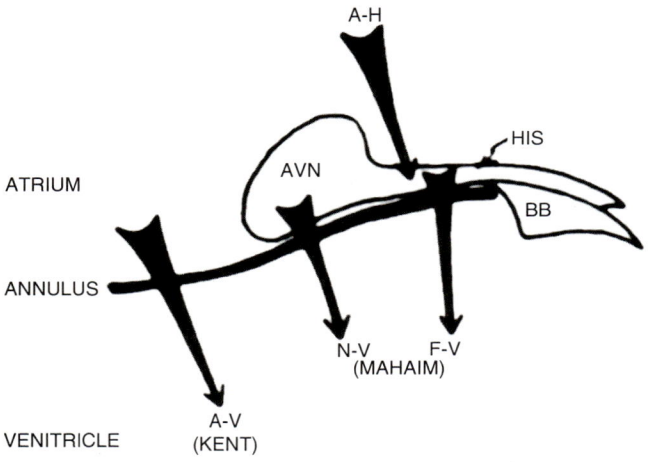

Fig. 30.1 Variants of preexcitation

3. Antidromic tachycardia where the NV/NF fiber is antegrade limb and AV node is the retrograde limb (Table 30.1) [4, 8–12].

Variable QRS morphologies can be seen in patients with manifest NF/NV fibers depending on the distal insertion site of the fiber (LBBB left inferior axis (Fig. 30.3), LBBB left superior axis and RBBB inferior axis) [8]. Presence of AV dissociation ruled out extranodal accessory pathway mediated antidromic tachycardia. Coexistent tachycardias were noted in these patients including AVNRT and AVRT. It is therefore critical to determine the mechanism critical for tachycardia maintenance because targeting the NFV may not eliminate tachycardia in cases where it is a bystander. Elimination of manifest NF/NV fibers conduction was noted after ablation

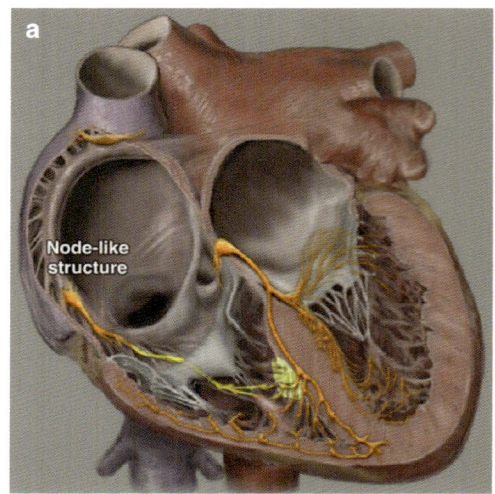
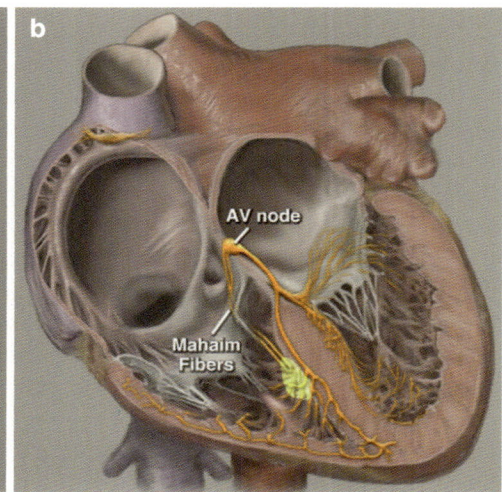

Fig. 30.2 (a) Atriofascicular fiber. (b) Nodofascicular pathway

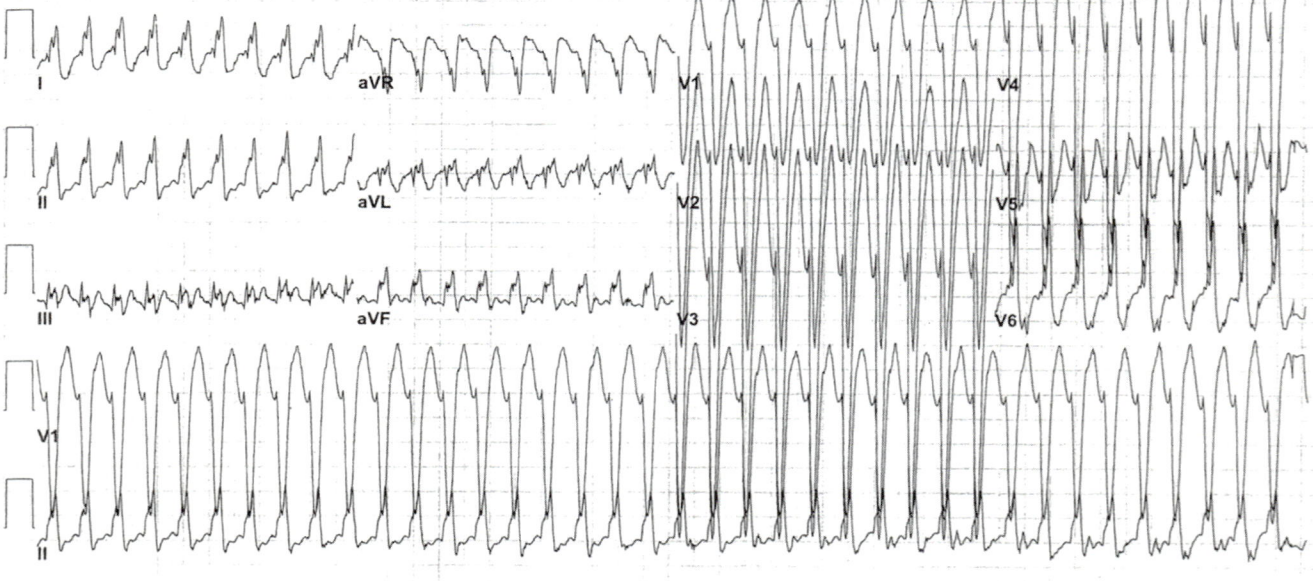

Fig. 30.3 Antidromic nodoventricular tachycardia

Table 30.1 Nodofascicular/ventricular tachycardia

- Manifest NF/NV tachycardia
  - Double fire
  - Preexcited bystander
  - Antidromic tachycardia
- Concealed NF/NV tachycardia

Table 30.2 SVT with VA block

- AVNRT with upper common pathway block
- Focal junctional tachycardia
- Concealed NFT/NVT tachycardia
- Intra-hisian reentry

Table 30.3 Diagnostic maneuvers for NF/NVT

- AV dissociation during SVT (spontaneous or pacing induced)
- His refractory PVC during SVT advanced / delayed the next His and V or terminated SVT
- Bundle branch block leads to prolongation of VA interval or tachycardia cycle length
- $VA_{RVPACE} - VA_{SVT} > 85$ ms
- $AH_{AOD} - AH_{SVT} > 40$ ms
- His overdrive pacing during SVT showing A capture in <2 beats
- Ventricular Fusion with VOD during SVT proves NVT
- Programmed RV extrastimuli showing antegrade His activation

at traditional slow pathway region in three patients and after surgical closure of atrial septal defect in one patient [8].

30.4 Concealed NFT/NVT

Concealed NF/NV tachycardia is more common than manifest NF/NV tachycardia [13–16]. It is an important differential diagnosis in patients who present with SVT and are noted to have VA dissociation or block (Table 30.2). The differential diagnosis includes AVNRT, focal junctional tachycardia, and intra-hisian reentrant tachycardia. The circuit for concealed NF/NV involves AV node His Bundle activation in antegrade manner and NF/NV fiber is the retrograde limb. This form of SVT shows a narrow QRS complex with His preceding every QRS. It can be wide complex tachycardia with typical bundle branch.

Recent description of this uncommon form of SVT shows that most of the patients have a critical AV delay (usually prolongation of infranodal and infra-hisian conduction) to sustain tachycardia. It is possible that the delay allows the concealed NF/NV fiber to conduct and sustain tachycardia. In a recent series, even though the His bundle potential could not be recorded in patients, infranodal disease was inferred because of PR prolongation and different PR with right versus left bundle branch block patterns during atrial pacing at the same rate. SVT was readily initiated by atrial programmed stimulation in all and by ventricular extrastimuli in two [16].

Table 30.3 shows various diagnostic maneuvers that can be done during SVT to make a diagnosis of NF/NV tachycardia [17]. The first step in differential diagnosis is to rule out orthodromic atrioventricular reentrant tachycardia (AVRT):

1. Most of the patients had A on V SVT that rules out AVRT (septal VA <60 ms).
2. In patients with short RP tachycardia presence of VA dissociation or block rules out extranodal accessory pathway participation. This can be noted spontaneously or can be induced by atrial pacing and dissociating it from the tachycardia.
3. Another differentiating finding is the presence of shorter AH during tachycardia as compared to atrial pacing at same cycle length from high right atrium. This argues for a parallel activation of atrium and His during tachycardia as noted in AV nodal tachycardia; AVRT has series activation and will have similar AH during tachycardia and atrial pacing [18].

Once that is done the next step is to rule out AVNRT with upper common pathway block and focal junctional tachycardia. This is done by proving that the ventricle is an integral part of the circuit. It is our practice to give V on His in patients even during A on V SVT.

1. Spontaneous or paced ventricular extrastimulus given when the His bundle is committed that pulls in (Fig. 30.4), pushes out the next His/V or terminates SVT proves the participation of accessory pathway and makes a diagnosis of concealed NF/NV tachycardia (typical AV accessory pathway was ruled out by AV dissociation).
2. Presence of bundle branch block or HV prolongation that prolongs the tachycardia cycle length also proves the participation of NF/NV fiber.
3. His overdrive pacing during SVT that leads to capture of atrium in less than or equal to two beats has also been shown to prove participation of accessory pathway in SVT [19].
4. Right ventricular extrastimulus delivered during sinus rhythm or SVT that shows antegrade activation of his bundle also proves participation of accessory pathway in SVT [17].

In a recent study, it was shown that patients with NV tachycardia showed a fused V during overdrive pacing or with the V on His that terminated tachycardia or pulled in or pushed out the next His and V. Fusion in the V argues for insertion of the fiber in the ventricle proving that most of the cases are NVT. It was also noted that the post pacing interval when doing overdrive pacing from RV apex was longer than when pacing from the base. This implies that most cases are NVT where the NV fiber is attached at the base of the ventricle [20]. This can also be used to map the distal insertion site of the Mahaim fiber and target that for successful ablation.

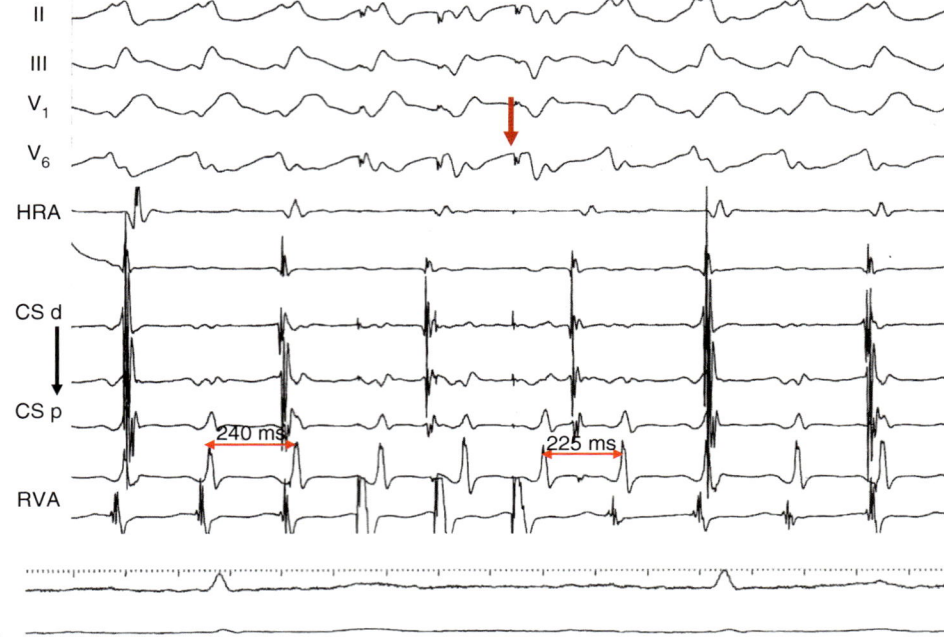

Fig. 30.4 PVC on His that advances the next V during wide complex tachycardia with VA block

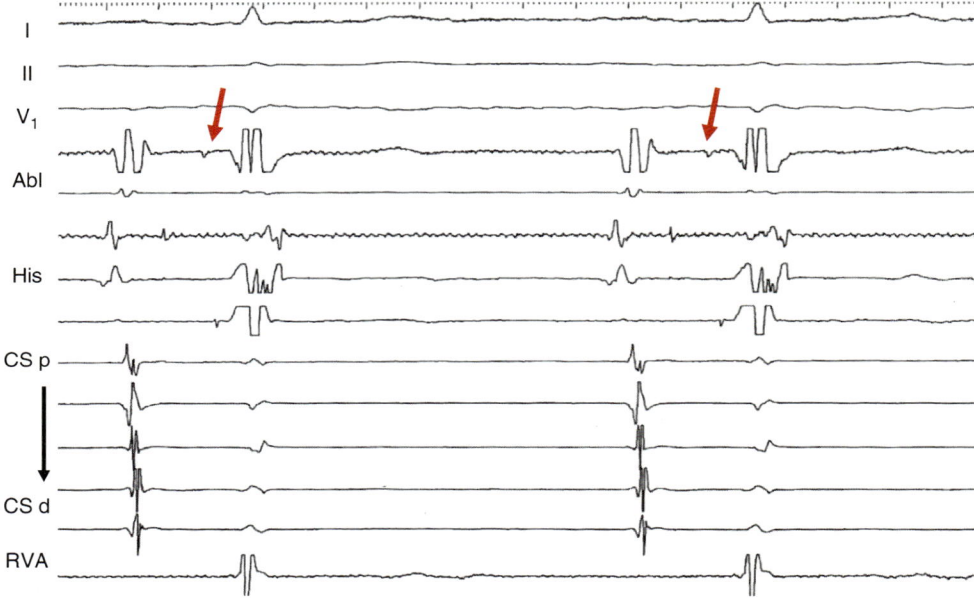

Fig. 30.5 Discrete potential on the ablator at the successful site within the coronary sinus

30.5 Catheter Ablation

Radiofrequency catheter ablation for NF/NV fibers was initially reported in 1994 by Wen. They failed in the ostium of the coronary sinus and were successful in the RV. Grogin et al. reported their experience in two patients with NVT where ablations at posterior septal region and anterior septal region were unsuccessful. PR prolongation was noted with ablation in the fast pathway region. Successful ablation was performed in the mid-septal region without AV block [8]. Haissaguerre et al. reported their result in a patient with NVT where they were unsuccessful in posterior, mid and anterior septal region. They were successful anteriorly below the tricuspid valve region [9]. Okishige et al. reported complete heart block while ablating in the mid-septal region for NVT [10]. Kottkamp et al. reported their experience with ablation of NVT in the fast pathway region that resulted in increased PR interval [11]. Hamdan et al. were not successful with ablation in mid-septal and posterior septal region in patient with right sided NVT [12]. Hluchy et al. reported successful ablation of concealed NVT in the mid-septal region guided by pathway potential without AV block [13].

We recently reported our experience in 15 patients from different centers. Three patients showed a discrete potential in the CS between the atrial (A) and the ventricular (V) electrograms during sinus rhythm that was recorded 3–4 cm in the CS (Fig. 30.5). In one patient this potential was mapped back to the proximal CS along the roof of the CS. Catheter ablation was successful at the site in the CS showing the largest potential. Mapping and ablation at distal insertion site in two patients with manifest NVT was not successful. Successful ablation sites in the other pts were the slow pathway region (10 pts) and fast pathway region (2 pt). PR prolongation was noted in ablation performed at the fast pathway region but no AV block was noted in this series. Junctional rhythm was noted at proximal insertion site in the AV node [21, 22].

30.6 Summary

So-called variant accessory pathways are increasingly recognized as being responsible for tachycardia circuits. Atriofascicular pathways have been well categorized by the work of Jackman and Haïssaguerre [23, 24]. Less well appreciated are pathways that bridge the AV node and fascicles or ventricles (true Mahaim tracts). These pathways are recognized by using maneuvers to exclude extranodal pathway but yet provide evidence that a pathway is present. We have also emphasized the diverse sites of ablation for these NF/NV pathways.

References

1. Mahaim I, Benatt A. Nouvelles recherches sur les connexions sperieures de la branche gauche du faisceau de His-Tawara avec cloison interventriculaire. Cariologia. 1938;1:61–120.
2. Klein GJ, Guiraudon GM, Kerr CR, Sharma AD, Yee R, Szabo T, Wah JA. "Nodoventricular" accessory pathway: evidence for a distinct accessory atrioventricular pathway with atrioventricular node-like properties. J Am Coll Cardiol. 1988;11:1035–40.
3. Tchou P, Lehmann MH, Jazayeri M, Akhtar M. Atriofascicular connection or a nodoventricular Mahaim fiber? Electrophysiologic elucidation of the pathway and associated reentrant circuit. Circulation. 1988;77:837–48.
4. Sternick EB. Mahaim fibre tachycardia: recognition and management. Indian Pacing Electrophysiol J. 2003;3:47–59.
5. Abbott JA, Scheinman MM, Morady F, Shen EN, Miller R, Ruder MA, Eldar M, Seger JJ, Davis JC, Griffin JC. Coexistent Mahaim and Kent accessory connections: diagnostic and therapeutic implications. J Am Coll Cardiol. 1987;10:364–72.
6. Gallagher JJ, Smith WM, Kasell JH, Benson DW Jr, Sterba R, Grant AO. Role of Mahaim fibers in cardiac arrhythmias in man. Circulation. 1981;64:176–89.
7. Quinn FR, Mitchell LB, Mardell AP, Dal Disler RN, Veenhuyzen GD. Entrainment mapping of a concealed nodoventricular accessory pathway in a man with complete heart block and tachycardia-induced cardiomyopathy. J Cardiovasc Electrophysiol. 2008;19(1):90–4.
8. Hoffmayer KS, Lee BK, Vedantham V, Bhimani AA, Cakulev IT, Mackall JA, Sahadevan J, Rho RW, Scheinman MM. Variable clinical features and ablation of manifest nodofascicular/ventricular pathways. Circ Arrhythm Electrophysiol. 2015;8:117–27.
9. Grogin HR, Lee RJ, Kwasman M, Epstein LM, Schamp DJ, Lesh MD, Scheinman MM. Radiofrequency catheter ablation of atriofascicular and nodoventricular Mahaim tracts. Circulation. 1994;90:272–81.
10. Haïssaguerre M, Campos J, Marcus FI, Papouin G, Clémenty J. Involvement of a nodofascicular connection in supraventricular tachycardia with VA dissociation. J Cardiovasc Electrophysiol. 1994;5:854–62.
11. Okishige K, Friedman PL. New observations on decremental atriofascicular and nodofascicular fibers: implications for catheter ablation. Pacing Clin Electrophysiol. May 1995;18(5 Pt 1):986–98.
12. Kottkamp H, Hindricks G, Shenasa H, Chen X, Wichter T, Borggrefe M, Breithardt G. Variants of preexcitation–specialized atriofascicular pathways, nodofascicular pathways, and fasciculoventricular pathways: electrophysiologic findings and target sites for radiofrequency catheter ablation. J Cardiovasc Electrophysiol. 1996;7:916–30.
13. Hamdan MH, Kalman JM, Lesh MD, Lee RJ, Saxon LA, Dorostkar P, Scheinman MM. Narrow complex tachycardia with VA block: diagnostic and therapeutic implications. Pacing Clin Electrophysiol. 1998;21:1196–206.
14. Hluchy J, Schickel S, Jörger U, Jurkovicova O, Sabin GV. Electrophysiologic characteristics and radiofrequency ablation of concealed nodofascicular and left anterograde atriofascicular pathways. J Cardiovasc Electrophysiol. 2000;11:211–7.
15. Ho RT, Frisch DR, Pavri BB, Levi SA, Greenspon AJ. Electrophysiological features differentiating the atypical atrioventricular node-dependent long RP supraventricular tachycardias. Circ Arrhythm Electrophysiol. 2013;6:597–605.
16. Badhwar N, Saarel EV, Germano JJ, Josephson ME, Scheinman MM. Concealed nodofascicular, (nodoventricular) tachycardia: electrophysiological characteristics and response to catheter ablation. Heart Rhythm. 2006;3(5):S196.
17. Badhwar N, Saarel EV, Dorostkar PC, Mehta D, Morady F, Stevenson WG, Josephson ME, Tchou PJ, Scheinman MM. Diagnostic maneuvers in patients with concealed nodofascicular, (nodoventricular) tachycardia. Heart Rhythm. 2013;10(5):S29.
18. Man KC, Niebauer M, Daoud E, Strickberger SA, Kou W, Williamson BD, Morady F. Comparison of atrial-His intervals during tachycardia and atrial pacing in patyients with long RP tachycardia. J Cardiovasc Electrophysiol. 1995;6:700–10.
19. Singh DK, Viswanathan MN, Tanel RE, Lee RJ, Lee BK, Marcus GM, Olgin JE, Han F, Vedantham V, Tseng ZH, Pellegrini C, Kawamura M, Gerstenfeld EP, Badhwar N, Scheinman MM. His overdrive pacing during supraventricular tachycardia: a novel maneuver for distinguishing atrioventricular nodal reentrant tachycardia from atrioventricular reciprocating tachycardia. Heart Rhythm. 2014;11(8):1327–35.
20. Badhwar N, Saarel EV, Kanj MH, Germano JJ, Dresing T, Tiyyagaru S, Roberts-Thompson KC, Jongnarangsin K, Mehta D, Morady F, Stevenson WG, Tchou PJ, Josephson ME, Scheinman MM. Role of ventricular pacing to elicit the distal insertion site in patients with concealed nodofascicular, (nodoventricular) tachycardia. Heart Rhythm. 2009;6(5):S103.
21. Badhwar N, Johnson CJ, Tchou PJ, Scheinman MM. Role of CS potential in successful mapping and ablation of left sided concealed nodofascicular/nodoventricular Tachycardia. Heart Rhythm. 2015;12(5):S172.
22. Badhwar N, Johnson CJ, Kalman JM, Stevenson WG, Tchou PJ, Mehta D, Saarel EV, Dorostkar PC, Sham'a RA, Birnie DH, Josephson ME, Scheinman MM. Successful site of ablation of nodoventricular tract: dustal vs proximal insertion. Heart Rhythm. 2016;13(5):S593.
23. Haïssaguerre M, Cauchemez B, Marcus F, Le Metayer P, Lauribe P, Poquet F, Gencel L, Clémenty J. Characteristics of the ventricular insertion sites of accessory pathways with anterograde decremental conduction properties. Circulation. 1995;91(4):1077–85.
24. Haïssaguerre M, Cauchemez B, Marcus F, Le Metayer P, Lauribe P, Poquet F, Gencel L, Clémenty J. Radiofrequency catheter ablation of right atriofascicular (Mahaim) accessory pathways guided by accessory pathway activation potentials. Circulation. 1994;89(6):2655–66.

Part VIII
Catheter Ablation of Ventricular Tachycardias

31. Outflow Tract Ventricular Tachycardias and Ventricular Premature Contractions: ECG-Based Prediction of Origin Sites

Hitoshi Hachiya

Keywords
ECG • Outflow tract • Ventricular arrhythmia • Catheter ablation

31.1 Introduction

Ventricular arrhythmias (VAs), such as ventricular premature contractions (VPCs) and ventricular tachycardia (VT) in patients without structural heart disease (idiopathic VA), mainly arise from the right and left ventricular outflow tracts (RVOT/LVOT) [1]. Prognosis in such patients is generally good, but there is a very small risk for malignant ventricular arrhythmias triggered in the RVOT-VAs [2, 3]. Moreover, it is known that a successful radiofrequency catheter ablation (RFCA) of outflow tract VA (OT-VA) improves the left ventricular dilation, ejection fraction, and clinical status in patients whose cardiac function is reduced due to increased OT-VA [4–7]. Therefore, RFCA is on its way to becoming treatment of choice for patients with OT-VA.

In approximately 70–80% of cases, the RVOT is the most common site for idiopathic VAs [8, 9]. RVOT-VAs occur more frequently in women than in men [10, 11], for example, with proportion of women cited as 59% in one study [11] (Table 31.1). Within RVOT-VAs, VPCs are more common than VTs [10]. Patients with RVOT-VAs are also younger than those with LVOT-VAs [11] (Fig. 31.1).

31.2 Which Patients Are Candidates for OT-VA Ablation?

31.2.1 Patients with Symptomatic VA

The vast majority of patients who have VPCs but no structural heart disease have a benign prognosis. Therefore, catheter ablation of VPCs is for the most part recommended for highly selected patients who remain very symptomatic despite conservative treatment, or for those with very high VPC burdens associated with a decline in LV systolic function [12]. Additionally, patients with short coupled VPCs may be at increased risk for malignant VAs [12, 13].

Although patients with only RVOT-VPCs are often treated conservatively, we believe that they should be periodically studied with Holter monitoring and referred for radiofrequency ablation if the short-coupled variant of RVOT-VT with polymorphic morphology is recognized [13] because of the potential (albeit unproven) role of short coupled VPCs in triggering more malignant arrhythmias.

Table 31.1 Gender differences in candidates for radiofrequency catheter ablation of RVOT-VAs and LVOT-VAs

Arrhythmia origin	No. (%)	VT	VPC	Male	Female
OT-VA	490	156	334	227	263
RVOT	331 (68)	105	226	135	196
LVOT (endocardial site, aortic sinus of Valsalva, epicardial site: the distal great cardiac vein, etc.)	159 (32)	51	108	92	67

Modified from Tanaka Y, et al. Circ J 75:1585-1591, 2011
OT-VA outflow tract ventricular arrhythmia, *RVOT* right ventricular outflow tract, *LVOT* left ventricular outflow tract, *VT* ventricular tachycardia, *VPC* ventricular premature contraction

H. Hachiya
Cardiovascular Center, Tsuchiura Kyodo Hospital,
4-1-1 Otsuno, Tsuchiura, Ibaraki 300-0028, Japan
e-mail: hh8814.cvm@tmd.ac.jp

31.2.2 Tachycardia-Induced Cardiomyopathy

A report published by Takemoto et al. suggests that frequent (>20%) RVOT-VPC may be a possible cause of LV dysfunction and/or heart failure, and RFCA produces clinical benefit in these patients [4]. Latchamsetty et al. studied 245 patients (21%) with an ejection fraction <50% who underwent VPC ablation. Independent predictors for VPC-induced cardiomyopathy by multivariate logistic regression analysis were male gender, lack of symptoms, high VPC burden, and an epicardial VPC location. After ablation, the mean VPC burden (VPC count/QRS count) in these patients decreased from 27% to 5% ($p < 0.01$), and mean ejection fraction increased from 38% to 50% [7].

31.3 ECG Algorithm for Identification of Origin Sites

Figure 31.2 shows an algorithm we developed [14] for identifying OT-VA origin sites based on VA ECG waveform analysis, by amalgamating findings in the literature. The sites are classified into the following five groups [14]:

Group 1: Right ventricular outflow tract (RVOT) excluding the pulmonary artery and His bundle regions.
Group 2: Pulmonary artery (PA).
Group 3: Near His bundle region (His).
Group 4: Endocardial left ventricular OT (LVOT).
Group 5: Difficult cases defined as those in which RFCA was unsuccessful at the best mapping site or which was successful on the coronary cusps or in the distal great cardiac vein (GCV)/anterior interventricular vein (AIV).

Step 1. Although it is always important to analyze the electrocardiographic precordial transition and frontal plane QRS axis of the spontaneous VA when determining site of

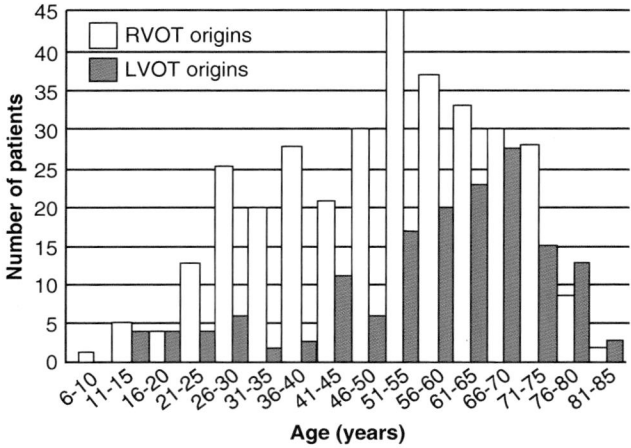

Fig. 31.1 Age distribution of patients with idiopathic ventricular arrhythmias arising from the RVOT and LVOT. In this graph, the difference in the age of the patients with RVOT and LVOT origins is shown; patients with LVOT were older than those with RVOT arrhythmias. *RVOT* right ventricular outflow tract, *LVOT* left ventricular outflow tract. From Tanaka Y, et al. Circ J. 2011; 75: 1585–1591

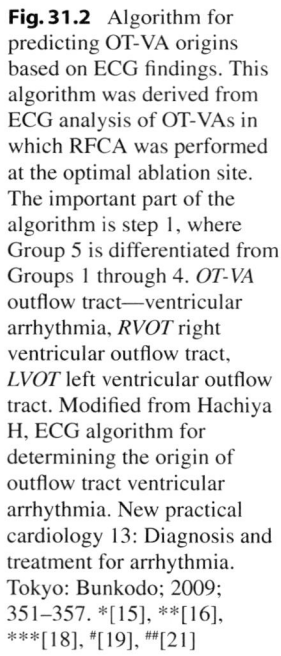

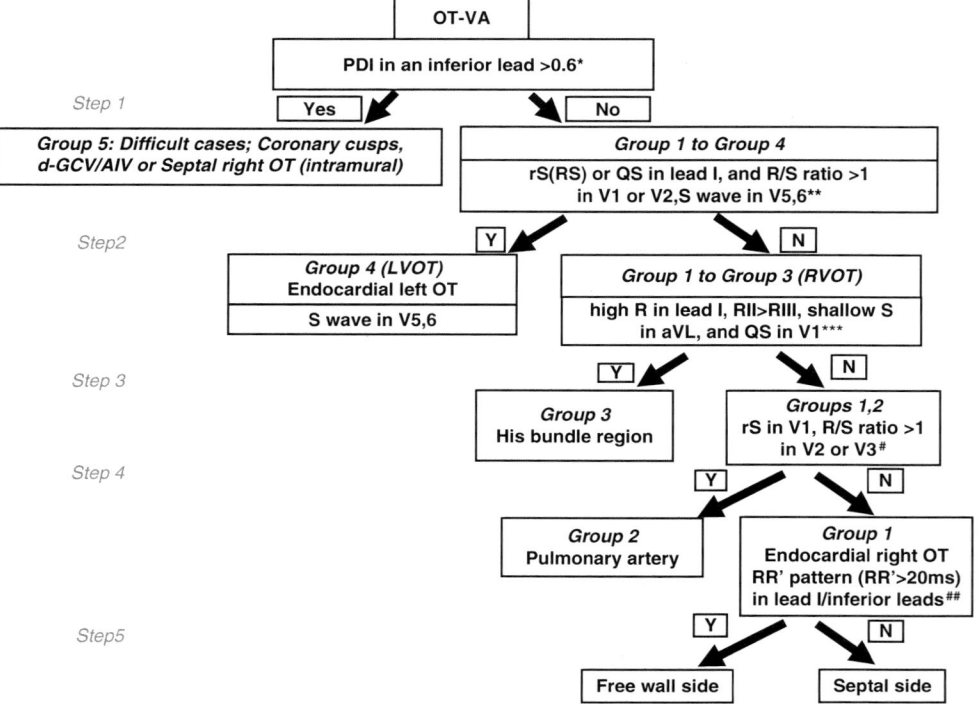

Fig. 31.2 Algorithm for predicting OT-VA origins based on ECG findings. This algorithm was derived from ECG analysis of OT-VAs in which RFCA was performed at the optimal ablation site. The important part of the algorithm is step 1, where Group 5 is differentiated from Groups 1 through 4. *OT-VA* outflow tract—ventricular arrhythmia, *RVOT* right ventricular outflow tract, *LVOT* left ventricular outflow tract. Modified from Hachiya H, ECG algorithm for determining the origin of outflow tract ventricular arrhythmia. New practical cardiology 13: Diagnosis and treatment for arrhythmia. Tokyo: Bunkodo; 2009; 351–357. *[15], **[16], ***[18], #[19], ##[21]

origin, we recommend calculating the PDI (peak deflection index, Fig. 31.3) first. PDI should be determined from the inferior limb lead that presents the tallest R wave by dividing the time from the QRS onset to the earliest peak deflection by the total QRS duration (PDI = T/QRS) [15].

A PDI of greater than 0.6 is more likely to be associated with ablation failure, suggesting that this ECG finding may be reflective of an intramural site or an epicardial site of origin [15].

Step 2 [16]. When an rS or QS pattern is seen in lead I, an R/S ratio is greater than 1 in V1 or V2, and an S wave is in V5 or V6, this categorizes the patient as group 4, endocardial LVOT. Although not a part of our VA waveform-based algorithm, comparison between the ECG of the VPC and that of the sinus beat is recommended at this step [17]. Specifically, if the VA transition (to R > S) occurs later than that of sinus beat QRS, then the VA origin is in the RVOT with 100% specificity. However, if the VA transition occurs at or earlier than that of the sinus beat, then the so-called V2 transition ratio* should be measured. If the transition ratio is <0.6, then RVOT origin is likely. If the transition ratio is ≥0.6, then LVOT origin is likely (sensitivity 95%, specificity 100%) [17]. *[transition ratio is defined as *R/(R + S) amplitudes for the VA beat divided by the same ratio for the sinus beat* [17]].

Step 3 [18]. begins subdivision of RVOT origins. If a high R in lead I, RII greater than RIII, shallow S in aVL, and QS in V1 are present, group 3: His bundle region is indicated.

Step 4 [19]. differentiates group 2 from group 1. An rS in V1 and an R/S ratio > 1 in V2 or V3 indicates group 2, pulmonary artery.

Regarding group 2, there is a report that claims to differentiate the right cusp (RC)-VAs from among the pulmonary sinus cusp (PSC)-VAs using ECG characteristics [20]. The manuscript reported that the successful ablation site was in the RC in ten patients (42%), the left cusp (LC) in eight (33%), and the anterior cusp (AC) in six (25%). ECG analysis showed that RC-VAs had significantly larger R-wave amplitude in lead I and a smaller aVL/aVR ratio of Q-wave amplitude compared with AC-VAs and LC-VAs, respectively. The R-wave amplitude in inferior leads was smaller in VAs localized in the RC than in the LC but did not differ between VAs from the AC and LC [20].

In **step 5** [21], RR' pattern (RR' > 20 ms) in lead I/inferior leads indicate free wall origin of the RVOT.

Examples of application of the algorithm (Fig. 31.2) to patient ECGs are shown in Figs 31.4a and 31.5a. In Fig 31.4a, the ECG of the female patient's OT-VPCs shows that PDI was 0.59. In step 1, the right arm is selected, a QS in lead I is seen, but there is an rS pattern with a deep S wave in the V1 lead which means R/S < 1. Therefore one goes to the right side in steps 2–4, and since there is no RR' pattern (RR' > 20 ms) in lead I/inferior leads in step 5, the origin is predicted to be at the septal RVOT.

In Fig. 31.5a, the PDI of the male patient's OT-VPCs was 0.74. The left arm should be selected in step 1 of the algorithm. The origin was predicted to be in Group 5.

31.4 Importance of Mapping

31.4.1 Electrophysiological Study

It is necessary to discontinue antiarrhythmic drugs before the procedure so electrophysiological study is performed in the absence of antiarrhythmic drug influence. Catheters are inserted under fluoroscopic guidance through the right femoral vein and positioned at the right ventricular apex or right ventricular outflow tract (RVOT). A 2- or 3.3-French multipolar electrode catheter inserted into the right subclavian or internal carotid vein is positioned in the proximal portion of

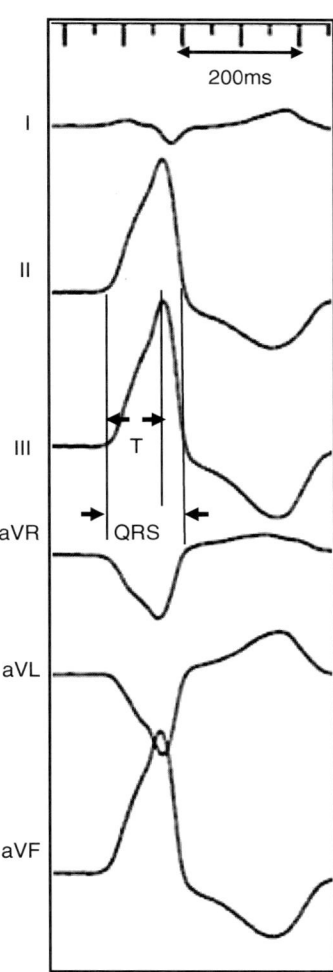

Fig. 31.3 Peak deflection index: PDI = T/QRS. The calculation of the PDI is determined from the 12-lead ECG in the inferior lead that presents the tallest R wave by dividing the time from the QRS onset to the earliest peak deflection by the total QRS duration. Modified from Hachiya H, et al. Circ J. 2010; 74: 256–261

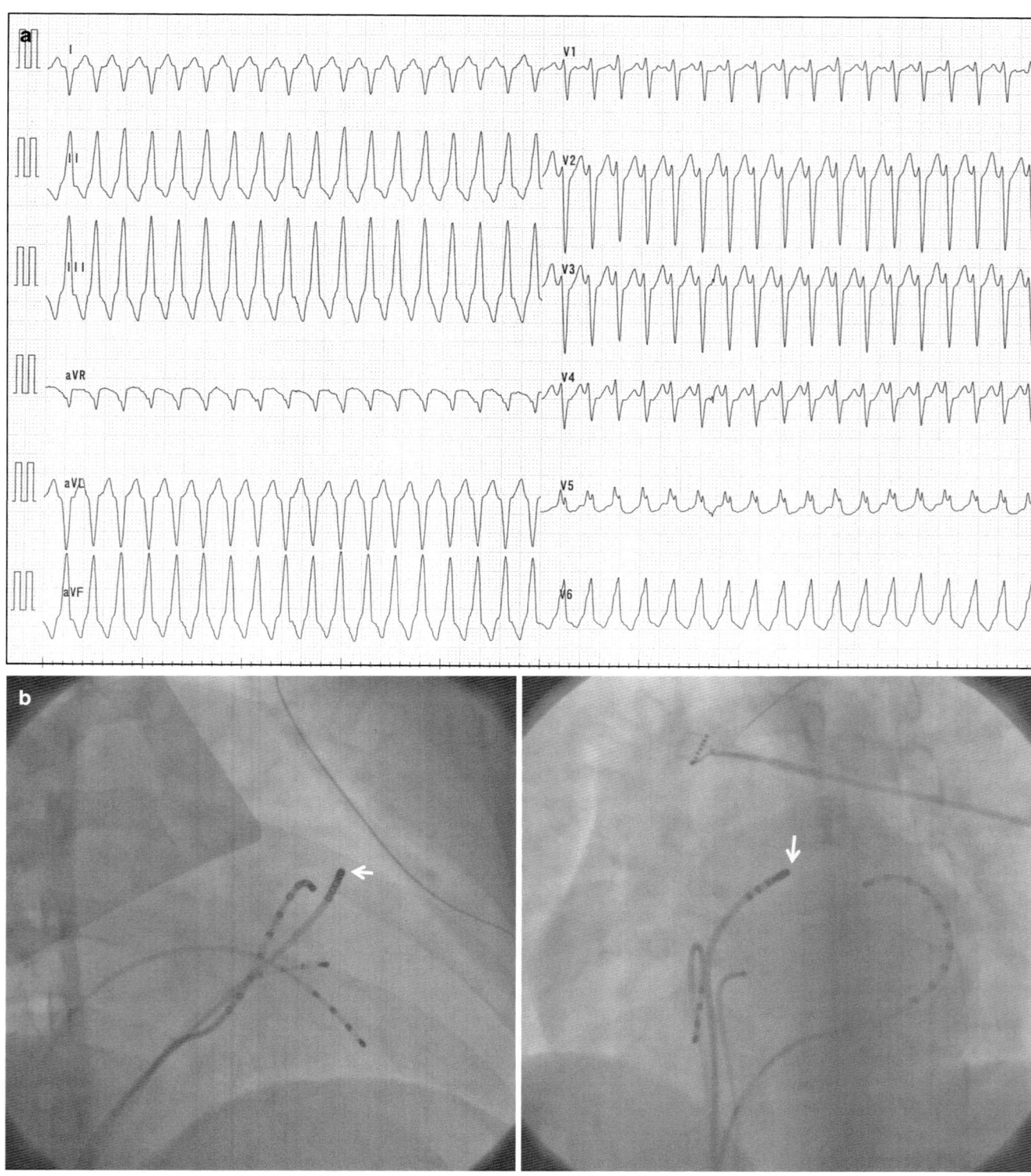

Fig. 31.4 (a) ECG of a ventricular tachycardia from a 20-year-old female patient. The PDI was 0.59. The ECG of her OT-VPCs shows a QS waveform in lead I and an LBBB pattern. However, note that in the V1 lead, there is an rS pattern with a deep S wave which means R/S < 1. The origin was predicted to be on the septal RVOT from the algorithm (Fig. 31.2). (b) Fluoroscopic image of the successful ablation site. The *white arrow* indicates the site. *RAO* right anterior oblique, *LAO* left anterior oblique. (c) The bipolar electrogram at the successful ablation site. The activation time was 38 ms. Note that the electrogram shows the initial deflection to be positive. Activation time is the interval from the onset of the local electrogram to the QRS onset of the VPC. (d) The unipolar electrogram at the successful ablation site. Note that the electrogram shows a distinctive QS pattern, and the stars mark the start of the downstroke

Fig. 31.4 (continued)

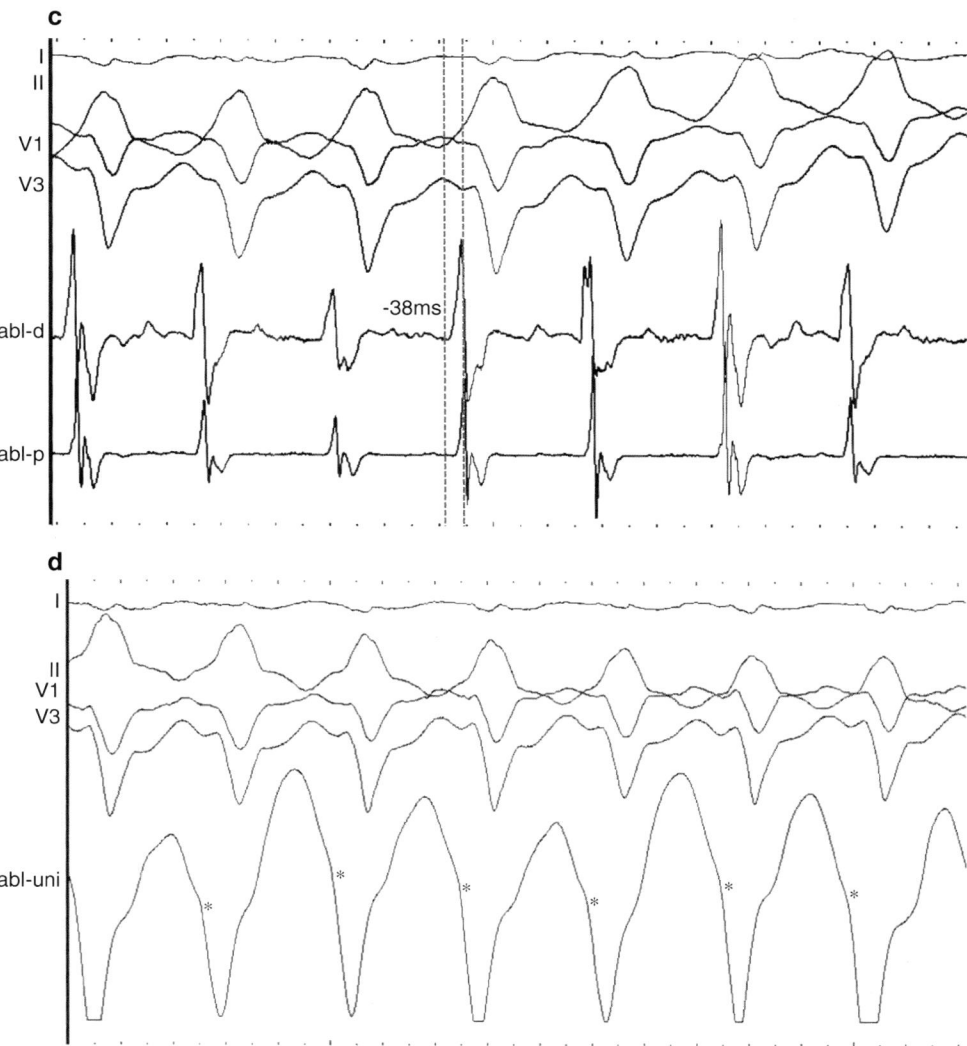

the AIV to the distal GCV. Initially, the RVOT area and pulmonary artery are mapped precisely, followed by careful mapping of the LVOT via the retrograde aortic approach. If pace mapping and activation mapping are thought to indicate that the VT does not originate from an endocardial LVOT site, the arterial mapping catheter is withdrawn from the left ventricle into the aorta and positioned just above the coronary cusps. A small-French multipolar electrode catheter which can be positioned in the proximal portion of the AIV to the distal GCV should be located to record ventricular activations along the anterior mitral annulus. When a ventricular activation recorded from the AIV-GCV catheter precedes the QRS onset or is earlier than that in the His bundle region, an LV ostial VA origin is suggested [10]. Care should be given to the local ventricular activation time relative to the QRS onset at the right ventricular His bundle region. During VAs with an origin in the right coronary cusp (RCC) and non-coronary cusp, a local ventricular activation recorded from the His bundle catheter precedes the QRS onset [10].

31.4.2 Induction Methods

We have sometimes experienced the inability to detect OT-VAs in the ablation session. In such cases, we perform ventricular burst pacing, standard programmed ventricular stimulation, and drug provocation such as infusion of isoproterenol (0.5-4 mg/min, i.v.), atropine (0.5–1 mg), and adenosine triphosphate (10–40 mg, i.v.) to induce OT-VAs.

When these additional procedures do not induce RVOT-VAs, the injection of edrophonium, 5–10 mg i.v., can sometimes induce RVOT-VAs if the development of RVOT-VAs seems to be correlated with an increase in the parasympathetic activity. A previous study found that the occurrence of

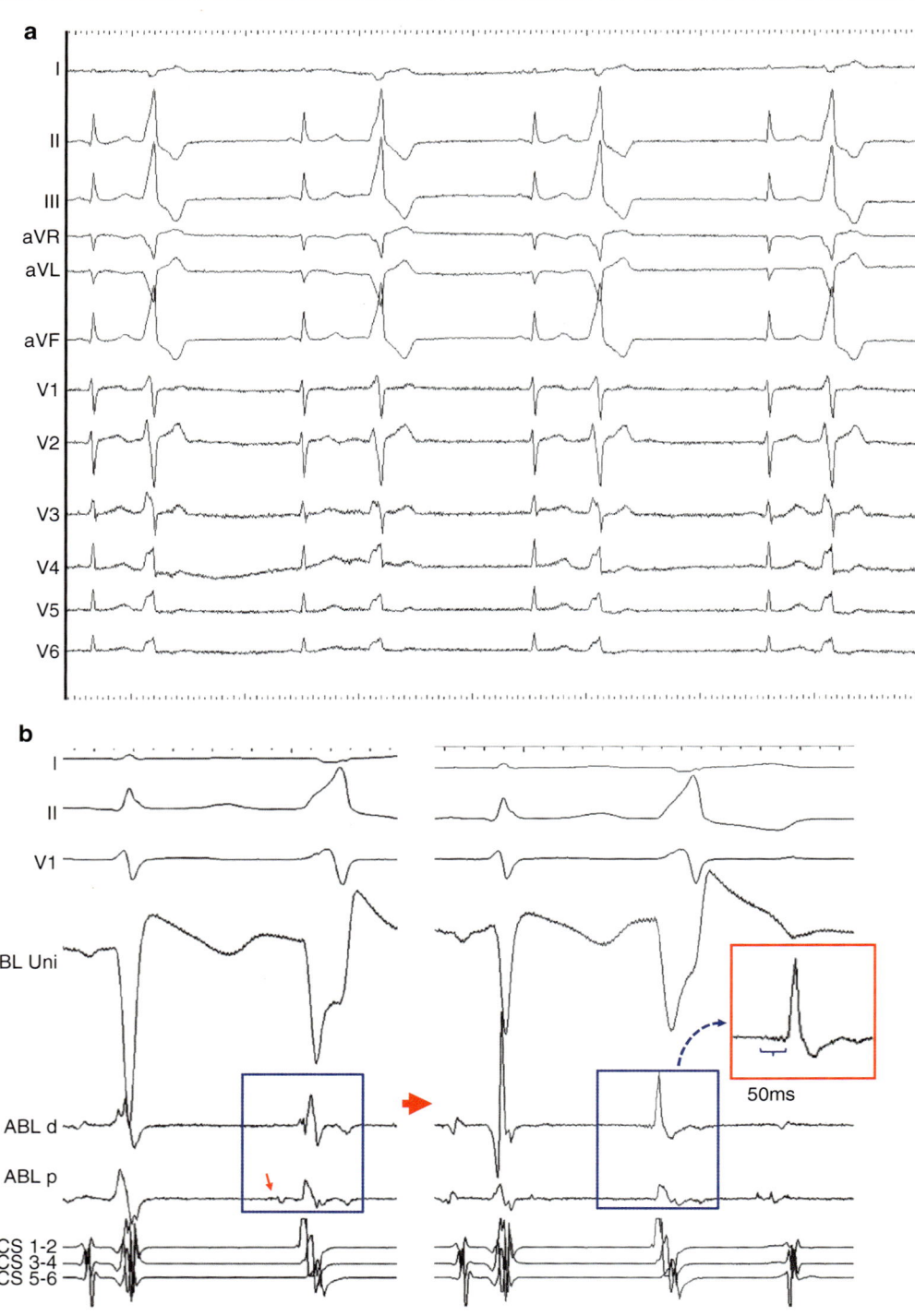

Fig. 31.5 (**a**) The ECG of this patient's OT-VPCs exhibits an rS in lead I and an LBBB pattern. Note that the PDI was 0.74, and the origin was predicted to be at the LCC from the algorithm (Fig. 31.2). (**b**) LCC mapping close to the RCC side. A fractionated continuous potential before the ventricular electrogram is marked with a *red open square*. The interval of the potential is 50 ms. The ECG shows leads I, II, and V1. ABL *Uni* unipolar electrogram recorded by the ablation catheter, *ABL d* distal bipolar electrogram recorded by the ablation catheter, *ABL p* proximal bipolar electrogram recorded by the ablation catheter, *CS* coronary sinus electrogram. CS1-2 is on the distal side. (**c**) The successful ablation site at the LCC. A discrete prepotential with an isoelectric line between the potential and ventricular electrogram was recorded by ABL-d as shown by the *red arrow*. Successful ablation was performed at the site where the activation time was 76 ms as indicated by the *red arrow*. In this case, ABL Uni did not reflect the discrete prepotential as indicated by the red star. (**d**) Pace mapping (PM) at the successful ablation site. PM at the LCC marked by the *red stars* exhibits an excellent PM with a 70 ms stimulus latency. On the other hand, the directly captured PM marked by the *blue stars* demonstrates a poor PM. A spontaneous clinical VPC is superimposed for comparison as shown by the *red rectangular frame*. The pacing output was 10 V/2 ms. *ABL* ablation. (**e**) The successful ablation site indicated by the *white arrows* at the LCC in the fluoroscopic images. Detailed mapping was needed to attain the optimal ablation site, but the LCC had only a small area. *RAO* right anterior oblique, *LAO* left anterior oblique. (**f**) CAG (coronary angiogram) after the successful ABL. There was no organic stenosis

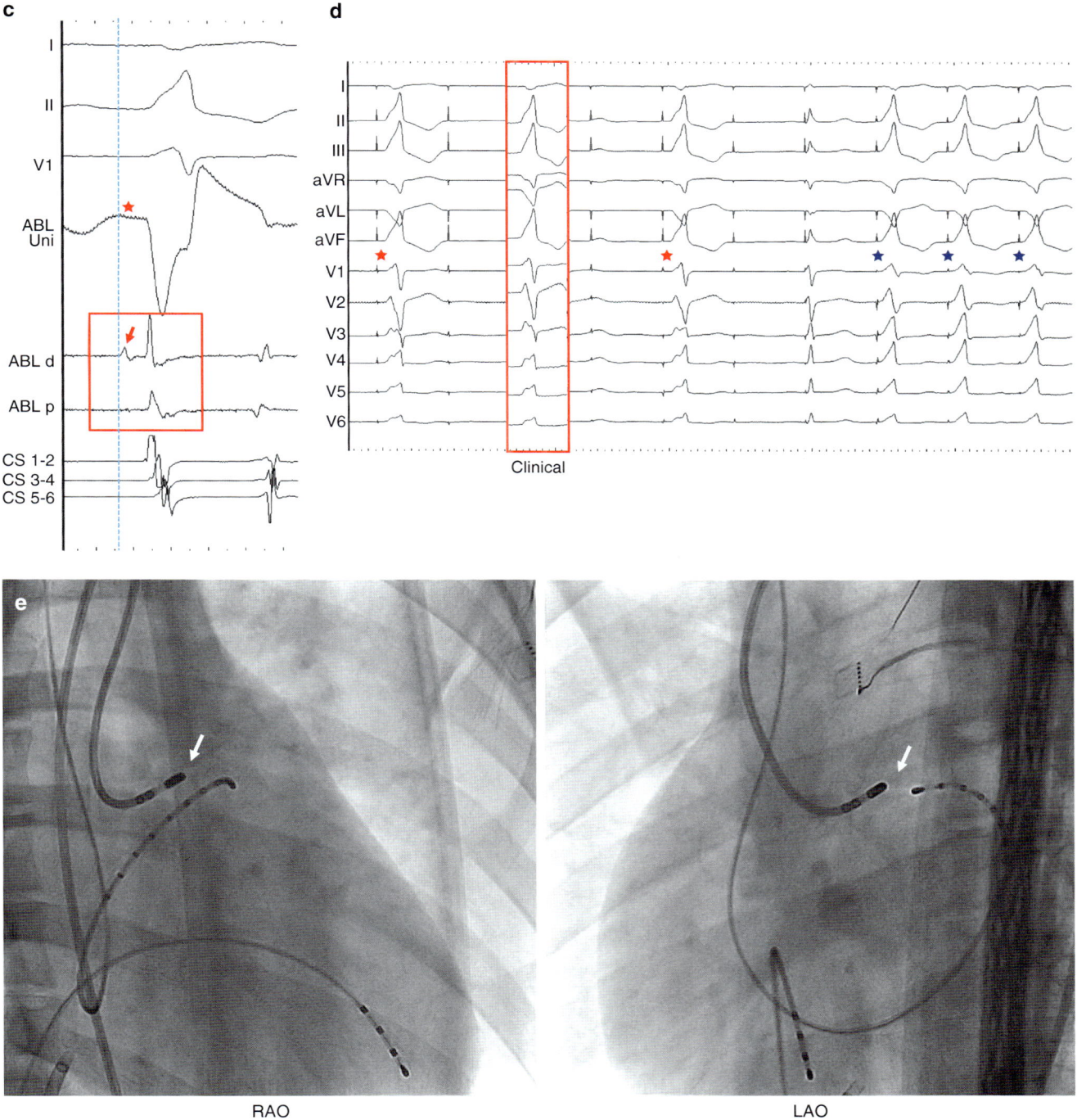

Fig. 31.5 (continued)

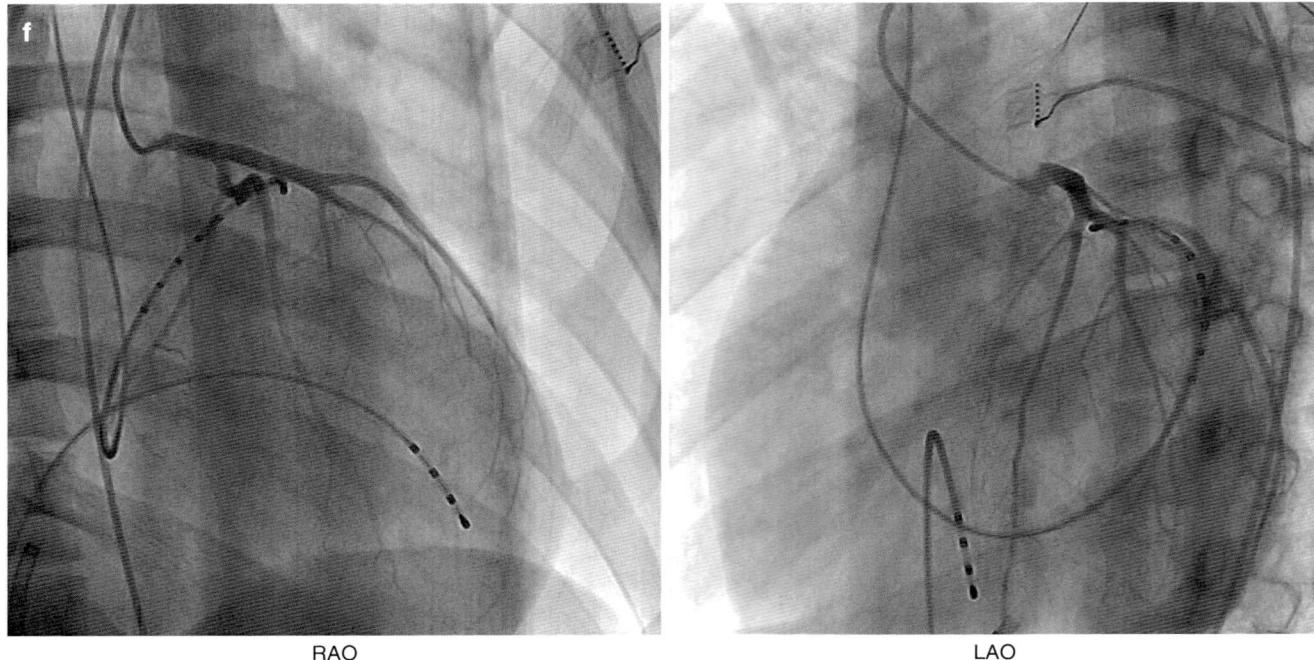

RAO   LAO

Fig. 31.5 (continued)

RVOT-VAs paralleled an increase in the parasympathetic activity in a small number (approximately 5%) of RVOT-VA patients [22]. In those patients, the average proportion of VPCs occurring at night was 74% of all VPCs in 24 h ambulatory monitoring. Furthermore, progressive increase in the high frequency (HF) parameter of hourly heart rate variability analysis coincided with an increase in the number of VPCs or development of RVOT-VT at night [22].

31.4.3 How to Determine the Optimal Ablation Site by Activation and Pace Mapping

VAs originating from the RVOT typically have local presystolic activation >20 ms and produce a near perfect pacemap match [23].

In the ablation of idiopathic VT, a QS pattern of ventricular unipolar electrogram (QS pattern V-uni) is simply and visually identifiable, is very useful, and should be given a high priority when determining the optimum target site [24]. An example of a QS pattern V-uni recorded at the successful ablation site is shown in Fig 31.4d. The successful ablation site (Fig 31.4b) preceded QRS onset by 38 ms (Fig 31.4c). In contrast, it does not always help to determine the optimal ablation site in CC-VA with discrete prepotential. This is because the QS pattern V-uni represents main ventricular activation, but does not always reflect the discrete prepotential like Fig. 31.5c. In Fig. 31.6, the QS pattern V-uni represents main ventricular activation and reflects the discrete prepotential. In Fig. 31.7, we give a flowchart of how to perform a fundamental electrophysiological study for determining optimal OT-VA ablation site.

31.4.4 Preferential Pathways

When RF applications at the exit sites are not effective, detailed mapping for finding discrete prepotentials and applying RF energy at a more proximal site of the preferential pathway would be highly effective [25]. Maruyama et al. reported an OT-VPC case in which VPC originating from the PA trunk was likely to propagate through preferential conduction pathways and exit from the proximal RVOT [26]. The report suggested that double potentials recorded in the RVOT may indicate the presence of preferential conduction that should be taken into account in identifying the ablation target in OT-VA [26].

VAs originating from the aortic sinus cusp often exhibit preferential conduction to the RVOT, which may render pace mapping or some algorithms using the electrocardiographic characteristics less reliable [27].

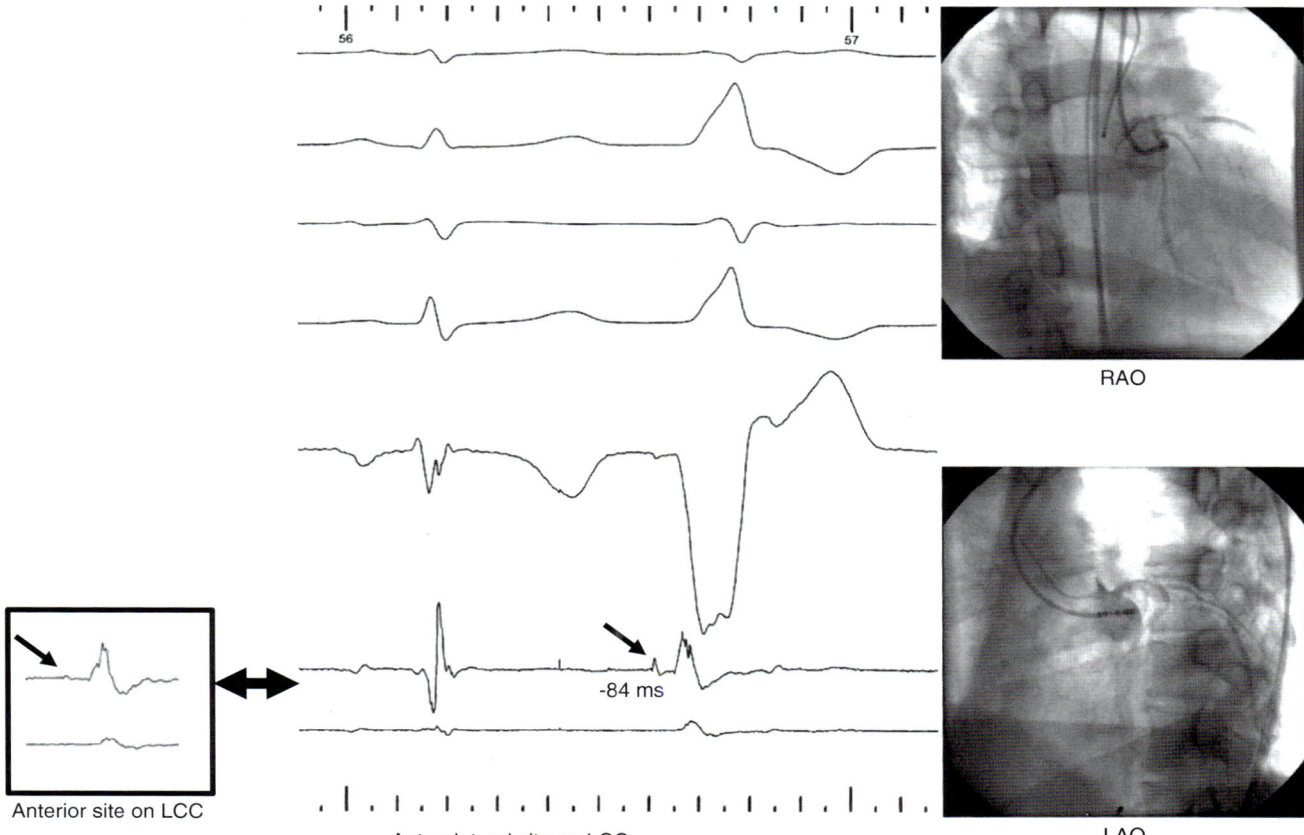

Fig. 31.6 Sensitivity of prepotential to catheter tip location. Detailed mapping on the LCC in a patient shows that when the tip of the mapping catheter was located at an anterior site on the LCC, a tiny blunt discrete prepotential was observed (*arrow, framed panel*). This became sharper and taller after the tip of the catheter was positioned at an anterolateral site, where the successful ablation was performed, as indicated by the *arrow* (*center panel*). In the fluoroscopic image, the tip of the ablation catheter is at the anterolateral site, where the successful ablation was performed, on the LCC. *LCC* left coronary cusp, *RAO* right anterior oblique, *LAO* left anterior oblique. From Hachiya H, et al. Circ Arrythm Electrophysiol. 2013; 6: 898–904

31.5 Ablation

31.5.1 Selection of the Ablation Catheter

An irrigation catheter is sometimes useful for avoiding thrombus formation but the shaft is stiffer than for non-irrigation catheters. Therefore, we recommend non-irrigation ablation catheters for OT-VA mapping and ablation at the present time. This is because flexibility of the shaft of the ablation catheter is needed to reach difficult sites (Fig. 31.8) and for detailed mapping, especially, on the CCs (Fig. 31.5e).

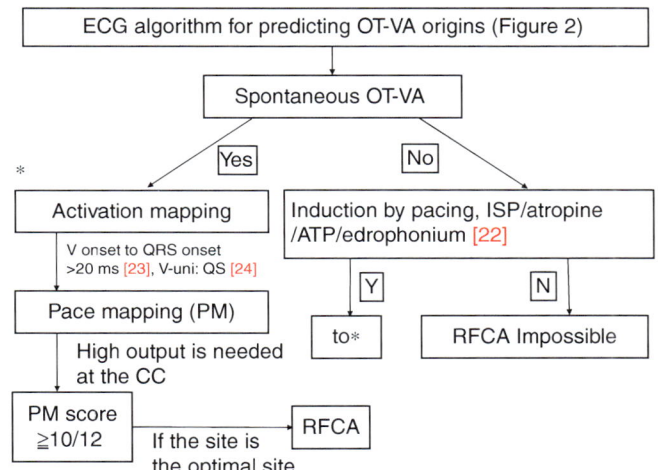

Fig. 31.7 How to perform an electrophysiological study for an OT-VA ablation. *V onset* onset of the local ventricular electrogram when VPCs appear, *V-uni* ventricular unipolar electrogram, *ISP* isoproterenol, *ATP* adenosine triphosphate

31.5.2 Coronary Cusp Ventricular Arrhythmia

A discrete prepotential was seen in nine (26%) of 35 patients with coronary cusp—ventricular arrhythmias (CC-VAs). In left or right CC-VA, the site of a discrete prepotential with

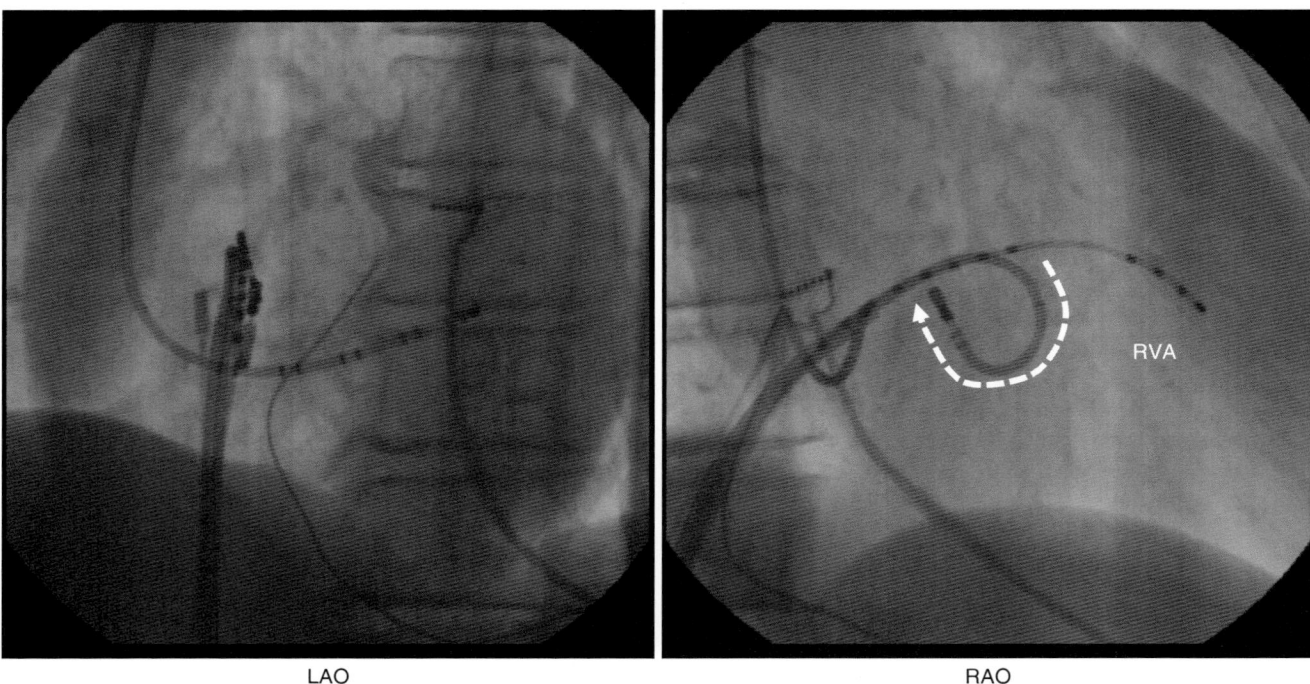

Fig. 31.8 The ablation catheter manipulation for a VPC near the His bundle. The site was targeted from the ventricular side as shown by the *dotted arrow*

≥50-ms activation time may be an indicator of a successful ablation site and facilitate successful ablation of CC-VAs [28].

31.5.3 Detailed Mapping Is Necessary for Coronary Cusp Ventricular Arrhythmia

Detailed mapping is required to reveal the critical discrete prepotential. We found that the discrete prepotential could easily become small and less defined if the mapping catheter was shifted a small distance (Fig. 31.6). We strongly believe that taking a few extra minutes to map the CCs carefully—they are small compared to that of the atrium and ventricle—is worth the effort because of the successful ablation it will lead to (Fig. 31.5b–d). That is not to say that one can find a discrete prepotential in all cases with higher sensitivity catheters and enough time, due to physical characteristics of the CC and spatial relationship between the CC and VT focus [28]. In the Fig. 31.5 case, the VPC disappeared 2.2 s after the RFCA was started with only one RF application.

RF energy should never be delivered more than three times to the same CC in any patient to avoid complications such as injury to the coronary arteries [28, 29].

A case report in which a discrete prepotential with an isoelectric line at the successful ablation site was recorded at the septal aspect of the RVOT-PA junction was also published in 2015 [30]. Therefore, detailed mapping is not only necessary for CC-VA but also for PA and RVOT-VA.

In CC-VAs with a discrete prepotential with an isoelectric line, one needs to assess pace mapping carefully. Note Fig 31.5d. Pace mapping at the LCC marked by the red stars exhibits excellent pace mapping with a 70 ms stimulus latency. On the other hand, the directly captured pace mapping marked by the blue stars demonstrates poor pace mapping. In pace mapping at the LCC marked by the red stars, we think it is likely that capture by the pacing stimulus was narrowly limited to the site of the discrete prepotential, the origin of the CC-VA. Conversely, it is probable that in the pace mapping marked by the blue stars, the score when pacing at the site of the successful ablation was poor because a greater area was captured than is desirable [28].

31.6 Endpoint of the Procedure

The endpoint of the catheter ablation is the elimination and noninducibility of the VT or VPCs during isoproterenol infusion (2–4 μg/min) and burst right ventricular pacing (to a cycle length as short as 300 ms) or programmed right ventricular stimulation. An acute success should be defined as complete elimination of the target VT or VPCs during continuous electrocardiogram monitoring in-hospital for at least 1 day after the ablation procedure.

31.7 Uncommon Origin Sites

When the catheter electrograms identify the distal great cardiac vein (d-GCV) as the earliest site, the LCC and coronary veins, which are the anterior interventricular vein (AIV) and d-GCV, should be considered as an epicardial OT-VA origin [31]. We reported that although the AIV follows the d-GCV anatomically, the R/S ratio in V1 and QRS duration may identify the site of origin as being either the AIV or d-GCV. That is, a low R/S ratio in V1 and shorter QRS duration may help identify AIV sites of epicardial OT-VA origins [31]. In another study of 189 patients with idiopathic VA, the site of origin of the ventricular arrhythmia was identified from within the coronary venous system in 27 of them (14 ± 5%; 95% confidence interval), either in the great cardiac vein ($n = 26$) or the middle cardiac vein ($n = 1$) [32]. Twenty of those 27 patients (74%) underwent successful ablation within the coronary venous system [32]. However, epicardial ablation targeting LVOT-VAs has several limitations. The first is that mapping in the GCV and AIV can generally result in a higher impedance, possible preventing or limiting radiofrequency energy delivery [33, 34]. The second is that due to the close proximity of the coronary arteries and the thick epicardial fat layer overlying those vessels, it is often not possible to perform an epicardial LVOT ablation [33, 35–38]. Last of all, radiofrequency ablation may cause inadvertent injury to the coronary arteries if the targeted ablation is within 5 mm of the coronary arteries [34–41].

VAs from the anterosuperior LVOT present with left bundle branch block morphology, inferior axis, and early transition in the precordial leads on surface ECG in the majority of patients. This region is not very easy to reach but is accessible with an antegrade approach via an anteroinferior transseptal puncture site using a reversed S curve on the ablation catheter. Clinically, only activation mapping is feasible because VA morphologies do not match QRS morphologies during pace mapping [42].

31.8 Complications

Although it is thought that cardiac tamponade, groin hematoma and AV block, etc. could occur, there are few reports regarding ablation complications in patients with OT-VA. In a report published by Latchamsetty et al. [7], among 1185 patients, a total of 62 complications occurred (5.2%), with 29 major complications (2.4%) and 33 minor complications (2.8%). The most common complications were related to vascular access, with 33 patients (2.8%) having groin-related complications, 15 (1.3%) of whom required transfusion or surgical intervention. Nine patients (0.8%) had pericardial tamponade requiring pericardiocentesis. Major complication rates were similar across different VPC locations but overall were highest for epicardial VPCs at 4.2%. Ablation of VPCs from the RVOT had the lowest major complication rate (2.1%) [7].

Yamada et al. described that in 44 patients with CC-VA, sinus bradycardia followed by complete AV block occurred in one patient with VPCs with an RCC origin, in whom an His bundle electrogram was not recorded at the successful ablation site [43]. Both sinus node function and AV conduction recovered soon after termination of radiofrequency delivery in this patient. A case of right coronary artery stenosis associated with idiopathic ventricular tachycardia ablation was reported in 2015 [44]. In CC-VA ablation, similar to these reports, AV block and coronary artery injury are raised as complications. It is essential to measure the distance from the ablation site to the area of the His bundle and determine the exact location of the coronary artery ostium using coronary angiograms (Fig 31.5e, f) or intracardiac echocardiography before and after RFCA to avoid AV block and coronary arterial damage.

Conclusion
Although the existence of a preferential pathway or discrete prepotential with an isoelectric line sometimes makes the ECG algorithm, QS pattern of ventricular unipolar electrogram, and pace mapping unreliable, in the majority of patients with OT-VA, ECG-based prediction of foci and detailed mapping of the OT facilitates an effective and safe RFCA.

References

1. Heeger CH, Hayashi K, Kuck KH, Ouyang F. Catheter ablation of idiopathic ventricular arrhythmias arising from the cardiac outflow tracts – recent insights and techniques for the successful treatment of common and challenging cases. Circ J. 2016;80:1073–86.
2. Takatsuki S, Mitamura H, Ogawa S. Catheter ablation of a monofocal premature ventricular complex triggering idiopathic ventricular fibrillation. Heart. 2001;86:e3.
3. Noda T, Shimizu W, Taguchi A, Aiba T, Satomi K, Suyama K, et al. Malignant entitiy of idiopathic ventricular fibrillation and polymorphic ventricular tachycardia initiated by premature extrasystoles originating from the right ventricular outflow tract. J Am Coll Cardiol. 2005;46:1288–94.
4. Takemoto M, Yoshimura H, Ohba Y, Matsumoto Y, Yamamoto U, Mohri M, et al. Radiofrequency catheter ablation of premature ventricular complexes from right ventricular outflow tract improves left ventricular dilation and clinical status in patients without structural heart disease. J Am Coll Cardiol. 2005;45:1259–65.
5. Sekiguchi Y, Aonuma K, Yamauchi Y, Obayashi T, Niwa A, Hachiya H, et al. Chronic hemodynamic effects after radiofrequency catheter ablation of frequent monomorphic ventricular premature beats. J Cardiovasc Electrophysiol. 2005;16:1057–63.

6. Bogun F, Crawford T, Reich S, Koelling TM, Armstrong W, Good E, et al. Radiofrequency ablation of frequent, idiopathic premature ventricular complexes: comparison with a control group without intervention. Heart Rhythm. 2007;4:863–7.
7. Latchamsetty R, Yokokawa M, Morady F, Kim HM, Mathew S, Tilz R, et al. Multicenter outcomes for catheter ablation of idiopathic premature ventricular complexes. J Am Coll Cardiol. 2015;1:116–23.
8. Authors/Task Force M, Priori SG, Blomstrom-Lundqvist C, Mazzanti A, Blom N, Borggrefe M, Camm J, et al. 2015 ESC guidelines for the management of patients with ventricular arrhythmias and the prevention of sudden cardiac death: The Task Force for the Management of Patients with Ventricular Arrhythmias and the Prevention of Sudden Cardiac Death of the European Society of Cardiology (ESC) Endorsed by: Association for European Paediatric and Congenital Cardiology (AEPC). Eur Heart J. 2015;36:2793–867.
9. Pytkowski M, Maciag A, Sterlinski M, Jankowska A, Kowalik I, Farkowski MM, et al. Novel algorithm for arrhythmogenic focus localization in patients with right ventricular outflow tract arrhythmias. Cardiol J. 2014;21:284–92.
10. Yamada T, Litovsky SH, Kay GN. The left ventricular ostium: An anatomic concept relevant to idiopathic ventricular arrhythmias. Circ Arrhythm Electrophysiol. 2008;1:396–404.
11. Tanaka Y, Tada H, Ito S, Naito S, Higuchi K, Kumagai K, et al. Gender and age differences in candidates for radiofrequency catheter ablation of idiopathic ventricular arrhythmias. Circ J. 2011;75:1585–91.
12. Pedersen CT, Kay GN, Kalman J, Borggrefe M, Della-Bella P, Dickfeld T, et al. EHRA/HRS/APHRS expert consensus on ventricular arrhythmias. Heart Rhythm. 2014;11:e166–96.
13. Viskin S, Rosso R, Rogowski O, Belhassen B. The 'short-coupled' variant of right ventricular outflow ventricular tachycardia: a not-so-benign form of benign ventricular tachycardia? J Cardiovasc Electrophysiol. 2005;16:912–6.
14. Hachiya H. ECG algorithm for determining the origin of outflow tract ventricular arrhythmia. In: Aonuma K, Matsuzaki M, editors. New practical cardiology 13: diagnosis and treatment for arrhythmia. Tokyo: Bunkodo; 2009. p. 351–7.
15. Hachiya H, Hirao K, Sasaki T, Higuchi K, Hayashi T, Tanaka Y, et al. Novel ECG predictor of difficult cases of outflow tract ventricular tachycardia: Peak deflection index on an inferior lead. Circ J. 2010;74:256–61.
16. Hachiya H, Aonuma K, yamauchi Y, Harada T, Igawa M, Nogami A, Iesaka Y, Hiroe M, Marumo F. Electrocardiographic characteristics of left ventricular outflow tract tachycardia. Pacing Clin Electrophysiol. 2000;23:1930–4.
17. Betensky BP, Park RE, Marchlinski FE, Hutchinson MD, Garcia FC, Dixit S, et al. The V2 transition ratio, a new electrocardiographic criterion for distinguishing left from right ventricular outflow tract tachycardia origin. J Am Coll Cardiol. 2011;57:2255–62.
18. Yamauchi Y, Aonuma K, Takahashi A, Sekiguchi Y, Hachiya H, Yokoyama Y, et al. Electrocardiographic characteristics of repetitive monophorphic right ventricular tachycardia originating near the His-bundle. J Cardiovasc Electrophysiol. 2005;16:1041–8.
19. Sekiguchi Y, Aonuma K, Takahashi A, Yamauchi Y, Hachiya H, Yokoyama Y, et al. Electrocardiographic and electrophysiologic characteristics of ventricular tachycardia originating within the pulmonary artery. J Am Coll Cardiol. 2005;45:887–95.
20. Liao Z, Zhan X, Wu S, Xue Y, Fang X, Liao H, et al. Idiopathic ventricular arrhythmias originating from the pulmonary sinus cusp: prevalence, ECG/electrophysiological characteristics, and catheter ablation. J Am Coll Cardiol. 2015;66:2633–44.
21. Tada H, Ito S, Naito S, Kurosaki K, Ueda M, Shinbo G, et al. Prevalence and electrocardiographic characteristics of idiopathic ventricular arrhythmia originating in the free wall of the right ventricular outflow tract. Circ J. 2004;68:909–14.
22. Hachiya H, Aonuma K, Yamauchi Y, Sekiguchi Y, Iesaka Y. Edrophonium-induced right ventricular outflow tract tachycardia. Pacing Clin Electrophysiol. 2005;28:S158–62.
23. Hutchinson MD, Garcia FC. An organized approach to the localization, mapping, and ablation of outflow tract ventricular arrhythmias. J Cardiovasc Electrophysiol. 2013;24:1189–97.
24. Soejima Y, Aonuma K, Iesaka Y, Isobe M. Ventricular unipolar potential in radiofrequency catheter ablation of idiopathic non-reentrant ventricular outflow tachycardia. Jpn Heart J. 2004;45:749–60.
25. Shirai Y, Goya M, Isobe M, Hirao K. Preferential pathway pacing within the aortic sinus of Valsalva: strong evidence for the existence of preferential conduction with different exit sites traversing the ventricular septum. J Cardiovasc Electrophysiol. 2015;26:805–8.
26. Maruyama M, Yamamoto T, Miyauchi Y, Mizuno K. Exit from the right ventricular outflow tract through the preferential conduction pathway in premature ventricular contractions originating from the pulmonary artery. Heart Rhythm. 2013;10:1407–8.
27. Yamada T, Murakami Y, Yoshida N, Okada T, Shimizu T, Toyama J, et al. Preferential conduction across the ventricular outflow septum in ventricular arrhythmias originating from the aortic sinus cusp. J Am Coll Cardiol. 2007;50:884–91.
28. Hachiya H, Yamauchi Y, Iesaka Y, Yagishita A, Sasaki S, Higuchi K, et al. Discrete prepotential as an indicator of successful ablation in patients with coronary cusp ventricular arrhythmia. Circ Arrythm Electrophysiol. 2013;6:898–904.
29. Hachiya H, Aonuma K, Yamauchi Y, Igawa M, Nogami A, Iesaka Y. How to diagnose, locate, and ablate coronary cusp ventricular tachycardia. J Cardiovasc Electrophysiol. 2002;13:551–6.
30. Miyazaki S, Hachiya H, Matsuda J, Takagi T, Watanabe T, Iesaka Y. Discrete prepotentials with an isoelectric segment at the successful ablation site in the right ventricular outflow tract and pulmonary artery junction in a case with a ventricular arrhythmia. Heart Rhythm Case Rep. 2015;1:348–51.
31. Hachiya H, Hirao K, Nakamura H, Taniguchi H, Miyazaki S, Komatsu Y, et al. Electrocardiographic characteristics differentiating epicardial outflow tract ventricular arrhythmias originating from the anterior interventricular vein and distal great cardiac vein. Circ J. 2015;79:2335–44.
32. Baman TS, Ilg KJ, Gupta SK, Good E, Chugh A, Jongnarangsin K, et al. Mapping and ablation of epicardial idiopathic ventricular arrhythmias from within the coronary venous system. Circ Arrhythm Electrophysiol. 2010;3:274–9.
33. Daniels DV, Lu YY, Morton JB, Santucci PA, Akar JG, Green A, Wilber DJ. Idiopathic epicardial left ventricular tachycardia originating remote from the sinus of Valsalva: electrophysiological characteristics, catheter ablation, and identification from the 12-lead electrocardiogram. Circulation. 2006;113:1659–66.
34. Yamada T, McElderry HT, Doppalapudi H, Okada T, Murakami Y, Yoshida Y, Yoshida N, Inden Y, Murohara T, Plumb VJ, Kay GN. Idiopathic ventricular arrhythmias originating from the left ventricular summit: anatomic concepts relevant to ablation. Circ Arrhythm Electrophysiol. 2010;3:616–23.
35. Jauregui Abularach ME, Campos B, Park KM, Tschabrunn CM, Frankel DS, Park RE, Gerstenfeld EP, Mountantonakis SE, Mountantonakis S, Garcia FC, Dixit S, Tzou WS, Hutchinson MD, Lin D, Riley MP, Cooper JM, Bala R, Callans DJ, Marchlinski FE. Ablation of ventricular arrhythmias arising near the anterior epicardial veins from the left sinus of Valsalva region: ECG features, anatomic distance, and outcome. Heart Rhythm. 2012;9:865–73.
36. Sacher F, Roberts-Thomson K, Maury P, Tedrow U, Nault I, Steven D, Hocini M, Koplan B, Leroux L, Derval N, Seiler J, Wright MJ, Epstein L, Haissaguerre M, Jais P, Stevenson WG. Epicardial

ventricular tachycardia ablation: a multicenter safety study. J Am Coll Cardiol. 2010;55:2366–72.
37. Koruth JS, Aryana A, Dukkipati SR, Pak HN, Kim YH, Sosa EA, Scanavacca M, Mahapatra S, Ailawadi G, Reddy VY, d'Avila A. Unusual complications of percutaneous epicardial access and epicardial mapping and ablation of cardiac arrhythmias. Circ Arrhythm Electrophysiol. 2011;4:882–8.
38. Roberts-Thomson KC, Steven D, Seiler J, Inada K, Koplan BA, Tedrow UB, Epstein LM, Stevenson WG. Coronary artery injury due to catheter ablation in adults: presentations and outcomes. Circulation. 2009;120:1465–73.
39. Sun Y, Arruda M, Otomo K, Beckman K, Nakagawa H, Calame J, Po S, Spector P, Lustgarten D, Herring L, Lazzara R, Jackman W. Coronary sinus-ventricular accessory connections producing posteroseptal and left posterior accessory pathways: incidence and electrophysiological identification. Circulation. 2002;106:1362–7.
40. Stavrakis S, Jackman WM, Nakagawa H, Sun Y, Xu Q, Beckman KJ, Lockwood D, Scherlag BJ, Lazzara R, Po SS. Risk of coronary artery injury with radiofrequency ablation and cryoablation of epicardial posteroseptal accessory pathways within the coronary venous system. Circ Arrhythm Electrophysiol. 2014;7:113–9.
41. Makimoto H, Zhang Q, Tilz RR, Wissner E, Cuneo A, Kuck KH, Ouyang F. Aborted sudden cardiac death due to radiofrequency ablation within the coronary sinus and subsequent total occlusion of the circumflex artery. J Cardiovasc Electrophysiol. 2013;24:929–32.
42. Ouyang F, Mathew S, Wu S, Kamioka M, Metzner A, Xue Y, et al. Ventricular arrhythmias arising from the left ventricular outflow tract below the aortic sinus cusps: mapping and catheter ablation via transseptal approach and electrocardiographic characteristics. Circ Arrhythm Electrophysiol. 2014;7:445–55.
43. Yamada T, McElderry HT, Doppalapudi H, Murakami Y, Yoshida Y, Yoshida N, et al. Idiopathic ventricular arrhythmias originating from the aortic root prevalence, electrocardiographic and electrophysiologic characteristics, and results of radiofrequency catheter ablation. J Am Coll Cardiol. 2008;52:139–47.
44. Kusa S, Hachiya H, Kakuta T, Iesaka Y. Right coronary artery ostial stenosis associated with idiopathic ventricular tachycardia ablation. Heart Rhythm Case Rep. 2015;1:13–7.

Idiopathic Left Fascicular Ventricular Tachycardia

Akihiko Nogami

Keywords

Ventricular tachycardia · Fascicular tachycardia · Purkinje · Verapamil · Catheter ablation

32.1 Introduction

Sustained monomorphic ventricular tachycardia (VT) is most often related to myocardial structure heart disease, including healed myocardial infarction and cardiomyopathies. However, no apparent structural abnormality is identified in about 10% of all sustained monomorphic VTs in the United States [1] and 20% of those in Japan [2]. These VTs are referred to as "idiopathic." Idiopathic VTs usually occur in specific locations and have specific QRS morphologies [3–8], whereas VTs associated with structural heart disease have a QRS morphology that tends to indicate the location of the scar. Idiopathic VT comprises multiple discrete subtypes that are best differentiated by their mechanism, QRS morphology, and site of origin. The most common idiopathic VT originates from a focus in the outflow tract of the right ventricle, and its mechanism is most likely triggered activity. In idiopathic left VT, four types of VT exist: verapamil-sensitive left fascicular VT (reentry), nonreentrant fascicular VT with a focal origin in the distal Purkinje system (abnormal automaticity), left ventricular outflow tract VT, and VT from the mitral annulus (triggered activity, reentry, or automaticity). This chapter focuses on the assessment and nonpharmacological treatment of idiopathic left fascicular VT including verapamil-sensitive left fascicular VT and nonreentrant fascicular VT.

32.2 Verapamil-Sensitive Left Fascicular VT

32.2.1 Classification and Pathophysiology

32.2.1.1 History and Classification

Verapamil-sensitive fascicular VT is the most common form of idiopathic left VT. It was first recognized as an electrocardiographic entity in 1979 by Zipes and colleagues [9], who identified the characteristic diagnostic triad: (1) induction with atrial pacing, (2) right bundle branch block (RBBB) and left-axis configuration, and (3) manifestation in patients without structural heart disease. In 1981, Belhassen and associates [10] were the first to demonstrate the verapamil sensitivity of the tachycardia, a fourth identifying feature. Ohe and coworkers [11] reported another type of this tachycardia, with RBBB and a right-axis deviation, in 1988. And we described the upper septal form of this tachycardia [12, 13]. According to the QRS morphology, verapamil-sensitive left fascicular VT can be classified into three subgroups: (1) left posterior fascicular VT, whose QRS morphology exhibits an RBBB configuration and inferior axis deviation (Fig. 32.1a); (2) left anterior fascicular VT, whose QRS morphology exhibits an RBBB configuration and right-axis deviation (Fig. 32.1b); and (3) upper septal fascicular VT, whose QRS morphology exhibits a narrow QRS configuration and normal or right-axis deviation (Fig. 32.1c). Left posterior fascicular VT is common, left anterior fascicular VT is uncommon, and left upper septal fascicular VT is very rare.

32.2.1.2 Substrate and Mechanism

The anatomic basis of this tachycardia has provoked considerable interest. Some data suggest that the tachycardia

A. Nogami, M.D., Ph.D.
Department of Cardiology, Faculty of Medicine,
Tsukuba University, 1-1-1 Tennodai, Tsukuba 305-8575, Japan
e-mail: akihiko-ind@umin.ac.jp

© Springer Nature Singapore Pte Ltd. 2018
K. Hirao (ed.), *Catheter Ablation*, https://doi.org/10.1007/978-981-10-4463-2_32

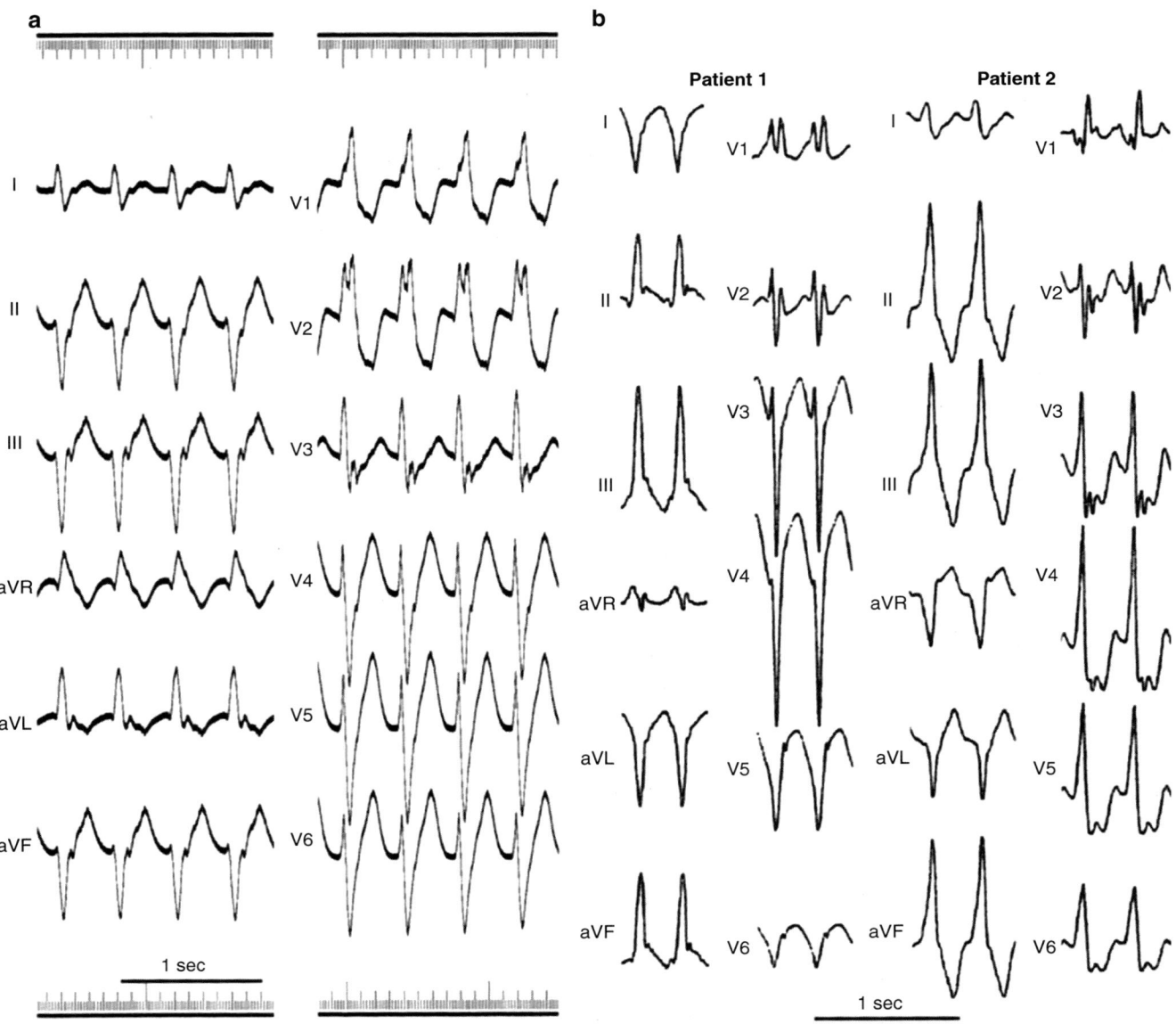

Fig. 32.1 Twelve-lead electrocardiograms of verapamil-sensitive left fascicular ventricular tachycardias (VTs). (**a**) Left posterior fascicular VT. (**b**) Left anterior fascicular VT. (**c**) Left upper septal VT (**a**, From Nogami A. Idiopathic left ventricular tachycardia: assessment and treatment. Card Electrophysiol Rev. 2002; 6: 448–457. **b**, From Nogami A, Naito S, Tada H, et al. Verapamil-sensitive left anterior fascicular ventricular tachycardia: results of radiofrequency ablation in six patients. J Cardiovasc Electrophysiol 1998; 9: 1269–1278. **c**, From Talib AK, Nogami A, Nishiuchi S, et al. Verapamil-sensitive upper septal idiopathic left ventricular tachycardia: Prevalence, mechanism, and electrophysiological characteristics. JACCCEP 2015; 1: 369–380)

may originate from a false tendon or fibromuscular band in the left ventricle [14–16]. Suwa and coworkers [15] described a false tendon in the left ventricle of a patient with idiopathic VT in whom the VT was eliminated by surgical resection of the tendon. Using transthoracic and transesophageal echocardiography, Thakur and colleagues [16] found false tendons extending from the posteroinferior left ventricle to the basal septum in 15 of 15 patients with idiopathic left VT but in only 5% of control patients. Maruyama and associates [17] reported a case with the

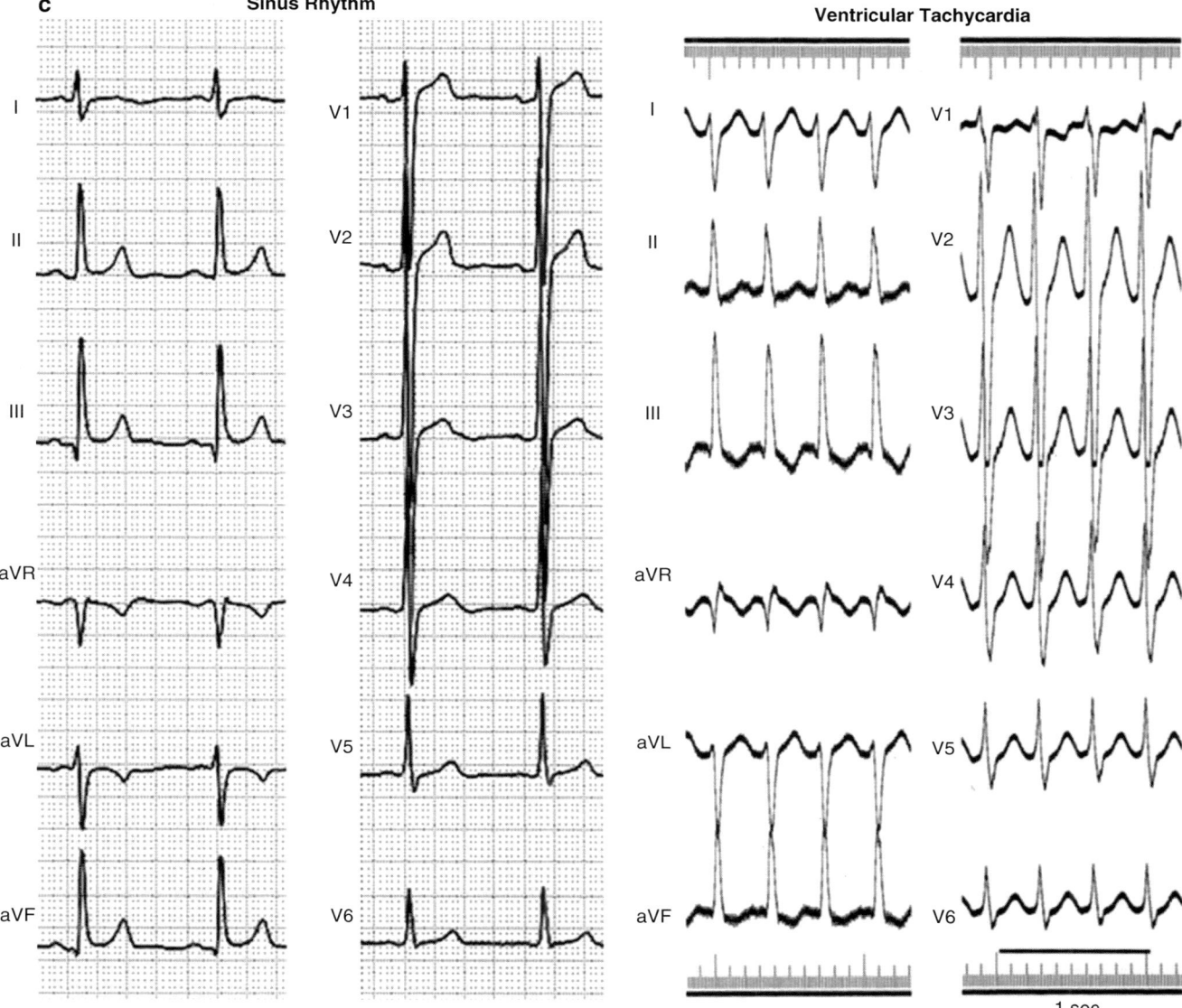

Fig. 32.1 (continued)

recording of sequential diastolic potentials bridging the entire diastolic period and a false tendon extending from the mid-septum to the inferoapical septum. Lin and colleagues [18] found that 17 of 18 patients with idiopathic VT had this fibromuscular band but also found it in 35 of 40 control patients. They concluded that the band was a common echocardiographic finding and was not a specific arrhythmogenic substrate for this tachycardia although they could not exclude the possibility that the band was a potential substrate of the VT. Small fibromuscular bands, trabeculae carneae, and small papillary muscles cannot be detected by transthoracic echocardiography. The Purkinje networks in these small anatomic structures are important when considering the mechanism of left fascicular VT. This circuit is not completely defined but may comprise fascicular tissue and ventricular myocardium.

The mechanism of verapamil-sensitive left VT is reentry because it can be induced, entrained, and terminated by programmed ventricle or atrial stimulation. To confirm its reentry circuit and the mechanism, my colleagues and I performed left ventricular septal mapping using an octapolar electrode catheter in 20 patients with left posterior fascicular VT [19]. In 15 of 20 patients (75%), two distinct potentials, P1 and P2, were recorded during the VT at the mid-septum (Fig. 32.2). Although the mid-diastolic potential (P1) was recorded earlier from the proximal rather than the distal electrodes, the fused presystolic Purkinje potential (P2) was recorded earlier from the distal electrodes. During sinus rhythm, recording at the same site demonstrated P2, which was recorded after the His bundle potential and before the onset of the QRS complex; however, the sequence of the P2 was the reverse of that seen during the VT. VT could be entrained from the atrium and from the ventricle. Entrainment pacing from the atrium or ventricle captured P1 orthodromically and reset the VT. The interval from the stimulus to P1 was prolonged as the pacing rate increased. These findings demonstrated that P1 is a critical potential in the circuit of the verapamil-sensitive left posterior fascicular VT and suggested the presence of a macroreentry circuit involving the normal Purkinje system and abnormal Purkinje tissue with decremental properties and verapamil sensitivity. Although P1 has proved to be a critical potential in the VT circuit, whether the left posterior fascicle or Purkinje fiber (P2) is involved in the retrograde limb of the reentrant circuit used to be unclear [17, 20, 21]. Morishima and I [21] reported a case with negative participation of the proximal left posterior fascicle to the VT circuit. Selective capture of left posterior fascicle by sinus beat did not affect the cycle length of VT, and the postpacing interval after the entrainment from left ventricular septal myocardium was equal to the cycle length

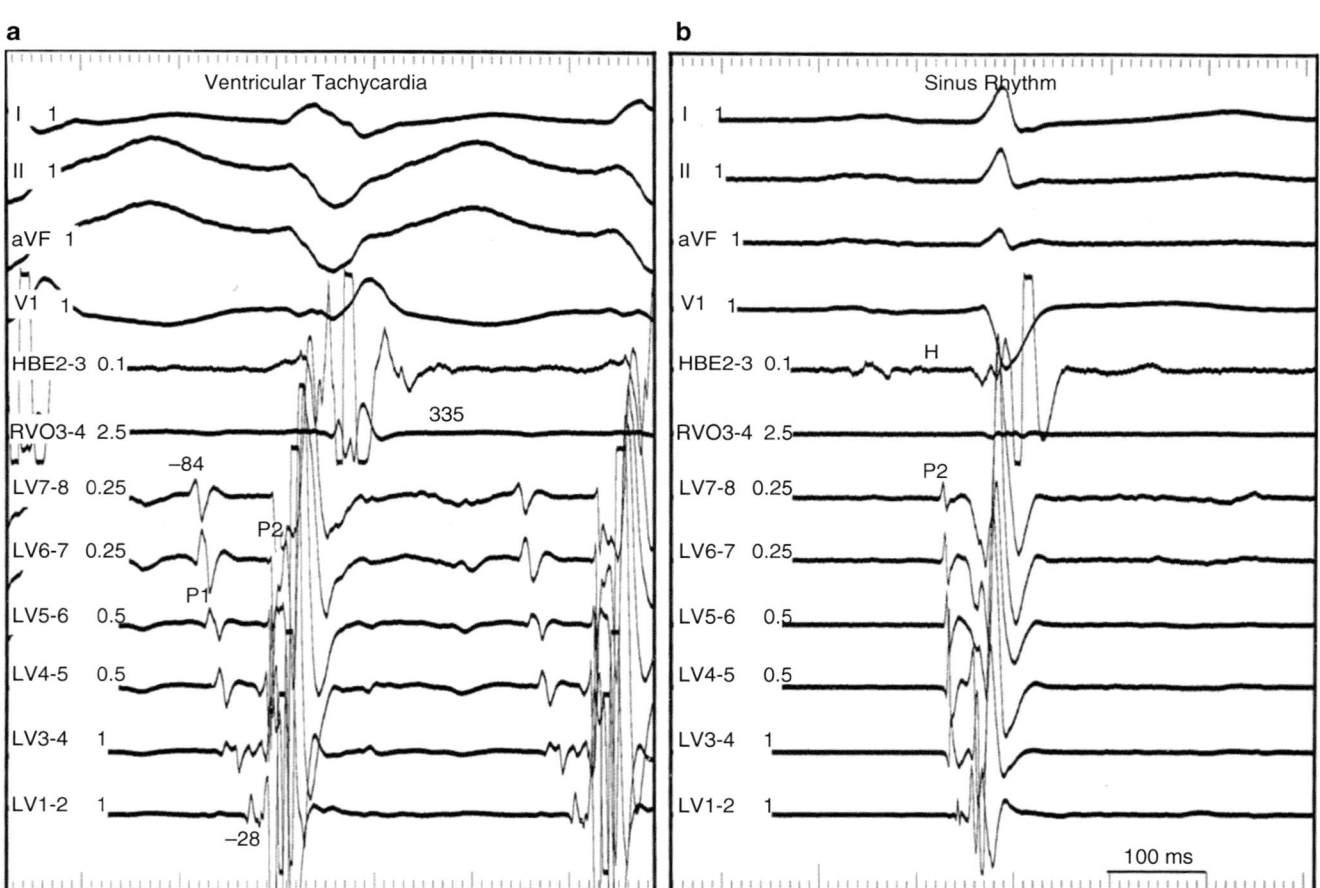

Fig. 32.2 Intracardiac recordings from an octapolar electrode catheter. (**a**) During left posterior fascicular ventricular tachycardia, a diastolic potential (P1) and a presystolic Purkinje potential (P2) were recorded. While P1 was recorded earlier from the proximal rather than the distal electrodes, P2 was recorded earlier from the distal rather than the proximal electrodes. (**b**) During sinus rhythm, recording at the same site demonstrated the P2, is now recorded before the onset of the QRS complex and is earliest on the proximal electrodes. *HBE* His bundle electrogram, *RVO* right ventricular outflow, *LV* left ventricle, *7–8* proximal bipole; *1–2* distal bipole, *H* His (From Nogami A, Naito S, Tada H, et al. Demonstration of diastolic and presystolic Purkinje potential as critical potentials on a macroreentry circuit of verapamil-sensitive idiopathic left ventricular tachycardia. J Am Coll Cardiol 2000; 36: 811–823)

of VT. These findings suggest that the retrograde limb of the circuit is not the proximal left posterior fascicle, but left ventricular septum itself. Maeda and associates [22] demonstrated the direct proof of the negative participation of P2 in the circuit. RF energy application was delivered at the site with P1 and P2 during VT. Just after RF energy delivery, an activation sequence of P2 changed from distal-to-proximal to proximal-to-distal, and the QRS configuration also changed. However, VT still continued with the same cycle length. This is the direct proof that P1 is bystander, but influences the QRS configurations. Ouyang and coworkers [23] suggested that idiopathic left VT reentry might be a small macroreentry circuit consisting of one anterograde Purkinje fiber with a Purkinje potential, one retrograde Purkinje fiber with retrograde Purkinje potential, and the ventricular myocardium as the bridge.

32.2.1.3 Tachycardia Circuit

The hypothesized circuit of left posterior fascicular VT is depicted in Fig. 32.3a. In this circuit, P1 represents the activation potential in the distal portion of the specialized Purkinje tissue; it has decremental properties and verapamil sensitivity. P2 represents the activation of the left posterior fascicle or Purkinje fiber near the left posterior fascicle, and it is a bystander during VT. P1 represents the antegrade limb of the circuit in VT and left ventricular septal muscle is the retrograde limb. During sinus rhythm, the activation goes from P2 to P1 at the point of the fusion; therefore, P1 is buried in the local ventricular activation. During VT, P1 and P2 activate in the reverse direction. This explains why the activation sequences of P2 are reversed during sinus rhythm and VT. Recently, Liu and colleagues [24] suggested that the circuit of the left posterior fascicular VT is the macroreentrant loop involving the ventricular myocardium, a part of the left posterior fascicle, a slow conduction zone, and a specially conducting P1 fiber (Fig. 32.4a). Of 14 patients with idiopathic left fascicular VT, P1 potential was recorded during VT in nine patients (64%) and RF ablation was successful at P1 sites. In the remaining four patients (36%) without a recorded P1 potential during VT, ablation was successful at the earliest P2 sites (Fig. 32.4b, c). They also suggested that the site of the connection of P1 and P2 can be speculated by HV interval during VT.

32.2.2 Diagnostic Criteria

32.2.2.1 Surface Electrocardiogram

Based on the QRS morphology, verapamil-sensitive fascicular VT can be classified into three subgroups. The

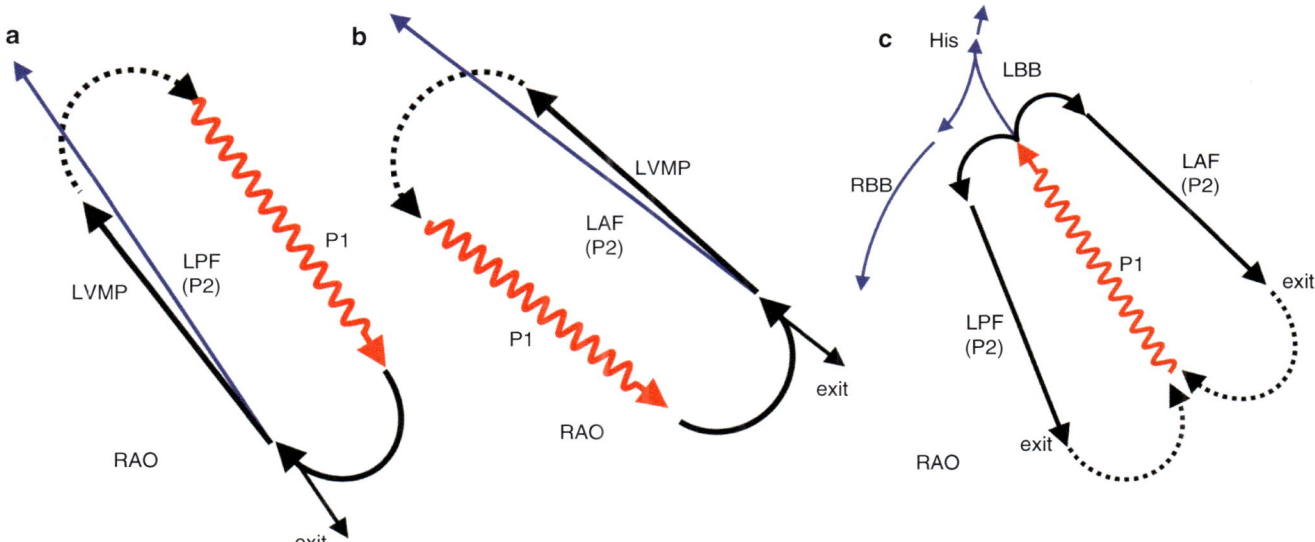

Fig. 32.3 Schematic representation of the reentrant circuits in verapamil-sensitive left fascicular ventricular tachycardias (VTs). (**a**) Left posterior fascicular VT. During the VT, P1 propagates from base to apex, P2 and left ventricular myocardial potentials (LVMP) activate in the reverse direction. The proposed upper turn-around area is shown by the *dotted line*. The undulating line represents a zone of slow conduction. Although the antegrade limb of the VT circuit consists of P1, the retrograde limb consists of LVMP, but not of P2. (**b**) Left anterior fascicular VT. During VT, the antegrade limb is the P1, the retrograde limb is the LVMP, and the exit to the ventricular muscle is near the distal portion of left anterior fascicle. (**c**) Left upper septal VT. P1 represents the activation potential of the specialized Purkinje tissue at left ventricular upper septum. P2 represents the activation of the left anterior and posterior fascicles. Both left anterior and posterior fascicles are the antegrade limbs of the reentrant circuit in VT. This explains why this VT exhibits a narrow QRS configuration and inferior axis. *LAF* left anterior fascicle, *LPF* left posterior fascicle, *LBB* left bundle branch, *LVMP* left ventricular myocardial potential, *P1* diastolic potential, *P2* presystolic Purkinje potential, *RAO* right anterior oblique view, *RBB* right bundle branch

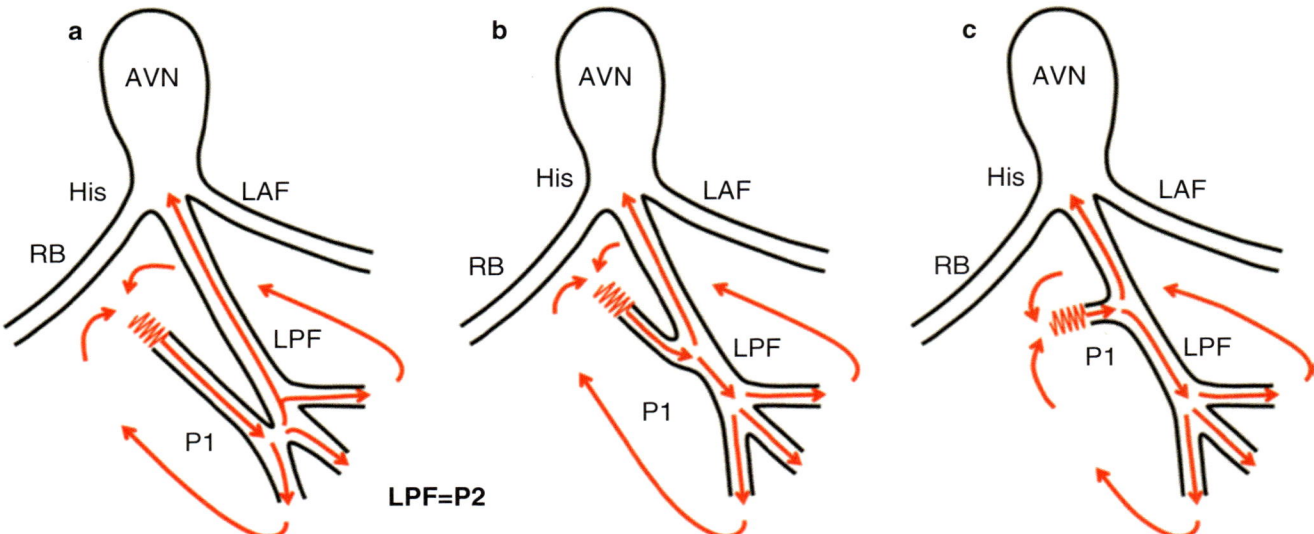

Fig. 32.4 Schematic representation of the reentrant circuits in the left posterior fascicular ventricular tachycardia (VT). The reentry circuit of LPF-VT includes ventricular myocardium, a part of the LPF, a P1 fiber, and a slow conduction zone connecting the ventricular myocardium and proximal P1. (**a**) In the cases with a recorded P1 and a more negative His-ventricular (HV) interval during LPF-VT, the P1 fiber is parallel and adjacent to the LPF, and the connection between P1 and the LPF (P2) is located at a more distal portion of the LPF. (**b**) In the cases with a recorded P1 and a slightly negative HV interval during LPF-VT, the P1 fiber is parallel and adjacent to the LPF, and the connection between P1 and the LPF (P2) is located at the middle or proximal portion of the LPF. (**c**) In the cases without a recorded P1, and HV interval that is slightly negative, the P1 fiber may be short in length or nonparallel in orientation to the LPF, or both. *AVN* atrioventricular node, *HIS* His bundle electrogram, *LAF* left anterior fascicle, *RB* right bundle (From Liu Q, Shehata M, Jiang R, et al. Macroreentrant loop in ventricular tachycardia from the left posterior fascicle: New implications for mapping and ablation. Circ Arrhythm Electrophysiol 2016; 9. pii: e004272)

12-lead ECG of the left posterior fascicular VT exhibits an RBBB and a superior axis (left-axis deviation or superior right-axis) (Fig. 32.1a). This is the common type of verapamil-sensitive fascicular VT and may account for up to 76–90% of cases [12, 13]. The uncommon type of this VT is a left anterior fascicular VT whose QRS morphology exhibits an RBBB configuration and inferior axis deviation (Fig. 32.1b) [11, 25]. The last type of VT is an upper septal fascicular VT, whose QRS morphology exhibits a relatively narrow QRS configuration and normal or right-axis deviation (Fig. 32.1c) [12, 26]. This type of VT is rare (2–6%) [12, 13].

32.2.2.2 Intracardiac Electrograms

With left posterior fascicular VT, the earliest ventricular activation is recorded from the apical septum, and diastolic potentials are recorded from the mid-septum. His activation follows QRS onset by 5–30 ms [27]. During sinus rhythm, recording from the same site demonstrates the Purkinje potentials after the His bundle potential and before the onset of the QRS complex.

With left anterior fascicular VT, the earliest ventricular activation is recorded from the anterolateral left ventricle, and diastolic potentials are recorded from the mid-septum. There have been several reports that describe a left VT with an RBBB configuration, right-axis deviation, and a different mechanism. Yeh and colleagues [28] reported four cases with an RBBB configuration and right-axis deviation. This VT was adenosine sensitive and was successfully ablated from the anterobasal left ventricle. The chest leads exhibited an atypical RBBB configuration with wide "R" morphology. Crijns and colleagues [29] reported a case of interfascicular reentrant VT with an RBBB configuration and right-axis deviation (bundle branch reentry tachycardia type B). In their patient, the VT circuit used the anterior fascicle as the anterograde limb and the posterior fascicle as the retrograde limb. Interfascicular VT usually has a His bundle potential recorded in the diastolic phase during the VT as well as posterior fascicular potentials. However, it may be difficult to distinguish between interfascicular VT and intrafascicular VT (verapamil-sensitive left anterior fascicular VT) [25]. The diagnostic criteria for left VTs are given in Table 32.1.

The differential diagnosis includes supraventricular tachycardias with bifascicular block aberrancy. With left upper septal fascicular VT, the retrograde activation of the His bundle is recorded before the onset of the QRS complex. If there is retrograde ventriculoatrial conduction during the tachycardia, it mimics atrioventricular nodal reentry tachycardia or atrioventricular reciprocating tachycardia. The response of these tachycardias to verapamil and the ability to initiate and entrain them by atrial pacing may also

Table 32.1 Diagnostic criteria for idiopathic left fascicular tachycardias

Verapamil-sensitive left fascicular tachycardia
1. Characteristic surface ECG appearance
• RBBB and superior axis configuration (common type)
• RBBB and inferior axis configuration (uncommon type)
• Narrow QRS and inferior axis configuration (rare type)
2. Electrophysiologic findings
• Tachycardia dependence on left ventricular fascicular reentry
• Purkinje potentials and diastolic potentials preceding ventricular activation
• Changes in tachycardia rate preceded by similar changes in Purkinje and diastolic potentials
• His activation follows QRS onset (short positive HV in rare type)
• Induction and entrainment with ventricular and/or atrial pacing
3. Drug response
• Verapamil-sensitive termination or slowing of tachycardia due to conduction slowing or block in fascicular system
Nonreentrant fascicular ventricular tachycardia
1. Characteristic surface ECG appearance
• RBBB and either superior or inferior axis deviation
• Faster VT is prone to exhibit wider QRS
2. Electrophysiologic findings
• Mechanism of tachycardia consistent with abnormal automaticity
• Induction by exercise and catecholamines
• Unable to induce or entrain by ventricular stimulation
• Transient suppression by adenosine and with overdrive pacing or faster supraventricular rhythm
• Negative HV interval in tachycardia
3. Drug response
• Responsive to lidocaine, β-blockers, and class Ia drugs
• No response to verapamil

ECG electrocardiogram, *HV* His-to-ventricular, *RBBB* right bundle branch block, *VT* ventricular tachycardia

lead to diagnostic confusion. To avoid a misdiagnosis, recognition of the retrograde sequence of the His bundle activation and measurement of a shorter His-to-ventricular (HV) interval during the tachycardia than in sinus rhythm is important. An earlier potential than the His bundle potential is recorded from the left ventricular upper septum, where the left bundle potential is recorded during sinus rhythm. VT can be slowed or terminated by the intravenous administration of verapamil; however, it is unresponsive to Valsalva maneuvers. Class Ia and class Ic drugs are also effective. Rare cases of adenosine responsiveness occur, but only if the tachycardia shows catecholamine dependency.

In bundle branch reentry, the His activation precedes activation of the left bundle to produce a RBBB QRS morphology. In idiopathic left VT, the HV interval is shorter (negative) and follows left fascicular activation.

32.2.3 Mapping and Ablation

RF catheter ablation may be considered a potential first-line therapy for patients with idiopathic VT because these VTs can be eliminated by ablation in a high percentage of patients.

32.2.3.1 Left Posterior Fascicular Ventricular Tachycardia

Conventional left ventricular septal mapping using a multipolar electrode catheter is useful in patients with left posterior fascicular VT [19]. Electroanatomic activation mapping is not typically required, but the ability to tag catheter positions of interest is often helpful. Two distinct potentials, P1 and P2, can be recorded during the VT from the mid-septum. Because the diastolic potential (P1) has been proved a critical potential in the VT circuit, this potential can be targeted to cure the tachycardia. Nakagawa and coworkers [27] first reported the importance of Purkinje potentials in the ablation of this VT, and Tsuchiya and associates [30] reported the significance of a late diastolic potential and emphasized the role of late diastolic and presystolic potentials in the VT circuit. However, the successful ablation sites identified by these two research groups were different. Whereas Nakagawa's ablation sites were at the apical-inferior septum of the left ventricle, Tsuchiya's ablation sites were at the basal septal regions close to the main trunk of the left bundle branch. These findings suggest that any P1 during VT can be targeted for catheter ablation. We usually target the apical third of the septum to avoid the creation of left bundle branch block (LBBB) or atrioventricular block.

Using the retrograde aortic approach, the ablation catheter crosses the aortic valve with a tight curve oriented to the right side of the fluoroscopic view in RAO. Once in the left ventricular chamber, the catheter is rotated toward the septum, then the curvature is opened, allowing the tip of the catheter to fall toward the inferior septum toward the apex. In our study, P1 was recorded during the VT in 15 of 20 patients (75%). RF ablation was successfully performed at this site in all 15 patients. During energy application, the P1-QRS interval was gradually prolonged, and the VT was terminated by block between P1 and QRS. After termination of the tachycardia, the P1 was noted to occur after the QRS complex during sinus rhythm, whereas the P2 was still observed before the QRS complex. After successful ablation, the P1 occurred after the QRS complex, with an identical activation sequence to that observed during the VT. When the distal segment of P1 is ablated, the P1 activation proceeds orthodromically around the circuit and subsequently blocks from a proximal to distal direction during sinus rhythm. The P1 that appears after ablation exhibits decremental properties during atrial pacing or ventricular pacing, or both, and the intravenous administration of verapamil significantly prolongs the His-to-P1 interval during sinus rhythm.

Pace-mapping at the successful ablation site is usually not good because the selective pacing of P1 is difficult, and there is an antidromic activation of the proximal P1 potential. Pace-mapping after successful ablation is sometimes better than before ablation because the antidromic activation of P1 is blocked [31].

In the remaining five of our 20 patients (25%), the diastolic potential (P1) could not be detected, and a single fused P2 was recorded only at the VT exit site. Successful ablation was performed at this site in all five patients. We can speculate that the circuit in these patients may have involved less of the Purkinje system or that the area of slow conduction may not have been close to the endocardial surface. Liu and colleagues [24] also reported that P1 potential could not be recorded during VT in 4 of 14 patients (36%), and RF ablation was successful at the earliest P2 sites. They speculated that the P1 fiber in the patients without a recorded P1 potential may be short in length or nonparallel in orientation to the left posterior fascicle, or both (Fig. 32.4).

32.2.3.2 Left Anterior Fascicular Ventricular Tachycardia

Figure 32.1b shows the 12-lead ECG of verapamil-sensitive left anterior fascicular VTs. In our series of this type VT [25], the mean cycle length of the VT was 390 ± 62 ms, and the mean electrical axis during the VT was 120 ± 16°. Left ventricular endocardial mapping during left anterior fascicular VT identified the earliest ventricular activation in the anterolateral wall of the left ventricle. RF current delivered to this site suppressed the VT in three patients (patient 1 in Fig. 32.1b). The fused Purkinje potential was recorded at that site and preceded the QRS complex by 20–35 ms, with pace-mapping exhibiting an optimal match between the paced rhythm and clinical VT. In the remaining three patients (patient 2 in Fig. 32.1b), RF catheter ablation at the site of the earliest ventricular activation was unsuccessful. In these patients, a Purkinje potential was recorded in the diastolic phase during the VT at the mid-anterior left ventricular septum. The Purkinje potential preceded the QRS during VT by 56 to 66 ms, and catheter ablation at these sites was successful.

One of our patients with the left anterior fascicular VT also had a typical left posterior fascicular VT. Kottkamp and colleagues [32] also reported one patient who had two left VT configurations with right- and left-axis deviation. In this patient, RF catheter ablation delivered to the single site between the left anterior and posterior fascicles successfully eliminated both VTs. This suggests that the antegrade limbs in these VTs are the common pathways.

The circuit of the left anterior fascicular VT was shown in Fig. 32.3b. In this circuit, P1 represents the activation potential in the proximal portion of the specialized Purkinje tissue with a decremental property. During VT, the antegrade limb is the P1, and the retrograde limb is the left ventricular muscle. This type of VT can be named as left anterior slow-fast type fascicular VT. The circuits of the left anterior and posterior fascicular VTs are mirror images (Fig. 32.3a, b).

32.2.3.3 Left Upper Septal Fascicular Ventricular Tachycardia

In the patients with the upper septal fascicular VT [12, 13], a fused Purkinje potential was recorded at left posterior fascicular area during sinus rhythm. And during VT, recording at the same site also demonstrated a fused presystolic Purkinje potential. The activation sequences of Purkinje potentials at left posterior fascicular area are similar during sinus rhythm and VT. This site is one of exit during VT because a fused presystolic ventricular potential was recorded. And the other exit site during VT might be left anterior fascicular area because the QRS morphology during VT is quite narrow and exhibited an inferior axis. This VT was successfully ablated at the left ventricular upper septum. At this site, a left bundle branch (left fascicle; LF) potential was recorded during sinus rhythm and the Purkinje potential preceded the QRS by 35 ms during the VT. The RF application eliminated the VT without creating an LBBB or atrioventricular block.

When the P1 is selectively captured during tachycardia, concealed entrainment can be obtained [13, 26]. Multipolar electrode catheter on the LV middle septum demonstrates articulate diastolic potential (P1) and presystolic potential (P2) during VT. Activation sequence of P1 is from distal to proximal, while the activation sequence of P2 is from proximal to distal. These activation sequences of P1 and P2 are reverse pattern of those in left posterior or anterior fascicular VT. Entrainment pacing from the middle septal area with P1 potential selectively captures P1 potential and produces an identical QRS complex to that of the VT with an S-QRS latency of 53 ms, equal to the P1-QRS interval during VT. The difference between the postpacing interval (S-P1) and the VTCL is 10 ms.

The hypothesized VT circuit is depicted in Fig. 32.3c. In this circuit, P1 represents the activation potential of the specialized Purkinje tissue at left ventricular upper septum. P2 represents the activation of the left anterior and posterior fascicles. Both left anterior and posterior fascicles are the antegrade limbs of the reentrant circuit in VT. This explains why this VT exhibits a narrow QRS configuration and inferior axis. DP represents the common retrograde limb of the circuit in VT and can be ablation target. This type of VT can be named as fast-slow type fascicular VT. The circuit of the left upper septal fascicular VT is the antidromic form of the left anterior and posterior fascicular VTs (Fig. 32.3).

32.2.3.4 End Point of Radiofrequency Ablation

With catheter ablation of verapamil-sensitive idiopathic left VT, no special mapping or ablation system is typically needed. We usually use a quadripolar steerable electrode catheter with irrigation. RF energy is delivered using maximum power of 40 W. We deliver RF energy during the tachycardia of left posterior and anterior fascicular VTs. If the VT is terminated or slowed within 15 s, additional current is applied for another 60–90 s. If the initial RF current is ineffective, ablation is directed to a more proximal site with the earlier diastolic potential. If the mid-diastolic potential cannot be detected, RF current is applied at the VT exit site showing a single fused presystolic Purkinje potential. With upper septal fascicular VT, we deliver RF energy for 30–60 s during sinus rhythm to avoid atrioventricular block. We perform catheter ablation in this region using a low power output (i.e., 10 W), which can gradually be increased while carefully monitoring for development of a junctional rhythm or atrioventricular block.

After the ablation, programmed stimulation should be repeated. Other than the noninducibility of VT, there are several electrophysiologic findings that can serve as end points of RF applications for left posterior fascicular VT. After ablation of the distal attachment between P1 and ventricular muscle, P1 appears after the QRS complex. However, this phenomenon is not sufficient for an end point because this only indicates conduction block in the direction from the left septal ventricular muscle to P1 only. This unidirectional block can be seen during the baseline state [23] or after an insufficient RF application [31]. To confirm the creation of bidirectional block between P1 and the ventricular muscle, we do atrial pacing with various cycle lengths after the ablation. If there is residual conduction from P1 to the ventricular muscle, a premature ventricular complex (i.e., ventricular echo beat) with a similar QRS morphology as that observed during the VT can be observed repeatedly.

32.2.4 Success and Recurrence Rates

Our experience at the time of this writing includes 160 patients with left posterior fascicular VT, 40 patients with left anterior fascicular VT, and 12 patients with left upper septal fascicular VT. The success and recurrence rates are 97% and 4.5%, respectively, for left posterior fascicular VT; 90% and 10% for left anterior fascicular VT; and 100% and 8% for left upper septal fascicular VT.

Aside from the complications that may result from any left ventricular electrophysiologic procedure (e.g., thrombophlebitis, damage to the femoral artery, ventricular perforation), the only complication that has been associated with catheter ablation of idiopathic left VT has been LBBB and atrioventricular block. Tsuchiya and associates [30] reported that two patients (12.5%) had transient LBBB after ablation in their series of 16 patients. They targeted the left basal septum, and the LBBB disappeared within 10 min without VT recurrence. In our experience, 1 (0.5%) of 198 patients had a transient atrioventricular block. This patient had a left posterior fascicular VT, and the diastolic potential (P1) at the mid-septum was targeted for the ablation. Before the ablation, the patient had catheter-induced RBBB. About 15 s into the RF delivery, the VT terminated, and second-degree atrioventricular block was observed. The atrioventricular block disappeared immediately after discontinuation of the RF energy delivery.

32.2.5 Troubleshooting the Difficult Case

Inability to reliably induce VT is a formidable obstacle to successful ablation. Isoproterenol facilitates induction of sustained VT in 60–70% of those patients without inducible sustained VT at baseline. In some patients, the administration of small doses of class Ia drugs enhances the slow conduction at the specialized Purkinje tissue and facilitates induction of stable sustained VT. Catheter mapping sometimes mechanically suppresses the conduction in the VT circuit ("bump" phenomenon). In such cases, a ventricular echo beat during sinus rhythm or atrial pacing is useful. If premature ventricular complexes with a similar QRS morphology to that observed during the VT are repeatedly seen, activation mapping can be performed. If no ventricular echo beats are inducible, the empirical anatomic approach can be an effective strategy for ablation of left posterior fascicular VT [33, 34]. First, the VT exit site is sought by pace-mapping during sinus rhythm, and RF energy is delivered to that site. Second, a linear lesion is placed at the mid-septum, perpendicular to the long axis of the left ventricle, about 10–15 mm proximal to the VT exit. During anatomic linear ablation, P1 suddenly appears after the QRS complex if the ablation site is on the descending limb of the VT circuit. This anatomic approach is also useful in patients in whom diastolic Purkinje potential cannot be recorded during VT [34].

If a good electrogram is not found at the septum, one possible reason is poor catheter contact with the septum. The left anterior oblique fluoroscopic view is used to guide the catheter toward the septum, and the right anterior oblique view to guide the catheter posteriorly and toward the apical third of the septum.

If ablation catheter stability is poor during the VT because of excessive heart motion, RF energy can be delivered during sinus rhythm. However, even during sinus rhythm, frequent ventricular premature beats (with a similar QRS morphology to that observed during the VT) and VT are sometimes induced during the RF energy application. In such cases, overdrive pacing or intravenous administration of verapamil is effective for suppressing the ventricular premature beats and VT during the RF energy application. However, after such an infusion, the noninducibility of the VT becomes invalid as an end point for the ablation. Cryoablation of left fascicular VT has been reported in a selected population [35]. Cryoablation is effective given the superficial nature of the reentrant circuit and may offer the advantages of no induction of premature ventricular complexes and extreme catheter stability during ablation.

32.3 Nonreentrant Fascicular VT

32.3.1 Clinical and Electrophysiologic Characteristics

Another type of idiopathic fascicular VT is the nonreentrant fascicular VT from the Purkinje system [36]. This VT is classified as propranolol-sensitive automatic VT [1]. Although nonreentrant fascicular VT is usually observed in patients with ischemic heart disease [37], it is also observed in patients with structurally normal hearts [38, 39]. Nonreentrant fascicular VT from the left ventricle can present with an RBBB configuration and either a left- or right-axis deviation on the 12-lead ECG, depending on the origin. It is difficult to distinguish this VT from reentrant fascicular VT by 12-lead ECG. This VT can be induced by exercise and catecholamines (e.g., isoproterenol and phenylephrine); however, it cannot be induced or terminated by programmed ventricular stimulation. Although this VT is responsive to lidocaine and β-blockers, it is usually not responsive to verapamil. This can be used as a differentiation from verapamil-sensitive fascicular VT. This VT is transiently suppressed by adenosine and with overdrive pacing. The clinical and electrophysiologic characteristics of this VT have not been well defined [38, 39]. Gonzalez and colleagues [38] reported the electrophysiologic spectrum of Purkinje-related VT in eight patients and showed the mechanism to be consistent with abnormal automaticity or triggered activity in five patients. The 12-lead ECG during VT in these patients showed RBBB with left-axis deviation. A distinct His deflection was recorded with an HV interval during VT that was shorter than that during sinus rhythm. Recently, we reported 15 patients (2.8%) with nonreentrant fascicular VT among 530 idiopathic VT patients who were referred for ablation [36]. This VT is usually originated from the left posterior fascicle, and less commonly from the left anterior fascicle and right ventricular Purkinje network. The diagnostic criteria for left VTs are given in Table 32.1.

Monomorphic premature ventricular complexes have been shown to initiate ventricular fibrillation (VF) in patients with no structural heart disease [40, 41] and ischemic heart disease [42, 43]. However, the difference in the clinical and electrophysiologic characteristic between VF triggered by premature ventricular complex from Purkinje system and monomorphic nonreentrant fascicular VT has been undetermined. Tsuchiya and associates [44] reported a patient who exhibited the transition from Purkinje-related polymorphic VT to monomorphic VT. The intravenous administration of pilsicainide (class Ic) provoked incessant nonsustained polymorphic VT, and the polymorphic VT changed to monomorphic VT after the additional administration of pilsicainide. RF current application to the Purkinje system at the left ventricular septum suppressed both polymorphic and monomorphic VTs.

32.3.2 Mapping and Ablation

The ablation target of nonreentrant fascicular VT is the earliest Purkinje activation during VT, whereas that of verapamil-sensitive fascicular VT is not necessarily the earliest Purkinje activation. Catheter ablation is effective, whereas pacemap-guided approach is less efficacious [36].

Because the VT could not be induced by ventricular stimulation and catecholamines, isolated premature ventricular complex with a similar QRS morphology to that observed during the VT was targeted. Left ventricular endocardial mapping during premature ventricular complex identified the earliest Purkinje activation in the anterolateral wall of the left ventricle. The fused Purkinje potential was also recorded at that site during sinus rhythm.

32.3.3 Complications

The complication that has been associated with catheter ablation of nonreentrant fascicular VT has been LBBB and atrioventricular block. In verapamil-sensitive fascicular VTs, the creation of LBBB or atrioventricular block as the complication is quite rare because the ablation target is the diastolic "abnormal" Purkinje potential (P1) during VT, and the abolition of the normal Purkinje or fascicle potential (P2) is not needed to suppress the VT. On the other hand, the abolition of the Purkinje network is usually necessary to suppress the nonreentrant fascicular VT. After successful ablation, the amplitude of the local myocardium has been diminished, and presystolic Purkinje potential was sometimes eliminated and appeared after the myocardial potential. Because this site was located at the distal portion of the left posterior fascicle, there has been no change in the surface QRS morphology or HV interval after ablation. If the VT arises from a more proximal portion of the fascicle, there is a potential risk for creating LBBB or atrioventricular block by ablation. Rodriguez and colleagues [39] reported the nonreentrant fascicular VT with an RBBB configuration and right-axis deviation in whom left anterior fascicular block occurred after the ablation. Lopera and associates [37] reported two nonreentrant fascicular VT cases with ischemic heart disease in whom complete atrioventricular block occurred after the successful ablation of VT. In our reported 15 patients [36], right-axis deviation was observed in 1 patient, and mild left-axis deviation was observed in another patient; however, neither atrioventricular block nor LBBB was found during or after RFCA.

32.3.4 Success and Recurrence Rates

Our experience at the time of this writing includes 16 patients with idiopathic nonreentrant fascicular VT. In all patients, VT and ventricular premature complex were suppressed by catheter ablation; however, the true acute success rate is unclear because this VT is difficult to induce. Therefore, the recurrence rate is high (25%).

References

1. Lerman BB, Stein KM, Markowitz SM. Mechanism of idiopathic ventricular tachycardia. J Cardiovasc Electrophysiol. 1997;8:571–83.
2. Okumura K, Tsuchiya T. Idiopathic left ventricular tachycardia: clinical features, mechanism and management. Card Electrophysiol Rev. 2002;6:61–7.
3. Coggins DL, Lee RJ, Sweeney J, Chein WW, et al. Radiofrequency catheter ablation as a cure for idiopathic tachycardia of both left and right ventricular origin. J Am Coll Cardiol. 1994;23:1333–41.
4. Daoud E, Morady F. Catheter ablation of ventricular tachycardia. Curr Opin Cardiol. 1995;10:21–5.
5. Ito S, Tada H, Naito S, et al. Development and validation of an ECG algorithm for identifying the optimal ablation site for idiopathic ventricular outflow tract tachycardia. J Cardiovasc Electrophysiol. 2003;14:1280–6.
6. Callans DJ, Menz V, Schwartzman D, et al. Repetitive monomorphic tachycardia from the left ventricular outflow tract: electrocardiographic patterns consistent with a left ventricular site of origin. J Am Coll Cardiol. 1997;29:1023–7.
7. Kanagaratnam L, Tomassoni G, Schweikert R, et al. Ventricular tachycardias arising from the aortic sinus of valsalva: an under-recognized variant of left outflow tract ventricular tachycardia. J Am Coll Cardiol. 2001;37:1408–14.
8. Ouyang F, Fotuhi P, Ho SY, et al. Repetitive monomorphic ventricular tachycardia originating from the aortic sinus cusp: electrocardiographic characterization for guiding catheter ablation. J Am Coll Cardiol. 2002;39:500–8.
9. Zipes DP, Foster PR, Troup PJ, Pedersen DH. Atrial induction of ventricular tachycardia: reentry versus triggered automaticity. Am J Cardiol. 1979;44:1–8.
10. Belhassen B, Rotmensch HH, Laniado S. Response of recurrent sustained ventricular tachycardia to verapamil. Br Heart J. 1981;46:679–82.
11. Ohe T, Shimomura K, Aihara N, et al. Idiopathic sustained left ventricular tachycardia: clinical and electrophysiological characteristics. Circulation. 1988;77:560–8.
12. Nogami A. Idiopathic left ventricular tachycardia: assessment and treatment. Card Electrophysiol Rev. 2002;6:448–57.
13. Talib AK, Nogami A, Nishiuchi S, Kowase S, Kurosaki K, Matsui Y, Kawada S, Watanabe A, Nozoe M, Uno K, Yagishita A, Yamauchi Y, Takahashi Y, Kuwahara T, Takahashi A, Kumagai K, Naito S, Asakawa T, Sekiguchi Y, Aonuma K. Verapamil-sensitive upper septal idiopathic left ventricular tachycardia: prevalence, mechanism, and electrophysiological characteristics. JACCCEP. 2015;1:369–80.
14. Gallagher JJ, Selle JG, Svenson RH, et al. Surgical treatment of arrhythmias. Am J Cardiol. 1988;61(27):44A.
15. Suwa M, Yoneda Y, Nagao H, et al. Surgical correction of idiopathic paroxysmal ventricular tachycardia possibly related to left ventricular false tendon. Am J Cardiol. 1989;64:1217–20.
16. Thakur RK, Klein GJ, Sivaram CA, et al. Anatomic substrate for idiopathic left ventricular tachycardia. Circulation. 1996;93:497–501.
17. Maruyama M, Terada T, Miyamoto S, Ino T. Demonstration of the reentrant circuit of verapamil-sensitive idiopathic left ventricular tachycardia: direct evidence for macroreentry as the underlying mechanism. J Cardiovasc Electrophysiol. 2001;12:968–72.
18. Lin FC, Wen MS, Wang CC, et al. Left ventricular fibromuscular band is not a specific substrate for idiopathic left ventricular tachycardia. Circulation. 1996;93:525–7.
19. Nogami A, Naito S, Tada H, et al. Demonstration of diastolic and presystolic Purkinje potential as critical potentials on a macroreentry circuit of verapamil-sensitive idiopathic left ventricular tachycardia. J Am Coll Cardiol. 2000;36:811–23.
20. Kuo JY, Tai CT, Chiang CE, et al. Is the fascicle of left bundle branch involved in the reentrant circuit of verapamil-sensitive idiopathic left ventricular tachycardia? Pacing Clin Electrophysiol. 2003;26:1986–92.
21. Morishima I, Nogami A, Tsuboi H, Sone T. Negative participation of the left posterior fascicle in the reentry circuit of verapamil-sensitive idiopathic left ventricular tachycardia. Heart Rhythm. 2012;23:556–9.
22. Maeda S, Yokoyama Y, Nogami A, Chik WW, Hirao K. First case of left posterior fascicle in a bystander circuit of idiopathic left ventricular tachycardia. Can J Cardiol. 2014;30(1460):e11–3.
23. Ouyang F, Cappato R, Ernst S, et al. Electroanatomic substrate of idiopathic left ventricular tachycardia: Unidirectional block and macroreentry within the Purkinje network. Circulation. 2002;105:462–9.
24. Liu Q, Shehata M, Jiang R, Yu L, Chen S, Zhu J, Ehdaie A, Sovari AA, Cingolani E, Chugh SS, Jiang C, Wang X. Macroreentrant loop in ventricular tachycardia from the left posterior fascicle: new implications for mapping and ablation. Circ Arrhythm Electrophysiol. 2016;9:pii:e004272.
25. Nogami A, Naito S, Tada H, et al. Verapamil-sensitive left anterior fascicular ventricular tachycardia: results of radiofrequency ablation in six patients. J Cardiovasc Electrophysiol. 1998;9:1269–78.
26. Nishiuchi S, Nogami A, Naito S. A case with occurrence of antidromic tachycardia after ablation of idiopathic left fascicular tachycardia: mechanism of left upper septal ventricular tachycardia. J Cardiovasc Electrophysiol. 2013;24:825–7.
27. Nakagawa H, Beckman KJ, McClelland JH, et al. Radiofrequency catheter ablation of idiopathic left ventricular tachycardia guided by a Purkinje potential. Circulation. 1993;88:2607–17.
28. Yeh SJ, Wen MS, Wang CC, et al. Adenosine-sensitive ventricular tachycardia from the anterobasal left ventricle. J Am Coll Cardiol. 1997;30:339–45.
29. Crijns HJ, Smeets JL, Rodriguez LM, Meijer A. Cure of interfascicular reentrant ventricular tachycardia by ablation to anterior fascicle of the left bundle branch. J Cardiovasc Electrophysiol. 1995;6:486–92.

30. Tsuchiya T, Okumura K, Honda T, et al. Significance of late diastolic potential preceding Purkinje potential in verapamil-sensitive idiopathic left ventricular tachycardia. Circulation. 1999;99:2408–13.
31. Tada H, Nogami A, Naito S, et al. Retrograde Purkinje potential activation during sinus rhythm following catheter ablation of idiopathic left ventricular tachycardia. J Cardiovasc Electrophysiol. 1998;9:1218–24.
32. Kottkamp H, Hindricks G, Willems S, et al. Idiopathic left ventricular tachycardia: new insights into electrophysiological characteristics and radiofrequency catheter ablation. Pacing Clin Electrophysiol. 1995;18:1285–97.
33. Lin D, Hsia HH, Gerstenfeld EP, et al. Idiopathic fascicular left ventricular tachycardia: linear ablation lesion strategy for noninducible or nonsustained tachycardia. Heart Rhythm. 2005;2:934–9.
34. Talib AK, Nogami A. Anatomical ablation strategy for noninducible fascicular tachycardia. Cardiac Electrophysiol Clin. 2016;8:115–20.
35. Timmermans C, Manusama R, Alzand B, Rodriguez LM. Catheter-based cryoablation of postinfarction and idiopathic ventricular tachycardia: initial experience in a selected population. J Cardiovasc Electrophysiol. 2010;21:255–61.
36. Talib AK, Nogami A, Morishima I, Oginosawa Y, Kurosaki K, Kowase S, Komatsu Y, Kuroki K, Igarashi M, Sekiguchi Y, Aonuma K. Non-reentrant fascicular tachycardia: clinical and electrophysiological characteristics of a distinct type of idiopathic ventricular tachycardia. Circ Arrhythm Electrophysiol. 2016;9:pii:e004177.
37. Lopera G, Stevenson WG, Soejima K, et al. Identification and ablation of three types of ventricular tachycardia involving the His-Purkinje system in patients with heart disease. J Cardiovasc Electrophysiol. 2004;15:52–8.
38. Gonzalez RP, Scheinman MM, Lesh MD, et al. Clinical and electrophysiologic spectrum of fascicular tachycardias. Am Heart J. 1994;128:147–56.
39. Rodriguez LM, Smeets JL, Timmermans C, et al. Radiofrequency catheter ablation of idiopathic ventricular tachycardia originating in the anterior fascicle of the left bundle branch. J Cardiovasc Electrophysiol. 1996;7:1211–6.
40. Haïssaguerre M, Shah DC, Jaïs P, et al. Role of Purkinje conducting system in triggering of idiopathic ventricular fibrillation. Lancet. 2002;359:677–8.
41. Nogami A, Sugiyasu A, Kubota S, Kato K. Mapping and ablation of idiopathic ventricular fibrillation from the Purkinje system. Heart Rhythm. 2005;2:646–9.
42. Bänsch D, Ouyang F, Antz M, et al. Successful catheter ablation of electrical storm after myocardial infarction. Circulation. 2003;108:3011–6.
43. Masuda K, Nogami A, Kuroki K, Igarashi M, Sekiguchi Y, Komatsu Y, Kowase S, Kurosaki K, Nishihara S, Niwa K, Tsuchiya T, Igawa M, Aonuma K. Conversion to Purkinje-related monomorphic ventricular tachycardia after ablation of ventricular fibrillation in ischemic heart disease. Circ Arrhythm Electrophysiol. 2016;9:pii:e004224.
44. Tsuchiya T, Nakagawa S, Yanagita Y, Fukunaga T. Transition from Purkinje fiber-related rapid polymorphic ventricular tachycardia to sustained monomorphic ventricular tachycardia in a patient with a structurally normal heart: a case report. J Cardiovasc Electrophysiol. 2007;18:102–5.

Bundle Branch Reentrant Ventricular Tachycardia

Mitsuhiro Nishizaki, Seiji Fukamizu, and Harumizu Sakurada

Keywords

Bundle branch reentrant ventricular tachycardia • Interfascicular reentrant ventricular tachycardia • His-Purkinje • Entrainment • Catheter ablation

33.1 Introductory Remarks

Reentry within His-Purkinje system was recognized as a normal electrophysiological response, which can produce isolated repetitive complexes. However, macroreentrant circuit involving the bundle branches or the fascicles can develop bundle branch reentrant ventricular tachycardia (BBR-VT) in patients with conduction disturbance within the His-Purkinje system, which is associated with organic heart diseases such as prior myocardial infarction, cardiomyopathy, and valvular heart diseases [1, 2].

33.2 Clinical Features and ECG Interpretation

BBR-VT rate is often very rapid, which may lead to hemodynamic compromise and syncope or cardiac arrest in patients with advanced structural heart disease. Patients with BBR-VT also have nonspecific intraventricular conduction delay, either complete or incomplete left bundle branch block pattern and prolonged HV interval in sinus rhythm on the 12-leads ECG. In particular, His-Purkinje conduction delay is essential for development of BBR-VT. BBR-VT is a ventricular tachyarrhythmia that is usually seen in patients with structural heart disease, reduced left ventricular (LV) ejection function and congestive heart failure. BBR-VT was more frequently encountered in patients with nonischemic cardiomyopathy who had inducible sustained monomorphic ventricular tachycardia, compared to patients with ischemic cardiomyopathy due to prior myocardial infarction. Moreover, His-Purkinje conduction delay degenerating into BBR-VT is observed in other disease including myotonic dystrophy, hypertrophic cardiomyopathy, and valvular heart disease [1–3].

BBR-VT usually exhibits the QRS morphology with a left bundle branch block (LBBB) configuration; however, a right bundle branch block (RBBB) pattern is rarely seen in patients with BBR-VT, in which it is often accompanied by a left hemiblock. In the patients, interfascicular reentry should be considered.

33.3 Mechanism

BBR-VT is a form of macroreentrant VT in which the reentry circuit includes the His bundle, the right and left bundles, the ventricular septum, and the Purkinje system. The most common form of BBR-VT induced during programmed extrastimulation exhibits a typical LBBB pattern. Especially, this tachycardia is initiated most frequently during right ventricular (RV) extrastimulation (Figs. 33.1 and 33.2).

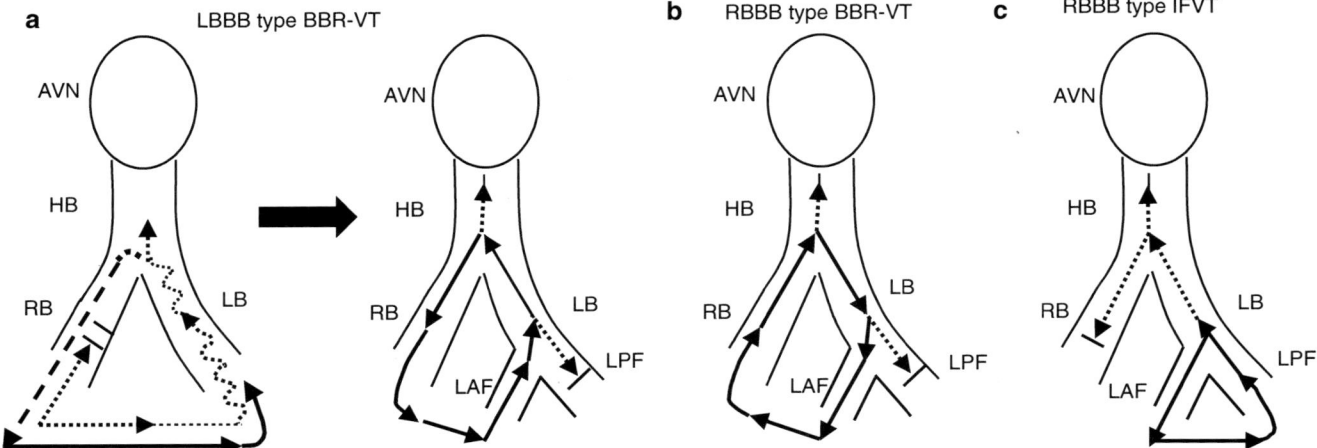

Fig. 33.1 Schematics of BBR-VT and IFVT. (**a**) Induction (*left panel*) and maintenance (*right panel*) of LBBB type BBR-VT. During RV stimulation, retrograde block occur in the RB with slow retrograde conduction through the LB, leading to the retrograde His bundle activation via the left bundle branch. Together with a critical degree of retrograde delay in left bundle conduction, the impulse can return down the RB to excite the ventricles producing the LBBB pattern. (**b**) Reentrant circuit in RBBB type BBR-VT. Antegrade conduction down the LB and retrograde conduction up the RB is observed in BBR-VT with the QRS morphology with an RBBB configuration. (**c**) Reentrant circuit in RBBB type IFVT: The impulse conducts anterogradely over the left anterior fascicle, and then conduct retrogradely over the left posterior fascicle, giving rise to RBBB type IFVT. *BBR-VT* bundle branch reentrant ventricular tachycardia, *IFVT* interfascicular reentrant ventricular tachycardia, *Arrowheads* site of activation wavefront, *AVN* atrioventricular node, *RB* right bundle branch, *LB* left bundle branch, *LAF* left anterior fascicle, *LPF* left posterior fascicle

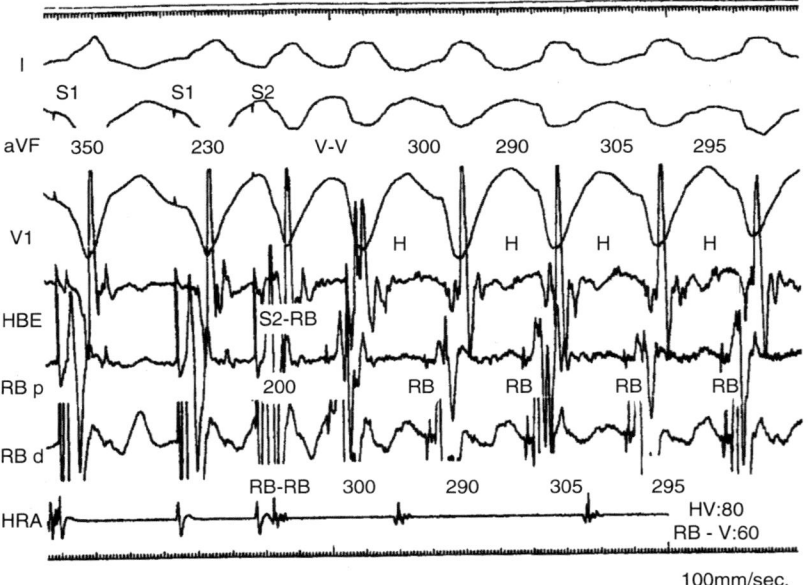

Fig. 33.2 Surface ECG and intracardiac electrograms during induction of LBBB type BBR-VT during RV stimulation at close coupling interval (230 ms). When the tachycardia is induced, the atrioventricular (A-V) dissociation is observed. During VT, changes in the V-V interval are preceded by changes in the H-H and RB-RB interval. *HBE* His bundle electrogram, *RB* right bundle branch, *HRA* high right atrium

In this tachycardia, the right bundle branch (RB) constitutes the antegrade limb of reentrant circuit, and the retrograde limb is the left bundle branch (LB). During RV stimulation at close coupling interval, retrograde conduction delay and block occur in the RB with slow retrograde conduction through the LB, leading to the retrograde His bundle activation via the LB. Together with a critical degree of retrograde delay in left bundle conduction, the impulse can return down the RB to excite the ventricles producing the LBBB pattern of similar morphology to the stimulated complex at the right ventricular apex. Therefore, in BBR-VT generating the QRS morphology with an LBBB configuration, the initial site of ventricular depolarization is at the right ventricular apex (Figs. 33.1 and 33.2). On the other hand, reentrant circuit with anterograde conduction down the LB and retrograde conduction up the RB is recognized in BBR-VT with the QRS morphology with an RBBB configuration, the so-called reverse BBR-VT. Therefore, conduction in the reentrant circuit occurs in the opposite direction [1–4] (Fig. 33.1). In particular, an RBBB type BBR-VT is often induced by the incremental atrial pacing in addition to ventricular pacing [4].

A variant form of BBR is interfascicular reentry [5–7]. Ventricular tachycardia due to interfascicular reentry is often observed in patients with an anterior infarction and RBBB together with either left anterior or posterior fascicular block on the ECG. The impulse conducts anterogradely down the anterior fascicle without conduction delay and retrogradely up the posterior fascicle to form macroreentry within the His-Purkinje system. The His bundle is activated retrogradely over the posterior fascicle during anterograde conduction, which produces a shorter H-V interval than during sinus rhythm. The QRS morphology exhibits the RBBB with left posterior fascicular block pattern (Fig. 33.1). On the other hand, the reentrant circuit may be depolarized in opposite direction, which gives rise to a QRS morphology of the RBBB with left anterior fascicle block pattern. This tachycardia shows a similar QRS morphology to verapamil-sensitive idiopathic left ventricular tachycardia in patients without structural heart disease, and it is necessary to differentiate between the two.

33.4 Electrophysiological Testing

The patients with BBR-VT commonly have prolongation of the QRS complex duration and the H-V interval in sinus rhythm. Induction of BBR-VT is often achieved with one or more premature ventricular beats or programmed stimulation of the ventricle, where retrograde activation is blocked due to refractoriness from the preceding normally conducted anterograde beat in the RB and into the LB with a shorter refractory period. As a result, the impulse conducts retrogradely up the LB to the His bundle and then conducts anterogradely down the RB, activating the ventricle at the termination of the RB. Therefore, the QRS during VT has an LBBB pattern and may closely resemble the sinus rhythm QRS if baseline LBBB is present.

Diagnostic features of BBR-VT are shown in Table 33.1.

(a) The QRS morphology of the tachycardia exhibited a typical LBBB or RBBB pattern. (b) Induction of BBR-VT during ventricular stimulation depends on His-Purkinje conduction delay (prolongation of V-H intervals). (c) The onset of the ventricular depolarization is preceded by the His potentials (d) The H-V, RB-V, or LB-V interval during the tachycardia is longer than or equal to each interval during sinus rhythm (Fig. 33.3). In some cases, if a very proximal His bundle is recorded, the H-V interval during the tachycar-

Table 33.1 Diagnostic features of BBR-VT

(a) The QRS morphology of the tachycardia exhibits a typical LBBB or RBBB pattern
(b) Induction of BBR-VT during ventricular stimulation depends on His-Purkinje conduction delay (prolongation of V-H intervals)
(c) The onset of the ventricular depolarization (QRS complex) is preceded by the His potentials
(d) The H-V, RB-V, or LB-V interval during the tachycardia is longer than or equal to each interval during sinus rhythm
(e) Variations in the H-H, RB-RB, or LB-LB interval during the tachycardia precede the changes in the V-V interval
(f) The RB and the LB deflection occurs after the His deflection during BBR-VT with an LBBB and an RBBB configuration, respectively
(g) The QRS morphology during atrial entrainment is identical to the QRS morphology during BBR-VT
(h) The difference between the postpacing interval after entrainment from the right ventricular apex and the tachycardia cycle length is less than 30 ms
(i) RBB-VT is no longer inducible after the RB ablation

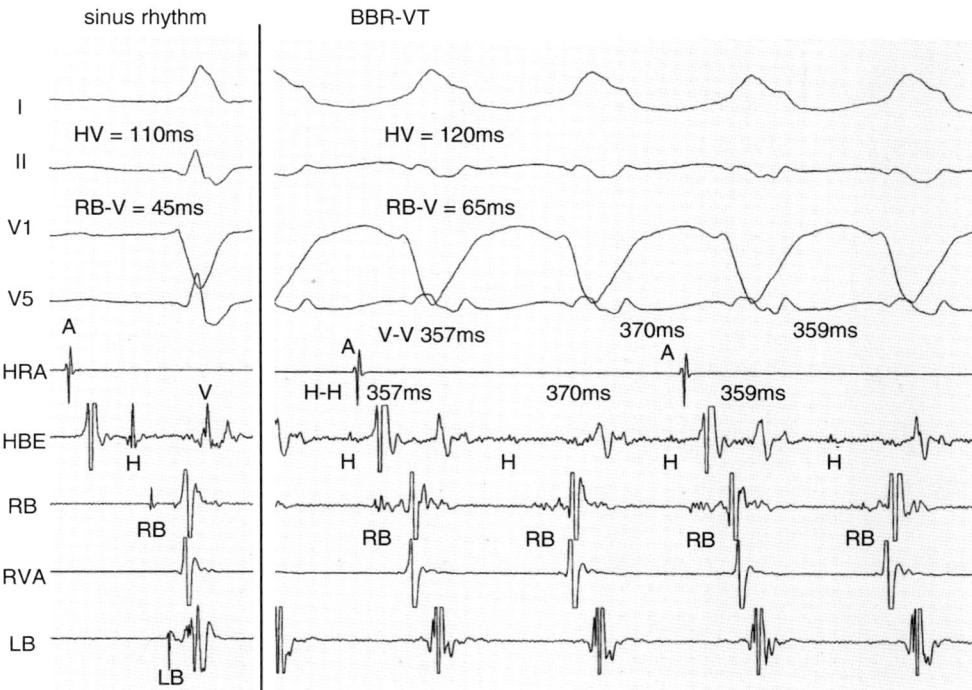

Fig. 33.3 An example of LBBB type BBR-VT. AV dissociation is present during BBR-VT (*right panel*). A His potential (H) is followed by right bundle branch potential (RB) and precedes each QRS complex. The H-V (120 ms) and RB-V (65 ms) interval during VT is longer than the H-V (110 ms) and RB-V (45 ms) during sinus rhythm (*left panel*). Variations in the H-H, RB-RB interval during the tachycardia precede the changes in the V-V interval

dia may be shorter than during sinus rhythm. (e) Variations in the H-H, RB-RB, or LB-LB interval during the tachycardia precede the changes in the V-V interval (Figs. 33.2 and 33.3). (f) The RB and the LB deflection occurs after the His deflection during BBR-VT with an LBBB and an RBBB configuration, respectively. (g) The QRS morphology during atrial entrainment is identical to the QRS morphology during BBR-VT. (h) The difference between the postpacing interval (PPI) after entrainment from the right ventricular apex (RVA) and the tachycardia cycle length (TCL) is less than 30 ms (1) RBB-VT is no longer inducible after the RB ablation.

The His-Purkinje system could be activated passively in the retrograde fashion and isn't involved in the reentrant circuit of BBR-VT. Therefore, the retrograde His deflection reflects passive activation of the His-Purkinje system. A change in cycle length of the tachycardia doesn't depend on the variation of V-H interval. Thus, even if tachycardia cycle length changes markedly, V-H interval can exhibit no change.

Especially, the diagnosis and mechanism of BBR-VT can be elucidated by demonstration of transient entrainment of BBR-VT by atrial and ventricular stimulation [8, 9]. During entrainment of BBR-VT with an LBBB configuration by atrial pacing, impulse is conducted from atrium to His bundle and the anterograde impulse is conducted orthodromically through the RB and resets the tachycardia. On the other hand, the impulse is anterogradely and antidromically through LB and collides with the previous orthodromic wavefront within LB, giving rise to concealed conduction block. Therefore, the QRS morphology during atrial entrainment is identical to the QRS morphology during the tachycardia (Fig. 33.4). However, during entrainment by pacing from right ventricular apex, the antidromic pacing wavefront

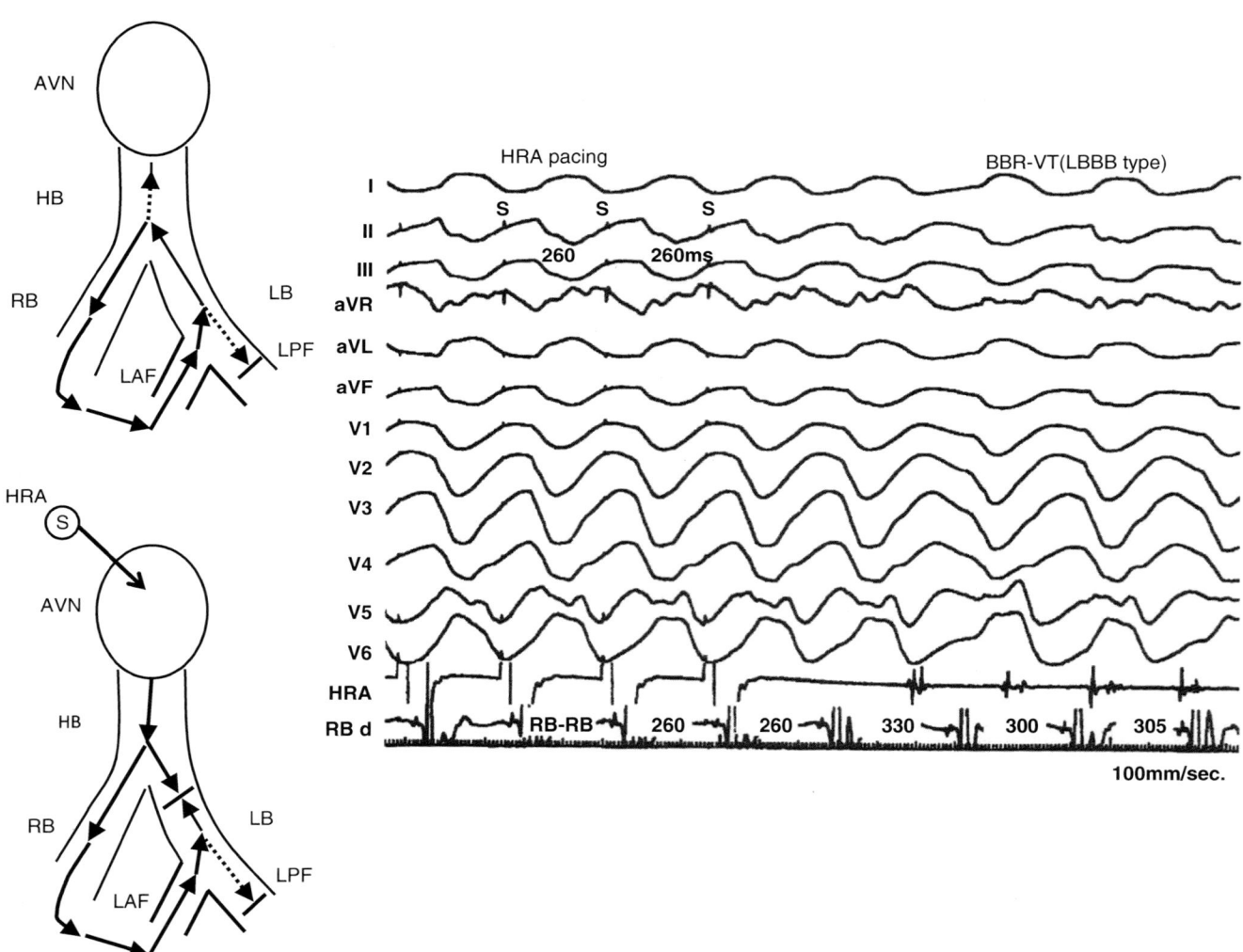

Fig. 33.4 Schematics (*left panels*) and surface ECG (*right panel*) during transient entrainment of BBR-VT by high right atrium (HRA) pacing. During entrainment of LBBB type BBR-VT (*left upper panel*) by HRA pacing, impulse is conducted from atrium to His bundle and the anterograde impulse is conducted orthodromically through the RB. On the other hand, the impulse is anterogradely and antidromically through LB and collides with the previous orthodromic wavefront within LB, giving rise to concealed conduction block (*left lower panel*). The QRS morphology during entrainment pacing from HRA at a pacing cycle length of 260 ms is identical to the QRS morphology during the tachycardia (*right panel*)

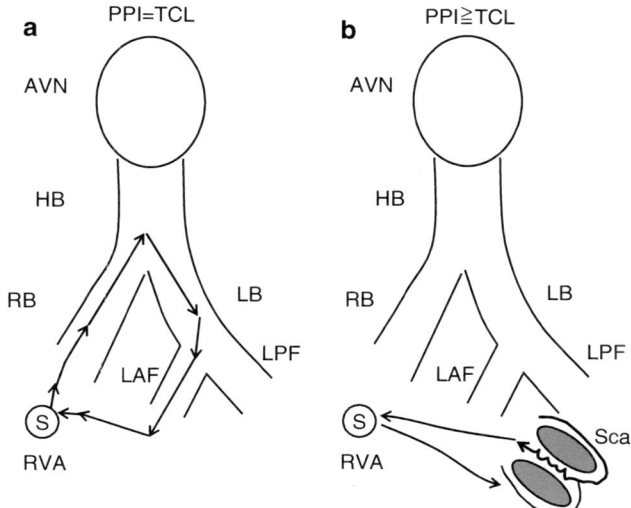

Fig. 33.5 Schematics of different activation wavefront between BBR-VT (**a**) and myocardial reentrant VT (**b**) during postpacing cycle after entrainment pacing from right ventricular apex (RVA). The postpacing interval (PPI) is similar to the tachycardia cycle length (TCL) because pacing site of RVA is close to reentrant circuit of BBRT-VT. However, when pacing site of RVA is remote from circuit of myocardial VT, the PPI is longer than the TCL

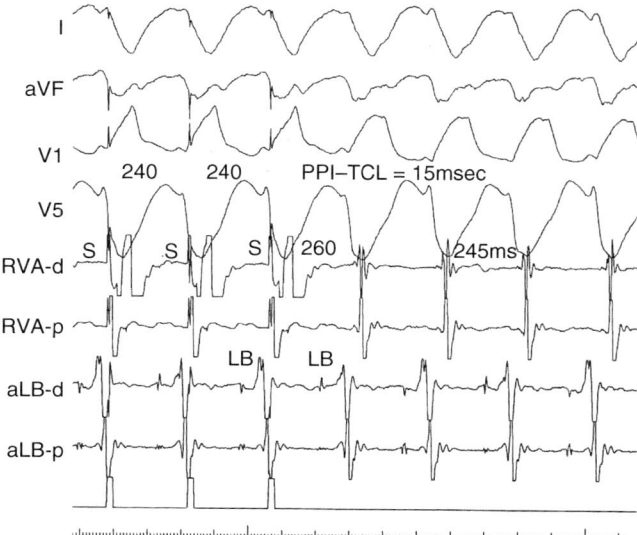

Fig. 33.6 Surface ECG and intracardiac electrograms during postpacing cycle after entrainment pacing from RVA in RBBB type BBR-VT. The PPI (260 ms) after entrainment pacing approximated the TCL of 245 ms

collides with the previous orthodromic wavefront within ventricular myocardium, which leads to the different QRS morphology from the morphology during the tachycardia.

The different components of activation wavefront between BBR-VT and ventricular myocardial reentrant VT during the postpacing cycle after entrainment pacing from RVA are shown in Fig. 33.5. The RB distal insertion is located mostly in the RVA. Therefore, the PPI is similar to the TCL because pacing site of RVA is close to reentrant circuit of BBRT-VT. Conversely, when pacing site of RVA is remote from circuit in myocardial reentrant VT, the PPI is longer than the TCL. Moreover, the PPI is similar to the TCL in BBRT-VT with either LBBB or RBBB QRS-complex configuration. Namely, a PPI-TCL < 30 ms is suggestive of BBR-VT. Figure 33.6 shows a representative case who had BBR-VT with RBBB QRS-complex configuration. In electrophysiological testing, the PPI after entrainment pacing from RVA in BBR-VT was 260 ms, which approximated the TCL of 245 ms.

33.5 The Differential Diagnosis

The differential diagnosis for BBR-VT includes (1) myocardial reentrant VT (2) interfascicular reentrant VT (3) a supraventricular tachycardia with aberrant conduction.

The differential diagnosis of BBR-VT can be made from the surface electrocardiogram (ECG). BBR-VT usually exhibits a "typical" LBBB pattern similar to the QRS morphology of a supraventricular tachycardia with preexisting or functional BBB [5–7]. On the other hand, an "atypical" LBBB pattern with slurring in the initial of QRS is frequently recognized in myocardial VT. In addition to the surface ECG finding, electrophysiological testing is ultimately required to differentiate BBR-VT from other tachycardias.

The tachycardias, except BBR-VT, don't necessarily show prolonged H-V interval. In myocardial reentrant VT, the His usually does not precede a ventricular activation. Moreover, in interfascicular reentrant VT, contrary to BBR-VT, the H-V interval during tachycardia is commonly the same as or shorter than the H-V interval during sinus rhythm. The difference between the PPI after entrainment of tachycardia by pacing from RVA and the TCL is less than 30 ms in BBR-VT, whereas myocardial reentrant VT, interfascicular VT, and a supraventricular tachycardia show mostly a PPI-TCL > 30 ms and probably excluded [8, 9] (Fig. 33.7).

In contrast to BBR-VT, VT due to interfascicular reentry is commonly observed in patients with anterior myocardial infarction and either left anterior or posterior hemiblock [5–7]. Because these patients often exhibit complete and bidirectional RBBB, BBR-VT cannot be induced. However, when retrograde slow conduction in apparently blocked fascicle is still present, the impulse conducts anterogradely over the healthy fascicle, and then conduct retrogradely over the blocked fascicle, giving rise to interfascicular reentrant VT. In such cases, the QRS morphology during VT is identical to that in sinus rhythm.

A representative case with interfascicular reentrant tachycardia is shown in Fig. 33.8 [10]. A 12-lead electrocardiogram during tachycardia showed wide QRS complex with

RBBB configuration and right axis deviation due to left posterior hemiblock, of which morphology was identical to that during sinus rhythm, except for the atrioventricular (A-V) dissociation (Fig. 33.8). In the electrophysiological testing, VT was repeatedly induced by programmed atrial and ventricular stimulation. During VT, the His potential constantly preceded the QRS complex (V) with the H-V interval of 27 ms, which was shorter than that during sinus rhythm (67 ms). In this patient, atrial tachycardia (AT) with irregular ventricular rates was also inducible by programmed atrial

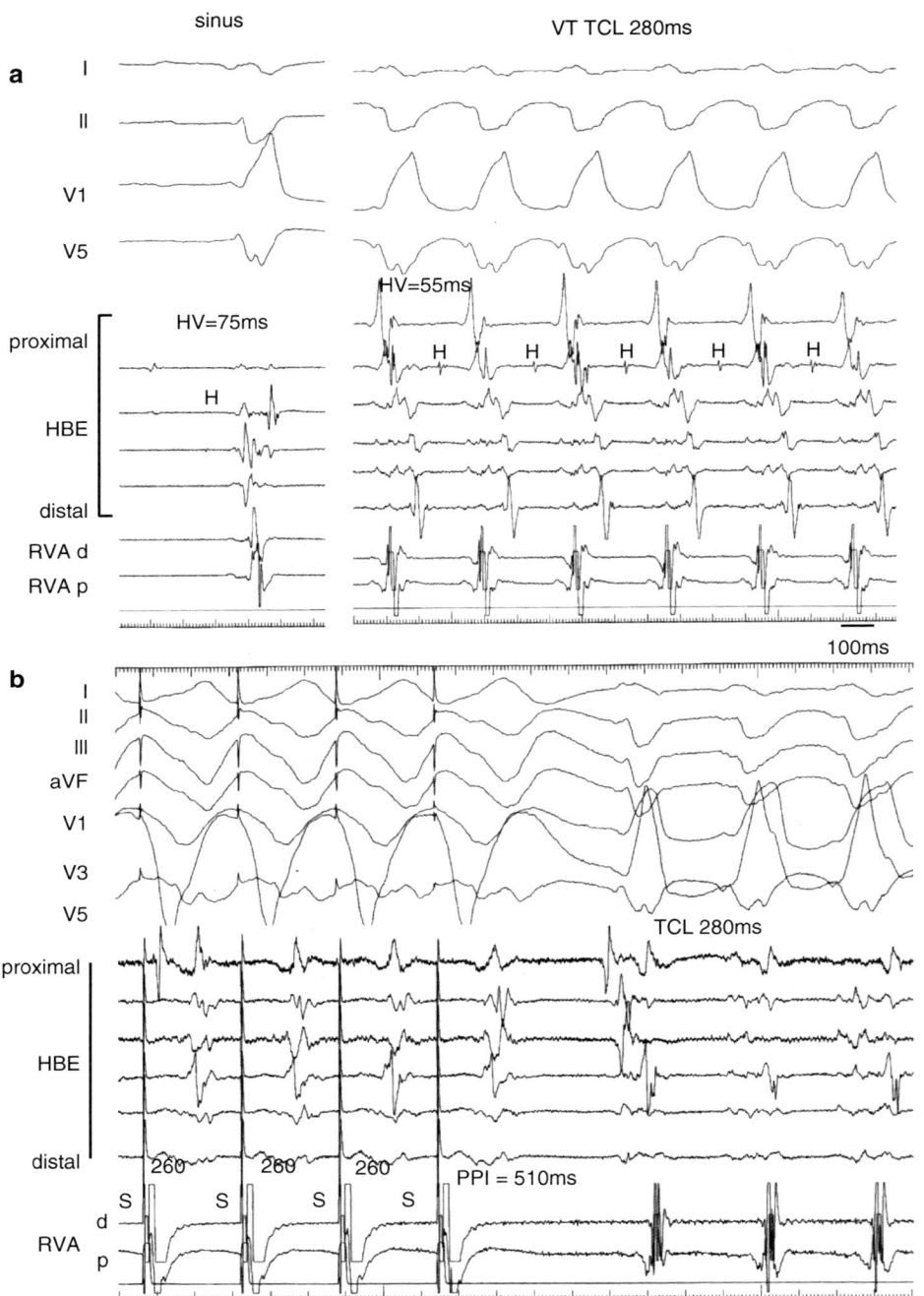

Fig. 33.7 Surface ECG and intracardiac electrograms during postpacing cycle after entrainment pacing from RVA in interfascicular VT. During interfascicular reentrant VT exhibiting QRS morphology with an RBBB configuration, the His potential (H) constantly precede the QRS complex with the H-V interval of 55 ms, which was shorter than that during sinus rhythm (75 ms) (**a**). The PPI (510 ms) after entrainment pacing from RVA is distinctly longer than the TCL of 280 ms (**b**)

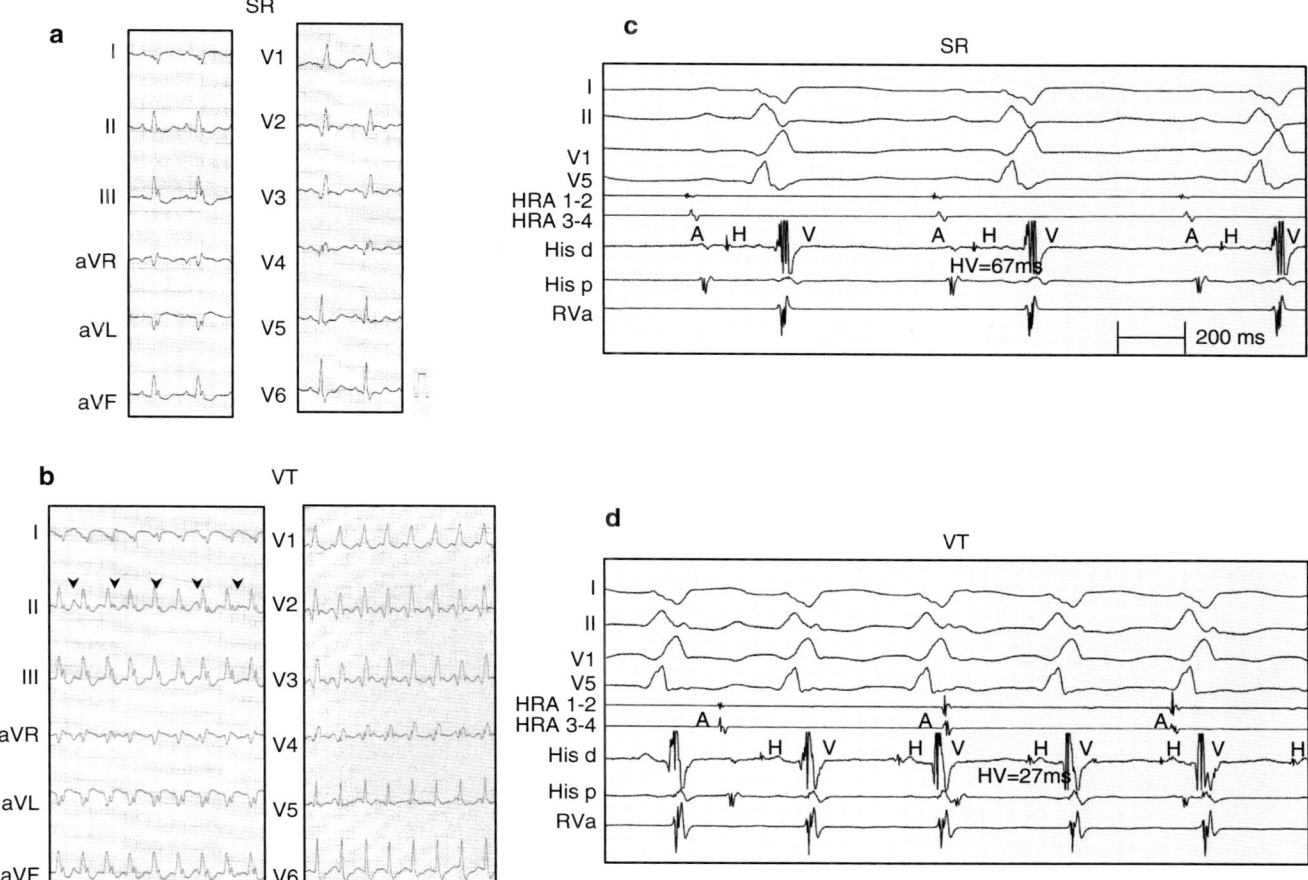

Fig. 33.8 A 12-lead electrocardiogram and intracardiac electrograms during sinus rhythm (SR) and interfascicular reentrant VT. VT (**b**) Showed wide QRS complex with RBBB and left posterior fascicular block, of which morphology was identical to that during sinus rhythm (**a**), except for the A-V dissociation (*arrowheads*). During VT (**d**), the His potential constantly preceded the QRS complex (V) with the H-V interval of 27 ms, which was shorter than that during sinus rhythm (67 ms) (**c**)

stimulation, and the ventricular cycle length spontaneously regularized during the tachycardia. The H-V interval shortened concurrently from 57–65 ms to 27 ms after achieving regular ventricular rate without changing the QRS morphology (Fig. 33.9) [10]. In this patient, the diagnosis of VT was an interfascicular reentrant tachycardia in which the VT excitation conducted anterogradely through the healthy left anterior fascicle and retrogradely through the blocked left posterior fascicle. The posterior fascicle was thought to have exclusively retrograde conductivity because of the same QRS morphology during sinus rhythm and VT. The abrupt regularization of the tachycardia cycle length during AT was considered as a spontaneous transition from AT to interfascicular reentrant tachycardia because of the shortened H-V interval in the latter. While an initiation of BBR-VT by rapid atrial stimulation was reported, an induction of interfascicular reentrant tachycardia from atrial tachyarrhythmia was very rare [4].

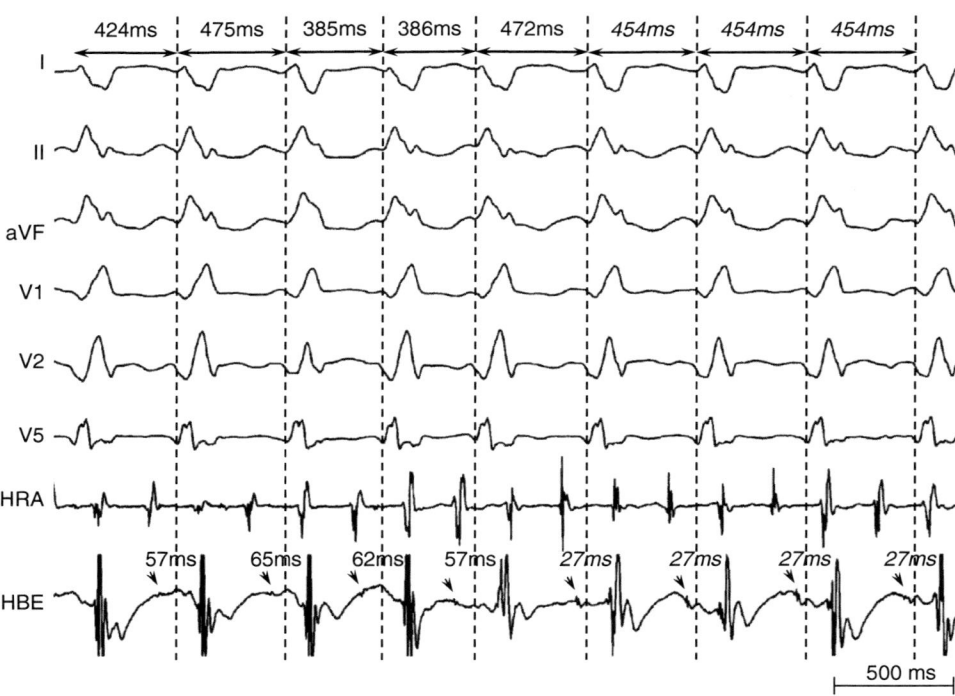

Fig. 33.9 Spontaneous regularization from irregular to regular ventricular rates during atrial tachycardia in the same patient as shown in Fig. 33.8 [10]. Every ventricular activity was preceded by His potential (*arrowheads*). The R-R intervals indicated at the top became regular from the sixth QRS complex. Note that H-V interval became shorter concurrently (27 ms) with regularization of ventricular rate than those during irregular ventricular rates (57–65 ms)

33.6 Treatment

33.6.1 Catheter Ablation

It is important to accurately diagnose BBR-VT and interfascicular VT in electrophysiological testing because they can be cured with catheter ablation. Successful elimination of BBRT-VT and interfascicular VT depends on whether accurate diagnosis of them is accomplished. Catheter ablation more effectively and safely eliminates BBR-VT compared to antiarrhythmic drug therapy [11, 12]. Moreover, the ablation therapy can be helpful in management of patients who have unacceptable frequent shocks from implantable cardioverter-defibrillator (ICD) and can be useful, if they qualify for an ICD and the device is refused or is contraindicated.

Catheter radiofrequency ablation of the RB is recommended and an effective therapy for treatment for BBR-VT [13, 14]. In this procedure, a catheter is inserted into the femoral vein and passed through the tricuspid valve until a right bundle electrogram is recorded. Most commonly, complete RBBB is made by ablation of the RB.

BBR-VT has also been reported to be treated by ablation of the LB, which may help to prevent cardiac pacing in some cases with relatively normal RB [15]. However, higher success rates were noted in ablation of the RB compared to that of the LB, which is more difficult than ablating the RB. Moreover, since the majority of patients with BBR-VT require ICD therapy, ablation of the RB is a first choice for BBR-VT.

Catheter ablation has been very successful in BBR-VT that characteristically has a left (rarely a right) bundle branch morphology, whereas ablation of the RB often prolong the preexisting abnormal HV interval and worsen infranodal conduction, thereby often leading to pacing therapy. However, the patients with BBR-VT and structured heart disease who are suitable candidates for ablation of the RB have mostly an indication for ICD implantation [14, 16].

VT due to interfascicular reentry is commonly seen in patients with anterior infarction and either left anterior or posterior hemiblock. In such patients with degenerating conduction system, ablation of the diseased fascicle is reasonable for treatment of VT although a pacemaker or ICD would likely be required. If the target of ablation is the diseased left posterior fascicule, this site is near the basal septum of LV where the fascicular potentials were recorded during sinus rhythm. In the patients requiring ICD or cardiac resynchronization therapy defibrillator (CRT-D), the left anterior fascicle is also occasionally chosen for the target site of ablation [5, 10] (Fig. 33.10).

33.6.2 ICD Therapy

The prognosis is often poor in patients followed after successful ablation of BBR-VT because they have underlying structural heart disease and severe LV dysfunction, which lead to development of congestive heart failure and sudden cardiac death due to other myocardial VTs. Therefore, implantation of a dual-chamber ICD or CRT-D should be

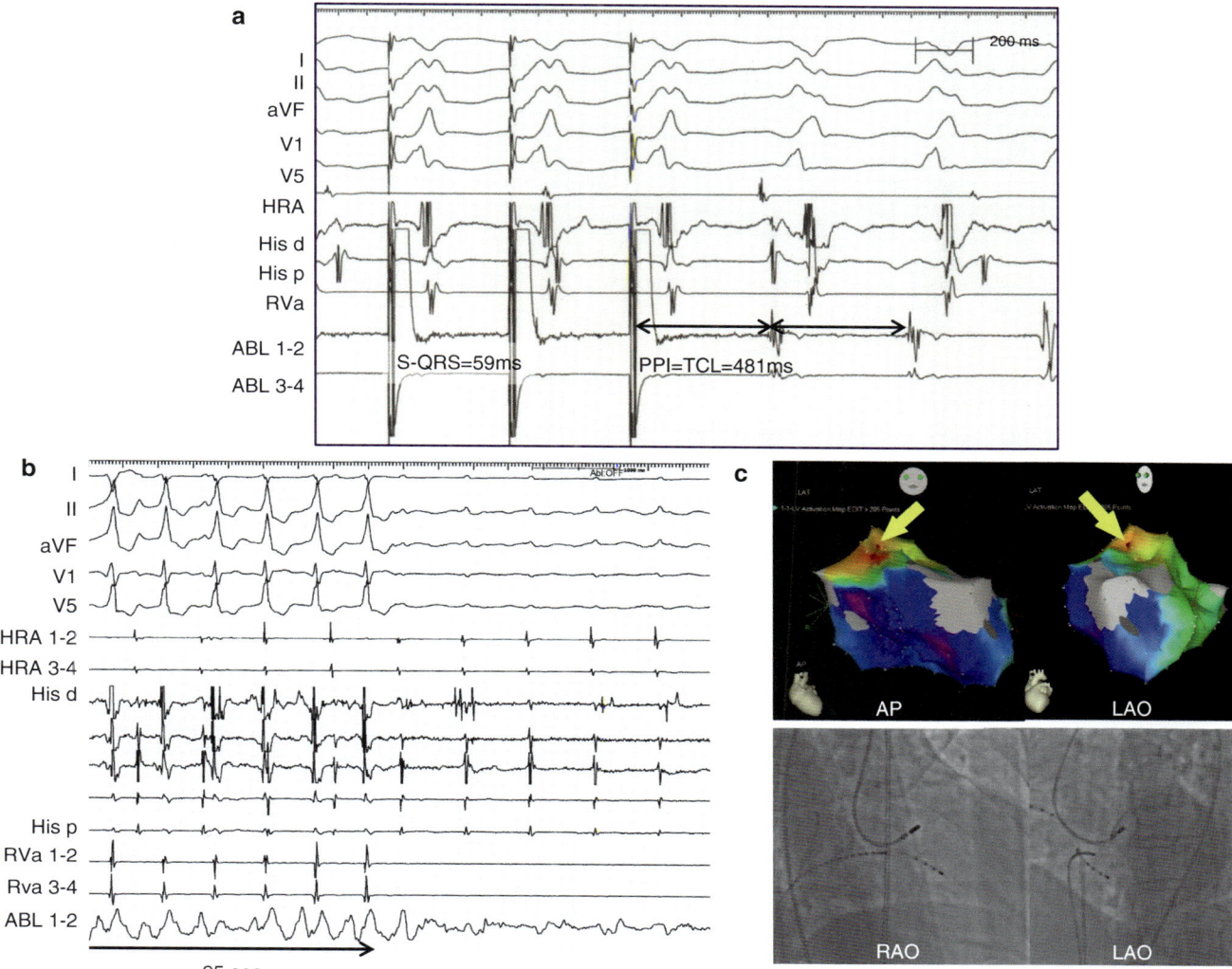

Fig. 33.10 Surface ECG and intracardiac electrograms during post-pacing cycle after entrainment pacing from proximal site of the left anterior fascicle in interfascicular reentrant VT in the same patient as shown in Fig. 33.8 (**a**). The PPI after concealed entrainment was identical to the TCL of 481 ms. Radiofrequency ablation at this site was performed during VT. VT was successfully terminated after 25 s of the energy application, which also resulted in complete A-V block (**b**). Fluoroscopic images and CARTO 3D mapping (*arrowheads*) showed the sites at radiofrequency energy application in proximal site of the left anterior fascicle (**c**). Implantation of a cardiac resynchronization therapy defibrillator (CRT-D) was mandatory in this patient because of significantly reduced left ventricular systolic function and dyssynchrony of ventricular contraction. Therefore, it was not considered essential to salvage the A-V conduction. After the ablation procedure and CRT-D implantation, the patient has been symptom-free for a follow-up period

considered for the primary or secondary prevention of sudden cardiac death in these patients after catheter ablation for BBR-VT [17].

References

1. Akhtar M, Gilbert C, Wolf FG, et al. Reentry within the His-Purkinje system. Elucidation of reentrant circuit using right bundle branch and His bundle recordings. Circulation. 1978;58:295–304.
2. Caceres J, Jazayeri M, McKinnie J, et al. Sustained bundle branch reentry as a mechanism of clinical tachycardia. Circulation. 1989;79:256–70.
3. Blanck Z, Dhala A, Deshpande S, et al. Bundle branch reentrant ventricular tachycardia: cumulative experience in 48 patients. J Cardiovasc Electrophysiol. 1993;4:253–62.
4. Mizusawa Y, Sakurada H, Nishizaki M, et al. Characteristics of bundle branch reentrant ventricular tachycardia with a right bundle branch block configuration: feasibility of atrial pacing. Europace. 2009;11:1208–13.
5. Crijns HJ, Smeets JL, Rodriguez LM, et al. Cure of interfascicular reentrant ventricular tachycardia by ablation of the anterior fascicle of the left bundle branch. J Cardiovasc Electrophysiol. 1995;6:486–92.
6. Delacretaz E, Stevenson WG, Ellison KE, et al. Mapping and radiofrequency catheter ablation of the three types of sustained monomorphic ventricular tachycardia in nonischemic heart disease. J Cardiovasc Electrophysiol. 2000;11:11–7.

7. Lopera G, Stevenson WG, Soejima K, et al. Identification and ablation of three types of ventricular tachycardia involving the his-purkinje system in patients with heart disease. J Cardiovasc Electrophysiol. 2004;15:52–8.
8. Merino JL, Peinado R, Fernández-Lozano I, et al. Transient entrainment of bundle-branch reentry by atrial and ventricular stimulation: elucidation of the tachycardia mechanism through analysis of the surface ECG. Circulation. 1999;100:1784–90.
9. Merino JL, Peinado R, Fernandez-Lozano I, et al. Bundle-branch reentry and the postpacing interval after entrainment by right ventricular apex stimulation: a new approach to elucidate the mechanism of wide-QRS-complex tachycardia with atrioventricular dissociation. Circulation. 2001;103:1102–8.
10. Nakamura T, Nishizaki M, Shimizu M, et al. Conversion from irregular to regular wide QRS tachycardia: What is the mechanism? J Cardiovasc Electrophysiol. 2014;25:553–5.
11. Tchou P, Jazayeri M, Denker S, et al. Transcatheter electrical ablation of right bundle branch. A method of treating macroreentrant ventricular tachycardia attributed to bundle branch reentry. Circulation. 1988;78:246–57.
12. Cohen TJ, Chien WW, Lurie KG, et al. Radiofrequency catheter ablation for treatment of bundle branch reentrant ventricular tachycardia: results and long-term follow-up. J Am Coll Cardiol. 1991;18:1767–73.
13. Blanck Z, Akhtar M. Ventricular tachycardia due to sustained bundle branch reentry: diagnostic and therapeutic considerations. Clin Cardiol. 1993;16:619–22.
14. European Heart Rhythm Association, Heart Rhythm Society, Zipes DP, et al. ACC/AHA/ESC 2006 guidelines for management of patients with ventricular arrhythmias and the prevention of sudden cardiac death: a report of the American College of Cardiology/American Heart Association Task Force and the European Society of Cardiology Committee for Practice Guidelines (Writing Committee to Develop Guidelines for Management of Patients With Ventricular Arrhythmias and the Prevention of Sudden Cardiac Death). J Am Coll Cardiol. 2006;48:e247–346.
15. Blanck Z, Deshpande S, Jazayeri MR, et al. Catheter ablation of the left bundle branch for the treatment of sustained bundle branch reentrant ventricular tachycardia. J Cardiovasc Electrophysiol. 1995;6:40–3.
16. Mehdirad AA, Keim S, Rist K, et al. Long-term clinical outcome of right bundle branch radiofrequency catheter ablation for treatment of bundle branch reentrant ventricular tachycardia. Pacing Clin Electrophysiol. 1995;18:2135.
17. Epstein AE, DiMarco JP, Ellenbogen KA, et al. ACC/AHA/HRS 2008 guidelines for device-based therapy of cardiac rhythm abnormalities: a report of the American College of Cardiology/American Heart Association Task Force on Practice Guidelines (writing committee to revise the ACC/AHA/NASPE 2002 guideline update for implantation of cardiac pacemakers and antiarrhythmia devices): developed in collaboration with the American Association for Thoracic Surgery and Society of Thoracic Surgeons. Circulation. 2008;117:e350–408.

Papillary Muscle Ventricular Tachycardia

34

Hiroshi Tada

Keywords

Papillary muscle • Ventricular tachycardia • Premature ventricular contraction • Ventricular fibrillation

34.1 Introductory Remarks

Idiopathic ventricular arrhythmias that originate from papillary muscles are not rare and account for 4–12% of idiopathic ventricular arrhythmias [1, 2]. Syncope and cardiac arrest due to papillary muscle arrhythmias are rare and generally non-life threatening. However, several cases of premature ventricular contractions (PVCs) from papillary muscles triggering ventricular fibrillation (VF) have been reported [3, 4]. The mechanism of the ventricular tachycardia (VT) is typically focal in nature and not reentrant. Catheter ablation may be required for symptomatic patients, patients with tachycardia-induced cardiomyopathy, or those with PVCs triggering ventricular fibrillation. Radiofrequency catheter ablation is challenging because of catheter instability during papillary muscle contractions and the thickened base of the papillary muscles, which might account for the variable success rate of this arrhythmia. The use of irrigation catheters with contact force sensing, intracardiac echocardiography, and image integration using 3-dimensional mapping systems can help to obtain acute success (elimination of targeted PVC/VTs). However, at present, the long-term prognosis after the ablation is unknown.

H. Tada, M.D., Ph.D.
Faculty of Medical Sciences, Department of Cardiovascular Medicine, University of Fukui, 23-3 Matsuokashimoaizuki, Eiheiji-cho, Yoshida-gun, Fukui 910-1193, Japan
e-mail: htada@u-fukui.ac.jp

34.2 Epidemiology and Anatomic Considerations

Recently, it has become known that idiopathic tachycardias (VTs) or premature ventricular contractions (PVCs) can originate from papillary muscles. Papillary muscle arrhythmias account for 4–12% of idiopathic arrhythmias [1, 2] and are generally non-life threatening. However, papillary muscle PVCs can trigger ventricular fibrillation (VF) [3, 4]. Patients with papillary muscle VT/PVCs seem to be older than those with VT/PVCs arising from the right ventricular (RV) OT and left ventricular (LV) fascicles [5, 6].

Papillary muscles support the subvalvular structures of the mitral and tricuspid valves. In the left ventricle (LV), the tension apparatus of both mitral leaflets inserts into two groups of papillary muscles. The anterior papillary muscle and posterior papillary muscle arise from a middle to apical site of the anterior or inferior wall of the LV, serving as an anatomic landmark for the beginning of the apical component of the LV. Their thickness (generally equal to the left ventricular [LV] wall [7]), prompt and dynamic movements, and contractions and relaxations with the cardiac cycles could cause difficulty for the catheter ablation of papillary muscle arrhythmias. Furthermore, variable exit sites from an intramural focus or its attachment to false cords may account for multiple QRS morphologies of papillary muscle arrhythmias [8]. Papillary muscle arrhythmias originate more commonly from the posterior papillary muscle than from the anterior papillary muscle [8]. This kind of arrhythmia can occur from papillary muscles in the right ventricle (RV) [9]. The right ventricular (RV) papillary muscle consists of the anterolateral, posteromedial, and septal (or medial) muscles. Papillary muscle arrhythmias can originate from each of the RV papillary muscles, but the septal muscle seems to be the most common site for arrhythmias [9, 10]. Because the septal muscle arises from the RV outflow tract [7], the ventricular arrhythmias of septal muscle origins may have similar QRS morphologies to those arising from the RV outflow tract [8].

34.3 Mechanism and Clinical Manifestation

Papillary muscle arrhythmias are usually exercise induced and catecholamine sensitive, requiring isoproterenol or epinephrine for their induction [9, 11]. The mechanism is typically focal in nature and not reentrant. This VT cannot be entrained and has a lack of late potentials at the ablation site [8]. PVCs and nonsustained VTs are more common than sustained VT, and the VTs are less likely to be sustained compared with fascicular tachycardias. Syncope and cardiac arrest are rare.

Frequent papillary PVCs can induce cardiomyopathy that is reversible if suppression of the PVCs is successful [9]. There are also reported cases of PVCs from papillary muscles triggering ventricular fibrillation (VF) [3, 4]. In patients with mitral valve prolapse syndrome, fascicular and papillary muscle PVCs of the LV often trigger VF and sudden cardiac death [12]. Catheter ablation may be required for symptomatic patients, those with tachycardia-induced cardiomyopathy, and those with PVCs triggering VF.

34.4 ECG Characteristics

Patients with papillary muscle arrhythmias usually have normal 12-lead ECGs during sinus rhythm. The 12-lead ECGs during arrhythmias may be similar to those of LV fascicular, mitral annular, and RV outflow tract VTs.

Arrhythmias from the LV papillary muscles have a right bundle branch block pattern (Fig. 34.1) [5, 11, 13]. Arrhythmias

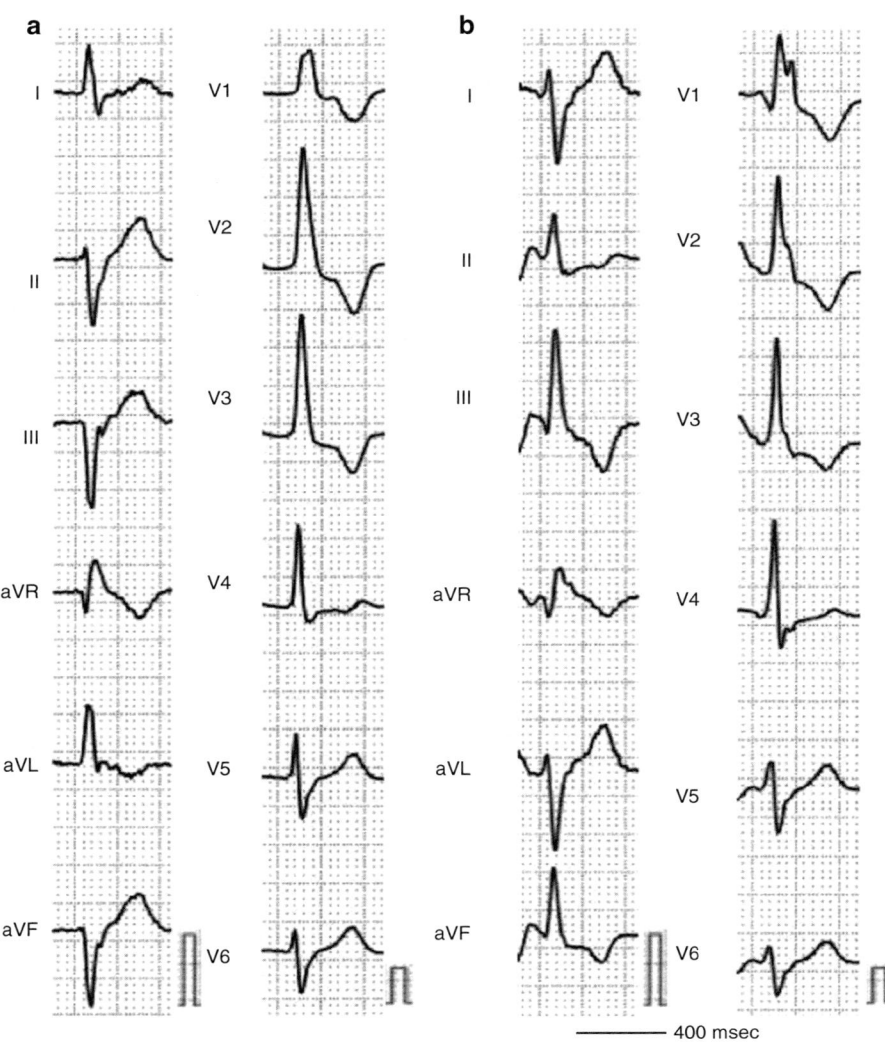

Fig. 34.1 12-Lead ECGs. (**a**) Premature ventricular contractions (PVCs) from the left ventricular (LV) posterior papillary muscle. (**b**) PVCs from the LV anterior papillary muscle

from the anterior and posterior papillary muscles usually have inferior and superior axes, respectively. The 12-lead ECGs during these arrhythmias may be similar to those of LV fascicular and mitral annular arrhythmias. However, some ECG characteristics can help differentiate papillary muscle arrhythmias from fascicular arrhythmias [13]: (1) Papillary muscle arrhythmias usually have a wider QRS (150 ± 15 vs. 127 ± 11 ms), and that is significantly greater in papillary muscle arrhythmias than idiopathic left verapamil-sensitive VTs (150 ± 15 ms vs. 127 ± 11 ms). (2) The V1 morphology of posterior papillary muscle VTs typically has a qR morphology or R compared with an rsR′ for fascicular VTs and will notably have the absence of Q-waves in leads I and aVL (Figs. 34.1 and 34.2a). (3) Papillary muscle arrhythmias often exhibit multiple QRS morphologies, with subtle changes seen spontaneously or during ablation. These subtle morphologic changes are thought to be from preferential conduction to different exit sites or multiple regions of origins within the complex structure of the papillary muscles [8]. The LV endocavitary structures that connect to the papillary muscles, such as the chordae tendineae and false tendons through which conducting fibers can run, may also be associated with multiple QRS morphologies. Thus, compared with fascicular arrhythmias, a wider QRS complex and the absence of an rR′ pattern are often observed in papillary arrhythmias [6, 13, 14]. A recent algorithm demonstrated a QRS width of >130 ms is the best cutoff value for differentiating these two arrhythmias [6]. Papillary muscles arrhythmias are less likely to exhibit a positive precordial lead concordance, which is a marked difference from mitral annular arrhythmias [6].

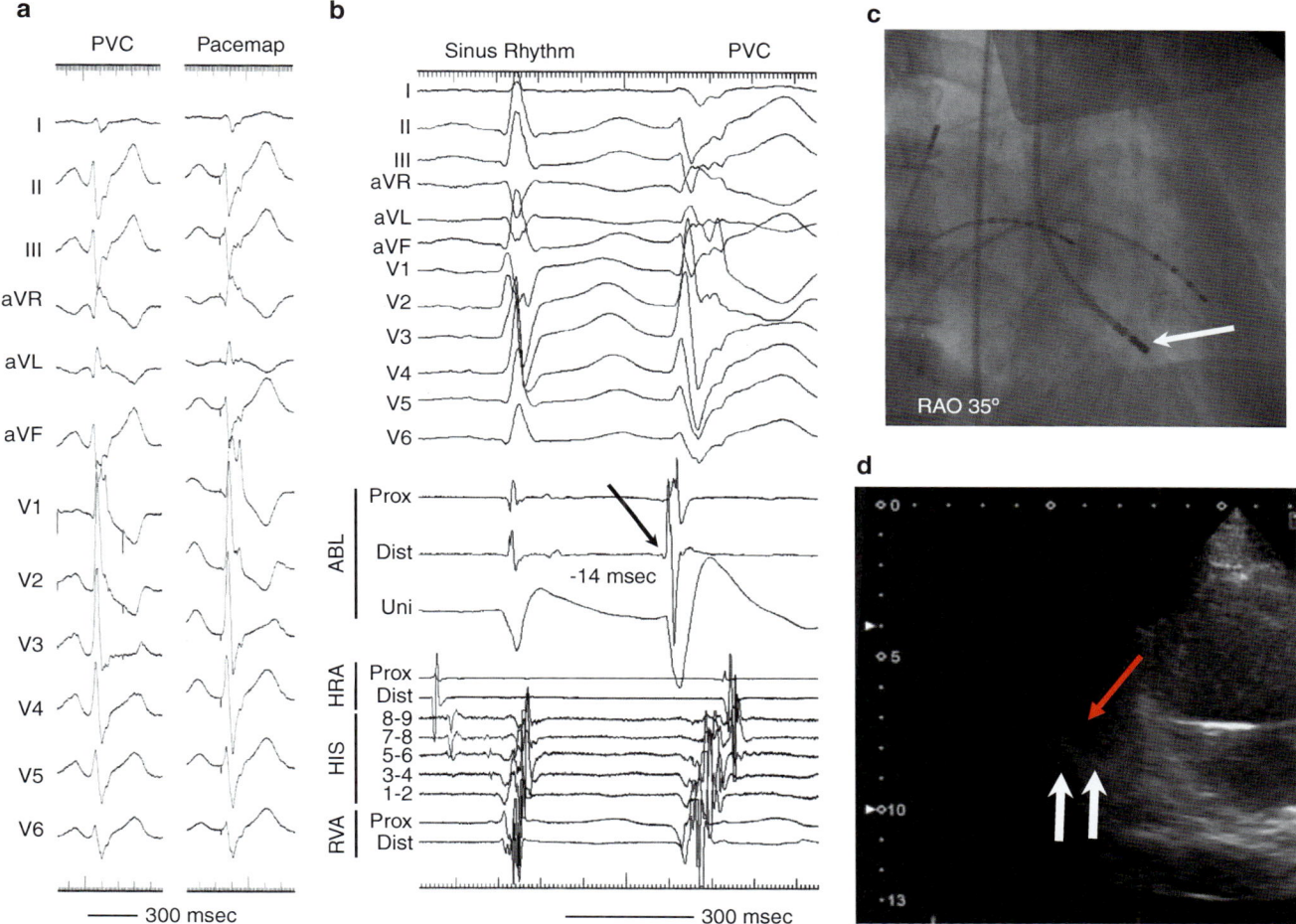

Fig. 34.2 Premature ventricular contractions (PVCs) arising from the left ventricular (LV) posterior papillary muscle. (**a**) A 12-lead ECG. A clinical PVC and pace map at the successful ablation site at the posterior papillary muscle. The QRS width is 163 ms. (**b**) Intracardiac recordings. During the PVC, a distinct local activation recorded by the ablation catheter (ABL) preceded the onset of the QRS complex by 14 ms (*arrow*). Note that no Purkinje potentials were found at the ablation site during sinus rhythm or the PVC. (**c**) A radiograph obtained in the right anterior oblique (RAO 35°) projection showing the ablation sites (*arrow*). (**d**) Transthoracic echocardiography demonstrates that the tip of the ablation catheter (*red arrow*) is attached to the posterior papillary muscle (*white arrows*). Successful catheter ablation was obtained with an irrigation catheter (ThermoCool®, Biosense Webster, Diamond Bar, CA, USA) at and around that site. The energy and duration were 30–40 W and 50–120 s for each application, respectively

A recent study reported that all RV papillary muscle arrhythmias had an LBBB morphology and rS or QS pattern in lead V1 [9]. Septal papillary PVCs had an earlier precordial transition (≤V4) and inferior axis. Meanwhile, anterior/posterior papillary muscle PVCs had a later R-wave transition (>V4) and superior axis. The QRS complex was broader for the RV papillary muscle arrhythmias and they had a wider QRS complex than arrhythmias arising from the RV outflow tract (163 ± 21 ms vs. 141 ± 22 ms). Another study of 29 patients with septal PVCs [15] reported that, in addition to an rS or QS pattern in lead V1 and an LBBB morphology, a monophasic R pattern in lead I and aVL was found among 29 (100%) and 23 (79.3%) patients with septal PVCs, respectively. Meanwhile, a QS or qs pattern was found in lead aVR in 25 (86.2%) patients. The precordial R-wave transition helped to distinguish the origin of the PVCs, in which an early transition (≤V4) occurred among tricuspid valvular RV septum PVCs and later precordial R-wave transition (>V4) among the basal RV septum PVCs.

34.5 Mapping and Catheter Ablation

Papillary muscle arrhythmias are usually induced only by isoproterenol or burst pacing, and not by programmed atrial or ventricular stimulation. Some papillary muscle arrhythmias (25–45%) have Purkinje potentials preceding the QRS during PVCs/VT at the ablation site [16]. Purkinje potentials can be found very close to or slightly after the QRS onset during sinus rhythm and the targeted arrhythmias. If Purkinje potentials present during sinus rhythm and the arrhythmia, they may have varied ventricular potentials (Fig. 34.3). They will also be late compared with the pre-QRS for fascicular VTs.

Catheter ablation of papillary muscle arrhythmias is typically performed at the site of the earliest endocardial activation (Figs. 34.2 and 34.3). Activation mapping is the most useful for ablation of papillary muscle arrhythmias [2, 8]. Some do not exhibit recordings with diastolic potentials during sinus rhythm or the VT, which suggests that the Purkinje network is not involved in these kinds of arrhythmias [2]. Pace mapping is also performed when PVCs are infrequent,

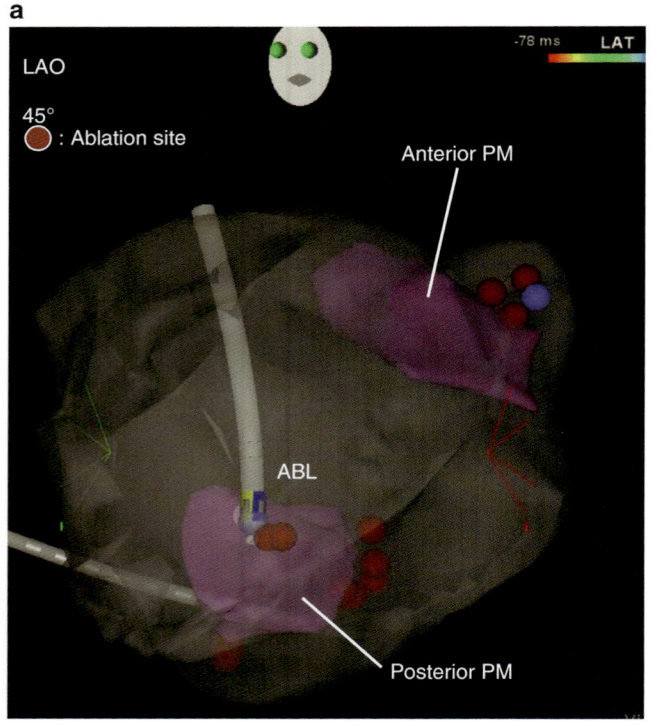

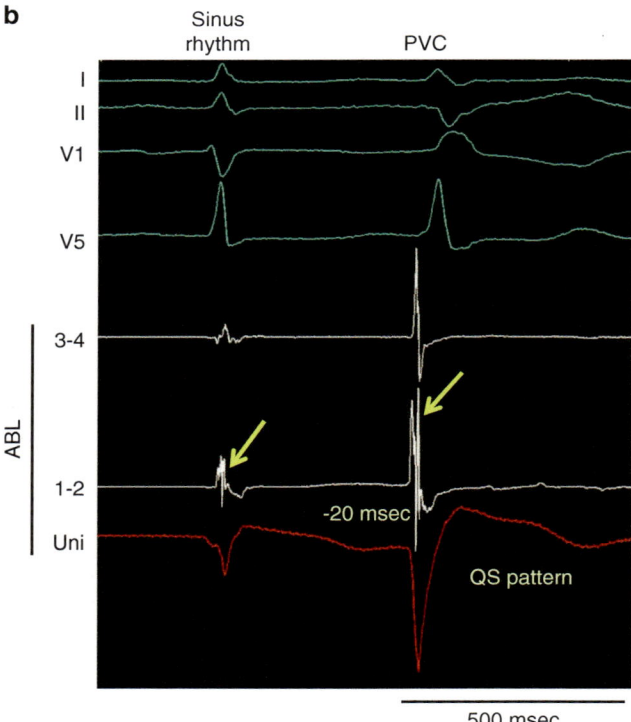

Fig. 34.3 Premature ventricular contractions (PVCs) arising from the left ventricular (LV) posterior papillary muscle. (**a**) Intracardiac echocardiography-defined LV endocardial surface and papillary muscles integrated into the 3-dimensional electroanatomical mapping (CARTO-3®, Biosense Webster). The ablation catheter (ABL) is positioned at the base of the posterior papillary muscle. (**b**) Intracardiac recordings at the ablation sites. The earliest activation during the PVC was found near the base of the posterior papillary muscle. The local activation time during the PVCs preceded the QRS onset by 20 ms. After 28 applications of radiofrequency energy at and around this site, no further PVCs spontaneously occurred. The ablation catheter was an irrigation catheter (ThermoCool®SMARTTOUCH™, Biosense Webster). The energy and duration were 30–45 W and up to 70 s for each application. In total, 28 radiofrequency energy applications were required for a cure

but pace mapping only correlates with the exit site [11]. Given the possibility of capturing more papillary muscle tissue beyond just the arrhythmogenic focus, pace mapping can be inaccurate or misleading.

Successful catheter ablation usually requires irrigated ablation catheters and intracardiac echocardiography (ICE) to visualize the direct contact with the papillary muscle (Figs. 34.2 and 34.3). Detailed 3-dimensional reconstruction of the ventricles, image integration by ICE and/or multi-detector computed tomography [16], and the use of contact-sensing ablation catheters are also useful and important for a successful ablation (Fig. 34.4). Furthermore, a trans-septal approach may be required to obtain good contact of the ablation catheter with the LV papillary muscles. In any case, radiofrequency catheter ablation is challenging because of catheter instability during papillary muscle contractions and the thickened base of the papillary muscles. The creation of a deep lesion may be necessary for a long-term success due to the distance between the VT origin and endocardial surface [2]. Energies during radiofrequency ablation of 30–70 W have been reported to be necessary to achieve impedance drops of up to 8–10 Ω [8]. A relatively wide area (approximately half) of the papillary muscle circumference and multiple ablation lesions may need to be targeted because of the potential for a deep intramural focus with multiple exits [8].

A recent study [16] reported that cryoablation has been used when traditional radiofrequency ablation has failed, and may be more effective than radiofrequency ablation because of the improved contact stability.

34.6 Acute Success and Recurrence Rates of Catheter Ablation

Acute procedural success for ablation of papillary muscle arrhythmias (i.e., elimination of targeted PVC/VTs during the procedure) is generally fair (60%- 100%) [8–10, 17]. A previous study [2] reported that the recurrence rates for

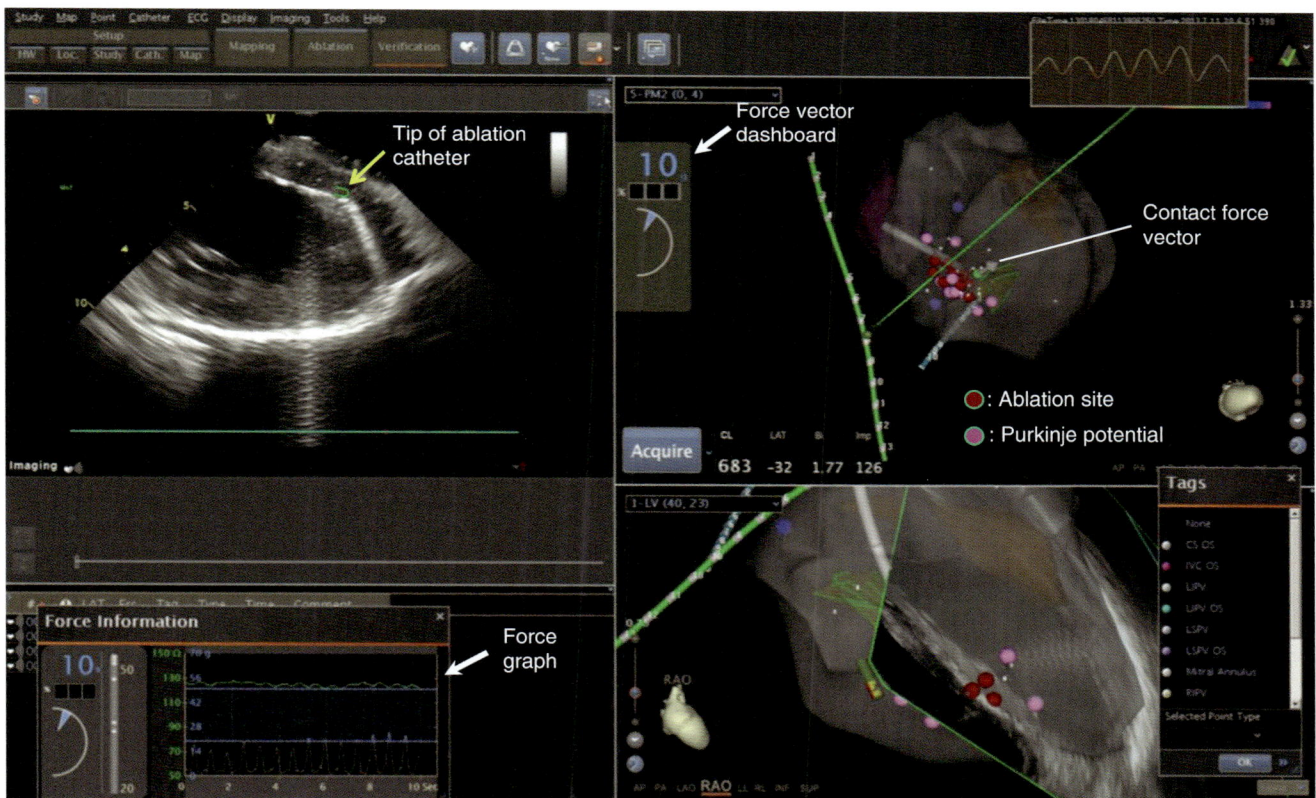

Fig. 34.4 Nonsustained ventricular tachycardia arising from the left ventricular posterior papillary muscle. Cartosound™ system (Biosense Webster) was used for image integration using intracardiac echography (ICE). The use of the specific ICE catheter Soundstar™ (Biosense Webster) allows integration of the ICE images in the Carto™ system, and thus a 3-dimensional "non-invasive" reconstruction of the chamber anatomy. The ablation catheter providing real-time contact force data on an integrated platform (ThermoCool® SmartTouch™, Biosense Webster) was used for ablation. Contact force data was particularly useful for mapping areas such as the base of posterior papillary muscle that is difficult to reach and ensuring good contact is essential. The energy and duration were 30–45 W and up to 120 s for each application. In total, 14 radiofrequency energy applications were required for a cure

arrhythmias originating from anterior papillary muscles and posterior papillary muscles are 71% and 50%, respectively, which are greater than those for left anterior fascicular (25%) and left posterior fascicular (13%) arrhythmias. Another study reported that the presence of Purkinje potentials at the site of the origin and a smaller size of the papillary muscles are associated with a successful ablation [17]. So far, the long-term prognosis after ablation is unknown.

34.7 Complications of Catheter Ablation

Injury to neighboring structures particularly the atrioventricular valves is of concern. Gradual titration of the power, careful manipulation of the catheter, and detailed observation using real-time ICE imaging are important to avoid any complications. Postablation follow-up should include echocardiography to rule out any mitral regurgitation [2], but its incidence is low.

References

1. Latchamsetty R, Yokokawa M, Morady F, Kim HM, Mathew S, Tilz R, et al. Multicenter outcomes for catheter ablation of idiopathic premature ventricular complexes. JACC Clin Electrophysiol. 2015;1:116–23.
2. Yamada T, McElderry HT, Okada T, Murakami Y, Doppalapudi H, Yoshida N, et al. Idiopathic focal ventricular arrhythmias originating from the anterior papillary muscle in the left ventricle. J Cardiovasc Electrophysiol. 2009;20:866–72.
3. Van Herendael H, Zado ES, Haqqani H, Tschabrunn CM, Callans DJ, Frankel DS, et al. Catheter ablation of ventricular fibrillation: importance of left ventricular outflow tract and papillary muscle triggers. Heart Rhythm. 2014;11:566–73.
4. Santoro F, Di Biase L, Hranitzky P, Sanchez JE, Santangeli P, Perini AP, et al. Ventricular fibrillation triggered by PVCs from papillary muscles: clinical features and ablation. J Cardiovasc Electrophysiol. 2014;25:1158–64.
5. Yamada T, Doppalapudi H, McElderry HT, Okada T, Murakami Y, Inden Y, et al. Idiopathic ventricular arrhythmias originating from the papillary muscles in the left ventricle: prevalence, electrocardiographic and electrophysiological characteristics, and results of the radiofrequency catheter ablation. J Cardiovasc Electrophysiol. 2010;21:62–9.
6. Al'Aref SJ, Ip JE, Markowitz SM, Liu CF, Thomas G, Frenkel D, et al. Differentiation of papillary muscle from fascicular and mitral annular ventricular arrhythmias in patients with and without structural heart disease. Circ Arrhythm Electrophysiol. 2015;8:616–24.
7. Hai JJ, Desimone CV, Vaidya VR, Asirvatham SJ. Endocavitary structures in the outflow tract: anatomy and electrophysiology of the conus papillary muscles. J Cardiovasc Electrophysiol. 2014;25:94–8.
8. Yamada T, Doppalapudi H, McElderry HT, Okada T, Murakami Y, Inden Y, et al. Electrocardiographic and electrophysiological characteristics in idiopathic ventricular arrhythmias originating from the papillary muscles in the left ventricle: relevance for catheter ablation. Circ Arrhythm Electrophysiol. 2010;3:324–31.
9. Cawford T, Mueller G, Good E, Jongnarangsin K, Chugh A, Pelosi F Jr, et al. Ventricular arrhythmias originating from papillary muscles in the right ventricle. Heart Rhythm. 2010;7:725–30.
10. Santoro F, DI Biase L, Hranitzky P, Sanchez JE, Santangeli P, Perini AP, et al. Ventricular tachycardia originating from the septal papillary muscle of the right ventricle: electrocardiographic and electrophysiological characteristics. J Cardiovasc Electrophysiol. 2015;26:145–50.
11. Doppalapudi H, Yamada T, McElderry HT, Plumb VJ, Epstein AE, Kay GN. Ventricular tachycardia originating from the posterior papillary muscle in the left ventricle: a distinct clinical syndrome. Circ Arrhythm Electrophysiol. 2008;1:23–9.
12. Syed FF, Ackerman MJ, McLeod CJ, Kapa S, Mulpuru SK, Sriram CS, et al. Sites of successful ventricular fibrillation ablation in bileaflet mitral valve prolapse syndrome. Circ Arrhythm Electrophysiol. 2016;9(5):pii:e004005. https://doi.org/10.1161/CIRCEP.116.004005.
13. Good E, Desjardins B, Jongnarangsin K, Oral H, Chugh A, Ebinger M, et al. Ventricular arrhythmias originating from a papillary muscle in patients without prior infarction: a comparison with fascicular arrhythmias. Heart Rhythm. 2008;5:1530–7.
14. Park KM, Kim YH, Marchlinski FE. Using the surface electrocardiogram to localize the origin of idiopathic ventricular tachycardia. Pacing Clin Electrophysiol. 2012;35:1516–27.
15. Lian-Pin W, Yue-Chun L, Jing-Lin Z, Cheng Z, Jun-Hua C, Jun H, et al. Catheter ablation of idiopathic premature ventricular contractions and ventricular tachycardias originating from right ventricular septum. PLoS One. 2013;8(6):e67038. https://doi.org/10.1371/journal.pone.0067038.
16. Rivera S, Ricapito Mde L, Tomas L, Parodi J, Bardera Molina G, Banega R, et al. Results of cryoenergy and radiofrequency-based catheter ablation for treating ventricular arrhythmias arising from the papillary muscles of the left ventricle, guided by intracardiac echocardiography and image integration. Circ Arrhythm Electrophysiol. 2016;9:e003874. https://doi.org/10.1161/CIRCEP.115.003874.
17. Yokokawa M, Good E, Desjardins B, Crawford T, Jongnarangsin K, Chugh A, et al. Predictors of successful catheter ablation of ventricular arrhythmias arising from the papillary muscles. Heart Rhythm. 2010;7:1654–9.

Ventricular Tachycardia in Non-ischemic Cardiomyopathy

Masahiko Goya

Keywords

Catheter ablation • Non-ischemic VT • Dilated cardiomyopathy • Cardiac sarcoidosis • Arrhythmogenic right ventricular cardiomyopathy/dysplasia

35.1 Introduction

Non-ischemic cardiomyopathy is defined as a cardiomyopathy characterized by mechanical dysfunction in the absence of significant coronary artery disease. Therefore, this category contains various kinds of heart disease. Patients with non-ischemic cardiomyopathy can present with different types of ventricular arrhythmias ranging from ventricular premature beats to sustained monomorphic ventricular tachycardia (VT) and ventricular fibrillation. Similar to those with ischemic cardiomyopathy, patients with non-ischemic cardiomyopathy and a severely impaired LV function (LVEF < 35%) have the risk of sudden death. Implantable cardioverter-defibrillators (ICDs) are the treatment of choice. However, the results of the Sudden Cardiac Death in Heart Failure Trial (SCD-HeFT) demonstrated that, compared with the patients with ischemic cardiomyopathy, mortality is less in patients with non-ischemic cardiomyopathy; the 5-year mortality was 43% for ischemic, but only 28% for non-ischemic cardiomyopathy (Figs. 35.1, 35.2, 35.3, 35.4, and 35.5).

According to the EHRA/HRS/APHRS expert consensus [1] on ventricular arrhythmias, the first-line therapy for non-ischemic VT is optimization of the ICD programming and antiarrhythmic drugs. However, ventricular tachyarrhythmias cannot be prevented by the ICD itself. Moreover, ICD shocks reduce the quality of life, and episodes of VT predict an increased risk of death and heart failure despite effective treatment with an ICD. Catheter ablation has been proven to be an effective choice of treatment for VT and may be indicated for some patients as either a primary therapy or an adjunct to an ICD implantation. This chapter will provide a summary of our current understanding of VT related to dilated cardiomyopathy (DCM), surgically repaired congenital heart disease, post cardiac valve surgery, arrhythmogenic right ventricular cardiomyopathy/dysplasia (ARVC/D), and cardiac sarcoidosis.

35.2 Dilated Cardiomyopathy

The term "dilated cardiomyopathy" refers to a heterogeneous group. An underlying etiology can be identified in only about 50% of patients, while the remaining 50% are considered to be idiopathic (so called DCM). VT occurs in only 5% of patients with DCM; 80% of those tachycardias are caused by scar-related reentry in the myocardium and 20% by bundle branch reentry (BBRT) and focal mechanisms.

M. Goya
Department of Cardiovascular Medicine, Tokyo Medical and Dental University,
1-5-45 Yushima, Bunkyo-ku, Tokyo 113-8510, Japan
e-mail: cameister58.cvm@tmd.ac

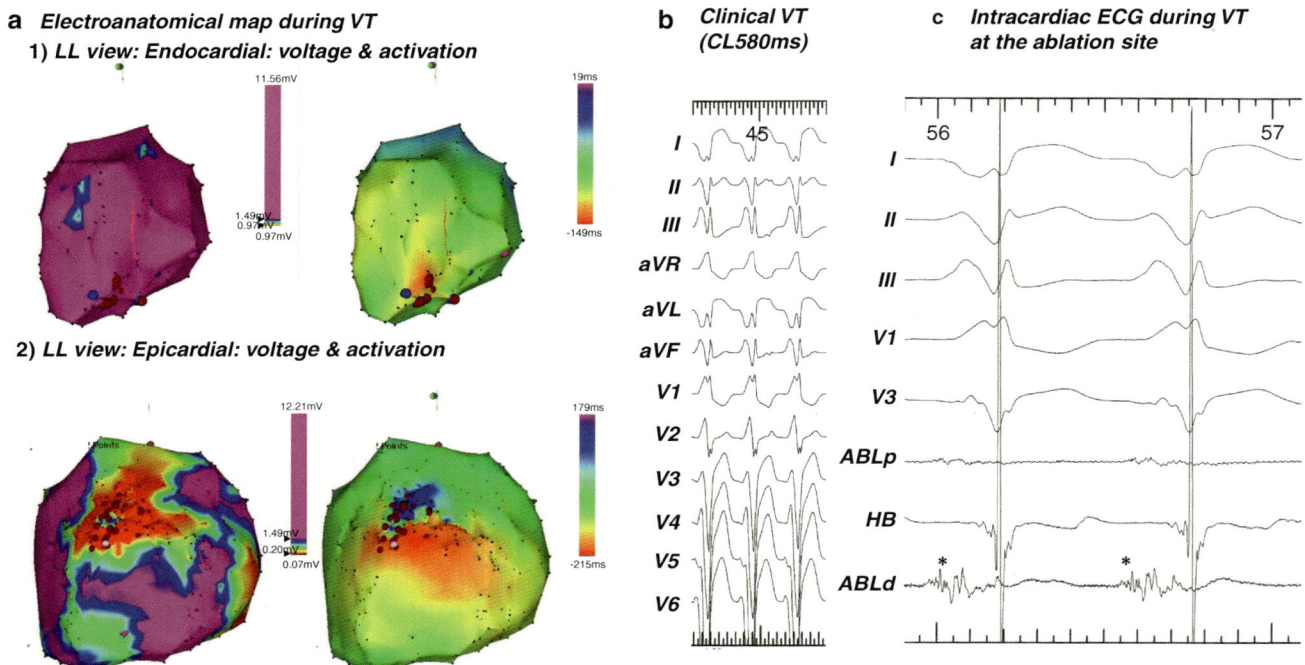

Fig. 35.1 Ablation of a VT in a patient with DCM. (**a**) Voltage and activation maps during the VT of the endocardium (*1*) and epicardium (*2*). There are no abnormal low-voltage areas on the endocardium. The VT exhibits a focal activation pattern. However, a low-voltage area is seen in the anterior region on the epicardium. The VT exhibits macro-reentry. (**b**) The surface ECG during the VT. (**c**) The intracardiac ECG at the ablation site during the VT. Diastolic potentials (**c**: *asterisk*) were recorded inside the low-voltage area. A radiofrequency application at this site terminated the VT. *LL* left lateral, *CL* cycle length, *ABL* ablation, *HB* His bundle, *p* proximal, *d* distal

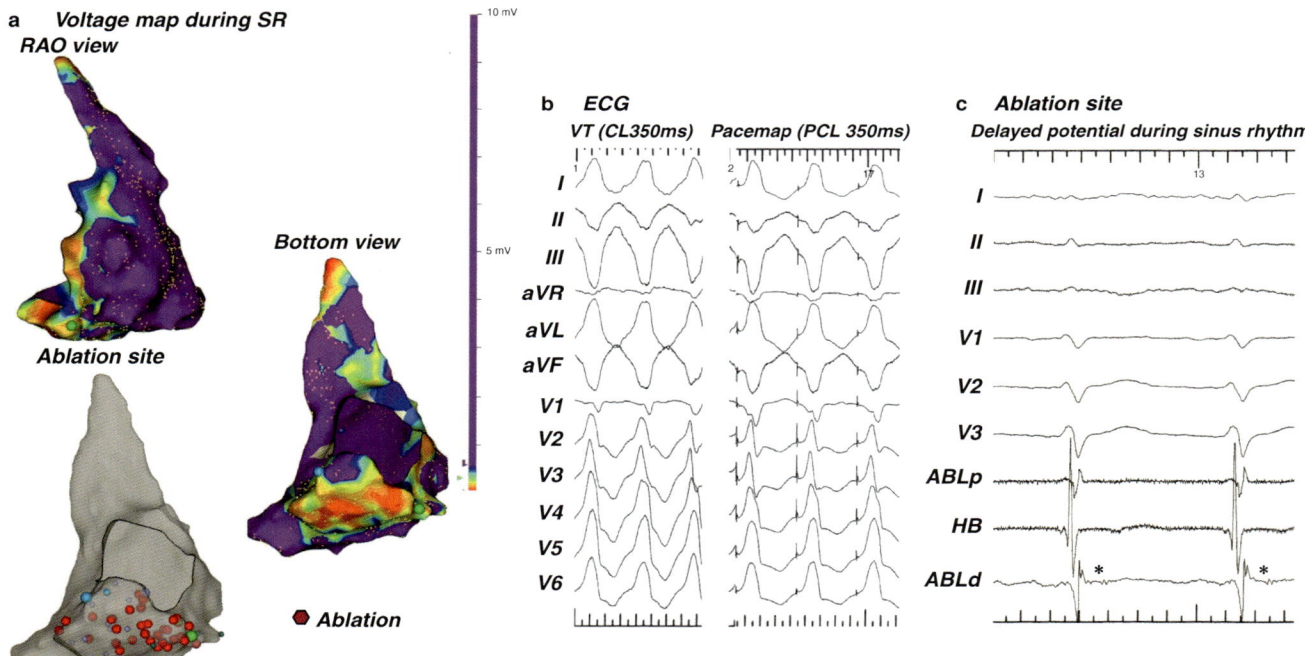

Fig. 35.2 Ablation of a VT in a patient with ARVC. (**a**) A voltage map of the RV in the RAO and bottom views during sinus rhythm. An abnormal low-voltage area is demonstrated in the inferior wall of the RV. (**b**) The surface ECG during the VT and a pacemap. (**c**) The intracardiac ECG at the delayed potential recording site inside the low-voltage area (**c**: *asterisk*). A pacemap at the delayed potential recording site shows an almost identical QRS morphology as the VT (**b**). All delayed potentials disappeared by repeated RF applications inside the abnormal low-voltage area (*red tag* in the gray chamber). RAO: right anterior oblique

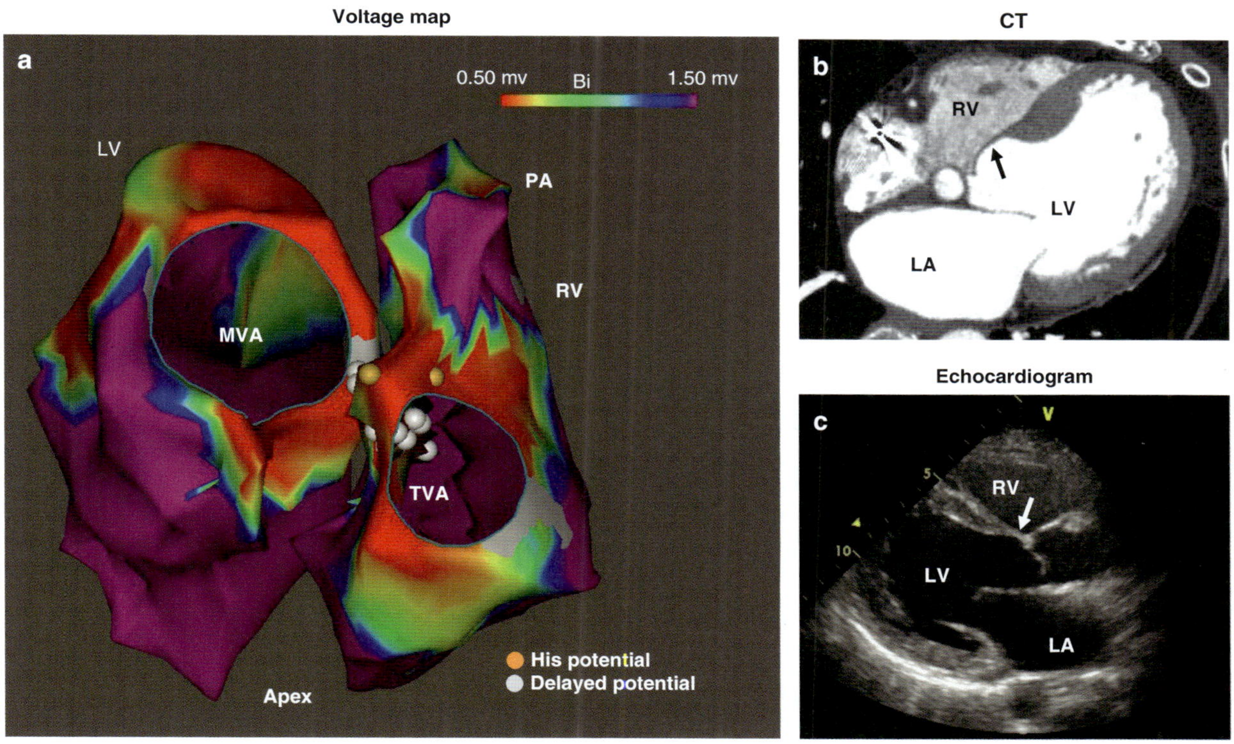

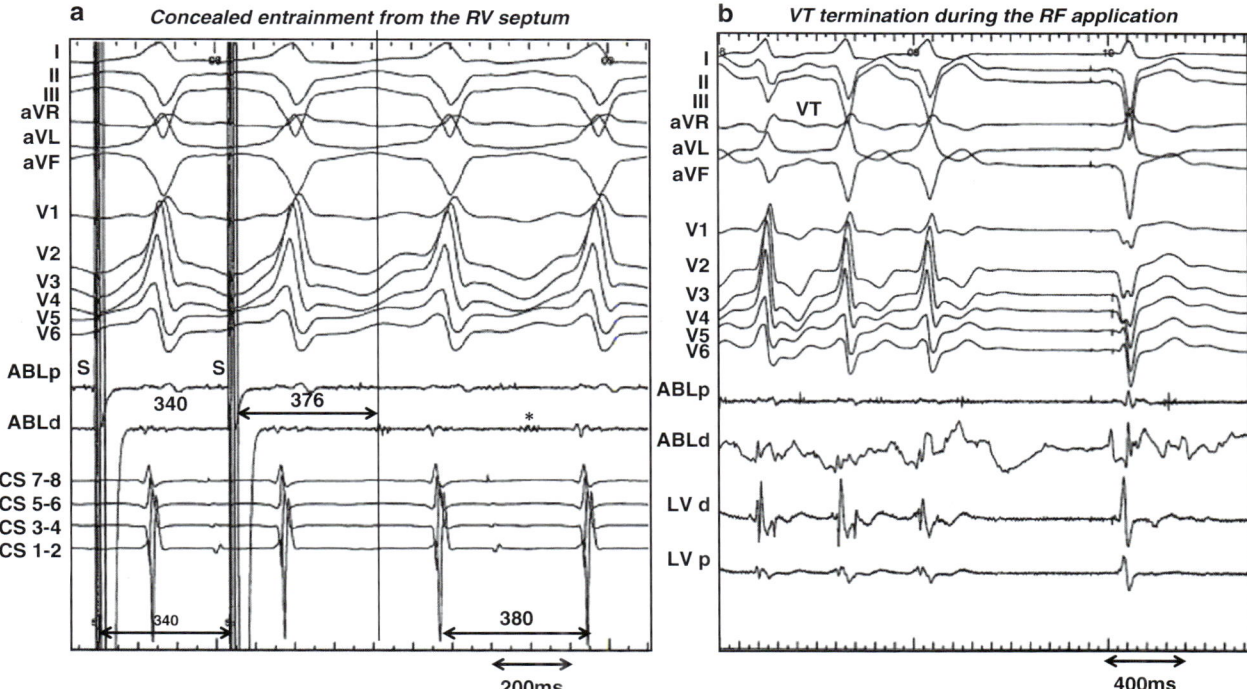

Fig. 35.3 Electroanatomical map, CT, and echocardiogram in a patient with cardiac sarcoidosis. (**a**) Voltage map of the RV and LV during sinus rhythm. An abnormal low-voltage area (<1.5 mV) is located in the perivalvular region. Delayed potentials are recorded at the basaloseptum. (**b**) An enhanced CT in the four chamber view. Wall thinning is observed in the basaloseptum (**c**: *black arrow*). (**c**) An echocardiogram also demonstrates wall thinning of the septum (**c**: *white arrow*). *LV* left ventricle, *PA* pulmonary artery, *RV* right ventricle, *MVA* mitral valve annulus, *TVA* tricuspid valve annulus, *LA* left atrium

Fig. 35.4 Entrainment from the delayed potential recording site is shown. (**a**) Pacing entrains the clinical VT without a QRS fusion. Two distinct potentials are recorded from the ablation site (ABLd). The local potential (*asterisk*) is captured during pacing. The post pacing interval is 376 ms, which approximates the tachycardia cycle length of 380 ms. (**b**) The VT is terminated by a radiofrequency energy application. *CS* coronary sinus, *LV* left ventricle

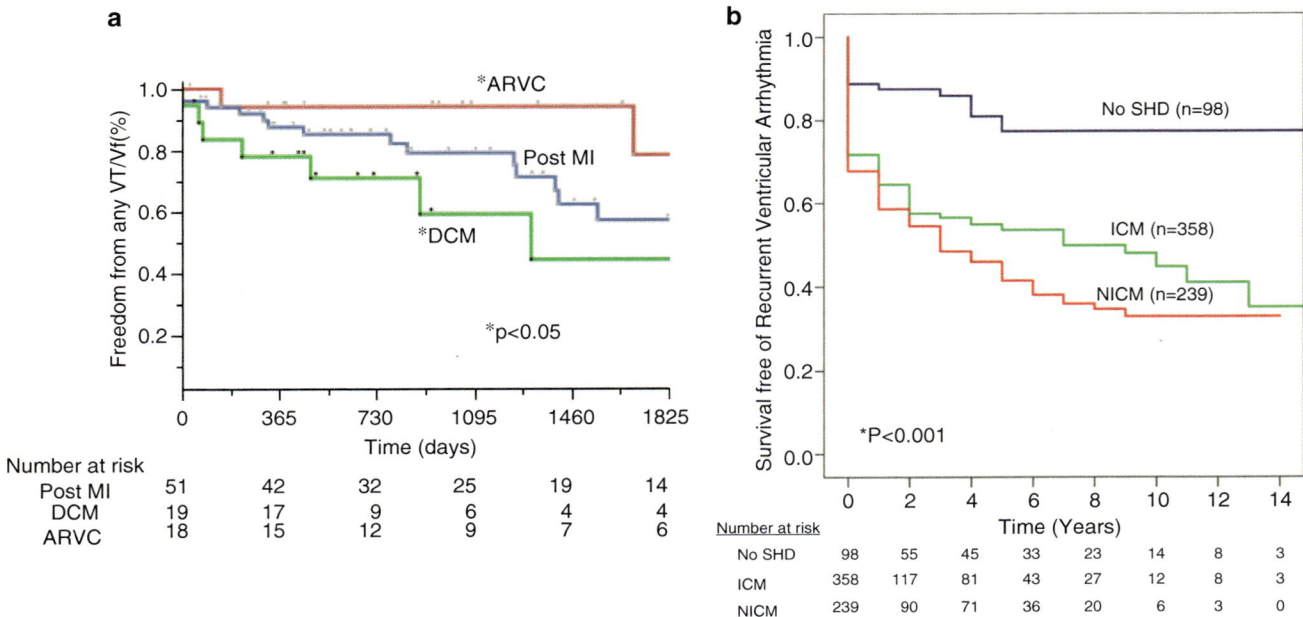

Fig. 35.5 Survival free of recurrent ventricular arrhythmias after ablation. (**a**) ARVC-VT ablation was associated with a better long-term prognosis than DCM. Post-infarction VT demonstrated a midrange outcome (from Goya et al. [28]). (**b**) An excellent prognosis is shown in the absence of structural heart disease. The highest recurrence is shown in patients with non-ischemic cardiomyopathy (from Kumar et al. [29]). *SHD* structural heart disease, *ICM* ischemic cardiomyopathy, *NICM* non-ischemic cardiomyopathy

35.2.1 Anatomic and Electrophysiologic Substrate of DCM-VT

In contrast to post-infarction VT, the anatomic and electrophysiological substrate of VT due to non-ischemic cardiomyopathy has not been well characterized. Histologically, the ventricular myocardium in DCM is characterized by multiple patchy areas of interstitial and replacement fibrosis and a myofiber disarray with variable degrees of myocyte hypertrophy and atrophy. An altered cellular function with abnormal membrane potentials is associated with myocyte hypertrophy and may be arrhythmogenic in experimental settings. Nonreentrant mechanisms of ventricular arrhythmias, like triggered activity arising from delayed afterdepolarizations (DADs) or early afterdepolarizations (EADs), have been reported in patients and animal models with DCM [2, 3]. In studies of explanted hearts, de Bakker et al. [4] found unexcitable fibrosis creating regions of conduction block and surviving myocardium creating potential reentry circuit paths in DCM. Slow conduction through muscle bundles separated by interstitial fibrosis can cause a zigzag path producing slow conduction that promotes reentry. Because of this complex pathological background, patients with DCM exhibit various kinds of ventricular arrhythmias.

Among patients with DCM, sustained monomorphic VT is not common. Compared with post-infarction VT, scars are probably due to progressive replacement fibrosis, and the areas of scar are smaller and transmural scar is rare and intramural scars are common. Further, scars are often located in the epicardial region [2] or adjacent to a valve annulus [5]. Detecting the location of the scar magnetic resonance imaging (MRI) with delayed Gd enhancement is useful.

35.2.2 Catheter Ablation of DCM-VT

These features account for the perception that ablation of DCM-VT is more difficult when compared with that of post-infarction VT. In 2004, Soejima et al. [5] reported a case series of 28 patients with DCM-VT. The VTs were due to focal VT, BBRT, and myocardial reentry VT in 5, 2, and 22 patients, respectively. Most (63%) endocardial scars were adjacent to a valve annulus. Epicardial mapping and ablation was performed if the endocardial ablation failed. Of the 19 VT circuit isthmuses identified, seven were associated with an epicardial scar. The scars were greater in extent on the epicardium than on the endocardium. At least one VT was abolished in 16 of 22 patients and all VTs were abolished in 12 of 22. During a mean follow-up of 334 days, VT recurred in 46% of the patients, one patient died of heart failure, and a cardiac transplantation was performed in two patients.

Oloriz et al. [6] categorized DCM-VT according to the scar predominance and the consequent arrhythmias as either anteroseptal or inferolateral. Delayed-enhanced imaging and a simple ECG analysis allowed the prediction of the scar location. Further, the VT recurrence and redo rates were particularly high for a setting with an anteroseptal substrate because of the involvement of an intramural septal substrate.

As for post-infarction VT, scar homogenization improves the long-term ventricular arrhythmia-free survival compared with a standard limited-substrate ablation. Recently Gokoglan et al. reported [7] a better long-term efficacy of an endoepicardial scar homogenization approach compared with that of a standard ablation also in DCM-VT.

The most frequent mechanism of DCM-VT is scar-related reentry, so catheter ablation is a useful and effective treatment choice. However, the success rate appears to be lower than that of a previously reported study with post-infarction VT even with an endocardial and epicardial approach, presumably because of the septal and mid-myocardial distribution of the scar in some cases.

35.3 Surgically Repaired Congenital Heart Disease

Congenital heart anomalies occur in almost 1% of births, and early surgical repair is required in 30–50% of patients. Although the life expectancy has improved, sudden cardiac death due to lethal ventricular arrhythmias remains one of the most important and unsolved clinical issues. The mechanism of the VT after a surgically repaired congenital heart disease (post CHD-VT) is also reentry. The substrate of the reentry is scar created by a ventriculotomy or patches. Myocardial hypertrophy occurs in a variety of malformations and also likely contributes to the arrhythmia risk. The approach to the catheter ablation of post-CHD-VT is the same as that for the other scar-related VTs. Understanding the anatomic complexities is the key to successful ablation results. An electroanatomical mapping system integrated with echocardiography, MRI, or CT is highly helpful. Identification of the region of scar and a substrate mapping approach to identify channels has been described. Data are mainly from case reports and small patient series. A report using a substrate mapping approach after a Tetralogy of Fallot or ventricular septal defect repair described common isthmuses supporting reentry between the tricuspid or pulmonic valve annuli and scar or a patch in the septum or RV free wall that could be targeted for ablation. In 2009, Zeppenfeld et al. reported [8] in 11 patients that 15 different VTs were inducible. Ablation abolished all inducible VTs. During an average follow-up of 30 months, 91% of the patients were free from VTs. In a series of ten patients with a Tetralogy of Fallot [9], mapping with a noncontact electrode array demonstrated macroreentry in 11 of 13 induced VTs. Ablation was performed in eight patients, six of whom were free of VT during the follow-up. In those small series, no serious complications were reported.

35.4 Post Cardiac Valve Surgery

Regarding VT after cardiac valve surgery, BBRT has been reported [10, 11] and is well known. Eckart et al. [12] analyzed 20 patients who had VT after aortic or mitral valve surgery in the absence of a known myocardial infarction. VT after cardiac valve surgery appears to be bimodal in presentation, occurring either early after surgery or years later. In this patient group, reentry in a region of scar predominantly located in the periannular region is more common than BBRT. Further, catheter ablation can be successful.

35.5 Arrhythmogenic Right Ventricular Cardiomyopathy/Dysplasia (ARVC/D)

Right ventricular diseases causing VT are infrequent. ARVC/D is probably the most common cause and has a prevalence of approximately one in 5000. ARVC/D is an inherited myocardial disease. Scar-related reentry is the most common mechanism of VT. Recently, the clinical course and predictors of arrhythmic risk were examined in 301 patients [13]. The high risk of life-threatening arrhythmias in patients with ARVC/D spans from adolescence to an advanced age, reaching its peak between ages 21 and 40 years. Atrial fibrillation, syncope, participation in strenuous exercise after the diagnosis of ARVC/D, hemodynamically tolerated sustained monomorphic ventricular tachycardia, and a male sex predicted lethal arrhythmias during the follow-up. The lack of efficacy of antiarrhythmic therapy and the lifesaving role of ICDs highlight the importance of risk stratification in the patient management.

35.5.1 Anatomic and Electrophysiologic Substrates of ARVC/D-VT

ARVC/D is characterized by fibrofatty replacement of the myocardium within the so-called triangle of dysplasia, which encompasses the RV inflow, outflow, and apex. The disease process usually begins in the epicardium or intramural layers and progresses to the endocardium. The left ventricle (LV) is affected in up to 76% of cases [14–16]. Pathologic regions are demonstrated as contiguous low-voltage, long-duration electrograms. Interestingly, there is a good correlation between low-voltage areas delineated by electroanatomical mapping and the histopathologic findings of myocyte loss and fibrofatty replacement [15]. The endocardial low-voltage abnormalities are adjacent to the tricuspid and/or pulmonic valve and extend for a variable distance toward the apex, involving both the RV wall and to a lesser extent the interventricular septum [16]. Scars adjacent to the mitral valve can be observed in patients with LV involvement.

35.5.2 Catheter Ablation of ARVC/D-VT

ARVC/D-VTs are inducible with programmed ventricular stimulation and can be entrained. The mechanism of the tachycardia is mainly reentry involving the regions of abnormal electrograms. Therefore, the same mapping and ablation techniques for post-infarction VT can be applied. Focal VTs in ARVC/D have been described, although some of those cases may represent epicardial reentry with a focal endocardial breakthrough. In the early 2000s, there were several reports concerning the catheter ablation of ARVC/D. According to those reports, catheter ablation can reduce the frequent episodes of VT, but the long-term follow-up has demonstrated a continued risk of recurrence. However, only an endocardial approach was used in most of the cases. Recently, Bai et al. [17] and Berruezo et al. [18] reported the endocardial and epicardial substrate based mapping and ablation of ARVC/D-VT. Bai et al. [17] reported a freedom from VT/VF or ICD therapy of 84.6% in patients who were mapped and ablated with an endocardial and epicardial approach during a follow-up of at least 3 years. Bai et al. [17] and Philip et al. [19] reported the importance of VPCs in patients with ARVC-VT. These reports might suggest that VT ablation of ARVC/D is highly effective during the short- and long-term follow-up period with an endocardial and epicardial approach.

35.6 Cardiac Sarcoidosis

Sarcoidosis is a granulomatous disease of an unknown etiology. Non-necrotizing granulomas are the pathological features and are most often associated with involvement of the lungs and thoracic lymph nodes. The heart is the third most commonly affected organ. Cardiac sarcoidosis occurs in 10–15% of patients with systemic sarcoidosis in Japan. Sudden cardiac death due to bradyarrhythmias or ventricular tachyarrhythmias can occur in patients with cardiac sarcoidosis [20].

35.6.1 Anatomic and Electrophysiologic Background of Sarcoidosis VT

Various ventricular arrhythmias induced by triggered activity or abnormal automaticity have been observed as a result of myocardial inflammation due to cardiac sarcoidosis. The most common mechanism of ventricular arrhythmias in sarcoidosis is macroreentry around areas of granulomatous scar [20]. Immunosuppression using corticosteroids is often used in patients with an active phase of cardiac sarcoidosis. As for ventricular arrhythmias, several studies have suggested beneficial results of immunosuppressive therapy [21], and on the contrary others have failed to show any benefit.

35.6.2 Catheter Ablation of Sarcoidosis VT

Cardiac sarcoidosis with RV involvement can mimic ARVC/D. Non-ischemic cardiomyopathy and myocardial infarctions also initiate some RV scar-related VTs. The methods for mapping and ablation are the same as those for scar-related VTs; activation mapping, entrainment mapping, substrate mapping, and combined approaches have been used. As in post-infarction VTs, large scars and reentry circuits with extensive areas of abnormal electrograms, evidence of slow conduction, and bystander regions can be demonstrated by electroanatomical mapping.

Jefic et al. [22] described the role of catheter ablation in nine patients with sarcoidosis VT after a failed immunosuppression therapy. The majority of the patients had either VT storms or incessant VT. The mechanism of the targeted VTs was predominantly reentry. Therefore, VTs could be mapped and analyzed using an electroanatomical mapping system and conventional electrophysiologic methods such as entrainment mapping and pace mapping. The most frequent location of the reentry circuit was the para-tricuspid area. In patients with epicardial scarring, an epicardial approach is required to eliminate the VT. Pre-procedural information of the location of scars detected by MRI might be helpful to decide the approach. Ablation outcomes in the study by Jefic et al. [22] were favorable, with either the elimination of VT recurrences or a reduction in the VT burden. In contrast, Koplan et al. [23] reported recurrences of VT in most patients. A more extensive arrhythmogenic substrate with more advanced cardiac disease at the time of the VT ablation may be the reason for this discrepancy.

Recently, several reports concerning sarcoidosis VT have been published. Naruse et al. [21] enrolled 37 patients with sarcoidosis VT and evaluated the clinical effects of medical therapy using steroid and antiarrhythmic agents in association with catheter ablation. Twenty-three (62%) patients were free from VTs with medications. Fourteen patients underwent catheter ablation. Sarcoidosis VTs were successfully suppressed by medications with or without catheter ablation in the majority of their patients. Kumar et al. [24] reported that multiple inducible VTs were observed with a mechanism consistent with scar-mediated reentry in all sarcoidosis VTs. After ≥1 procedure, ablation abolished ≥1 inducible VT in 90% and eliminated VT storms in 78% of the patients; however, multiple residual VTs remained inducible. Therefore, they concluded that catheter ablation was effective in terminating VT storms and eliminating ≥1 inducible VT in the majority of patients, but recurrences were common. Ablation in conjunction with antiarrhythmic drugs could help palliate the VT in this high-risk population [24]. Muser et al. [25] evaluated 31 patients with sarcoidosis VT that underwent catheter ablation and reported favorable results. Overall the VT-free survival was 55% at 2 years of follow-up. Among the 16 (52%) patients with VT recurrences, ablation resulted in a significant reduction of the VT burden, with eight (50%) having only isolated [1–3] VT episodes and only one patient with a recurrent VT storm.

Catheter ablation is effective to reduce the VT burden and is useful for bailing-out of VT storms in patients with cardiac sarcoidosis. Still many of the patients require a combination therapy of immunosuppressive agents and antiarrhythmic drugs.

35.7 Long-Term Results of Catheter Ablation of Non-ischemic VT

Several papers on the long-term follow-up outcomes after VT ablation in patients with non-ischemic cardiomyopathy have been published. In addition to the results of the SCD-HeFT, Sacher et al. [26] reported that ischemic cardiomyopathy had a 2-fold increased risk of mortality compared with non-ischemic heart disease, despite a lower VT recurrence. Tokuda et al. [27] reported the long-term follow-up outcomes of VT ablation in patients with non-ischemic heart disease. In that study, the ARVC/D-VT ablation outcomes were significantly better than the DCM-VT ablation outcomes, which is consistent with our study results [28]. Kumar et al. [29] estimated the long-term outcomes after catheter ablation of VT in patients with and without structural heart disease. Complete procedural success was higher in the patients with no structural heart disease than in those with ischemic cardiomyopathy and non-ischemic cardiomyopathy (79%, 56%, and 60%, respectively; $P < 0.001$). At 6 years, the ventricular arrhythmia-free survival was higher in the patients with no structural heart disease (77%) than in those with ischemic cardiomyopathy (54%) and non-ischemic cardiomyopathy (38%) ($P < 0.001$), and the overall survival was lowest in the patients with ischemic cardiomyopathy (48%), followed by those with non-ischemic cardiomyopathy (74%) and no structural heart disease (100%) ($P < 0.001$).

The above suggests that catheter ablation is effective in patients with ischemic and non-ischemic heart disease, but regarding the recurrence rate of VT/Vf, non-ischemic VT has a higher recurrence rate. Furthermore, the mortality of non-ischemic VT is less compared to that of ischemic VTs. In a matter of speaking, catheter ablation of non-ischemic VTs is more important in clinical medicine than that for ischemic VTs. Further developments are required to improve the ablation results of non-ischemic VTs.

References

1. Pedersen CT, Kay GN, Kalman J, et al. EHRA/HRS/APHRS expert consensus on ventricular arrhythmias. Europace. 2014;16:1267–83.
2. Hsia HH, Marchlinski FE. Characterization of the electroanatomic substrate for monomorphic ventricular tachycardia in patients with nonischemic cardiomyopathy. Pacing Clin Electrophysiol. 2002;25:1114–27.
3. Pogwizd SM, McKenzie JP, Cain ME. Mechanisms underlying spontaneous and induced ventricular arrhythmias in patients with idiopathic dilated cardiomyopathy. Circulation. 1998;98:2404–14.
4. de Bakker JM, van Capelle FJ, Janse MJ, et al. Slow conduction in the infarcted human heart. 'Zigzag' course of activation. Circulation. 1993;88:915–26.
5. Soejima K, Stevenson WG, Sapp JL, et al. Endocardial and epicardial radiofrequency ablation of ventricular tachycardia associated with dilated cardiomyopathy. The importance of low-voltage scars. J Am Coll Cardiol. 2004;43:1834–42.
6. Oloriz T, Silberbauer J, Maccabelli G, et al. Catehter ablation of ventricular arrhythmia in nonischemic cardiomyopathy. Anterosptal versus inferolateral scar sub-types. Circ Arrhythm Electrophysiol. 2014;7:414–23.
7. Gokoglan Y, Mohanty S, Gianni C, et al. Scar homogenization versus limited-substrate ablation in patients with nonischemic cardiomyopathy and ventricular tachycardia. J Am Coll Cardiol. 2016;68:1990–8.
8. Zeppenfeld K, Schalij MJ, Bartelings MM, et al. Catheter ablation of ventricular tachycardia after repair of congenital heart disease: electroanatomic identification of the critical right ventricular isthmus. Circulation. 2007;116:2241–52.
9. Kriebel T, Saul JP, Schneider H, Sigler M, Paul T. Noncontact mapping and radiofrequency catheter ablation of fast and hemodynamically unstable ventricular tachycardia after surgical repair of tetralogy of Fallot. J Am Coll Cardiol. 2007;50:2162–8.
10. Fedgchin B, Pavri BB, Greenspon AJ, Ho RT. Unique self-perpetuating cycle of atrioventricular block and phase IV bundle branch block in a patient with bundle branch reentrant tachycardia. Heart Rhythm. 2004;1:493–6.
11. Lewalter T, Jung W, Preusse CJ, Lickfett L, Wolpert C, Yang A, Welz A, Luderitz B. Radiofrequency catheter ablation of an incessant ventricular tachycardia following valve surgery. Pacing Clin Electrophysiol. 2002;25:105–8.
12. Eckart RE, Hruczkowski TW, Tedrow UBZ, Koplan ZBA, Epstein LM, Stevenson WG. Sustained ventricular tachycardia associated with correctrive valve surgery. Circulation. 2007;116:2005–11.
13. Mazzanti A, Ng K, Faragli A, Maragna R, Chiodaroli E, et al. Arrhythmogenic right ventricular cardiomyopathy. Clinical course and predictors of arrhythmic risk. J Am Coll Cardiol. 2016;68:2540–50.
14. Kies P, Bootsma M, Bax J, Schalij MJ, van der Wall EE. Arrhythmogenic right ventricular dysplasia/cardiomyopathy: screening, diagnosis, and treatment. Heart Rhythm. 2006;3:225–34.
15. Liuba I, Marchlinski FE. The substrate and ablation of ventricular tachycardia in patients with nonischemic cardiomyopathy. Circ J. 2013;77:1957–66.
16. Marra MP, Leoni L, Bauce B, Corbetti F, Zorzi A, Migliore F, et al. Imaging study of ventricular scar in arrhythmogenic right ventricular cardiomyopathy: comparison of 3D standard electroanatomical

voltage mapping and contrast-enhanced cardiac magnetic resonance. Circ Arrhythm Electrophysiol. 2012;5:91–100.
17. Bai R, Di Biase L, Shivkumar K, et al. Ablation of ventricular arrhythmias in arrhythmogenic right ventricular dysplasia/cardiomyopathy arrhythmia-free survival after endo-epicardial substrate based mapping and ablation. Circ Arrhythm Electrophysiol. 2011;4:478–85.
18. Berruezo A, Fern'andez-Armenta J, Mont L, et al. Combined endocardial and epicardial catheter ablation in arrhythmogenic right ventricular dysplasia incorporating scar dechanneling technique. Circ Arrhythm Electrophysiol. 2012;5:111–21.
19. Philips B, Madhavan S, James C, et al. High prevalence of catecholamine-facilitated focal ventricular tachycardia in patients with arrhythmogenic right ventricular dysplasia/cardiomyopathy. Circ Arrhythm Electrophysiol. 2013;6(1):160–6.
20. Birnie DH, Sauer WH, Bogun F, Cooper JM, Culver DA, et al. HRS expert consensus statement on the diagnosis ans management of arrhythmias associated with cardiac sarcoidosis. Heart Rhythm. 2014;11(7):1304–23.
21. Naruse Y, Sekiguchi Y, Nogami A, Okada H, Yamauchi Y, et al. Systemic treatment approach to ventricular tachycardia in cardiac sarcoidosis. Circ Arrhythm Electrophysiol. 2014;7:407–13.
22. Jefic D, Joel B, Good E, et al. Role of radiofrequency catheter ablation of ventricular tachycardia in cardiac sarcoidosis: report from a multicenter registry. Heart Rhythm. 2009;6:189–95.
23. Koplan BA, Soejima K, Baughman K, Epstein LM, Stevenson WG. Refractory ventricular tachycardia secondary to cardiac sarcoid: electrophysiologic characteristics, mapping, and ablation. Heart Rhythm. 2006;3:924–9.
24. Kumar S, Barbhaiya C, Nagashima K, Choi EK, Epstein LM, et al. Ventricular tachycardia in cardiac sarcoidosis. Characterization of ventricular substrate and outcomes of catheter ablation. Circ Arrhythm Electrophysiol. 2015;8:87–93.
25. Muser D, Santangeli P, Pathak RK, Castro SA, Liang JJ, et al. Long-term outcomes of catheter ablation of ventricular tachycardia in patients with cardiac sarcoidosis. Circ Arrhythm Electrophysiol. 2016;9:e004333. https://doi.org/10.1161/CIRCEP.111.004333.
26. Sacher F, Tedrow UB, Field ME, et al. Ventricular tachycardia ablation: evolution of patients and procedures over 8 years. Circ Arrhythm Electrophysiol. 2008;1:153–61.
27. Tokuda M, Tedrow UB, Kojodjojo P, et al. Catheter ablation of ventricular tachycardia in nonischemic heart disease. Circ Arrhythm Electrophysiol. 2012;5:992–1000.
28. Goya M, Fukunaga M, Hiroshima K, Hayashi K, Makihara Y, et al. Long-term outcomes of catheter ablation of ventricular tachycardia in patients with structural heart disease. J Arrhythm. 2015;31(1):22–8.
29. Kumar S, Romero J, Mehta N, Fujii A, Kapur S, et al. Long-term outcome after catheter ablation of ventricular tachycardia in patients with and without structural heart disease. Heart Rhythm. 2016;13:1957–63.

Ventricular Tachycardia in Ischemic Heart Disease

Kyoko Soejima and Akiko Ueda

Keywords

Ventricular tachycardia · Ischemic cardiomyopathy · Infarction · Isthmus

36.1 Mechanisms for Ventricular Tachycardia Associated with Ischemic Cardiomyopathy

36.1.1 Myocardial Scar-Related Reentry

Scar-related reentry is a leading cause of ventricular tachycardia (VT) associated with chronic ischemic cardiomyopathy (ICMP), which involves scar and the surrounding border zone as part of a macro-reentrant circuit. After an acute myocardial infarction, mechanical and electrical remodeling occurs to support the reentry; alteration of the ionic current in myocardial cells causes a change in action potential duration and amplitude, and nonuniform refractoriness yields unidirectional block. Replacement of necrotic tissue with fibrotic tissue develops over several days to months following acute infarction and creates a heterogeneous three-dimensional (3D) structure, in which activation propagates in a zigzag fashion [1]. Adipose tissue deposition in the infarct area results in further conduction delay. Redistribution of the gap junction results in nonuniform and slow conduction. Diminished membrane voltage in the damaged area yields premature complexes, and deleterious neural remodeling in the peri-infarct region probably contributes to the electrophysiological heterogeneity of the myocardium, altering excitability and creating a substrate for ventricular arrhythmias.

This histopathological remodeling favors conditions for the initiation and maintenance of sustained monomorphic reentrant VTs.

36.1.2 Substrates in the Conduction System

Another form of ICMP-related VT involves the His-Purkinje system (HPS). Lopera et al. reported that 11 of 153 patients (7.1%) with ICMP-related VT showed HPS involvement: bundle branch reentry, interfascicular VT, and focal VT originating in the distal HPS [2]. VT involving the left posterior fascicle, being analogous to idiopathic VT, has also been reported [3].

36.2 Substrate Evaluation

The substrate for ICMP-VT exists in the infarction and border zone, mostly in the endocardium, but sometimes involving mid-myocardial or epicardial areas. Evaluation of the substrate prior to catheter ablation is useful for planning the procedure.

36.2.1 MRI

Late gadolinium-enhancement cardiac magnetic resonance (LGE-CMR) has been used to visualize the 3D structure of the complex substrate and provides clinical information that is useful for locating the target substrate for ablation. This information can help plan the approach: endocardial vs. epicardial ablation for free wall substrate, or left vs. right

K. Soejima (✉) · A. Ueda
Department of Cardiology, Kyorin University School of Medicine, 6-20-2 Shinkawa, Mitaka, Tokyo 181-8611, Japan
e-mail: skyoko@ks.kyorin-u.ac.jp; akiko.ut23@gmail.com

ventricle ablation for septal VT, according to the LGE distribution [4]. A 3D color-coded shell map based on the pixel signal intensity is reconstructed by LGE-CMR to depict the scar core and border zone distribution, and is compared with the 3D electroanatomical mapping (EAM). A CMR-defined border zone channel is able to identify 74% of the critical VT isthmus [5], suggesting the possibility of using LGE-CMR prior to the ablation procedure to depict the clinically relevant VT channels.

Although the majority of ICMP-VT patients can be ablated endocardially, some require epicardial ablation. Acosta et al. showed that patients with a transmural infarct who underwent endocardial ablation had a greater risk of recurrence compared with non-transmural infarct patients and suggested that infarct transmurality by LGE-CMR might be a useful criterion for the selection of a first-line combined endo-epicardial approach [6].

36.2.2 Intracardiac Echo

An abnormal substrate can be depicted by intracardiac echo in patients who are not able to undergo an MRI examination [7]. Areas with increased echogenicity or wall thinning can be tagged and displayed on the 3D EAM, which helps to focus on the mapping of the region of interest.

36.3 Mapping

The majority of the VTs associated with structural heart disease are hemodynamically unstable; therefore, activation or entrainment mapping cannot be performed. Usually, substrate and pace mapping during stable rhythm are performed to identify the circuit.

36.3.1 Entrainment Mapping

Entrainment refers to the continuous interaction between the wavefront of the paced activation and the VT, and the specific response to multiple stimuli delivered during VT. Usually, pacing at a cycle length (CL) 10–20 ms shorter than the VTCL is delivered to entrain the VT, as rapid pacing is likely to cause slow conduction, change the conduction path, or terminate VT. It is used to define the mechanism of the VT and to determine the relation between the location of the pacing site and that of the reentrant circuit. During entrainment, premature stimuli enter the excitable gap and propagate orthodromically and collide antidromically with the preceding tachycardia wavefront, resetting the VT. Pacing from outside the circuit will result in QRS fusion, as the myocardium is activated from two different directions: from the exit of the VT circuit and from the pacing site. Entrainment is mandatory to define the reentrant circuit by its response and to guide successful catheter ablation. Figure 36.1 summarizes the interpretation steps [8].

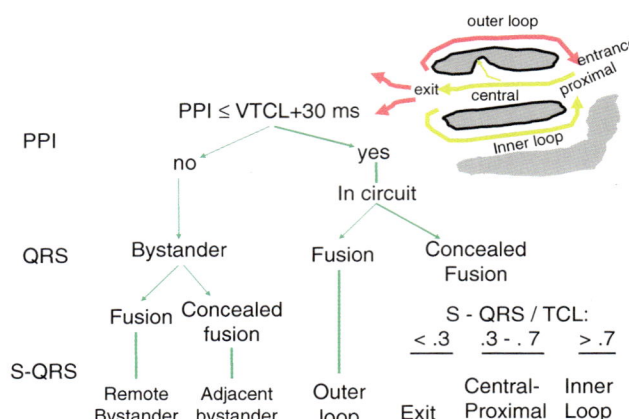

Fig. 36.1 Entrainment mapping. If the PPI–VTCL difference is within 30 msec, the site is in the circuit. Then if the QRS morphology shows concealed fusion, Stimulus-QRS is compared to the TCl. If it is 30% or less, the site is exit, 31–70% is central to proximal portion of the isthmus

36.3.1.1 Step 1: Post-pacing Interval (PPI) Following Entrainment

The PPI following entrainment analyzes the proximity of the pacing site to the reentry circuit. The stimulated wavefront requires time to reach the circuit, traverse it, and return to the pacing site. If the pacing site is within the reentry circuit, the time to and from the circuit is zero, and the PPI differs from the VTCL by 30 ms or less.

36.3.1.2 Step 2: QRS Configuration During Entrainment

The next step is to compare the paced QRS morphology to the VT. During entrainment, the QRS complex is the result of fusion between the wavefront propagating directly away from the pacing site and those emerging from the VT circuit. If the pacing site is within the isthmus of the reentry circuit, pacing accelerates the VT rate to the pacing rate without any change in the QRS (concealed fusion). In the outer loop of the reentry circuit, however, the pacing stimulus directly captures the surrounding myocardium, which causes a change in QRS morphology (manifest fusion).

36.3.1.3 Step 3: S-QRS Interval During Entrainment

During entrainment with concealed fusion, the interval from the pacing stimulus to the onset of QRS indicates the conduction time from the pacing site to the VT exit. If the previous two steps were positive, then the evaluation of Step 3 is performed to identify the exact location of the pacing site in relation to the reentry circuit. If the S-QRS interval is 0.3 of the VTCL or less, the site is considered as an exit of the isthmus; if it is from 0.31 to 0.50 of the VTCL, it is the central isthmus; while if it is 0.51–0.70 of the VTCL, it is the proximal isthmus.

Another important use of entrainment mapping is to identify the local electrogram. Fractionated or delayed isolated potentials are often recorded during ICMP-VT and assessment of the local activation electrogram is important, to measure the PPI and to reconstruct the precise activation map. Figure 36.2 shows the captured local electrogram in contrast to the non-captured far-field potential.

36.3.2 Pace Mapping

Pace mapping is frequently used to identify the circuit exit during the stable rhythm. Pacing at a rate similar to the VT might produce a similar functional block during VT and help to identify the isthmus site. It is possible to infer the possible site of origin based on the ECG, which helps to guide pace mapping (Fig. 36.3). In addition, pace mapping in sinus rhythm also provides a measure of slow conduction, indicated by a stimulus-to-QRS interval of more than 40 ms [9, 10]. During the substrate mapping, pace mapping is performed at sites with abnormal electrograms or at the scar border to identify the exit. Occasionally, pace mapping deeper into the scar demonstrates a longer S-QRS interval with matched QRS and the isthmus can be tracked by the pace mapping. However, pace mapping often creates different QRS morphologies, even at the isthmus, due to the functional block. A functional response to pace mapping has been reported; pacing at a single site creates multiple QRS morphologies (multiple exit site) or induces VT by pacing. Pacing can propagate through the isthmus and may exit at different site, creating the different QRS morphology. If there is sufficiently slow conduction in the critical isthmus area, pace mapping itself can induce VT. Radiofrequency ablation targeting sites with these findings has been reported to be successful [11].

Pace match is usually evaluated by visually analyzing the 12-lead ECG. For a quantitative analysis, the Paso Module in the CARTO 3 system automatically compares

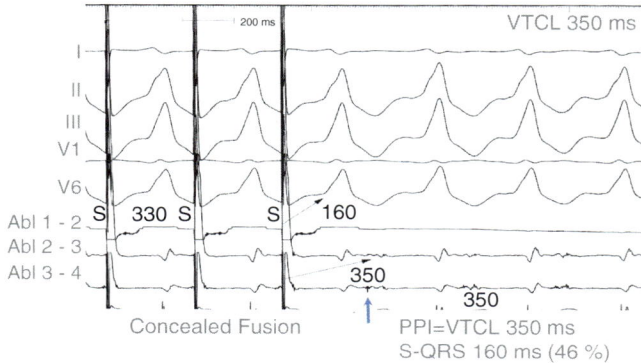

Fig. 36.2 At this site pacing was performed at 330 ms. PPI is same as VTCL and S-QRS is 46% of the VTCL. The site was at the central portion of the isthmus

Fig. 36.3 Exit determines QRS morphology. For focal VT, the QRS morphology is its origin. For reentrant VT, QRS suggests the location of the exit. As the activation goes in between the scar, QRS is not formed. Once the activation comes out of the circuit at the exit, QRS is formed. To identify the exit site of the reentrant circuit, 12-lead EKG is very important. You can decide where to map before you start the ablation. If V1 is LBBB, the exit is either in the RV or on the septum. If II, III, aVF shows inferior axis, the exit is located superior, or superior axis, it is located in the inferior wall. Also precordial leads tell you the basal or apical origin of VT

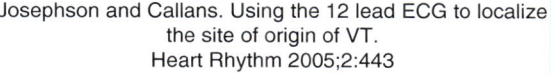

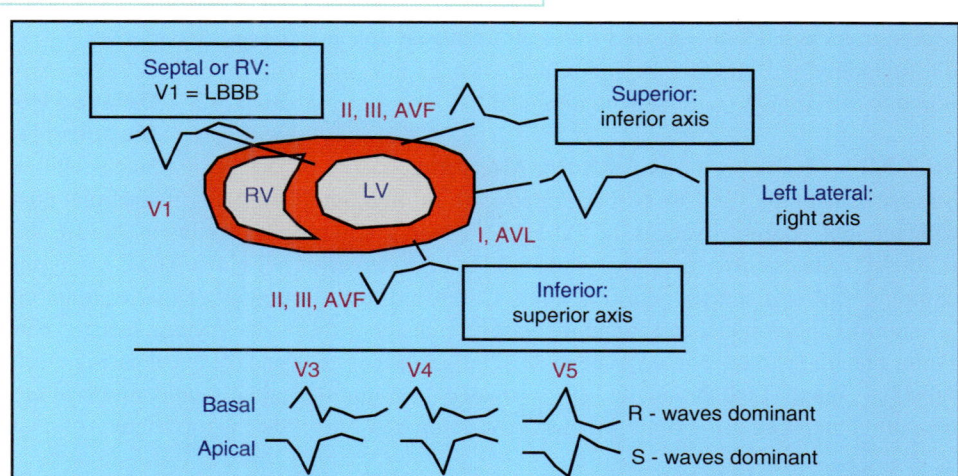

12 ECG signals of paced beats with targeted PVC/VT ECG signals, calculating the correlation values, and generates a good pace match tag when the value meets the correlation threshold. The default correlation threshold to discriminate matched from unmatched is 0.80, but it can be customized.

36.3.3 Substrate Mapping

Substrate-based ablation strategies have become the mainstay for VT associated with structural heart disease. The relationship between the VT substrate and an abnormal electrogram has been studied extensively in the past, using animal models as well as surgically resected myocardium. The amplitude of the local electrogram reflects the number of surviving myocardial bundles, and the fractionation reflects the slow propagation of an impulse through the region. Miller et al. evaluated the results of subendocardial resection: the origin of the VT was mapped and large regions with abnormal electrograms—such as late, split, and fractionated potentials—were found during sinus rhythm; these became mid-diastolic potentials during VT. By subendocardial resection, these potentials were eradicated and the VT became non-inducible. These findings suggest that subendocardial resection removes the critical areas of slow conduction that constitute the reentry circuit [12]. Linear lesions guided by pace mapping may interrupt the potential for reentry, in a similar way to subendocardial resection.

3D-EAM systems are used for substrate mapping. Usually, 1.5 mV is used as the cutoff for normal myocardium on the bipolar voltage map.

36.3.3.1 Unipolar Voltage Map for Deeper Myocardial Information

Unipolar electrogram recording has a large field of view compared to bipolar recording. It has been reported to provide valuable clues suggesting the presence of an epicardial or intramyocardial substrate and the need to pursue epicardial mapping and ablation [13]. A cutoff of 8.27 mV was found to differentiate normal from infarcted tissue.

36.3.3.2 Multielectrode Catheter Mapping

Substrate mapping used to be performed with an ablation catheter, but recent advances in 3D-EAM systems allow multielectrode catheter mapping, which yields high-density mapping during a shorter period of time. Compared to the 3.5-mm tip ablation catheter, a multielectrode catheter with 1-mm electrodes can provide a more detailed and accurate substrate map. Tschabrunn et al. evaluated the high-resolution mapping using both catheters, and compared substrate maps with pathological specimens and CMR findings [14]. As a larger electrode has a larger field of view, the electrogram is influenced by the nearby tissue: a thin layer of surviving subendocardial tissue and a thicker layer of scar, resulting in a low bipolar voltage. Therefore, surviving myocardium can be overlooked by the 3.5-mm tip catheter substrate map.

Many studies have evaluated methods for identifying the isthmus of the reentrant circuit by substrate mapping.

36.3.4 Identification of the Isthmus

36.3.4.1 Electrically Unexcitable Scar Mapping [15]

The borders of the reentrant circuit isthmus are defined by conduction block, functional or fixed. Pace mapping using a high stimulus strength (10 mA, 2 ms pulse width) identified the dense electrically unexcitable scars (EUS), and circuit isthmuses were identified adjacent to the EUS. Radiofrequency (RF) ablation lines between the EUS, or from the EUS to anatomical boundaries, successfully eliminated VTs. This method is usually useful for patients with transmural ischemic scar.

36.3.4.2 Voltage Channel [16]

Optimal adjustment for the voltage definition of non-conducting scar was evaluated based on the hypothesis that conducting bundles have larger voltage amplitude compared to the non-conducting scar. A voltage limit of <0.2 mV for scar definition identified the conducting channels. Conducting channels were not found in 24% of patients; reasons for this could be: (1) the scar areas might have been too narrow to detect; (2) the boundaries of the isthmus could be functional block, not detected during right ventricular apical (RVA) pacing or sinus rhythm; or (3) the dispersion of voltage in some scar areas may appear only during the VT rate. The electrode size may determine the extension of the local recording area.

36.3.4.3 Delayed Isolated Potential Mapping [17]

Delayed isolated potentials are considered to reflect activity in surviving myocardial bundles that might serve as a reentrant circuit isthmus, but are also present at bystander sites for target VTs [18]. These are bystander myocardial bundles that do not constitute the reentrant circuit for targeted VT. Compared to sinus rhythm, isolated potentials were more frequently identified by apical pacing. Areas with isolated delayed components and a multicomponent electrogram were highly predictive of the central isthmus of reentrant circuits.

36.4 Catheter Ablation in ICMP-VTs

36.4.1 Different Ablation Approaches in ICM-Related VTs

Various substrate-based approaches for targeting unmappable VT have been reported (Table 36.1). Recently, more extensive ablation to target all potential VT substrates has been reported. Practically, most approaches share similar general principles for identifying areas of interest, such as low voltage and late potentials (LPs).

36.4.2 Ablation for Mappable VTs

36.4.2.1 Conventional Mapping Techniques
For hemodynamically stable VT, activation and entrainment mapping can be fully performed. 3D EAM yields a visualization of the circuit by color-coded activation timing, and a critical isthmus can be identified. When the endocardial activation timing covers >90% of the VTCL, the activation map usually depicts a single- or dual-loop reentrant circuit around a scar area, a line of block, or an anatomical structure such as the mitral annulus [19]. However, if the endocardial activation map covers only a part of the VTCL, a review must be performed to check the correct annotation of the local electrogram. If all sites are found to have been correctly annotated, the circuit could be a micro-reentry, or may involve the mid-myocardium, epicardium, or the opposite chamber, which cannot be mapped from the endocardium of the mapped chamber.

The response to entrainment pacing demonstrates the relationship of the individual site to the reentrant circuit [20]. Pace mapping is also used to identify the VT isthmus exit. A recent report showed that the best pace match was at the exit and the worst at the entrance of the isthmus, showing the usefulness of pace mapping in identifying an appropriate ablation site [21]. Since these mapping techniques target an exact site that will interrupt the VT circuit, a single RF energy application, or a small number of them, can normally terminate the VT.

36.4.2.2 VT Isthmus Ablation After Termination
Successful VT termination during RF energy application, however, is not sufficient to prevent recurrence; therefore, a transection of the critical isthmus is usually necessary. For instance, ablation of a perimitral VT following inferior myocardial infarction requires conduction block through the isthmus between the mitral annulus and the inferior scar, which could be confirmed by a multielectrode catheter in the coronary sinus [22]. If the isthmus lacks an anatomical boundary, isthmus transection is more challenging, as the identified scar area may be functional. The size of the reentrant circuit isthmus can vary depending on the size of the mapping catheter electrode: 31 ± 7 mm long and 16 ± 8 mm wide by conventional mapping using an ablation catheter [19], but 15 mm long and 7 mm wide according to a novel ultra-high-resolution mapping system (Rhythmia, Boston Scientific) [14]. Substrates identified with a larger tip ablation catheter and a 1-mm electrode showed different sizes and characteristics. These findings suggest that the lower-resolution mapping could over- and/or underestimate the size of the isthmus.

36.4.3 Substrate-Based Ablation

36.4.3.1 Ablation Guided by Voltage and Pace Mapping
Hemodynamic intolerance in the vast majority of ICMP-related VTs precludes activation mapping, and the aforementioned substrate-based approaches are usually chosen.

36.4.3.2 Ablation of Late Potentials and Local Abnormal Ventricular Activities
LPs are a sensitive marker of a VT substrate and have been targeted for ablation. In the early days of substrate-based ablation, the target was limited to clinically relevant LPs [17, 23]. Recently, a more extensive approach targeting all LPs has been reported to be more effective [24, 25]. Jaïs et al. reported a similar approach that targeted local abnormal ventricular activities (LAVAs). They concluded that elimination of LAVAs was achieved in 70% of patients and was associated with a better long-term outcome [26]. They recently updated the result for 850 days follow-up as a VT recurrence rate of 36% [27].

Other groups reported the efficacy of ablation targeting earlier LPs, based on the hypothesis that there is an interconnection between the channel and later LPs that could be eliminated by ablation of the earlier LPs located at the entrance of the channel. Ablation targeting only the earlier LPs could sometimes complete "scar dechanneling" without the need for extensive ablation [28, 29].

36.4.3.3 Core Isolation
Areas of interest that are relevant to clinical and/or induced VTs within the low voltage zone (LVZ) could be identified by several techniques, including entrainment, voltage channels, LPs, or pace mapping. Tzou et al. reported a method that targeted these critical areas with contiguous lesions, aiming at electrical isolation of the region of interest [30].

Table 36.1 Procedure details and clinical outcomes in different substrate-based approaches for unstable VTs

Type of ablation/author (year)	Detail	ICMP patients/total number	Mapping catheter	Mapping points	Epicardial mapping	RF lesion (or time)	Procedural endpoint (% achieved)
Linear ablation							
Marchlinski (2000)	Linear ablation from scar to anatomical boundary/normal endocardium guided by PM	16–9	4-mm-tip	298 ± 72	No	59 ± 34	Non-inducibility (47%)
Soejima (2001)	Linear ablation parallel to scar border guided by PM/entrainment mapping	40/40	4- or 3.5-mm-tip	NR	No	21 ± 10	Non-inducibility (58%)
Channel ablation							
Arenal (2004)	Clinical VT related channel	26/26	4-mm-tip	142 ± 53	No	14 ± 8	Non-inducibility (96%)
Functional pacemap							
Tung (2012)	Sites with multiple exit sites/PM induction	26/44	NR	442(213–1604) (endo) 637(350–841) (epi)	Yes	4 ± 21 min	Non-inducibility (70%)
Late potential							
Arenal (2003)	LP related to target VT	21/24	4-mm-tip	111 ± 27	No	11 ± 8	Non-inducibility, VT related LP elimination (88%)
Volkmer (2006)	LP related to target VT	25/25	4- or 3.5-mm-tip	217 ± 87	No	14 ± 6	Non-inducibility, elimination of LPs (81%)
Vergara (2012)	All LP elimination	36/50	1.35- or 2-mm multielectrodes	407 ± 127(endo and epi)	Yes	NR	Elimination of LPs (84%)
Arenal (2013)	All LP elimination	59/59	4- or 3.5-mm-tip	NR	No	11 ± 5 min	Elimination of LPs (78%)
LAVA							
Jais (2012)	All LAVA abolishment	56/70	3.5- or 1-mm-tip multielectrodes	NR	Yes	23 ± 11 min	Elimination of LAVA (70%)
Yamashita (2016)	All LAVA abolishment	125/125	3.5- or 1-mm-tip multielectrodes	370(228–747) (endo) 432(328–758) (epi)	Yes	32 (20–50) min	Elimination of LAVA (60%) and non-inducibility (83%)
Dechanneling							
Tung (2013)	Earliest LPs in the CCs	15/21	2-mm-tip multielectrode	641(417–833)	Yes	7(4–14)	LP change/elimination Non-inducibility (84%)
Berruezo (2015)	CCs based on timing of delayed EGM	75/101	NR	481 ± 187(endo), 486 ± 218(epi)	Yes	28 ± 16 min	Elimination of all CCs (84%)

Core isolation					
Tzou (2015)	Isolation of low voltage scar involving putative VT isthmuses	32/44	3.5-mm-tip	522 ± 317 (endo) 456 ± 499 (epi)	Yes	111 ± 91	Isolation with exit block (84%)
Scar homogenization					
Di Biase (2012)	Empirically extended throughout the entire scar	43/43	3.5-mm-tip	NR	Yes	74 ± 21 min	Non-inducibility, abnormal EGM elimination, (NR)
Di Biase (2015)	Empirically extended throughout the entire scar	58/58	3.5-mm-tip	NR	Yes	68 ± 21 min	Non-inducibility, abnormal EGM elimination

CC conduction channel, *EGM* electrogram, *ICMP* ischemic cardiomyopathy, *IQR* interquartile range, *LP* late potential, *NR* not reported, *PM* pace mapping, *VT* ventricular tachycardia

36.4.3.4 Scar Homogenization

Scar homogenization is an approach that targets all abnormal electrograms in the scar area defined by voltage mapping. Di Biase et al. first compared this approach with the conventional method, and found a lower VT recurrence rate in the scar homogenization group (19% vs. 47%, $p = 0.006$) [31]. More recently, the same group reported the results of a multicenter randomized study that compared the scar homogenization approach and ablation limited to clinical and mappable VTs, showing the superiority of scar homogenization in terms of VT recurrence and mortality at 12-month follow-up [32].

36.4.3.5 Limitations of Current Substrate-Based Ablation

Voltage-based isthmus detection has been considered as an established methodology, but high-resolution mapping systems have revealed that the boundaries forming the VT isthmus are not always present as a fixed line of block, but rather as a functional block. Given that the functional block depends on the heart rate, the coupling interval of the premature impulse, or the direction of wavefront propagation, the substrate-based technique could have significant limitations [23]. Furthermore, there are no established criteria to confirm complete block in the setting of linear ablation.

Another limitation is the sampling bias of LPs, LAVAs, and abnormal electrograms in the LVZ. It is so far unclear how detailed the mapping needs to be in order to record these signals adequately. Electrode size and interelectrode distance may affect the ability to record abnormal signals. In addition, elimination of all LPs or LAVAs could be difficult in proximity to anatomical structures such as coronary arteries and phrenic nerves, because of safety concerns. In addition, remapping is required to validate the ablation effect.

36.4.4 Comparison of Different Ablation Approaches and Post-ablation Prognostic Factors

36.4.4.1 Comparison of Different Ablation Approaches

Head-to-head comparisons of conventional vs. substrate-based or among substrate-based approaches are limited. Two reports on scar homogenization vs. ablation limited to clinical/mappable VTs showed that more extensive ablation resulted in a better outcome. However, it is unclear whether these "bystander areas" with abnormal signals could develop clinical VTs in the future or not.

36.4.4.2 Impact of Ablation Endpoint on Long-Term Prognosis

Non-inducibility has mostly been used to define the acute success of VT ablation. Recent studies evaluating the impact of non-inducibility on long-term outcomes showed that VT non-inducibility after ablation is an independent predictor of lower all-cause mortality and improved VT-free survival [33, 34]. However, the ablation strategy used in these studies was limited to clinically relevant substrates and extensive substrate modification was not performed. In the latter approaches, completion of substrate elimination, i.e., abolition of all LPs and LAVAs, is an independent predictor of better long-term outcomes, rather than VT non-inducibility.

36.4.4.3 Endocardial-Only vs. Endo-epicardial Ablation

The majority of ICMP-related VT reentrant circuits are endocardial, but 15% of inferior infarctions have an epicardial circuit [35]. However, a recent report demonstrated that a combination of endo- and epicardial ablation as first-line therapy led to a lower rate of VT recurrence as compared to endocardial-only ablation [36]. Acosta and coworkers demonstrated the usefulness of infarct transmurality detected by CMR for the selection of patients who require endo- and epicardial ablation. The presence of transmural infarction is associated with an increased risk of VT recurrence, which suggests that endocardial-only ablation in such patients might not be sufficient [6].

36.4.5 Clinical Considerations

36.4.5.1 Pre-procedural Planning

Preoperative procedural planning regarding the access and types of catheter is important for safe and successful VT ablation. For accessing the left ventricle, a retrograde and/or antegrade approach is used. Prior to the procedure, calcification of the aorta and aortic valve needs to be checked for. In cases with aortic calcification and aortic valve stenosis or calcification, an antegrade approach is preferred to avoid possible atherosclerotic embolism or valve damage. In elderly patients, the aorta frequently becomes tortuous and elongated, resulting in difficult catheter manipulation. A long (80 cm) metallic 8-Fr sheath (Superflex®, Arrow international Inc., PA, USA) is often useful for overcoming these problems. A long deflectable sheath is often used for the transseptal approach. For left ventricular mapping with a multielectrode or basket type catheter, a transseptal approach is preferable.

The diagnostic catheter is usually placed at the right ventricular apex and/or outflow tract for VT induction. When involvement of a bundle branch or fascicle is suspected, His-bundle electrogram recording is crucial. A multielectrode catheter in the coronary sinus provides important information, especially for a mitral isthmus VT; it may be used for the detection of epicardial involvement and confirmation of bidirectional block following the ablation. A 2-Fr electrode catheter in a branch of the coronary sinus, such as the anterior interventricular vein, also provides important information. Deep mid-myocardial data can be obtained using a non-coated coronary guidewire.

36.4.5.2 Intra- and Post-procedural Considerations

An open irrigated catheter is usually used for VT related to structural heart disease. The volume load needs to be carefully monitored, especially in patients with reduced cardiac function or during a lengthy procedure, and a diuretic should be given if necessary. From the safety point of view, a contact force sensing catheter might be better when targeting a left ventricle with an aneurysm.

References

1. de Bakker JM, van Capelle FJ, Janse MJ, Tasseron S, Vermeulen JT, de Jonge N, Lahpor JR. Slow conduction in the infarcted human heart. 'Zigzag' course of activation. Circulation. 1993;88:915–26.
2. Lopera G, Stevenson WG, Soejima K, Maisel WH, Koplan B, Sapp JL, Satti SD, Epstein LM. Identification and ablation of three types of ventricular tachycardia involving the His-Purkinje system in patients with heart disease. J Cardiovasc Electrophysiol. 2004;15:52–8. https://doi.org/10.1046/j.1540-8167.2004.03189.x.
3. Hayashi M, Kobayashi Y, Iwasaki YK, Morita N, Miyauchi Y, Kato T, Takano T. Novel mechanism of postinfarction ventricular tachycardia originating in surviving left posterior Purkinje fibers. Heart Rhythm. 2006;3:908–18. https://doi.org/10.1016/j.hrthm.2006.04.019.
4. Andreu D, Ortiz-Pérez JT, Boussy T, Fernández-Armenta J, de Caralt TM, Perea RJ, Prat-González S, Mont L, Brugada J, Berruezo A. Usefulness of contrast-enhanced cardiac magnetic resonance in identifying the ventricular arrhythmia substrate and the approach needed for ablation. Eur Heart J. 2014;35:1316–26. https://doi.org/10.1093/eurheartj/eht510.
5. Fernández-Armenta J, Berruezo A, Andreu D, et al. Three-dimensional architecture of scar and conducting channels based on high resolution ce-CMR: insights for ventricular tachycardia ablation. Circ Arrhythm Electrophysiol. 2013;6:528–37. https://doi.org/10.1161/CIRCEP.113.000264.
6. Acosta J, Fernández-Armenta J, Penela D, et al. Infarct transmurality as a criterion for first-line endo-epicardial substrate-guided ventricular tachycardia ablation in ischemic cardiomyopathy. Heart Rhythm. 2016;13:85–95. https://doi.org/10.1016/j.hrthm.2015.07.010.
7. Bala R, Ren JF, Hutchinson MD, et al. Assessing epicardial substrate using intracardiac echocardiography during VT ablation. Circ Arrhythm Electrophysiol. 2011;4:667–73. https://doi.org/10.1161/CIRCEP.111.963553.
8. Stevenson WG, Friedman PL, Sager PT, Saxon LA, Kocovic D, Harada T, Wiener I, Khan H. Exploring postinfarction reentrant ventricular tachycardia with entrainment mapping. J Am Coll Cardiol. 1997;29:1180–9.
9. Brunckhorst CB, Delacretaz E, Soejima K, Maisel WH, Friedman PL, Stevenson WG. Identification of the ventricular tachycardia isthmus after infarction by pace mapping. Circulation. 2004;110:652–9. https://doi.org/10.1161/01.CIR.0000138107.11518.AF.
10. Stevenson WG, Sager PT, Natterson PD, Saxon LA, Middlekauff HR, Wiener I. Relation of pace mapping QRS configuration and conduction delay to ventricular tachycardia reentry circuits in human infarct scars. J Am Coll Cardiol. 1995;26:481–8.
11. Tung R, Mathuria N, Michowitz Y, Yu R, Buch E, Bradfield J, Mandapati R, Wiener I, Boyle N, Shivkumar K. Functional pace-mapping responses for identification of targets for catheter ablation of scar-mediated ventricular tachycardia. Circ Arrhythm Electrophysiol. 2012;5:264–72. https://doi.org/10.1161/CIRCEP.111.967976.
12. Miller JM, Tyson GS, Hargrove WC III, Vassallo JA, Rosenthal ME, Josephson ME. Effect of subendocardial resection on sinus rhythm endocardial electrogram abnormalities. Circulation. 1995;91:2385–91.
13. Hutchinson MD, Gerstenfeld EP, Desjardins B, et al. Endocardial unipolar voltage mapping to detect epicardial ventricular tachycardia substrate in patients with nonischemic left ventricular cardiomyopathy. Circ Arrhythm Electrophysiol. 2011;4:49–55. https://doi.org/10.1161/CIRCEP.110.959957.
14. Anter E, Tschabrunn CM, Buxton AE, Josephson ME. High-resolution mapping of postinfarction reentrant ventricular tachycardia: electrophysiological characterization of the circuit. Circulation. 2016;134:314–27. https://doi.org/10.1161/CIRCULATIONAHA.116.021955.
15. Soejima K, Stevenson WG, Maisel WH, Sapp JL, Epstein LM. Electrically unexcitable scar mapping based on pacing threshold for identification of the reentry circuit isthmus: feasibility for guiding ventricular tachycardia ablation. Circulation. 2002;106:1678–83.
16. Arenal A, del Castillo S, Gonzalez-Torrecilla E, Atienza F, Ortiz M, Jimenez J, Puchol A, García J, Almendral J. Tachycardia-related channel in the scar tissue in patients with sustained monomorphic ventricular tachycardias: influence of the voltage scar definition. Circulation. 2004;110:2568–74. https://doi.org/10.1161/01.CIR.0000145544.35565.47.
17. Arenal A, Glez-Torrecilla E, Ortiz M, Villacastín J, Fdez-Portales J, Sousa E, del Castillo S, Perez de Isla L, Jimenez J, Almendral J. Ablation of electrograms with an isolated, delayed component as treatment of unmappable monomorphic ventricular tachycardias in patients with structural heart disease. J Am Coll Cardiol. 2003;41:81–92.
18. Harada T, Stevenson WG, Kocovic DZ, Friedman PL. Catheter ablation of ventricular tachycardia after myocardial infarction: relation of endocardial sinus rhythm late potentials to the reentry circuit. J Am Coll Cardiol. 1997;30:1015–23.
19. de Chillou C, Lacroix D, Klug D, Magnin-Poull I, Marquié C, Messier M, Andronache M, Kouakam C, Sadoul N, Chen J, Aliot E, Kacet S. Isthmus characteristics of reentrant ventricular tachycardia after myocardial infarction. Circulation. 2002;105:726–31.
20. Stevenson WG, Khan H, Sager P, Saxon LA, Middlekauff HR, Natterson PD, Wiener I. Identification of reentry circuit sites during catheter mapping and radiofrequency ablation of ventricular tachycardia late after myocardial infarction. Circulation. 1993;88:1647–70.
21. de Chillou C, Groben L, Magnin-Poull I, et al. Localizing the critical isthmus of postinfarct ventricular tachycardia: the value of pace-mapping during sinus rhythm. Heart Rhythm. 2014;11:175–81. https://doi.org/10.1016/j.hrthm.2013.10.042.
22. Hayashi M, Kobayashi Y, Miyauchi Y, Morita N, Iwasaki Y, Yashima M, Atarashi H, Takano T, Nitta T, Tanaka S. Analysis of posterior mitral annular activation during entrainment and catheter ablation of mitral isthmus ventricular tachycardia using a coronary sinus catheter. J Interv Card Electrophysiol. 2000;4:427–34.
23. Volkmer M, Ouyang F, Deger F, Ernst S, Goya M, Bänsch D, Berodt K, Kuck KH, Antz M. Substrate mapping vs. tachycardia mapping using CARTO in patients with coronary artery disease and ventricular tachycardia: impact on outcome of catheter ablation. Europace. 2006;8:968–76. https://doi.org/10.1093/europace/eul109.
24. Vergara P, Trevisi N, Ricco A, Petracca F, Baratto F, Cireddu M, Bisceglia C, Maccabelli G, Della Bella P. Late potentials

abolition as an additional technique for reduction of arrhythmia recurrence in scar related ventricular tachycardia ablation. J Cardiovasc Electrophysiol. 2012;23:621–7. https://doi.org/10.1111/j.1540-8167.2011.02246.x.
25. Arenal Á, Hernández J, Calvo D, et al. Safety, long-term results, and predictors of recurrence after complete endocardial ventricular tachycardia substrate ablation in patients with previous myocardial infarction. Am J Cardiol. 2013;111:499–505. https://doi.org/10.1016/j.amjcard.2012.10.031.
26. Jaïs P, Maury P, Khairy P, et al. Elimination of local abnormal ventricular activities: a new end point for substrate modification in patients with scar-related ventricular tachycardia. Circulation. 2012;125:2184–96. https://doi.org/10.1161/CIRCULATIONAHA.111.043216.
27. Yamashita S, Cochet H, Sacher F, et al. Impact of new technologies and approaches for post-myocardial infarction ventricular tachycardia ablation during long-term follow-up. Circ Arrhythm Electrophysiol. 2016;9:1–12. https://doi.org/10.1161/CIRCEP.116.003901.
28. Tung R, Mathuria NS, Nagel R, Mandapati R, Buch EF, Bradfield JS, Vaseghi M, Boyle NG, Shivkumar K. Impact of local ablation on interconnected channels within ventricular scar: mechanistic implications for substrate modification. Circ Arrhythm Electrophysiol. 2013;6:1131–8. https://doi.org/10.1161/CIRCEP.113.000867.
29. Berruezo A, Fernandez-Armenta J, Andreu D, et al. Scar dechanneling: new method for scar-related left ventricular tachycardia substrate ablation. Circ Arrhythm Electrophysiol. 2015;8:326–36. https://doi.org/10.1161/CIRCEP.114.002386.
30. Tzou WS, Frankel DS, Hegeman T, Supple GE, Garcia FC, Santangeli P, Katz DF, Sauer WH, Marchlinski FE. Core isolation of critical arrhythmia elements for treatment of multiple scar-based ventricular tachycardias. Circ Arrhythm Electrophysiol. 2015;8:353–61. https://doi.org/10.1161/CIRCEP.114.002310.
31. Di Biase L, Santangeli P, Burkhardt DJ, et al. Endo-epicardial homogenization of the scar versus limited substrate ablation for the treatment of electrical storms in patients with ischemic cardiomyopathy. J Am Coll Cardiol. 2012;60:132–41. https://doi.org/10.1016/j.jacc.2012.03.044.
32. Di Biase L, Burkhardt JD, Lakkireddy D, et al. Ablation of stable VTs versus substrate ablation in ischemic cardiomyopathy: the VISTA randomized multicenter trial. J Am Coll Cardiol. 2015;66:2872–82. https://doi.org/10.1016/j.jacc.2015.10.026.
33. Yokokawa M, Kim HM, Baser K, et al. Predictive value of programmed ventricular stimulation after catheter ablation of post-infarction ventricular tachycardia. J Am Coll Cardiol. 2015;65:1954–9. https://doi.org/10.1016/j.jacc.2015.02.058.
34. de Riva M, Piers SR, Kapel GF, Watanabe M, Venlet J, Trines SA, Schalij MJ, Zeppenfeld K. Reassessing noninducibility as ablation endpoint of post-infarction ventricular tachycardia: the impact of left ventricular function. Circ Arrhythm Electrophysiol. 2015;8:853–62. https://doi.org/10.1161/CIRCEP.114.002702.
35. Svenson RH, Littmann L, Gallagher JJ, Selle JG, Zimmern SH, Fedor JM, Colavita PG. Termination of ventricular tachycardia with epicardial laser photocoagulation: a clinical comparison with patients undergoing successful endocardial photocoagulation alone. J Am Coll Cardiol. 1990;15:163–70.
36. Izquierdo M, Sánchez-Gómez JM, Ferrero de Loma-Osorio A, Martínez A, Bellver A, Peláez A, Núñez J, Núñez C, Chorro J, Ruiz-Granell R. Endo-epicardial versus only-endocardial ablation as a first line strategy for the treatment of ventricular tachycardia in patients with ischemic heart disease. Circ Arrhythm Electrophysiol. 2015;8:882–9. https://doi.org/10.1161/CIRCEP.115.002827.

Ablation of Brugada Syndrome

Yasuya Inden

Keywords

Brugada syndrome · Depolarization · Repolarization · Ventricular fibrillation · Ventricular premature beat · Epicardial approach · Substrate ablation

37.1 Introduction

Brugada syndrome is a hereditary arrhythmia with characteristic electrocardiographic findings and is associated with lethal arrhythmias. An ion channel abnormality induces an action potential difference/potential gradient between the endocardium and epicardium, which causes ST elevation and a negative T wave, and is thought to induce ventricular fibrillation (VF) [1]. However, the prevention of VF is difficult with medical therapy, and the treatment of ventricular fibrillation has been entrusted to an implantable cardioverter defibrillator (ICD). Meanwhile, some reports of ablation for Brugada syndrome have been published. Haissaguerre et al. reported that the ventricular premature beat (VPB) that triggers VF in the right ventricular outflow tract (RVOT) was identified, and was terminated by ablation, thereby preventing VF attacks [2]. Nademanee et al. reported that application of radiofrequency (RF) energy over the RVOT epicardium resulted in a normalized electrocardiogram (ECG) and inability to induce VF [3]. Abnormal potentials are detected over the RVOT epicardium in Brugada syndrome patients, but it is unclear whether the potentials are due to a depolarization or repolarization abnormality. However, we have been able to advance the management of Brugada syndrome with epicardial substrate ablation. In this chapter, I described the method of ablation for Brugada syndrome and the characteristic potentials recorded over the epicardium of the RVOT in Brugada patients.

Y. Inden
Department of Cardiology, Nagoya University Graduate School of Medicine, 65 Tsurumaicho, Showaku, Nagoya 466-8550, Japan
e-mail: inden@med.nagoya-u.ac.jp

37.2 The Targets for Brugada Syndrome Ablation

The typical ECG in Brugada syndrome has an incomplete right bundle branch block pattern QRS complex or a coved wave with ST elevation in the right precordial V1–3 leads [4]. It is extremely similar to the findings observed when the right coronary artery conus branch is occluded with a catheter; therefore, the substrate of Brugada syndrome may be present in the RVOT myocardium. Most patients with Brugada syndrome are in sinus rhythm in the outpatient clinic, but sometimes experience VPBs as a warning of a VF attack; these VPBs become a trigger, and VF is induced. Thus, two targets of ablation for Brugada syndrome have been proposed: the trigger VPB and the RVOT myocardium, which is believed to be a substrate.

37.3 Ablation of the VPB That Triggers VF

In 2003, Haissaguerre et al. reported that they performed ablation using an endocardial approach to the VPB that triggered VF in three patients with Brugada syndrome, and were able to inhibit VF [2]. The origins of the VPB were in the RVOT in two cases and the right ventricular Purkinje network in one case. The application times were very long (7–10 min), and might have modified the substrate of the VF. Nakagawa et al. also reported ablation of VPBs originating in the lateral free wall of the RVOT to prevent VF storm in a Brugada syndrome patient [5]. If unifocal VPBs are frequent, ablation targeting the trigger VPB is possible, and is useful for suppression of VF. When VPBs fail to develop during an ablation session, an effective VPB induction method will be necessary, or ablation must be performed while frequent VPBs are present. However, VF can still be induced if VPBs from another origin develop after ablation of the target trigger VPB. The approach to the target is simple and easy in VPB ablation, and VF attacks can be inhibited with a high success rate if the trigger is ablated.

37.4 Ablation of the Epicardial Myocardium in the RVOT Substrate of Brugada Syndrome

In 2011, Nademanee et al. reported ablation for Brugada syndrome. Abnormal potentials were observed over a wide area of the epicardium of the RVOT, and RF energy was delivered to this area to ablate all these potentials, with good effect [3]. They achieved ECG normalization in eight of nine patients, and had VF attack in one patient after ablation.

We also performed ablation in nine Brugada syndrome patients in the past 4 years (Fig. 37.1a). No abnormal potential was observed in the mapping of the endocardium of the right ventricle in most cases (Fig. 37.2a). Some cases showed a limited low-voltage area in the epicardium of the RVOT (Fig. 37.2b), but other cases showed no low-voltage areas. In all Brugada syndrome cases that we treated, the abnormal delayed potentials were detected over a wide range of the RVOT and right lateral ventricular wall (Fig. 37.3). The abnormal potentials had a fractionated, spiky, dull wave, or a split wave, and included a low-frequency component. The potential had an extremely long duration and extended beyond the QRS width to the onset of the T wave (Fig. 37.3). The ST segment was elevated and presented with a typical Brugada type ECG when we administered Ic antiarrhythmic drugs such as pilsicainide; moreover, the epicardial abnormal potential was extended even more, and the region where the abnormal potential was detected was enlarged. The delivery of RF energy targeted this abnormal potential (Fig. 37.4a–c), and the endpoint was ablation of all abnormal potentials in the right ventricular epicardium after infusion of an Ic drug. Potentials with prolonged continuation disappeared after RF application (Fig. 37.4d, e). Application regions were very wide (10.1–37.0 cm^2), and the total application time was 30–60 min. After RF application, a Brugada ECG pattern was not observed (Fig. 37.1b), and there were no further ST elevations with administration of an Ic drug. VF was induced in all nine cases before ablation, but could not be induced after ablation by the same protocol as before RF application in eight patients. The ECG was normalized in seven cases; we have followed all patients without medication, and eight have had no recurrence of VF. We were able to identify a wider arrhythmic substrate of Brugada syndrome

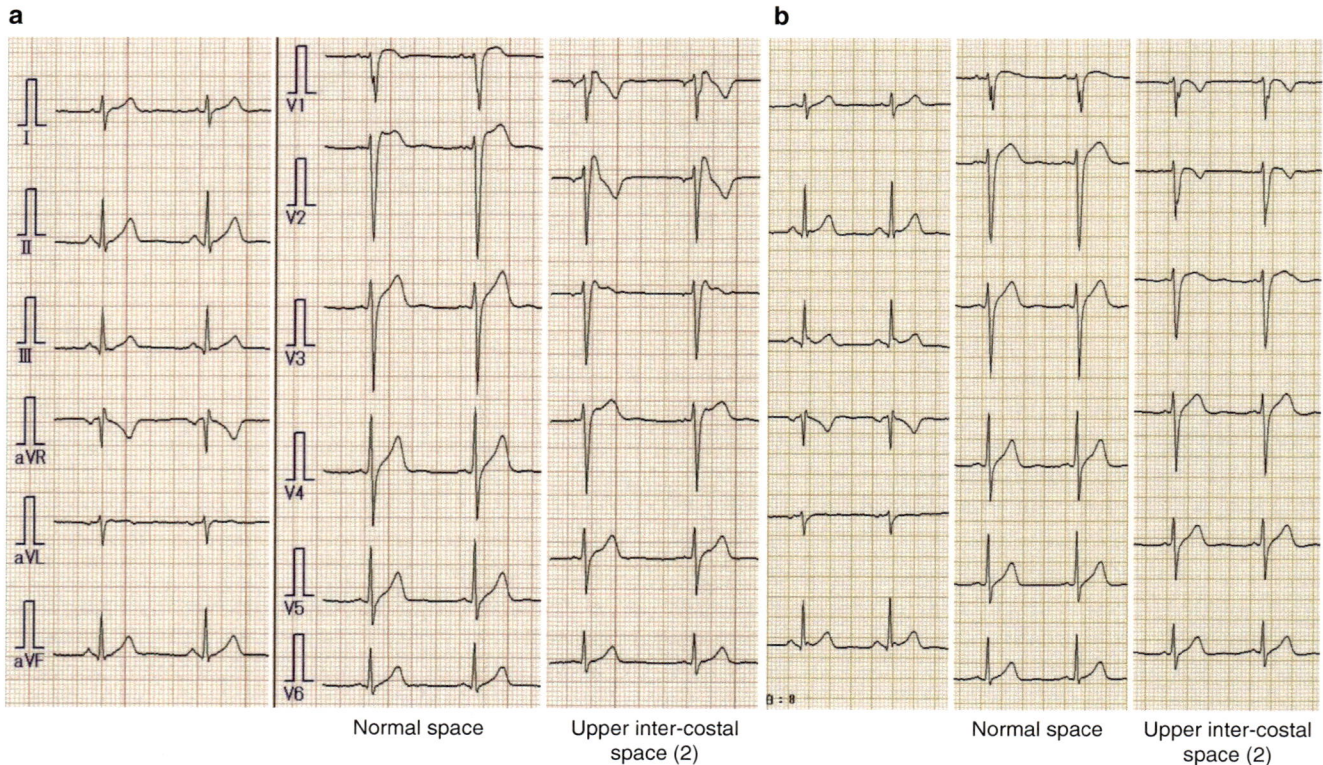

Fig. 37.1 Electrocardiogram (ECG) of a Brugada patient. Panel (**a**) showed ECG before ablation and Panel (**b**) showed ECG 1 year after ablation

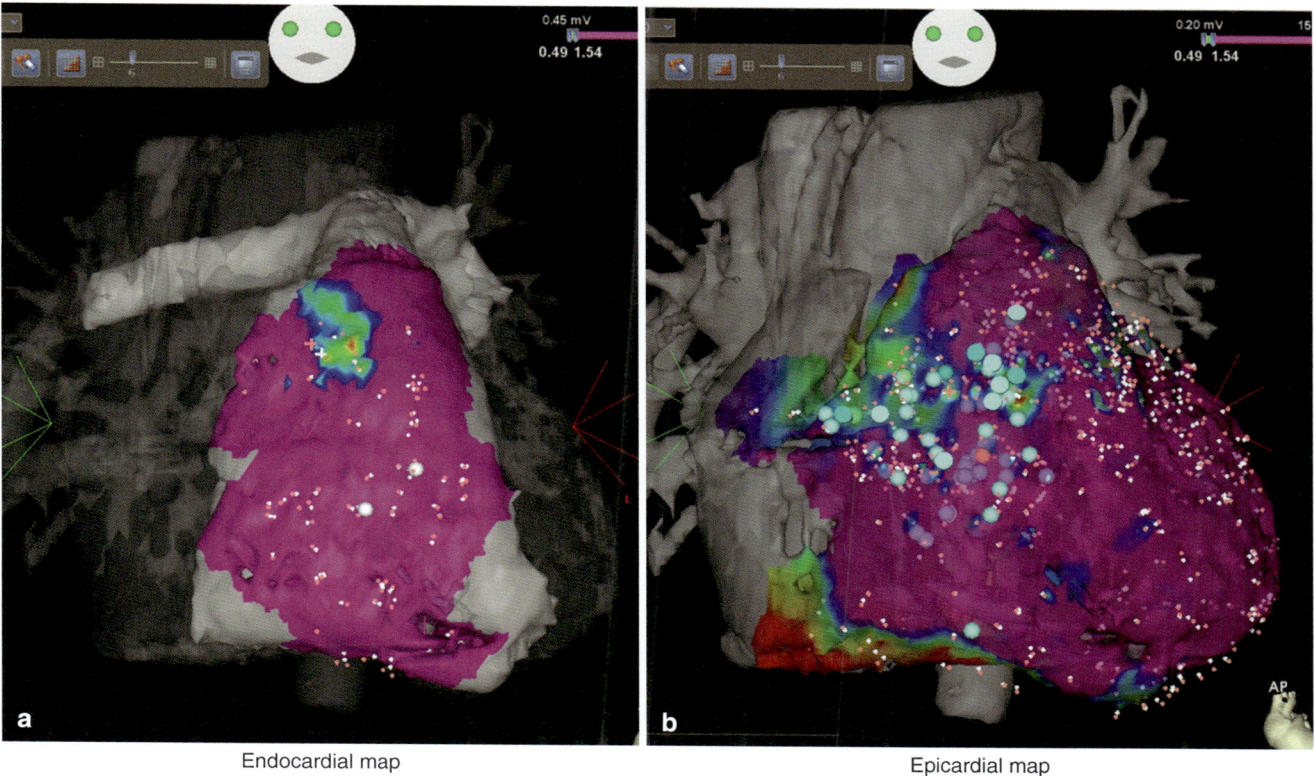

Fig. 37.2 Voltage map of a Brugada patient. Panel (**a**) showed a voltage map of the right ventricular endocardium and Panel (**b**) showed a voltage map of the right ventricular epicardium

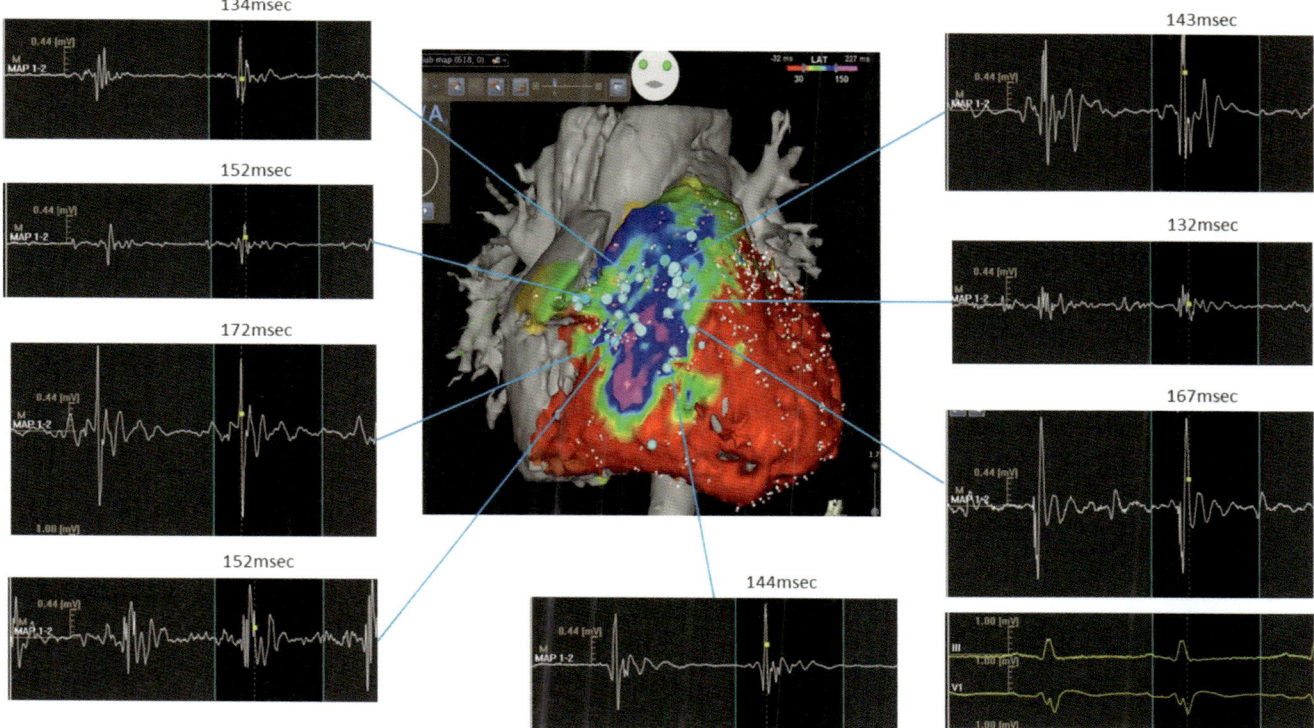

Fig. 37.3 Abnormal electrograms over the right ventricular epicardium

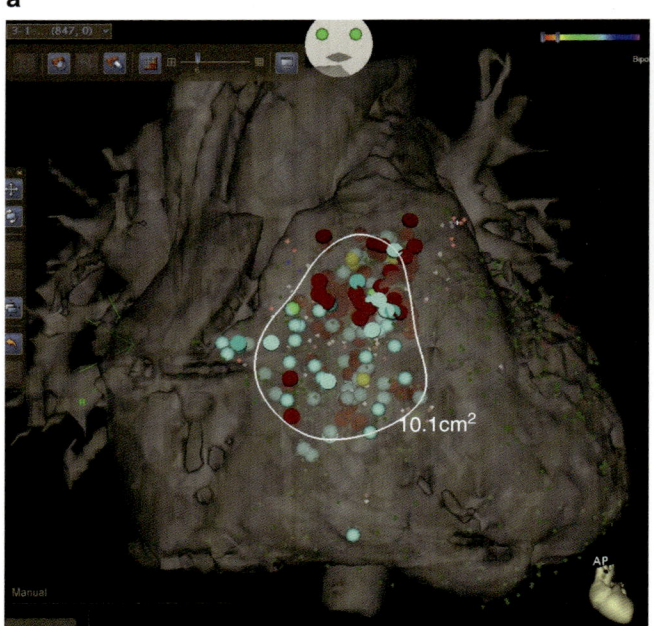

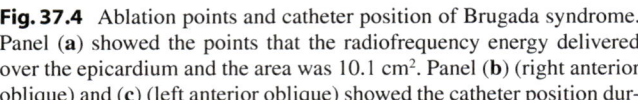

Fig. 37.4 Ablation points and catheter position of Brugada syndrome. Panel (**a**) showed the points that the radiofrequency energy delivered over the epicardium and the area was 10.1 cm². Panel (**b**) (right anterior oblique) and (**c**) (left anterior oblique) showed the catheter position during ablation procedure in the epicardium. Panel (**d**) was the electrogram before radiofrequency energy application, and the delayed potential disappeared after application (Panel **e**)

with administration of an Ic antiarrhythmic drug and could deliver RF energy to the entire abnormal area. As a result, the ST segment of the Brugada ECG normalized; we speculated that the epicardium of the RVOT was the region responsible for ST elevation and was associated with development and maintenance of VF.

After the report of Nademanee et al., other publications also showed the efficacy of epicardial ablation for Brugada syndrome. Brugada et al. reported 14 cases of Brugada ablation [6]. They used flecainide in all cases before RF application, and low-voltage areas over the epicardium in the RVOT broadened, with even more prolonged potentials. After ablation, no patients developed VF during a 5-month follow-up. Zhang et al. reported 11 cases of epicardial ablation, and eight had no recurrence of VF [7]. However, one patient without an ICD had cardiac sudden death. Therefore, an ICD is necessary after substrate ablation for Brugada syndrome, even though ablation is very effective.

37.5 Substrate Ablation of the RVOT by an Endocardial Approach

Epicardial ablation of the RVOT has been effective in Brugada syndrome patients, but there have also been reports of an endocardial approach. Shah et al. reported in 2011 that RF energy was delivered from the endocardial side around two origins of the VPB for 56 min in total; the VPB disappeared and the ECG also normalized [8]. The origin of the VPB was in the free wall of the RVOT and the development of VPB may have been associated with the substrate of the Brugada syndrome. Sunsaneewitayakul et al. reported RF energy was delivered to the delayed conduction region in the right ventricle using a noncontact mapping system in four Brugada syndrome patients with VF storm, and three showed normalization of the ECG [9]. However, abnormal potentials detected in the epicardium were not found in the endocardium; therefore, the identification of the application sites may be difficult with the endocardial approach. If we can identify an arrhythmic substrate from the endocardial side, we might be able to deliver RF energy deeply to the epicardial surface from the endocardial side.

37.6 Is the Abnormally Delayed Potential Caused by Delayed Conduction or a Repolarization Abnormality?

The abnormal electrogram recorded over the epicardium of the right ventricle shows fractionated delay potentials, and these potentials usually show delayed conduction. However, the potential often presented with a dull, low-frequency wave as well as with spiky, high-frequency waves. Sometimes, a split potential is observed. Moreover, we experienced some

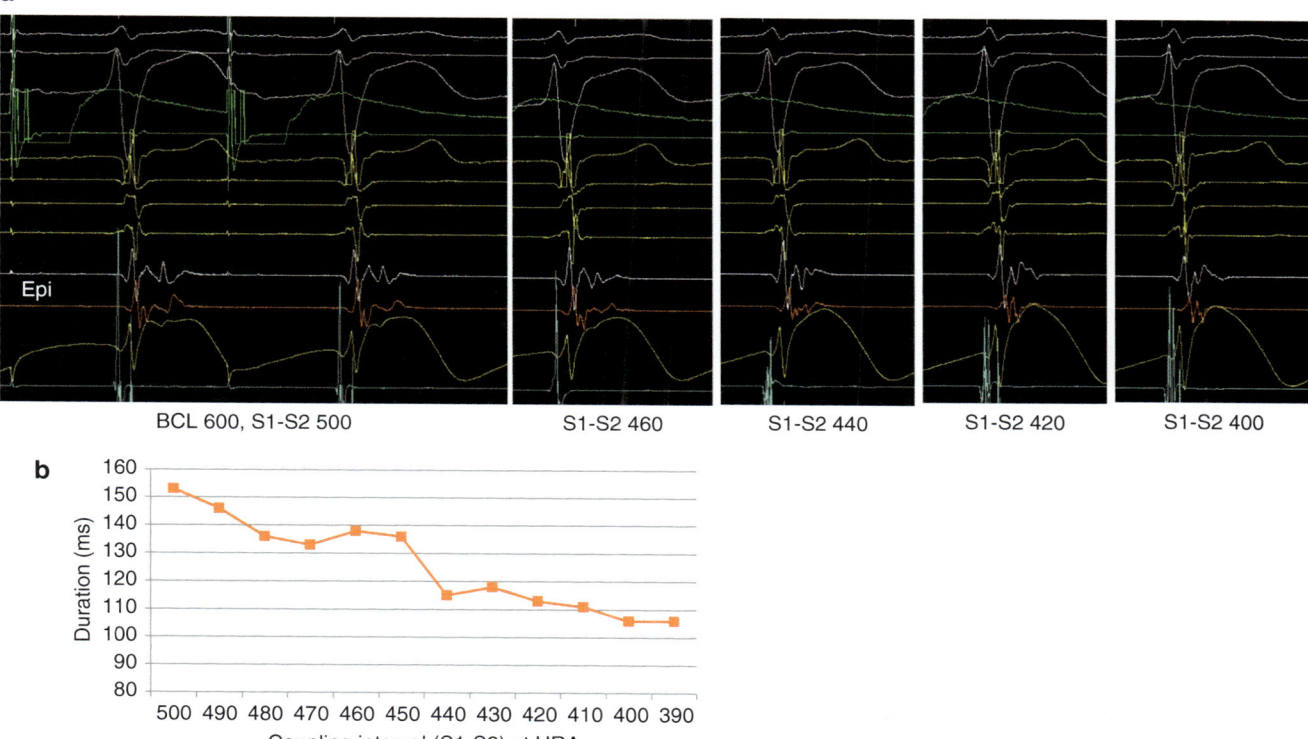

Fig. 37.5 The changes of the right ventricular epicardial potentials by extra stimulation from right atrium. Panel (**a**) showed the epicardial electrograms during stimulation. At the basic cycle length (BCL) of 600 ms, the potential was split, and the interval of the split potential shortened at S1–S2 interval of 500 ms. The duration of the delayed potential shortened gradually according to the shorter coupling interval. Panel (**b**) showed the relationship between the S1–S2 interval and the duration of the epicardial potential

cases in which the abnormal potential duration shortened according to shorter cycle length stimulation (Fig. 37.5). Delayed conduction should have resulted in an abnormal potential extended by a shorter coupling interval stimulation; therefore, this phenomenon was different from normal delayed conduction, although it might represent conduction block. The mechanism of the dull potentials over the epicardium is also unknown. Antzelevitch et al. reported that in wedge models of Brugada syndrome, the deep notch and Phase 2 reentry in the action potential of the epicardium induced VPB and VF [1], and that the delayed potential was recorded on the epicardial electrogram at this time [10]. The typical ST elevation and coved type electrocardiogram of Brugada syndrome was explained by transmural dispersion between the right ventricular endocardium and epicardium.

Meanwhile, a delayed potential is usually detected in delayed conduction. The depolarization theory of Brugada syndrome relies on right ventricular conduction slowing and involvement of structural abnormalities [11]. Fatty degeneration and fibrosis in the epicardial myocardium has been detected in Brugada syndrome patients [12, 13]. Furthermore, there are many reports of late potentials in signal-averaged ECGs, and right ventricular malformations [14] suggest the presence of a depolarizing abnormality. Nademanee et al. showed an increase in epicardial and interstitial fibrosis and a reduced gap junction in the RVOT [15]. It seems reasonable that ablation of all abnormal potentials over the epicardial RVOT abolished the coved Brugada ECG.

The abnormal potentials recorded over the epicardium are more likely to reflect both abnormalities of depolarization and repolarization in the RVOT, and a careful interpretation will be necessary for understanding of the abnormal potential in Brugada syndrome.

37.7 Current Status of Ablation for Brugada Syndrome

Following ablation for Brugada syndrome, the recurrence of VF has been reported, although many reports have indicated ablation was effective and could prevent VF in short-term follow-up. The long-term results of ablation for Brugada syndrome are unknown. Brugada syndrome associated with early repolarization syndrome has been reported. Successful ablation in such cases is rare. Furthermore, by performing CARTO mapping of Brugada syndrome twice in a 2-year interval, expansion of the right ventricular low-voltage area was observed, with one case demonstrating progressive change [16]. The current goal of ablation for Brugada syndrome is to reduce the frequency of VF in cases with frequent attacks. Brugada syndrome is an inherited disease, so even if ablation is successful, ICD placement is strongly recommended. Investigation of long-term results after ablation of a lot of Brugada cases is necessary.

References

1. Yan GX, Antzelevitch C. Cellular basis for the Brugada syndrome and other mechanisms of arrhythmogenesis associated with ST-segment elevation. Circulation. 1999;100:1660–6.
2. Haissaguerre M, Extramiana F, Hocini M, Cauchemez B, Jais P, Cabrera JA, et al. Mapping and ablation of ventricular fibrillation associated with long-QT and Brugada syndromes. Circulation. 2003;108(8):925.
3. Nademanee K, Veerakul G, Chandanamattha P, Chaothawee L, Ariyachaipanich A, Jirasirirojanakorn K, et al. Prevention of ventricular fibrillation episodes in Brugada syndrome by catheter ablation over the anterior right ventricular outflow tract epicardium. Circulation. 2011;123:1270–9. https://doi.org/10.1161/CIRCULATIONAHA.110.972612.
4. Brugada P, Brugada J. Right bundle branch block, persistent ST segment elevation and sudden cardiac death: a distinct clinical and electrocardiographic syndrome. A multicenter report. J Am Coll Cardiol. 1992;20(6):1391.
5. Nakagawa E, Takagi M, Tatsumi H, Yoshiyama M. Successful radiofrequency catheter ablation for electrical storm of ventricular fibrillation in a patient with Brugada syndrome. Circ J. 2008;72:1025–9.
6. Brugada J, Pappone C, Berruezo A, Vicedomini G, Manguso F, Ciconte G, et al. Brugada syndrome phenotype elimination by epicardial substrate ablation. Circ Arrhythm Electrophysiol. 2015;8:1373–81. https://doi.org/10.1161/CIRCEP.115.003220.
7. Zhang P, Tung R, Zhang Z, Sheng X, Liu Q, Jiang R, et al. Characterization of the epicardial substrate for catheter ablation of Brugada syndrome. Heart Rhythm. 2016;13:2151–8. https://doi.org/10.1016/j.hrthm.2016.07.025.
8. Shah AJ, Hocini M, Lamaison D, Sacher F, Derval N, Haissaguerre M. Regional substrate ablation abolishes Brugada syndrome. J Cardiovasc Electrophysiol. 2011;22:1290–1. https://doi.org/10.1111/j.1540-8167.2011.02054.x.
9. Sunsaneewitayakul B, Yao Y, Thamaree S, Zhang S. Endocardial mapping and catheter ablation for ventricular fibrillation prevention in Brugada syndrome. J Cardiovasc Electrophysiol. 2012;23:S10–6. https://doi.org/10.1111/j.1540-8167.2012.02433.x.
10. Szél T, Antzelevitch C. Abnormal repolarization as the basis for late potentials and fractionated electrograms recorded from epicardium in experimental models of Brugada syndrome. J Am Coll Cardiol. 2014;63:2037–45. https://doi.org/10.1016/j.jacc.2014.01.067.
11. Meregalli PG, Wilde AA, Tan HL. Pathophysiological mechanisms of Brugada syndrome: depolarization disorder, repolarization disorder, or more? Cardiovasc Res. 2005;67:367–78.
12. Tada H, Aihara N, Ohe T, Yutani C, Hamada S, Miyanuma H, et al. Arrhythmogenic right ventricular cardiomyopathy underlies syndrome of right bundle branch block, ST-segment elevation, and sudden death. Am J Cardiol. 1998;81:519–22.
13. Coronel R, Casini S, Koopmann TT, Wilms-Schopman FJ, Verkerk AO, de Groot JR, et al. Right ventricular fibrosis and conduction delay in a patient with clinical signs of Brugada syndrome: a combined electrophysiological, genetic, histopathologic, and computational study. Circulation. 2005;112:2769–77.
14. Takagi M, Aihara N, Kuribayashi S, Taguchi A, Shimizu W, Kurita T, et al. Localized right ventricular morphological abnormalities detected by electron-beam computed tomography represent arrhythmogenic substrates in patients with the Brugada syndrome. Eur Heart J. 2001;22:1032–41.
15. Nademanee K, Raju H, de Noronha SV, Papadakis M, Robinson L, Rothery S, et al. Fibrosis, connexin-43, and conduction abnormalities in the Brugada syndrome. J Am Coll Cardiol. 2015;66:1976–86. https://doi.org/10.1016/j.jacc.2015.08.862.
16. Notarstefano P, Pieroni M, Guida R, Rio T, Oliva A, Grotti S, et al. Progression of electroanatomic substrate and electric storm recurrence in a patient with Brugada syndrome. Circulation. 2015;131:838–41. https://doi.org/10.1161/CIRCULATIONAHA.114.013773.

Ablation of Catecholaminergic Polymorphic Ventricular Tachycardia

Keita Masuda, Takashi Kaneshiro, and Kazutaka Aonuma

Keywords
Catecholaminergic polymorphic ventricular tachycardia • Bidirectional VT • Sudden cardiac death

38.1 Introduction

Catecholaminergic polymorphic ventricular tachycardia (CPVT) is a lethal arrhythmogenic disease characterized by adrenergic-induced polymorphic ventricular tachycardia (VT) leading to syncope or sudden cardiac death during exercise or emotional stress in individuals without organic heart disease [1]. The cause of CPVT is reported to be a genetic abnormality of intracellular calcium handling. There are several subtypes [2], and the most common type of CPVT is caused by a gene mutation in ryanodine receptor 2 (*RYR2*, 35–79% of all cases) [3] and in calsequestrin 2 (*CASQ2*, 3–5%) [4]. The prognosis of patients diagnosed as having CPVT is poor as the 10-year mortality rate is ~40% [2]. Therefore, the successful management of fatal arrhythmias that may result in sudden cardiac death is particularly important.

38.2 Characteristics of the ECG and Arrhythmias in CPVT

CPVT is known to be associated with various types of arrhythmias. An electrocardiogram (ECG) at rest exhibits normal sinus rhythm or sinus bradycardia and may be sporadically accompanied by sick sinus syndrome [5]. Emotional stress, exercise, or catecholamine administration increases the number of premature ventricular contractions (PVCs) and induces polymorphic PVCs, polymorphic VT, bidirectional VT, or ventricular fibrillation (VF) (Fig. 38.1). CPVT is caused by an abnormality of intracellular calcium handling, which results in delayed after depolarization (DAD) and subsequent ventricular arrhythmias. Bidirectional VT is the most characteristic arrhythmia of this disease, and the "pingpong" mechanism has been reported as the possible mechanism of bidirectional VT, in which if there are DAD-induced PVCs with a different threshold of occurrence in more than two different sites of the heart, the initial PVC induces another PVC, and they provoke each other and progress to VT [6]. Exercise-induced supraventricular arrhythmias including atrial fibrillation (AF), atrial tachycardia (AT), and atrial flutter are also common.

38.3 Diagnostic Criteria

The diagnostic criteria according to the HRS/EHRA/APHRS guidelines are shown in Table 38.1 [7]. The diagnosis of CPVT is considered definitive if one of criteria (1–3) is satisfied and as suspected if criterion (4) is satisfied.

38.4 Therapy of CPVT

The therapeutic management of CPVT is shown in Table 38.2 [7]. Initially, to suppress the occurrence of arrhythmias, exercise restriction and the administration of beta-blockers should be considered. If the disease activity cannot be

K. Masuda • T. Kaneshiro • K. Aonuma (✉)
Department of Cardiology, Faculty of Medicine, University of Tsukuba, 1-1-1 Tennodai, Tsukuba, Ibaraki 305-8575, Japan
e-mail: masuda-k@umin.ac.jp; tskyt_kaneshiro@yahoo.co.jp; kaonuma@md.tsukuba.ac.jp

Fig. 38.1 Various types of ventricular arrhythmias seen in a CPVT patient. (**a**) Polymorphic VT. (**b**) Bidirectional VT. (**c**) PVC and subsequent VF [2]

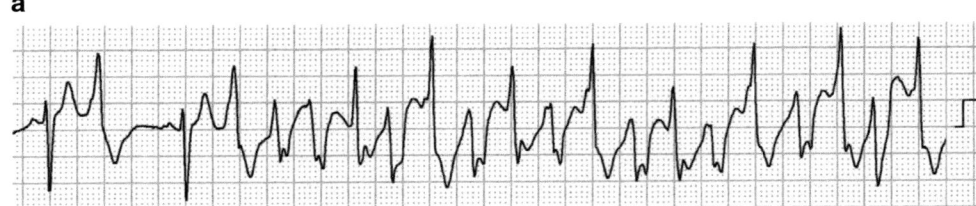

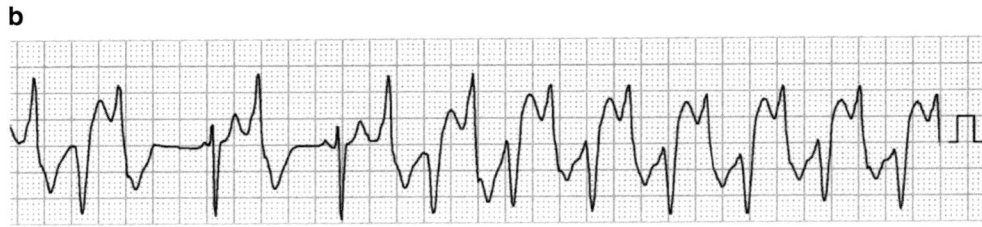

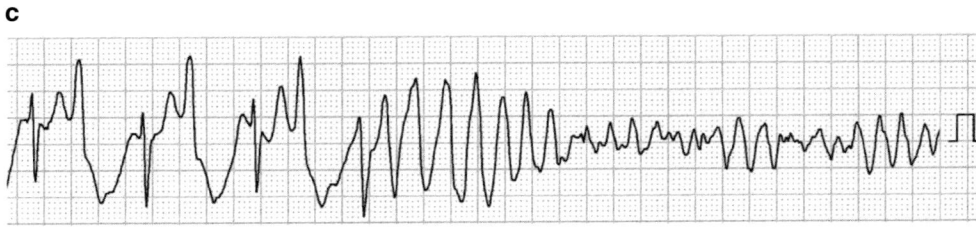

Table 38.1 Catecholaminergic polymorphic ventricular tachycardia (CPVT) expert consensus recommendations for CPVT diagnosis [7]

1. CPVT is diagnosed in the presence of a structurally normal heart, normal ECG, and unexplained exercise- or catecholamine-induced bidirectional VT or polymorphic PVCs or VT in an individual aged <40 years
2. CPVT is diagnosed in patients (index case or family member) who have a pathogenic mutation
3. CPVT is diagnosed in family members of a CPVT index case with a normal heart who exhibit exercise-induced PVCs or bidirectional/polymorphic VT
4. CPVT can be diagnosed in the presence of a structurally normal heart and coronary arteries, normal ECG, and unexplained exercise- or catecholamine-induced bidirectional VT or polymorphic PVCs or VT in an individual aged >40 years

Table 38.2 Expert consensus recommendations for CPVT therapeutic interventions [7]

Class I

1. The following lifestyle changes are recommended in all patients with a diagnosis of CPVT:
   (a) Limit/avoid competitive sports
   (b) Limit/avoid strenuous exercise
   (c) Limit exposure to stressful environments
2. Beta-blockers are recommended in all symptomatic patients with a diagnosis of CPVT
3. ICD implantation is recommended in patients with a diagnosis of CPVT who experience cardiac arrest, recurrent syncope, or polymorphic/bidirectional VT despite optimal medical management, and/or LCSD

Class IIa

4. Flecainide can be a useful addition to beta-blockers in patients with a diagnosis of CPVT who experience recurrent syncope or polymorphic/bidirectional VT while receiving beta-blockers
5. Beta-blockers can be useful in carriers of a pathogenic CPVT mutation without clinical manifestations of CPVT (concealed mutation-positive patients)

Class IIb

6. LCSD may be considered in patients with a diagnosis of CPVT who experience recurrent syncope or polymorphic/bidirectional VT/several appropriate ICD shocks while receiving beta-blockers and in patients who are intolerant to or have a contraindication to beta-blockers

Class III

7. ICD as a stand-alone therapy is not indicated in asymptomatic patients with a diagnosis of CPVT
8. Programmed electrical stimulation is not indicated in CPVT patients

controlled by these therapies alone, the addition of a calcium antagonist [8, 9], flecainide [10], or left cardiac sympathetic denervation (LCSD) [11] may be effective as the next step. The implantation of an implantable cardioverter defibrillator (ICD) is particularly important to avoid sudden cardiac death if the arrhythmic episodes persist despite medical therapy. However, delivery of a shock by an ICD, even when either appropriate or inappropriate, induces the release of endogenous catecholamine and may lead to an electrical storm of ventricular arrhythmias [12]. To avoid the delivery of an ICD shock as much as possible, catheter ablation has been proposed as an alternative method to the abovementioned treatment.

38.5 Ablation for CPVT

Although no large cohort studies investigating ablation for CPVT have been conducted to date, a few case studies have reported notable results [13–15]. The findings of these studies suggest that catheter ablation may be a useful therapeutic method for suppressing both ventricular and supraventricular arrhythmias in CPVT patients.

38.5.1 VT Ablation

Ablation for ventricular arrhythmias in patients with CPVT appears to be particularly difficult because the PVCs induced by catecholamine are multifocal. However, if the origin of the PVCs triggering polymorphic VT or VF can be precisely identified in the 12-channel ECG, catheter ablation may be feasible. Therefore, careful ECG monitoring is particularly important for the elimination of the arrhythmias. Notably, one case report described successful ablation for the suppression of ventricular arrhythmias in CPVT [13].

This case report describes a 38-year-old woman with recurrent episodes of syncope during exercise or emotionally exciting situations who had experienced VF induced by an exercise stress test and had been successfully resuscitated by electrical defibrillation. Her daughter had also exhibited the same syncopal episodes, and a detailed medical evaluation that included genetic testing revealed that she and her daughter had familial CPVT with a mutation in the *RyR2* gene. Administration of an intravenous infusion of epinephrine caused multifocal PVCs to develop that subsequently induced VF. Two types of PVCs, PVC1 and PVC2, which are shown in Fig. 38.2, accounted for a large portion of all PVCs and triggered the VF; therefore, catheter ablation was performed for these PVCs. The origin of the PVCs was identified by confirming the local bipolar and unipolar electrograms from the ablation catheter and comparing the PVC morphology with the QRS configuration obtained by pace mapping. The origin of PVC1 was located in the inferior left ventricular septum near the posterior papillary muscle (Fig. 38.3), where a perfect match of pace mapping was obtained and a Purkinje potential that preceded the onset of PVC1 by 18 ms was recorded. It was suggested that the Purkinje network may have an important role as an arrhythmic substrate in CPVT. PVC1 was successfully eliminated by radiofrequency energy application at this site. The successful site of PVC2 ablation was located in the left coronary cusp (Fig. 38.4), and PVC2 was eliminated in the same way as PVC1. Following ablation, an epinephrine infusion test revealed no recurrence of PVC1 or PVC2, and no VF was induced despite the observation of additional different PVCs.

In our institution, catheter ablation has been performed in 4 cases of CPVT so far, including the case described above (unpublished data). Although the ventricular arrhythmias in all cases were successfully suppressed in the acute phase, the long-term results were not favorable. Newly emerging arrhythmias were observed in all four cases despite the suppression of the arrhythmias targeted by catheter ablation. This result may imply that the arrhythmogenic substrate remained and that subsequent new arrhythmias can occur in CPVT. According to these data obtained at our institution, catheter ablation should be regarded not as a curative therapy but as an adjunctive therapy to rescue the patient from a fatal arrhythmia during the acute phase.

38.5.2 AF Ablation

The majority of inappropriate ICD shocks may be caused by atrial arrhythmias with rapid ventricular conduction [16]. Pizzale et al. reported a case of CPVT with paroxysmal AF, which led to polymorphic VT and an inappropriate ICD shock that resulted in sudden cardiac death [17]. Because ICD shock causes endogenous catecholamine secretion and a subsequent electrical storm, even an appropriate ICD shock

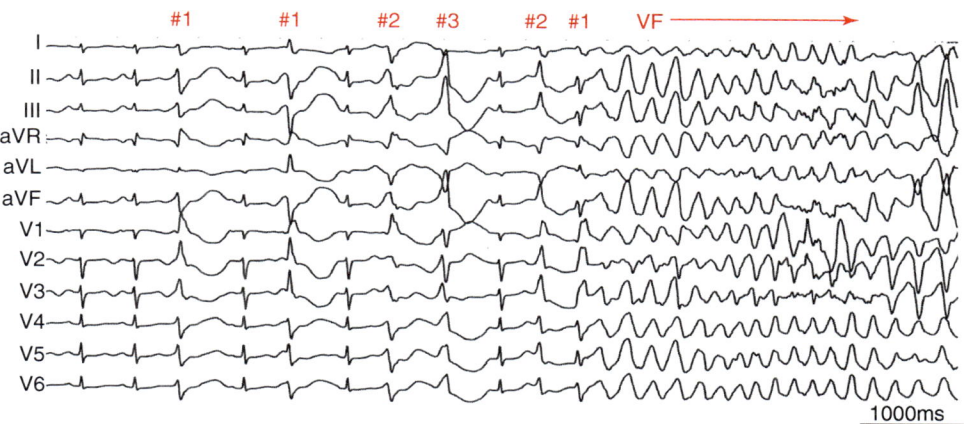

Fig. 38.2 Three types of PVC were seen in this patient. PVC1 (*#1*) and PVC2 (*#2*) accounted for the majority of all PVCs, and VF was triggered by PVC1 following PVC2 [13]

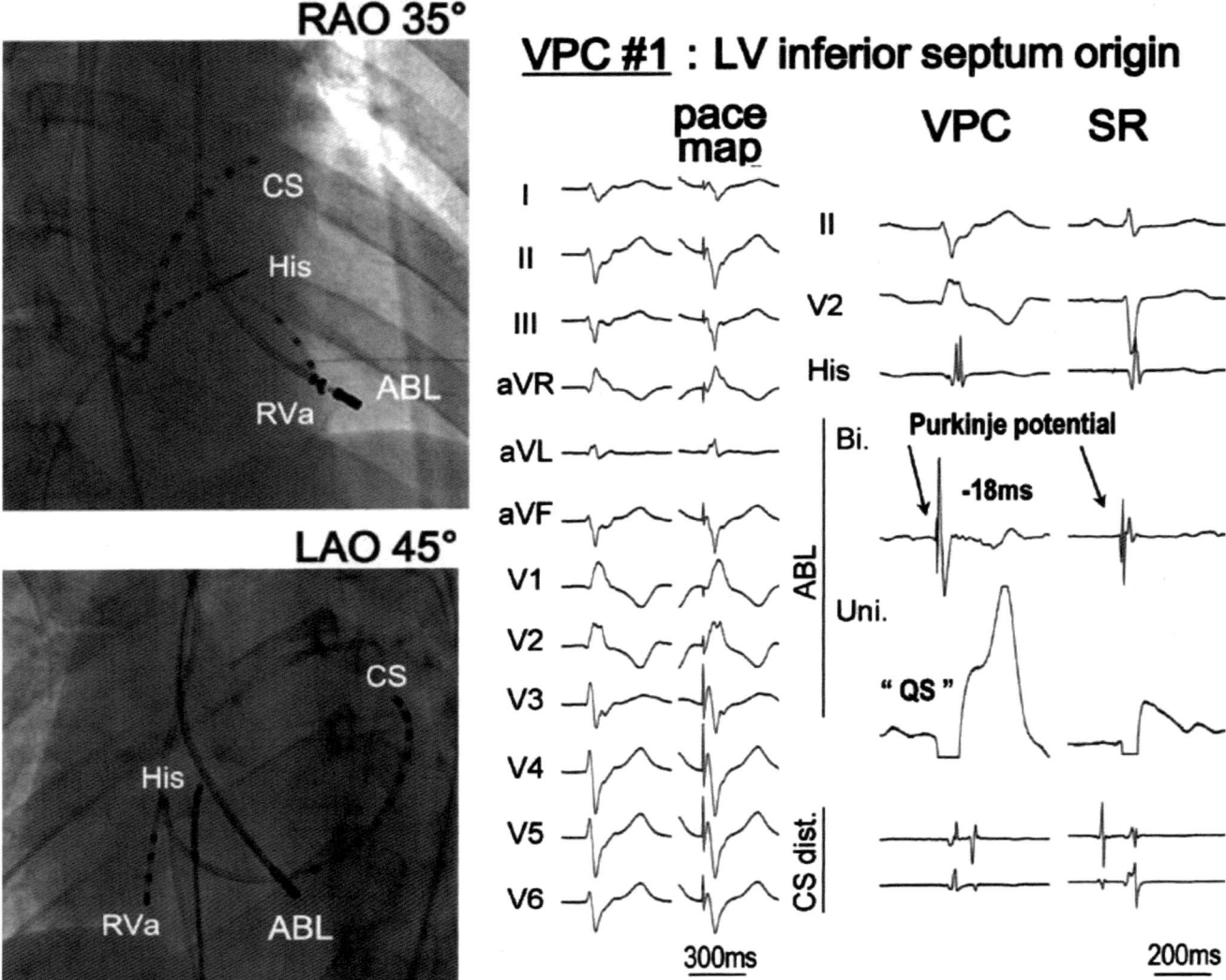

Fig. 38.3 Successful ablation site for PVC1. PVC1 was located in the inferior septum, as demonstrated by the fluoroscopic images. The pace map was consistent with the QRS morphology of this PVC, and bipolar and unipolar electrograms preceding the PVC by 18 ms were recorded. A Purkinje potential was also recorded [13]

can be one reason for sudden cardiac death [12]. Therefore, it is important that paroxysmal AF is managed to decrease the burden of ICD discharge and thus prevent sudden cardiac death in CPVT patients.

Two case reports show the successful treatment of paroxysmal AF accompanied by CPVT by catheter ablation. Catheter ablation for drug-refractory AF causing inappropriate ICD discharges may be an effective therapy in patients with CPVT.

The first case was that of an 18-year-old woman with CPVT who suffered from frequent inappropriate ICD shocks due to drug-refractory paroxysmal AF with a rapid ventricular response [14]. Although pulmonary vein isolation (PVI) was successfully performed that did not completely suppress the AF induced by isoproterenol at the end of this session, a decrease in the clinical events of AF and PVCs was achieved and resulted in the suppression of ICD shock delivery after this procedure. Wilde et al. reported that sympathetic denervation suppressed VT events by reducing the input for the internal release of catecholamine in CPVT patients [18], and this report demonstrated that PVI modified the cardiac sympathetic nerve activity because heart rate variability analysis

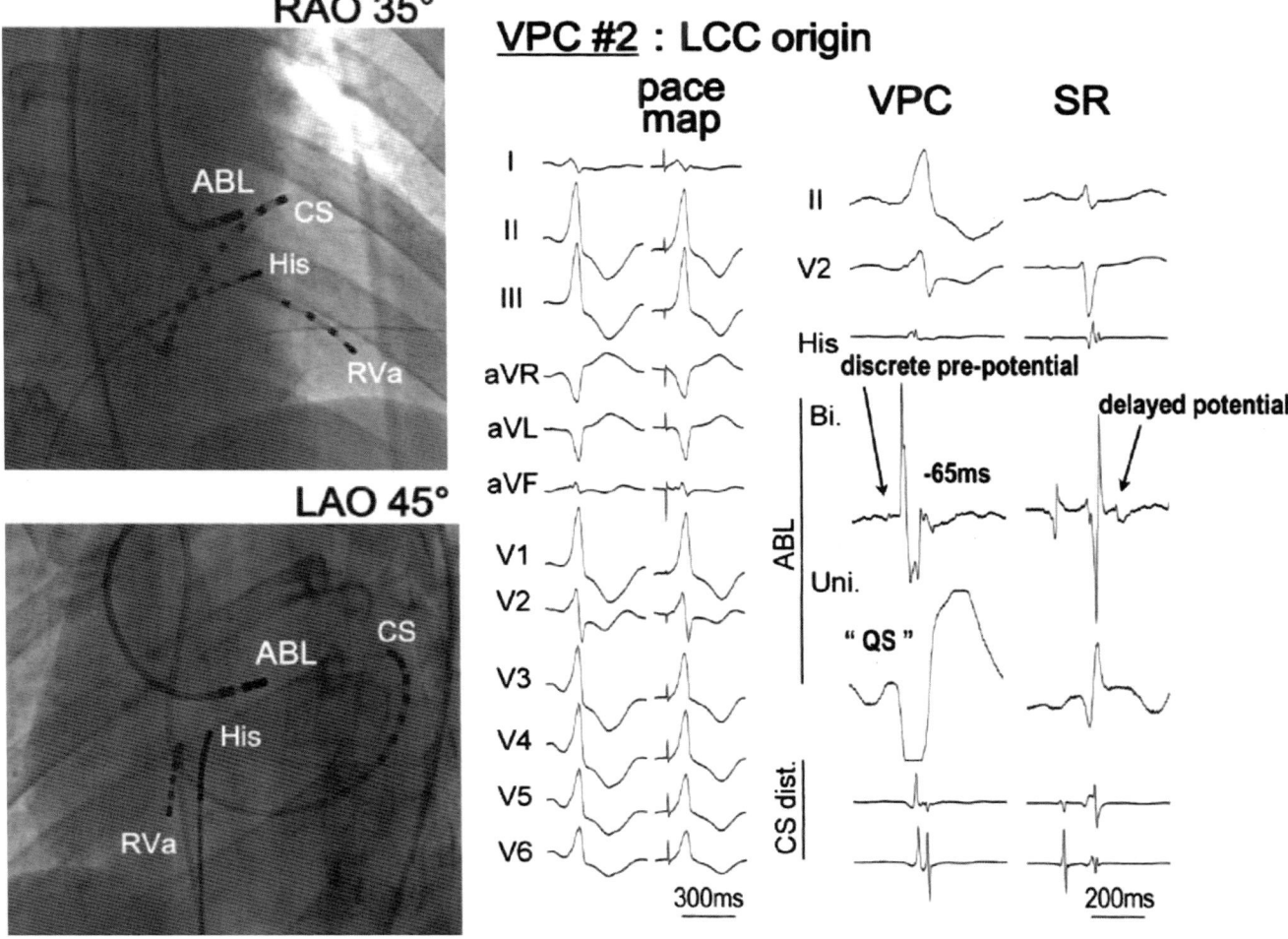

Fig. 38.4 Successful ablation site for PVC2. Fluoroscopic images show the origin of PVC2. A perfect pace map was obtained, and a discrete prepotential preceding the QRS complex by 65 ms was recorded in the bipolar electrogram [13]

during the 24-h Holter ECG showed a decrease in the high-frequency component and in the low-frequency/high-frequency ratio.

The second case, reported by Sugiyasu et al., involved a 13-year-old girl with exercise-induced multifocal ATs mimicking AF [15]. She underwent isolation of the PVs and focal ablation of the CS ostium that achieved complete elimination of AT/AF after the procedure. Although polymorphic VT was still induced by emotional stress or exercise, it was suppressed by the oral administration of atenolol.

There are some reports that ryanodine receptor dysfunction may have a role in the triggering and maintenance of AF in the PV or atrium [19, 20]. However, it remains unknown whether the arrhythmogenic substrates of AF in patients with CPVT originating from the pulmonary veins, or whether PVI alone is enough as an ablation strategy. Further investigations are required to elucidate the mechanism of AF in CPVT patients.

References

1. Leenhardt A, Lucet V, Denjoy I, Grau F, Ngoc DD, Coumel P. Catecholaminergic polymorphic ventricular tachycardia in children. A 7-year follow-up of 21 patients. Circulation. 1995;91:1512–9.
2. Sumitomo N. Current topics in catecholaminergic polymorphic ventricular tachycardia. J Arrhythm. 2016;32:344–51.
3. Priori SG, Napolitano C, Tiso N, Memmi M, Vignati G, Bloise R, Sorrentino V, Danieli GA. Mutations in the cardiac ryanodine receptor gene (hRyR2) underlie catecholaminergic polymorphic ventricular tachycardia. Circulation. 2001;103:196–200.
4. Lahat H, Eldar M, Levy-Nissenbaum E, Bahan T, Friedman E, Khoury A, Lorber A, Kastner DL, Goldman B, Pras E. Autosomal

recessive catecholamine- or exercise-induced polymorphic ventricular tachycardia: clinical features and assignment of the disease gene to chromosome 1p13–21. Circulation. 2001;103:2822–7.
5. Sumitomo N, Sakurada H, Taniguchi K, Matsumura M, Abe O, Miyashita M, Kanamaru H, Karasawa K, Ayusawa M, Fukamizu S, Nagaoka I, Horie M, Harada K, Hiraoka M. Association of atrial arrhythmia and sinus node dysfunction in patients with catecholaminergic polymorphic ventricular tachycardia. Circ J. 2007;71:1606–9.
6. Baher AA, Uy M, Xie F, Garfinkel A, Qu Z, Weiss JN. Bidirectional ventricular tachycardia: ping pong in the His-Purkinje system. Heart Rhythm. 2011;8:599–605.
7. Priori SG, Wilde AA, Horie M, Cho Y, Behr ER, Berul C, Blom N, Brugada J, Chiang CE, Huikuri H, Kannankeril P, Krahn A, Leenhardt A, Moss A, Schwartz PJ, Shimizu W, Tomaselli G, Tracy C. HRS/EHRA/APHRS expert consensus statement on the diagnosis and management of patients with inherited primary arrhythmia syndromes: document endorsed by HRS, EHRA, and APHRS in May 2013 and by ACCF, AHA, PACES, and AEPC in June 2013. Heart Rhythm. 2013;10:1932–63.
8. Swan H, Laitinen P, Kontula K, Toivonen L. Calcium channel antagonism reduces exercise-induced ventricular arrhythmias in catecholaminergic polymorphic ventricular tachycardia patients with RyR2 mutations. J Cardiovasc Electrophysiol. 2005;16:162–6.
9. Rosso R, Kalman JM, Rogowski O, Diamant S, Birger A, Biner S, Belhassen B, Viskin S. Calcium channel blockers and beta-blockers versus beta-blockers alone for preventing exercise-induced arrhythmias in catecholaminergic polymorphic ventricular tachycardia. Heart Rhythm. 2007;4:1149–54.
10. Watanabe H, van der Werf C, Roses-Noguer F, Adler A, Sumitomo N, Veltmann C, Rosso R, Bhuiyan ZA, Bikker H, Kannankeril PJ, Horie M, Minamino T, Viskin S, Knollmann BC, Till J, Wilde AA. Effects of flecainide on exercise-induced ventricular arrhythmias and recurrences in genotype-negative patients with catecholaminergic polymorphic ventricular tachycardia. Heart Rhythm. 2013;10:542–7.
11. De Ferrari GM, Dusi V, Spazzolini C, Bos JM, Abrams DJ, Berul CI, Crotti L, Davis AM, Eldar M, Kharlap M, Khoury A, Krahn AD, Leenhardt A, Moir CR, Odero A, Olde Nordkamp L, Paul T, Roses I Noguer F, Shkolnikova M, Till J, Wilde AA, Ackerman MJ, Schwartz PJ. Clinical management of catecholaminergic polymorphic ventricular tachycardia: the role of left cardiac sympathetic denervation. Circulation. 2015;131:2185–93.
12. Mohamed U, Gollob MH, Gow RM, Krahn AD. Sudden cardiac death despite an implantable cardioverter-defibrillator in a young female with catecholaminergic ventricular tachycardia. Heart Rhythm. 2006;3:1486–9.
13. Kaneshiro T, Naruse Y, Nogami A, Tada H, Yoshida K, Sekiguchi Y, Murakoshi N, Kato Y, Horigome H, Kawamura M, Horie M, Aonuma K. Successful catheter ablation of bidirectional ventricular premature contractions triggering ventricular fibrillation in catecholaminergic polymorphic ventricular tachycardia with RyR2 mutation. Circ Arrhythm Electrophysiol. 2012;5:e14–7.
14. Sumitomo N, Nakamura T, Fukuhara J, Nakai T, Watanabe I, Mugishima H, Hiraoka M. Clinical effectiveness of pulmonary vein isolation for arrhythmic events in a patient with catecholaminergic polymorphic ventricular tachycardia. Heart Vessel. 2010;25:448–52.
15. Sugiyasu A, Oginosawa Y, Nogami A, Hata Y. A case with catecholaminergic polymorphic ventricular tachycardia unmasked after successful ablation of atrial tachycardias from pulmonary veins. Pacing Clin Electrophysiol. 2009;32:e21–4.
16. Poole JE, Johnson GW, Hellkamp AS, Anderson J, Callans DJ, Raitt MH, Reddy RK, Marchlinski FE, Yee R, Guarnieri T, Talajic M, Wilber DJ, Fishbein DP, Packer DL, Mark DB, Lee KL, Bardy GH. Prognostic importance of defibrillator shocks in patients with heart failure. N Engl J Med. 2008;359:1009–17.
17. Pizzale S, Gollob MH, Gow R, Birnie DH. Sudden death in a young man with catecholaminergic polymorphic ventricular tachycardia and paroxysmal atrial fibrillation. J Cardiovasc Electrophysiol. 2008;19:1319–21.
18. Wilde AA, Bhuiyan ZA, Crotti L, Facchini M, De Ferrari GM, Paul T, Ferrandi C, Koolbergen DR, Odero A, Schwartz PJ. Left cardiac sympathetic denervation for catecholaminergic polymorphic ventricular tachycardia. N Engl J Med. 2008;358:2024–9.
19. Vest JA, Wehrens XH, Reiken SR, Lehnart SE, Dobrev D, Chandra P, Danilo P, Ravens U, Rosen MR, Marks AR. Defective cardiac ryanodine receptor regulation during atrial fibrillation. Circulation. 2005;111:2025–32.
20. Wongcharoen W, Chen YC, Chen YJ, Chen SY, Yeh HI, Lin CI, Chen SA. Aging increases pulmonary veins arrhythmogenesis and susceptibility to calcium regulation agents. Heart Rhythm. 2007;4:1338–49.

Epicardial Ablation for Ventricular Tachycardia

39

Shiro Nakahara

Keywords

Ventricular tachycardia · Catheter ablation · Epicardium

39.1 Introduction

The pericardial space has been historically viewed as a region accessed only in the clinical event of a hemodynamically significant effusion to treat tamponade or sample fluid for a therapeutic diagnosis. The pioneering work of Sosa and colleagues, first reported in 1996, opened up this new frontier to interventional cardiac electrophysiology and ablation [1]. The recent European Heart Rhythm Association/Heart Rhythm Society consensus document reported that an epicardial access is obtained in 17% of ventricular tachycardia (VT) ablation procedures, based on a survey of VT tertiary referral centers [2]. A recent multicenter study from referral centers found an overall epicardial access rate of 19% for patients undergoing VT ablation procedures [3]. This ranged from 6% in normal hearts, to 16% for ischemic cardiomyopathy, 35% for dilated cardiomyopathy, and 41% for arrhythmogenic right ventricular cardiomyopathy (ARVC). However, as techniques become more widely available, these numbers are likely to increase. This chapter focuses on the epicardial interventions in electrophysiology, and presents the recent knowledge in the field of epicardial VT ablation, and outlines the latest advances in this area.

S. Nakahara, M.D., Ph.D., F.A.C.C.
Department of Cardiology, Dokkyo Medical University Koshigaya Hospital, 2-1-50 Minami Koshigaya, Koshigaya, Saitama 343-8555, Japan
e-mail: nshiro@dokkyomed.ac.jp

39.2 Obtaining Access to the Pericardial Space

39.2.1 Subxiphoid Access

The subxiphoid approach has the advantage of allowing free access to the entire area of both the ventricular and atrial surfaces. Although the procedure is usually performed in the electrophysiological laboratory, it is more ideal to perform percutaneous pericardial procedures in a hybrid laboratory where cardiac surgery can be performed promptly. Generous sedation is required, and sometimes general anesthesia is used. Before puncturing the pericardial space, it is best to position the intracardiac catheters, as these act as anatomical landmarks of the right ventricular (RV) apex if no RV pacing or ICD leads are located in the right ventricular apex. After the delivery of local anesthesia, the skin entry site is placed approximately 2 cm below the subxiphoid process. A 17 G × 6 in (152 mm, Hakko Co., Ltd., Tokyo, Japan) Tuohy epidural needle with a soft-tipped wire is used. A shallow entry initially directed to the left shoulder is preferred to minimize the chance of puncturing the liver with an increased angle toward 45° after entering several centimeters. Manual pressure over the right upper quadrant may be applied to minimize the chance of a hepatic puncture. Biplane fluoroscopy is useful to assess the approach of the needle for the two approaches, namely, the anterior and posterior (inferior) approaches. If an anterior puncture is desired, the needle track is continued along a shallow course (<30°) and a steep lateral projection is helpful for assessing that the needle track is just posterior to the sternum as it approaches the anterior RV. A posterior approach requires steepening of the angle of needle course (>45°) to aim for the basal portion of the heart, which is fluoroscopically marked by the coronary sinus catheter. The right anterior oblique projection is useful for determining a basal versus apical approach angle. The left anterior oblique (LAO) projection is helpful to identify the RV free wall that forms the right heart border (Fig. 39.1a, b).

When the needle approaches the cardiac border, small volumes of contrast are injected using a 5-mL syringe attached to the needle. The fluid is seen to pool in the extrapericardial tissue until the needle enters the potential pericardial space, when further injection of contrast outlines the pericardium as a thin film surrounding the cardiac silhouette. Tenting of the pericardium is usually seen fluoroscopically before the puncture (Fig. 39.1c). A lack of blood on aspiration at this stage

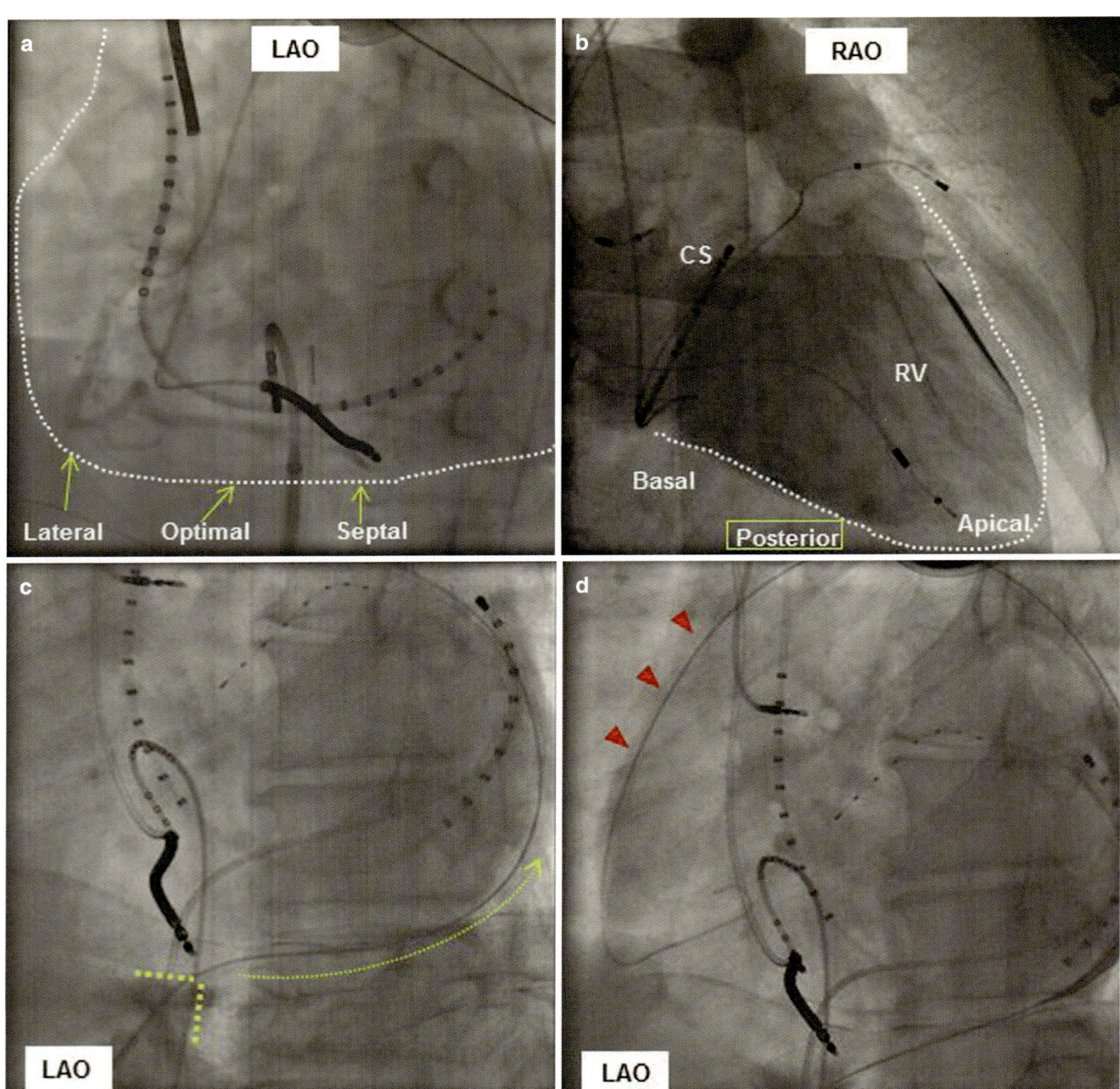

Fig. 39.1 (a, b) Relevant anatomy in the fluoroscopic views during the percutaneous access. In the left anterior oblique (LAO) view, a lateral approach increases the risk of a right ventricular (RV) puncture as the angulation is more perpendicular to the inferior surface of the heart, and the septal approach increases the risk of a posterior descending branch puncture as shown. In the right anterior oblique (RAO) view, steepening the angle of the entry allows the operator to adjust the depth of the puncture from apical to basal. (c, d) Optimal guidewire course within the pericardial space that crosses multiple chambers along the outermost cardiac border on fluoroscopy in the left anterior oblique (LAO) projection

confirms that the right ventricle has not been punctured; however, this is usually identified on contrast injection. Once in the pericardial space, the needle is stabilized with one hand while the syringe is removed and the wire advanced through the bevel. Guidewire placement is monitored fluoroscopically to ensure that inadvertent entry into the RV or the extrapericardial space has not occurred. Pericardial placement is confirmed by the wire wrapping around the cardiac silhouette, traversing the chamber boundaries as it traverses both right and left cardiac borders (Fig. 39.1c, d).

Inadvertent RV punctures are not rare occurrences, but are usually benign if only the needle or wire has entered the chamber in a patient who is not anticoagulated. When the RV is inadvertently entered with the needle (indicated by aspiration of blood or a contrast injection passing to the pulmonary artery), the needle can be pulled slightly; a contrast injection can then show silhouetting of the heart, and at that point the guidewire is advanced into the pericardial space. The small hole in the RV usually seals without incident. If the dilator and sheath have passed into the RV, the larger hole may require a surgical repair. In our hospital, an SL-0 sheath is always used for epicardial mapping and ablation. When advancing the sheath into the pericardial space, it is also important to ensure pericardial wire placement before the needle is withdrawn over the wire and the sheath introduced.

39.2.2 Mapping and Ablation Tools

After pericardial access is obtained, catheter movement is typically smooth and undeterred in the pericardial space. The long sheath can be advanced and torqued to assist in accessing regions outside of the catheter range. During mapping of the epicardium, the same techniques employed during endocardial mapping are performed (e.g., pacemapping, entrainment, and electroanatomic mapping). The two main commercially available electroanatomic mapping systems can be used for the epicardial mapping and ablation [4]. There are important advantages and disadvantages for both the electrofield (NavX; St. Jude Medical, Minneapolis, MN) and magnet-based (CARTO; Biosense-Webster, Diamond Bar, CA) systems. Because of the difference in the impedance between the pericardial space and blood pool, the epicardial geometry constructed with the electrofield system may appear less spherical. However, when compared with histopathologic scar, the correlation between both of these mapping systems is excellent [4]. Regardless of the mapping system choice, the use of a multipolar mapping catheter increases the sampling density and number of late potentials identified in a shorter period. Further, a recent advanced mapping module combined with multipolar catheter use also can facilitate faster and higher-density epicardial mapping (Fig. 39.2).

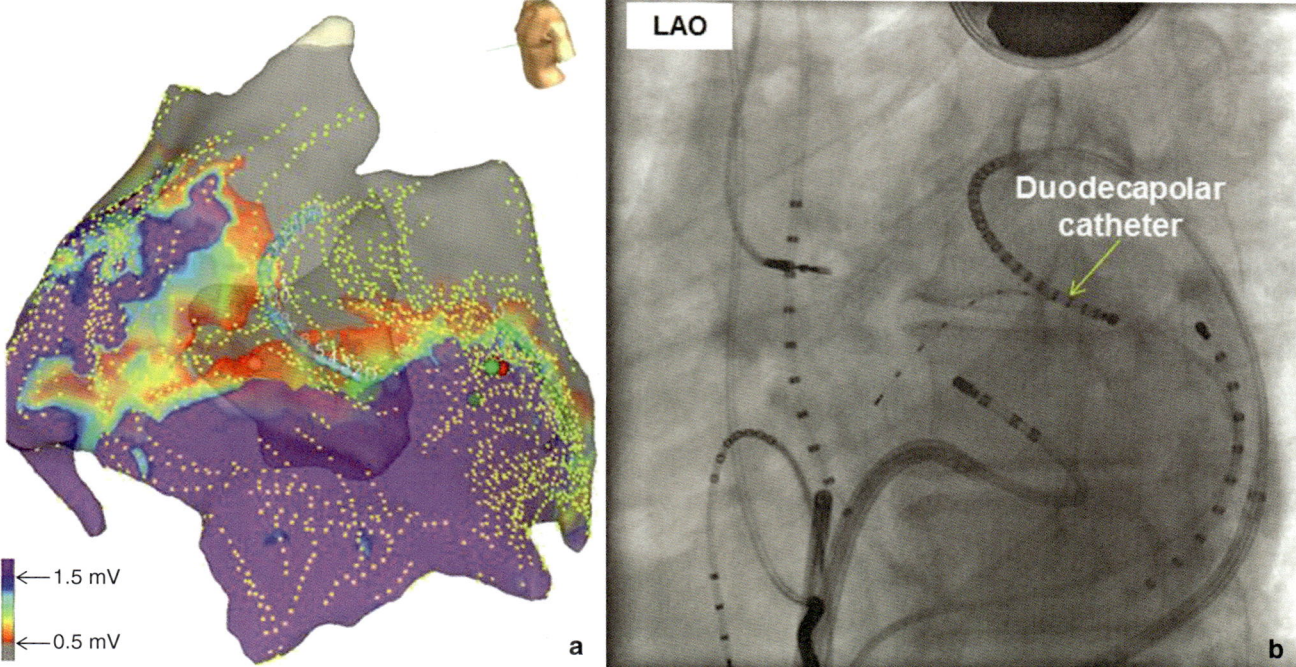

Fig. 39.2 (a) Combined endocardial and epicardial electroanatomical maps in a patient with nonischemic cardiomyopathy. (b) Left anterior oblique fluoroscopic view with a duodecapolar (DD) catheter positioned within the pericardium where a low-voltage area is demonstrated. The *yellow dots* indicate the electrogram sampling points. The multipolar catheter combined with the recent advanced mapping module (EnSite™ AutoMap Module) facilitates a faster and high-density mapping

The actual power settings for the epicardial ablation tend to be more tolerant than those used for endocardial ablation. However, the optimal power settings have not yet been defined. A titrated irrigated radiofrequency energy with a flow rate of 10–30 mL/min with up to 50 W and a temperature limit of 45–50 °C has been used for epicardial ablation [3, 5]. The concern for steam pops and char formation is mitigated by lesser chance of such in the pericardial space.

39.3 Clinical Indications for Epicardial Mapping

Several groups have used their clinical studies to propose ECG criteria that would indicate an epicardial focus or circuit of VT. The general criteria are related to the morphology of the QRS. They are all based on the presumed slower conduction during the initial part of the QRS as the depolarization wave traverses slowly from the epicardium to the endocardium and then spreads faster using the endocardial Purkinje fibers. Representative ECG criteria are shown in Table 39.1. Although some ECG criteria suggest an epicardial VT origin, other factors significantly influence their validity, most importantly the type of cardiomyopathy and region of the VT origin. These limitations have to be considered when applying the abovementioned ECG criteria for the assessment of the VT origin.

The implementation of epicardial mapping and ablation is more commonly performed at highly experienced centers [3, 6]. Wider adoption of epicardial mapping is justifiable at centers with a sufficiently low risk of complications. A combined epicardial-endocardial approach is associated with improved freedom from VT recurrence when compared to more limited endocardial strategies [7]. Furthermore, various practice patterns range from using epicardial ablation only in the case of a previously failed endocardial ablation to using an epicardial approach as part of a combined comprehensive initial strategy. However, randomized prospective

Table 39.1 Proposed electrocardiogram criteria and cutoff values for epicardial ventricular tachycardia origin

ECG criteria	Abbreviation	Explanation	Cutoff
Interval criteria			
QRS duration	QRSd	Interval measured from the earliest ventricular activation to the offset of the QRS in the precordial leads.	121 ms
Pseudo-delta wave	PdW	Interval measured from the earliest ventricular activation to the onset of the earliest fast deflection in any precordial lead	≥34 ms
Intrinsicoid deflection time	IDT	Interval measured from the earliest ventricular activation to the peak of the R wave in lead V2	≥85 ms
Shortest RS complex	SRS	Interval measured from the earliest ventricular activation to the nadir of the first S wave in any precordial lead	≥121 ms
Maximum deflection index	MDI	Interval measured from the earliest ventricular activation to the peak of the largest amplitude deflection in each precordial lead (taking the lead with the shortest time) divided by the QRSd	≥0.59
Morphology criteria (site-specific)			
Q wave in lead 1	–	Q wave in lead 1 during VT	–
Q wave in inferior leads	–	Q wave in the inferior leads during VT	–
No Q wave in inferior leads	–	No Q wave in the inferior leads during VT	–
QS in lead V2	–	QS complex in lead V2 during VT	–

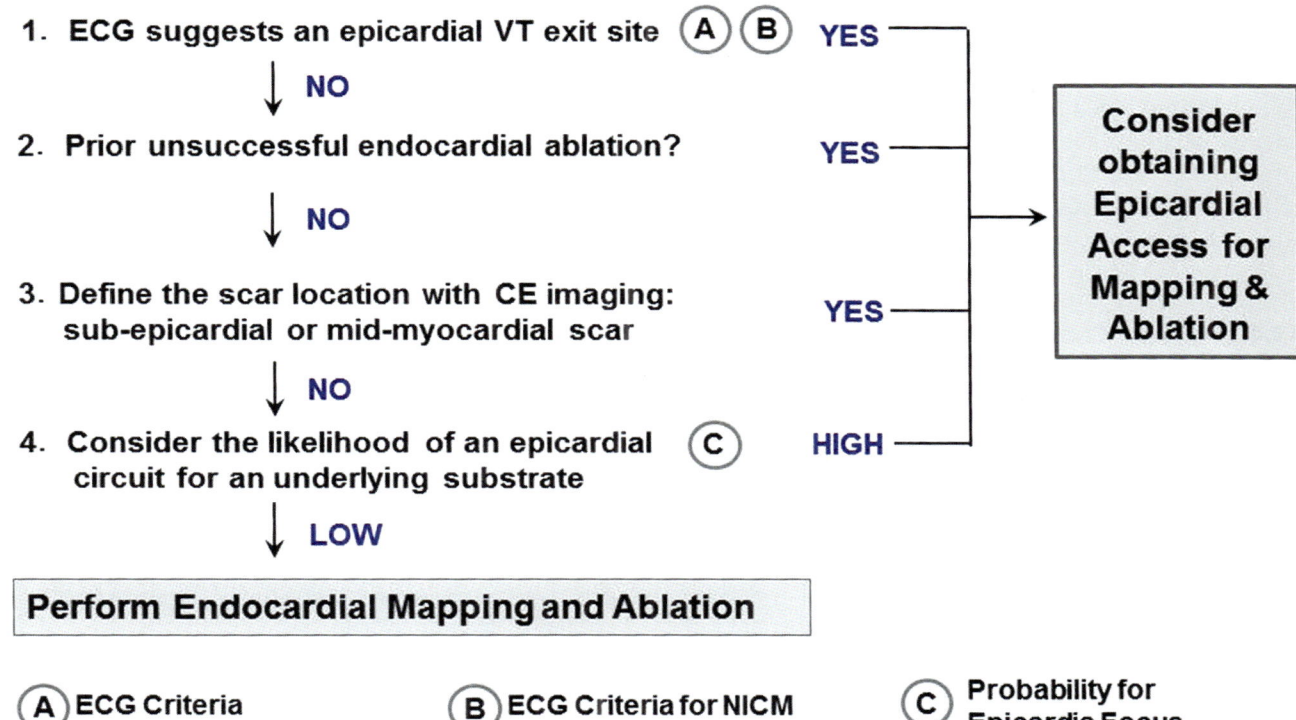

Fig. 39.3 Summary of the clinical indications for epicardial mapping and ablation. Modified from Boyle et al. Circulation. 2012;126:1752–69. Flowchart for the suggested approach to assess the need for an epicardial access and/or ablation. *VT* ventricular tachycardia, *CE* contrast enhanced MRI, *Pseudodelta* interval from the onset of the ventricular activation to the onset of the earliest rapid deflection in any precordial lead, *IDT* intrinsicoid deflection time, *MDI* maximal deflection, *ICM* ischemic cardiomyopathy, *NICM* nonischemic cardiomyopathy, *ARVC* arrhythmogenic right ventricular cardiomyopathy

data are lacking. A proposed strategy for clinical decision-making to assess a patient for an epicardial access is shown in Fig. 39.3.

39.4 Epicardial Substrate According to the Type of Cardiomyopathy

The substrate responsible for VT origins varies widely among the different types of cardiomyopathies. Consequently, the rate by which a successful VT ablation requires epicardial mapping and ablation is highly dependent on the type of cardiomyopathy. Of all the information available prior to the first VT ablation procedure, the type of cardiomyopathy is probably the best predictor for the necessity of an epicardial approach and we will discuss this in the next section.

39.4.1 Ischemic Cardiomyopathy

Patients with ischemic heart disease tend to have larger endocardial than epicardial scars, usually confined to a specific coronary vascular territory. Although there is a predilection for a subendocardial location of the VT substrate, epicardial circuits can be observed in a significant portion of patients. In tertiary centers, epicardial ablation has been required in up to 10% of post-MI VTs, and appears to be more frequently required for inferior wall infarct VTs than for those with anterior wall infarcts.

Sosa et al. were the first to show the feasibility of epicardial ablation in post-infarct patients [8]. Several studies have since reported good success rates of a combined endo- and epicardial ablation in patients with ischemic cardiomyopathy, mainly after a failed endocardial VT ablation [6, 9, 10].

Detailed endo- and epicardial mapping of stable VT circuits in post-myocardial infarction patients has revealed a putative epicardial isthmus in a minority of them [11]. The prevalence of an epicardial circuit may be higher in patients with inferior or infero-lateral rather than anterior myocardial infarctions [2, 10, 12]. Therefore, epicardial VT ablation in patients with ischemic cardiomyopathy should be considered after a failed endocardial ablation.

39.4.2 Dilated Cardiomyopathy

The main mechanism of VT in patients with dilated cardiomyopathy is myocardial reentry. Bundle branch reentry, inter-fascicular reentry, and focal automaticity are also possible mechanisms [13, 14]. Although endocardial ablation of myocardial reentry has a modest success rate, it is very successful for the remaining tachycardia mechanisms [13, 14]. Scar tissue is uniformly present in cases with myocardial reentry and mostly located with a predilection to a valve annulus and septal region [9, 14, 15]. Detailed epicardial electroanatomical substrate mapping has identified large confluent low-voltage areas consistent with myocardial scar (Fig. 39.4). Contrast-enhanced cardiac magnetic resonance imaging of patients with dilated cardiomyopathy also shows mid-wall fibrosis in up to one-third of cases, which differs from the subendocardial/transmural pattern found in ischemic cardiomyopathy [16]. The presence of mid-myocardial fibrosis has been found to be a predictive factor for an arrhythmic event [16]. Thus, epicardial ablation is needed more often in patients with sustained monomorphic VT associated with dilated, nonischemic CMP than in patients with a prior MI. Combined endo- and epicardial ablation in patients with dilated cardiomyopathy and VT results in high rates of arrhythmia-free outcomes [14, 15, 9]. However, the patient populations in those studies are highly selected as most had failed a previous endocardial VT ablation, favoring the presence of an epicardial circuit. Therefore, it cannot be generalized to all patients with dilated cardiomyopathy and VT; however, epicardial ablation should be considered in patients with a failed endocardial ablation.

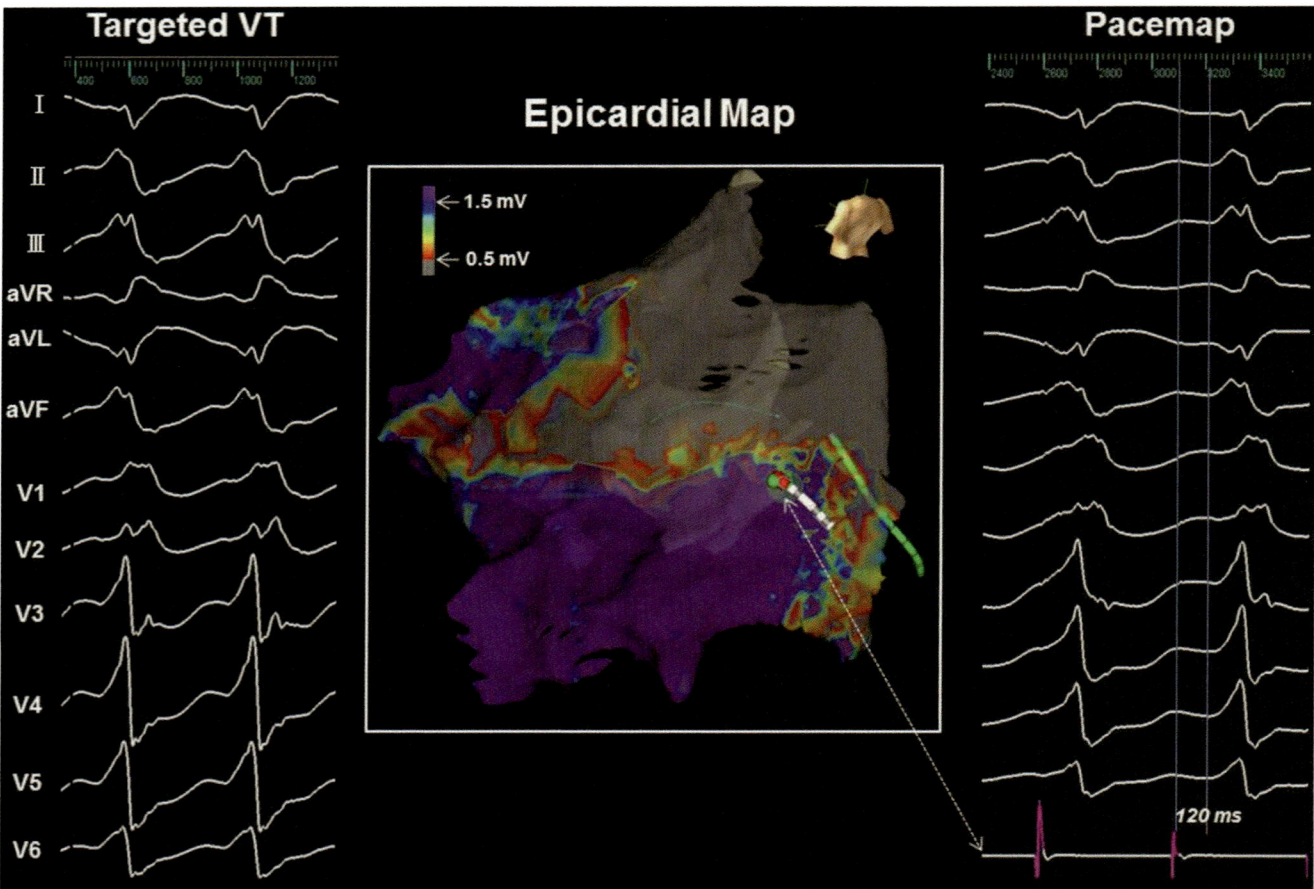

Fig. 39.4 Epicardial electroanatomical LV voltage maps. The 12-lead ECG recording of VT and pace-mapping data is shown. Pacing from a border zone site demonstrates the best pace-map match at an exit site. The stimulus to QRS interval was 120 ms, suggesting the existence of a slow conduction property at this site

39.4.3 Arrhythmogenic Right Ventricular Dysplasia

In patients with ARVC/D, sizable low-voltage areas often involve the infundibulum, free wall, and basal perivalvular regions, constituting the endocardial substrate. Recently, extensive epicardial low-voltage areas, often with fractionated and late electrographic recordings, have been identified. Epicardial scar is consistently larger than that on the endocardial surface. Histopathological studies in the hearts of ARVC/D patients also show transmural myocardial atrophy with fatty or fibro-fatty infiltration that is much more extensive on the epicardial side [17]. Garcia et al. also reported that ARVC/D has a predilection for scar in the basal perivalvular, apical, and outflow tract areas with the use of epicardial mapping. In a study of 13 patients who underwent endocardial and epicardial mapping after a failed endocardial ablation, this group reported that areas of low voltage (<1 mV for epicardium and 1.5 mV for endocardium) were more extensive on the epicardium and demonstrated multicomponent and late potentials [18]. The approach combined activation, entrainment, and pace mapping with focal or linear lesions targeting late potentials. During an average of 18 months of follow-up, 10 of 13 patients (77%) had no VT. Two non-randomized, multicenter studies compared the outcomes of ARVC/D patients treated with a combined endo-epicardial ablation versus exclusive endocardial ablation; both found a significantly higher long-term freedom from recurrent VT in the groups treated with the combined ablation [19, 20]. Taken together, recent insight has suggested that a combined endocardial and epicardial approach should be considered in ARVC/D patients.

39.5 Surgical Approach

In patients who had a prior cardiac surgery, dense adhesions decrease the operator's ability to determine if the puncture is in the pericardial space, limit the ability to access all epicardial regions, and increase the risk of bleeding because adhesions are bluntly dissected without direct visualization [21]. Although a percutaneous access has been reported in such patients, dense adhesions are often encountered limiting the mappable regions [21]. Thus, it is general practice not to attempt a percutaneous access due to the limited access and increased risk of complications. Rather, a minimally invasive surgical access can be obtained via a subxiphoid window or limited anterior thoracotomy to facilitate the catheter access in patients who have undergone prior cardiac surgery [22, 23].

39.6 Collateral Damage and Complications

Pericardial bleeding is the most frequent complication of a pericardial puncture and can be present to some degree in up to 30% of patients [2, 3]. Hepatic or intra-abdominal bleeding may also occur after accidental puncture of the liver or a subdiaphragmatic vessel [24]. Prior to delivering radiofrequency energy on the epicardial surface, the regional anatomy must be carefully considered for any potential collateral damage. The irrigated ablation technology has been shown to improve the lesion size in the epicardial space compared to standard catheters [25]. Acute and chronic coronary arterial injury from radiofrequency energy deliveries over or adjacent to vessels has been shown in an animal model [26]. The consensus statement recommends a distance greater than 5 mm from a coronary artery for a safe ablation throughout all phases of the cardiac cycle; however, many centers implement a larger safety margin of 1 cm [2]. When ablation is performed on the lateral wall of the epicardial left ventricle, the course of the left phrenic nerve should be assessed. High output pacing (>10 mA) is useful for characterizing the course of the phrenic nerve on the electroanatomic map [27]. If a targeted region is in close proximity to the phrenic nerve, separation of the epicardium from the parietal pericardium can be achieved by several methods, including the injection of water or air, or displacement with a balloon [28, 29]. Symptomatic pericarditis has been reported in up to 29% of patients after an epicardial ablation and may manifest as a major pericardial inflammatory reaction in some patients [3].

In two large multicenter experiences, Della Bella et al. observed major complications in 4% (eight tamponade and one abdominal bleed) of 222 cases, and Sacher et al. described a 5% (seven hemopericardium [>80 cc] and one coronary stenosis) incidence of acute major complications out of 156 procedures [3, 6]. Knowledge of the pericardial anatomy, adjacent anatomic structures, and adverse effects is helpful in avoiding and managing complications.

39.7 Epicardial Fat

Epicardial fat presents two unique challenges for mapping and ablation of ventricular tachycardia. As fat insulates the myocardium during contact mapping, low-voltage regions are frequently detected and can be difficult to distinguish from scar [30]. Additionally, when ablation is required in these regions, interposed fat impairs the efficacy of the radiofrequency delivery. Figure 39.5 demonstrates a situation in which when an extensive thickness of fat is suspected over a critical site, an open surgical approach for dissection may be necessary.

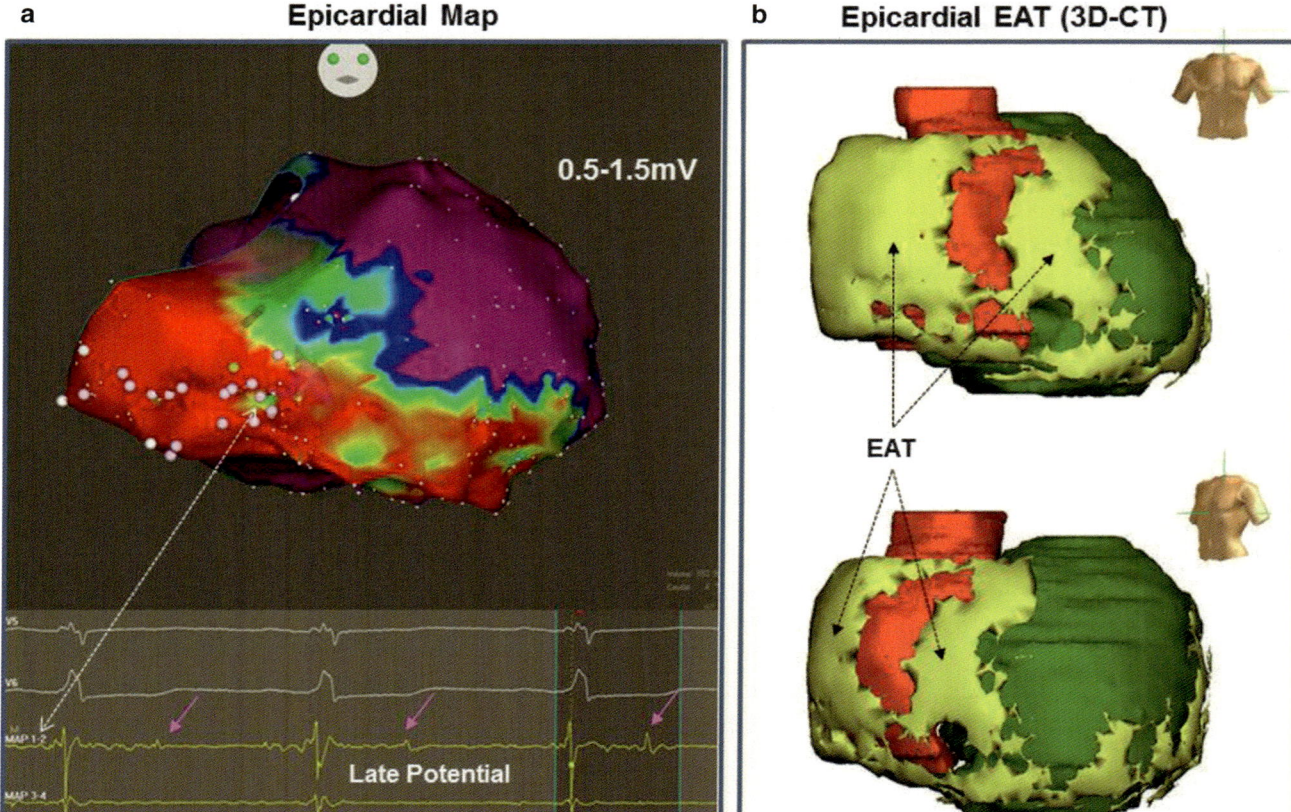

Fig. 39.5 (**a**, **b**) Comparison of an epicardial electroanatomical map and epicardial adipose tissue (EAT) detected by multidetector computed tomography (MDCT) in a patient with nonischemic cardiomyopathy. The correlation of the epicardial low-voltage areas on the CARTO system with EAT is demonstrated. Late potentials are recorded in the RV epicardial low-voltage areas where the EAT distribution also has been confirmed by MDCT. The spatial proximity between ideal ablation targets and the deposition of EAT are suggested

Conclusions

Epicardial mapping and ablation accessing the pericardial space via a percutaneous access has improved the understanding of the mechanism of scar substrates and has allowed the treatment of patients with VTs refractory to endocardial ablation. Although transthoracic epicardial mapping and ablation are relatively safe, complications can and do occur. Therefore, the possible complications associated with this technique should be well understood before the procedure. As this technique becomes more broadly adopted worldwide, further future prospective studies are needed to evaluate the role of epicardial ablation as a first-line therapeutic strategy in patients with recurrent VT.

References

1. Sosa E, Scanavacca M, d'Avila A, Pilleggi F. A new technique to perform epicardial mapping in the electrophysiology laboratory. J Cardiovasc Electrophysiol. 1996;7(6):531–6.
2. Aliot EM, Stevenson WG, Almendral-Garrote JM, Bogun F, Calkins CH, Delacretaz E, et al. EHRA/HRS expert consensus on catheter ablation of ventricular arrhythmias: developed in a partnership with the European Heart Rhythm Association (EHRA), a registered branch of the European Society of Cardiology (ESC), and the Heart Rhythm Society (HRS); in collaboration with the American College of Cardiology (ACC) and the American Heart Association (AHA). Europace. 2009;11(6):771–817. https://doi.org/10.1093/europace/eup098.
3. Sacher F, Roberts-Thomson K, Maury P, Tedrow U, Nault I, Steven D, et al. Epicardial ventricular tachycardia ablation – a multicenter safety study. J Am Coll Cardiol. 2010;55(21):2366–72. https://doi.org/10.1016/j.jacc.2009.10.084.
4. Tung R, Nakahara S, Ramirez R, Gui D, Magyar C, Lai C, et al. Accuracy of combined endocardial and epicardial electroanatomic mapping of a reperfused porcine infarct model: a comparison of electrofield and magnetic systems with histopathologic correlation. Heart Rhythm. 2011;8(3):439–47. https://doi.org/10.1016/j.hrthm.2010.10.044.
5. Tung R, Michowitz Y, Yu R, Mathuria N, Vaseghi M, Buch E, et al. Epicardial ablation of ventricular tachycardia: an institutional experience of safety and efficacy. Heart Rhythm. 2013;10(4):490–8. https://doi.org/10.1016/j.hrthm.2012.12.013.
6. Della Bella P, Brugada J, Zeppenfeld K, Merino J, Neuzil P, Maury P, et al. Epicardial ablation for ventricular tachycardia: a European multicenter study. Circ Arrhythm Electrophysiol.

2011;4(5):653–9. https://doi.org/10.1161/CIRCEP.111.962217. CIRCEP.111.962217 [pii]
7. Di Biase L, Santangeli P, Burkhardt DJ, Bai R, Mohanty P, Carbucicchio C, et al. Endo-epicardial homogenization of the scar versus limited substrate ablation for the treatment of electrical storms in patients with ischemic cardiomyopathy. J Am Coll Cardiol. 2012;60(2):132–41. https://doi.org/10.1016/j.jacc.2012.03.044. S0735-1097(12)01421-0 [pii]
8. Sosa E, Scanavacca M, d'Avila A, Oliveira F, Ramires JA. Nonsurgical transthoracic epicardial catheter ablation to treat recurrent ventricular tachycardia occurring late after myocardial infarction. J Am Coll Cardiol. 2000;35(6):1442–9. doi:S0735-1097(00)00606-9 [pii]
9. Nakahara S, Tung R, Ramirez RJ, Michowitz Y, Vaseghi M, Buch E, et al. Characterization of the arrhythmogenic substrate in ischemic and nonischemic cardiomyopathy implications for catheter ablation of hemodynamically unstable ventricular tachycardia. J Am Coll Cardiol. 2010;55(21):2355–65. https://doi.org/10.1016/j.jacc.2010.01.041. S0735-1097(10)01085-5 [pii]
10. Schmidt B, Chun KR, Baensch D, Antz M, Koektuerk B, Tilz RR, et al. Catheter ablation for ventricular tachycardia after failed endocardial ablation: epicardial substrate or inappropriate endocardial ablation? Heart Rhythm. 2010;7(12):1746–52. https://doi.org/10.1016/j.hrthm.2010.08.010. S1547-5271(10)00820-9 [pii]
11. Verma A, Marrouche NF, Schweikert RA, Saliba W, Wazni O, Cummings J, et al. Relationship between successful ablation sites and the scar border zone defined by substrate mapping for ventricular tachycardia post-myocardial infarction. J Cardiovasc Electrophysiol. 2005;16(5):465–71. https://doi.org/10.1046/j.1540-8167.2005.40443.x. JCE40443 [pii]
12. Santangeli P, Di Biase L, Burkhardt JD, Natale A. Lesion recovery, epicardial substrate, or new circuit? Exploring the dark side of recurrent ventricular tachycardia after endocardial ablation. Heart Rhythm. 2011;8(10):1523–4. https://doi.org/10.1016/j.hrthm.2011.07.002. S1547-5271(11)00791-0 [pii]
13. Delacretaz E, Stevenson WG, Ellison KE, Maisel WH, Friedman PL. Mapping and radiofrequency catheter ablation of the three types of sustained monomorphic ventricular tachycardia in nonischemic heart disease. J Cardiovasc Electrophysiol. 2000;11(1):11–7.
14. Soejima K, Stevenson WG, Sapp JL, Selwyn AP, Couper G, Epstein LM. Endocardial and epicardial radiofrequency ablation of ventricular tachycardia associated with dilated cardiomyopathy: the importance of low-voltage scars. J Am Coll Cardiol. 2004;43(10):1834–42. https://doi.org/10.1016/j.jacc.2004.01.029. S0735109704004590 [pii]
15. Cano O, Hutchinson M, Lin D, Garcia F, Zado E, Bala R, et al. Electroanatomic substrate and ablation outcome for suspected epicardial ventricular tachycardia in left ventricular nonischemic cardiomyopathy. J Am Coll Cardiol. 2009;54(9):799–808. https://doi.org/10.1016/j.jacc.2009.05.032. S0735-1097(09)01896-8 [pii]
16. Assomull RG, Prasad SK, Lyne J, Smith G, Burman ED, Khan M, et al. Cardiovascular magnetic resonance, fibrosis, and prognosis in dilated cardiomyopathy. J Am Coll Cardiol. 2006;48(10):1977–85. https://doi.org/10.1016/j.jacc.2006.07.049. S0735-1097(06)02111-5 [pii]
17. Basso C, Thiene G, Corrado D, Angelini A, Nava A, Valente M. Arrhythmogenic right ventricular cardiomyopathy. Dysplasia, dystrophy, or myocarditis? Circulation. 1996;94(5):983–91.
18. Garcia FC, Bazan V, Zado ES, Ren JF, Marchlinski FE. Epicardial substrate and outcome with epicardial ablation of ventricular tachycardia in arrhythmogenic right ventricular cardiomyopathy/dysplasia. Circulation. 2009;120(5):366–75. https://doi.org/10.1161/CIRCULATIONAHA.108.834903. CIRCULATIONAHA.108.834903 [pii]
19. Bai R, Di Biase L, Shivkumar K, Mohanty P, Tung R, Santangeli P, et al. Ablation of ventricular arrhythmias in arrhythmogenic right ventricular dysplasia/cardiomyopathy: arrhythmia-free survival after endo-epicardial substrate based mapping and ablation. Circ Arrhythm Electrophysiol. 2011;4(4):478–85. https://doi.org/10.1161/CIRCEP.111.963066. CIRCEP.111.963066 [pii]
20. Philips B, Madhavan S, James C, Tichnell C, Murray B, Dalal D, et al. Outcomes of catheter ablation of ventricular tachycardia in arrhythmogenic right ventricular dysplasia/cardiomyopathy. Circ Arrhythm Electrophysiol. 2012;5(3):499–505. https://doi.org/10.1161/CIRCEP.111.968677. CIRCEP.111.968677 [pii]
21. Tschabrunn CM, Haqqani HM, Cooper JM, Dixit S, Garcia FC, Gerstenfeld EP, et al. Percutaneous epicardial ventricular tachycardia ablation after noncoronary cardiac surgery or pericarditis. Heart Rhythm. 2013;10(2):165–9. https://doi.org/10.1016/j.hrthm.2012.10.012.
22. Soejima K, Couper G, Cooper JM, Sapp JL, Epstein LM, Stevenson WG. Subxiphoid surgical approach for epicardial catheter-based mapping and ablation in patients with prior cardiac surgery or difficult pericardial access. Circulation. 2004;110(10):1197–201. https://doi.org/10.1161/01.CIR.0000140725.42845.90.
23. Michowitz Y, Mathuria N, Tung R, Esmailian F, Kwon M, Nakahara S, et al. Hybrid procedures for epicardial catheter ablation of ventricular tachycardia: value of surgical access. Heart Rhythm. 2010;7(11):1635–43. https://doi.org/10.1016/j.hrthm.2010.07.009.
24. Sosa E, Scanavacca M. Epicardial mapping and ablation techniques to control ventricular tachycardia. J Cardiovasc Electrophysiol. 2005;16(4):449–52. https://doi.org/10.1046/j.1540-8167.2005.40710.x.
25. d'Avila A, Houghtaling C, Gutierrez P, Vragovic O, Ruskin JN, Josephson ME, et al. Catheter ablation of ventricular epicardial tissue: a comparison of standard and cooled-tip radiofrequency energy. Circulation. 2004;109(19):2363–9. https://doi.org/10.1161/01.CIR.0000128039.87485.0B.
26. D'Avila A, Gutierrez P, Scanavacca M, Reddy V, Lustgarten DL, Sosa E, et al. Effects of radiofrequency pulses delivered in the vicinity of the coronary arteries: implications for nonsurgical transthoracic epicardial catheter ablation to treat ventricular tachycardia. Pacing Clin Electrophysiol. 2002;25(10):1488–95.
27. Fan R, Cano O, Ho SY, Bala R, Callans DJ, Dixit S, et al. Characterization of the phrenic nerve course within the epicardial substrate of patients with nonischemic cardiomyopathy and ventricular tachycardia. Heart Rhythm. 2009;6(1):59–64. https://doi.org/10.1016/j.hrthm.2008.09.033.
28. Buch E, Vaseghi M, Cesario DA, Shivkumar K. A novel method for preventing phrenic nerve injury during catheter ablation. Heart Rhythm. 2007;4(1):95–8. https://doi.org/10.1016/j.hrthm.2006.09.019.
29. Di Biase L, Burkhardt JD, Pelargonio G, Dello Russo A, Casella M, Santarelli P, et al. Prevention of phrenic nerve injury during epicardial ablation: comparison of methods for separating the phrenic nerve from the epicardial surface. Heart Rhythm. 2009;6(7):957–61. https://doi.org/10.1016/j.hrthm.2009.03.022.
30. Tung R, Nakahara S, Ramirez R, Lai C, Fishbein MC, Shivkumar K. Distinguishing epicardial fat from scar: analysis of electrograms using high-density electroanatomic mapping in a novel porcine infarct model. Heart Rhythm. 2010;7(3):389–95. https://doi.org/10.1016/j.hrthm.2009.11.023.

Ablation of Electrical Storm

Yoshinori Kobayashi

Keywords

Electrical storm • Catheter ablation • Acute myocardial infarction • Idiopathic ventricular fibrillation • Ventricular tachycardia

40.1 Introduction

Electrical storm (ES) is commonly defined as the clustering of hemodynamically deteriorated ventricular tachycardia (VT) or ventricular fibrillation (VF) which requires the repeated applications of direct current shocks to save the life [1–4]. The ES has been shown to occur in a variety of cardiac conditions, including cardiac ischemia, reperfusion, severe inflammation, heart failure, and genetic electrophysiological abnormalities such as long QT syndrome and Brugada syndrome. Since the defibrillation threshold is certainly increased with the every repeated DC cardioversion, it is essential to suppress the emergence of the lethal arrhythmias as quickly as possible. To date, deep sedation and intravenous administration of amiodarone and beta blockers have been the first-line therapies for the ES associated with the structural heart disease. In the patients with the reduced cardiac function associated with ischemic heart disease, the intra-aortic balloon pump is effective to suppress the ES [5]. The stellate ganglion block and the renal sympathetic denervation [6] are occasionally applied in patients with drug-refractory ES. Meanwhile, for the VF storm in Brugada syndrome, isoproterenol has been shown to be effective. However, these urgent therapies often result in the failure in the suppression of the ES, consequently giving rise to a further lethal condition.

It is well known that catheter ablation is also a potent therapeutic modality to eliminate the incessant emergence of lethal arrhythmias in various clinical setting [2–4]. In this chapter, first the clinical background and prognosis of ES will be reviewed, then the indication, the targeted arrhythmia and substrate, and the methods and results of catheter ablation applied to suppress the ES will be described.

40.2 Clinical Background and Prognosis of the ES

40.2.1 Structural Heart Disease

The ES occurs in a variety of clinical setting. The underlying heart diseases of the ES include structural heart disease such as acute and subacute phase of myocardial infarction, ischemic cardiomyopathy, dilated cardiomyopathy, and inflammatory diseases [2, 3].

In the acute or subacute phase of MI, a variety of clinical factors are associated with the emergence of ES. These are the acute ischemia, spontaneous or interventional coronary reperfusion, pump failure, electrolytes abnormalities, and so on. Tokyo Coronary Care Unit (CCU) Network database has been conducted as an ongoing multicenter registry collecting clinical information in the acute and subacute phase of MI for the patients admitted to the CCU/ICU of the leading hospitals capable of advanced cardiac cares in the Tokyo metropolitan area (67 facilities). Using the database of 2011 and 2012, we have evaluated the clinical background and prognosis of the ES which occurred in the acute or subacute phase of MI and was first documented after the hospital arrival [7]. Thus, the patients with out-of-hospital cardiac arrest or VT/VF first documented before the hospitalization were excluded from this study. When ES is defined as more

Y. Kobayashi, M.D.
Division of cardiology, Tokai University Hachioji-hospital, 1838 Ishikawa-machi, Hachioji-shi, Tokyo 192-0032, Japan
e-mail: yoshikoba@tokai-u.jp

than three times of DC cardioversion during 24 h, there were 67 patients eligible to be included in this study. The incidence of ES is 67/6003 patients (1.1%) in this multicenter registry. With regard to the background of ES, it was revealed that the ES was associated with broad MI as the peak creatinine phosphokinase (CK) was significantly higher than the control group reduced cardiac function as Killip classification is worse, and frequent use of cardiac supporting devices (IABP and PCPS). These patients with ES are divided into two groups: the patients with ES first documented within 24 h from the onset of MI (Group-E: 46 patients) and the patients with ES first documented more than 24 h after the onset of MI (Group-D: 21 patients) and clinical parameters are compared between the two groups. The clinical condition was more critical in group-D than group-E, as group-D has more elderly people, higher prevalence of various complications, and higher mortality, as compared to group-E.

There have been several clinical investigations on the characteristics, treatment, and prognosis of the patients with ES who have undergone ICD implantation for both primary and secondary prevention [8–14]. The incidence of the ES distributed in the wide range (4–40%), presumably because of the heterogeneity of the clinical background such as the aim of ICD implantation (primary prevention or secondary prevention) and basic heart diseases, difference in the definition of the ES (two or three sustained ventricular arrhythmias within 24 h), and difference in the observational period (average 94–1417 days). The time of the emergence of ES also widely scattered from few months to years after the implantation of ICD. Approximately 70 % of the documented arrhythmias are VT, whereas the rest were VF or both VT and VF. The triggers of the ES were acute ischemia, congestive heart failure, electrolyte disturbances, and acute inflammation. It seems to be problematic that the predisposing factor of the ES could be clarified only in 10–40% of the patients while in the rest of patients it remained unknown [8–14]. With regard to the pharmacological treatment for the ES, there are several drugs, including beta blockers, amiodarone, azimilide [12], and nifekalant [15], which have been shown to be effective to suppress the storm. Out of these, amiodarone and beta blockers are most commonly used for this purpose [8, 10, 11, 16]. It should be emphasized that sedation is the most important treatment of the first priority to remove the pain due to repeated ICD shocks. Whether the prognosis of the patients with the documentation of an ES is worse or not, as compared to those without ES, has been a controversial issue in this category of patients. In several reports [9–11, 14], the ES is shown to cause an ominous prognosis with an increased future risk of arrhythmias and cardiac death (Hazard ratio 2.4–7.4), whereas the other reports did not show significant difference in the prognosis between the patients with and without ES. A recent meta-analysis on the role of ES as a mortality and morbidity risk factor and its clinical predictors revealed that the patients with ES have nearly threefold increased risk of death as compared to those without ES [17] (Fig. 40.1). It was also shown that ICD implantation for secondary prevention, class I antiarrhythmic drug use, monomorphic VT, and low EF are all associated with the ES and could be the significant predictors for future ES occurrence.

With regard to the role of catheter ablation in the patients with ES occurring after the ICD implantation, the catheter

Study or subgroup	Electrical storm Events	Total	No Electrical storm Events	Total	Weight	Risk ratio Random, 95% CI
Fries et al. 1997	10	34	1	23	2.5%	6.76 [0.93, 49.31]
Credner et al. 1998	2	14	6	122	3.8%	2.90 [0.65, 13.04]
Bansch et al. 2000	16	30	5	76	6.9%	8.11 [3.26, 20.16]
Greene et al. 2000	10	40	18	182	8.6%	2.53 [1.26, 5.06]
Exner et al. 2001	34	90	69	367	11.5%	2.01 [1.43, 2.82]
Verma et al. 2004	57	208	159	1796	12.0%	3.10 [2.37, 4.04]
Stuber et al. 2005	11	51	12	163	8.1%	2.93 [1.38, 6.24]
Gatzoulis et al. 2005	17	32	19	137	10.0%	3.83 [2.26, 6.50]
Hohnloser et al. 2006	4	148	16	485	5.8%	0.82 [0.28, 2.41]
Brigadieau et al. 2006	25	123	28	184	10.3%	1.34 [0.82, 2.18]
Sesselberg et al. 2007	15	27	82	692	11.1%	4.69 [3.16, 6.95]
Nord beck et al. 2010	13	40	24	684	9.4%	9.26 [5.11, 16.79]
Total (95% CI)		837		4911	100.0%	3.15 [2.22, 4.48]
Total events	213		439			

Heterogeneity: $\tau^2 = 0.25$; $\chi^2 = 47.93$, df = 11 ($P < 0.00001$); $I^2 = 77\%$

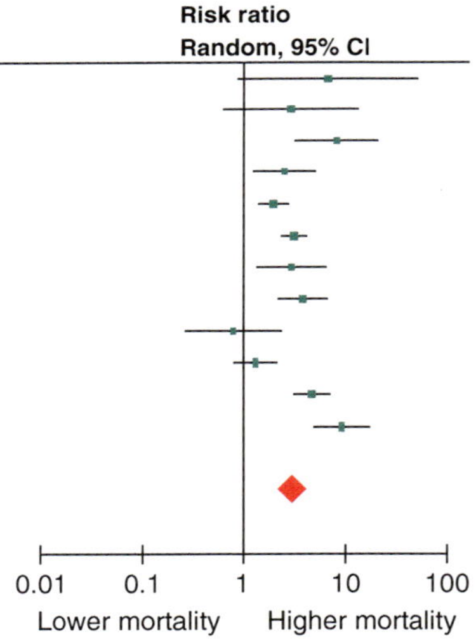

0.01 0.1 1 10 100
Lower mortality Higher mortality

Fig. 40.1 From the ref. [17] (Guerra et al.). Effect of ES on all-cause mortality. *CI* confidence interval, *df* degree of freedom. A meta-analysis of 12 studies comparing the mortality between the patients with and without ES during a median follow-up of 32 months: the ES accounts for a nearly threefold increased risk of death (Relative Risk 3.15)

ablation has been shown to be effective in acute or long-term suppression of ventricular arrhythmia and ES recurrence [18–21]. The largest scale study [19] demonstrated that even though the overall favorable effects of advanced strategies of catheter ablation on both the short-term and long-term recurrence of the ventricular arrhythmias and ES are clearly observed, the net protective efficacy is depending on how successful the catheter ablation is. In detail, the patients with complete success defined as achieving the prevention of inducibility of any VT by the procedures can predict a greater arrhythmia and event free survival t-han those with partial success defined as the successful ablation of only the clinical VTs with persistent inducibility of nonclinical sustained VTs, or failure. A similar result was obtained by another report [20]. According to a most recent single-center study [22] which investigated the underlying arrhythmia substrate using 186 ES patients associated with ischemic cardiomyopathy (ICM) and 101 patients associated with non-ischemic cardiomyopathy (NICM) demonstrated that the storm patients had different electrophysiologic substrate compared with non-storm patients in the extent and distribution of LV scar. In ICM, the storm patients had greater number of scarred LV segments and higher incidence of anterior, septal, and apical endocardial LV scar than the non-storm patients, On the contrary, in NICM, the extent and distribution of scar was similar except for the higher incidence of lateral scar in storm patients. Interestingly, the storm patients associated with NICM had a higher incidence of epicardial ablation than those associated with ICM. It was also revealed that the storm itself did not confer adverse long-term outcomes in ICM patients, but the recurrence of storm had worse outcomes than those without the storm recurrence, in patients with NIHD regardless of cardiomyopathy type.

40.2.2 Structurally Normal Heart

40.2.2.1 Idiopathic Ventricular Fibrillation

In Brugada syndrome, hypokalemia, high vagal tone, bradycardia, and fever can be predisposing factors of the ES [23]. Kaneko et al. [24] reported the clinical characteristics and management for Brugada syndrome with ES defined as ≥3 episodes (mean 25 times) of VF (22 patients) as compared with 110 age-matched patients without ES in a multicenter study. J wave in inferior or lateral leads, a spontaneous type I ECG pattern are significantly relating to the ES emergence, and horizontal or descending ST elevation tends to be associated with ES. Thus, a high prevalence of the early repolarization was found in the ES patients. During follow-up, the VF recurrence rate was significantly higher in Brugada with ES than without ES. Isoproterenol seemed to be effective in the acute phase and bepridil and quinidine in the long-term prevention. A simultaneous observation of the ECG features of both Brugada and J wave syndrome has been shown to be a predictor of VF recurrence by some other reports [25, 26]. In a clinical report evaluating the pattern of fibrillatory events in non-Brugada-type idiopathic ventricular fibrillation, J waves, a notch or slur in terminal portion of QRS complex >0.1mv above the isoelectric line in at least two contiguous inferior and/or lateral leads, are shown to be associated with the VF storm and the long-term arrhythmia recurrence [27].

40.2.2.2 Long QT Syndrome (LQTS), Catecholaminergic Polymorphic Ventricular Tachycardia (CPVT), and the ES in Children

The severity of ventricular arrhythmia is shown to be determined by genetic predisposition in both LQTS and CPVT [28–30]. A review article entitled "electrical storm in children" [31] showed that the ES is a rare medical emergency in children with a variety of etiologies including the primary electrical diseases (CPVT, LQTS, and Brugada syndrome), cardiomyopathies, and postoperative state of congenital heart diseases. Thus the individualized diagnosis and management is essential to protect sudden cardiac death.

40.3 Electrophysiology and Catheter Ablation in the ES of Polymorphic VT or VF (pVT/VF)

40.3.1 Acute or Subacute Phase of MI and Ischemic Cardiomyopathy

It has been shown that the ES occurring in the patients with ischemic heart disease could be successfully suppressed by catheter ablation targeting the origin of VPCs triggering the sustained arrhythmias at which discrete surviving Purkinje potential could be detected in the local electrogram [32–34]. It was also shown that additional RF deliveries applied at the surviving Purkinje fibers located in the extensive infarction zone may have resulted in the non-inducibility of the sustained arrhythmias themselves [34]. The Purkinje fiber can survive in the event of coronary occlusion in experimental studies [35, 36]. Such strength of Purkinje fiber to the ischemic events can attribute to its location at surface endocardium, much nutrition stores in the cytoplasm and less myofibrils, therefore Purkinje fiber shows less oxygen demand [37]. Although Purkinje cells survive over the ischemic event, it causes unignorable histological changes, leading to the formation of arrhythmogenic substrates including conduction and automatic abnormalities.

Table 40.1 Clinical demographic data of the seven patients with ES associated with ischemic heart disease

	Patient 1	Patient 2	Patient 3	Patient 4	Patient 5	Patient 6	Patient 7
Age	67	71	74	81	60	67	66
Gender	Male	Male	Male	Male	Male	Male	Male
Diagnosis	AMI	AMI	AMI	AMI	ICM	ICM	ICM
LVEF (%)	32	20	29	30	32	33	27
Killip class	III	III	I	II	–	–	–
NYHA class	–	–	–		III	II	III
Infarction	Anterior	Inferior	Anterior	Anterior	–	–	–
CA status	LAD closure RCA closure	LAD closure RCA, LCX stenosis	LAD stenosis LCX stenosis	LAD stenosis LCX stenosis	LAD stenosis LCX stenosis	LAD stenosis LCX stenosis	RCA closure LCD stenosis
Intervention	PCI	CABG	PCI	PCI	PCI	CABG	PCI
Interval (MI-VT/VF)	4 h	1 day	4 days	14 days	–	–	–
VT or VF	PVT and VF	PVT and VF	PVT and VF	PVT and VF	PVT and MVT	PVT and MVT	PVT and VF
No. of VT/VF	45	8	>200	4	10	6	40
No. of DC	48	10	185	7	5	4	45
AAs	–	AMD, CARV	AMD, MEX	AMD, MEX	AMD, MEX	AMD, CARV	AMD, MEX, NIX
Prognosis	D (1 month sepsis)	D (1 year, stomach carcinoma)	S (2 years)	S (2 weeks)	S (2 years)	D (5 months pneumonia)	S (4 months)

Seven cases with the ES
AMI acute myocardial infarction, *ICM* ischemic cardiomyopathy, *CA* coronary artery, *LAD* left anterior descending artery, *RCA* right coronary artery, *LCX* left circumflex artery, interval, *MI-VT* interval between the onset of MI and VT/VF, *PVT* polymorphic VT, *MVT* monomorphic VT, *DC* direct current shock, *AAs* antiarrhythmics, *AMD* amiodarone, *CARV* carvedilol, *MEX* mexiletine, *NIF* nifekarant, *D* dead, *S* survived

We have evaluated the clinical characteristics of the seven patients with ES associated with ischemic heart disease (Table 40.1), and the electrocardiographic and electrophysiologic features of the VPCs triggering the sustained pVT/VF (Table 40.2). In four patients the ES emerged in acute or subacute phase of MI (4 h to 14 days after the MI), while the remaining three patients experienced the ES in the remote phase. All patients had multivessel diseases and had severely reduced LV systolic function (LVEF 20–33%). The average number of the total pVT/VF and direct current shocks were 45 ± 70 and 43 ± 65, respectively. Although the ES was successfully eliminated without a recurrence by the catheter ablation targeting the survived Purkinje networks, the prognosis of the patients was rather worse, as three out of seven patients died due to severe inflammatory diseases or malignant disease. In four of the seven patients, two or more morphologies of the VPCs were confirmed to induce pVT/VF (Patient 1–4 in Table 40.2). The remaining three patients had only single morphology of the triggering VPC. A total of 12 morphologies of trigger VPCs were documented to have induced pVT/VF. Eleven VPCs exhibited a right bundle branch block (RBBB) morphology suggesting left ventricular origin with either a superior axis (seven VPCs) or inferior axis (four VPCs). The remaining one VPC showed LBBB pattern with inferior axis. The mean QRS duration was 130 ± 25 ms (range 100–170 ms), suggesting relatively narrow QRS complex. In Fig. 40.2, representative ECG recordings of VPCs followed by the induction of pVT are shown. In five patients, catheter ablation was performed exclusively targeting the origin of the VPCs, and the triggering VPCs were totally eliminated by small number of RF deliveries in three patients with single triggering VPC, whereas in the two patients with bi-morphologies of triggering VPCs (patient Nos. 1 and 3), a significant number of RF deliveries were necessary. In the remaining two patients (patient Nos. 2 and 4), with two or three morphologies of triggering VPCs, the successive RF deliveries targeting not merely the origin of VPCs (see Fig. 40.3) but also the surrounding surviving Purkinje fiber where the P potential was clearly detectable over the extensive MI zone proved by the low voltage of ventricular potential, successfully rendered VT/VF no longer inducible by the aggressive programmed pacing (see

Table 40.2 ECG and electrophysiological data of the seven patients

	Patient 1	Patient 2	Patient 3	Patient 4	Patient 5	Patient 6	Patient 7
VPCs triggering VA							
No. of VPCs	2	3	2	2	1	1	1
ECG morphology							
VPC 1	RBBB, sup	RBBB, inf	RBBB, sup	RBBB, sup	RBBB, sup	RBBB, sup	LBBB, inf
VPC 2	RBBB, sup	RBBB, sup	RBBB, inf	RBBB, inf	–	–	–
VPC 3	–	RBBB, inf	–	–	–	–	–
VPCs origin	VPC1:MS VPC2:PS	VPC1:MS VPC2:PS VPC3:AS	VPC1:PS VPC2:PS	VPC1:PS VPC2:MS	VPC1:PS	VPC1:MS	VPC1:LVOT
Pacemap score	VPC1:12 VPC2:10.5	VPC1:12 VPC2:11.5 VPC1:12	VPC1:11 VPC2:11	NA	VPC1:12	NA	VPC1:11.5
No. of RF	10	24	61	43	4	4	5
CA endpoint	VPC elimination	Non-inducibility	VPC elimination	Non-inducibility	VPC elimination	VPC elimination	VPC elimination
Purkinje potential							
Pp-QRS interval (during PVCs)	VPC1: 55 VPC2: 45	VPC1: 40 VPC2: 60 VPC3: 90	VPC1: 62 VPC2: 99	VPC1: NA VPC2: 55	VPC1: 58	VPC1: 100	VPC1: NA

The PVCs triggering the VTs were polymorphic in four patients and monomorphic in the remaining three patients. All the PVCs except one showed RBBB morphology with either superior or inferior axis and relatively narrow QRS configurations (average 135 ms). The successful ablation sites for the PVCs were widely distributed along the left ventricular septal area. At the successful ablation site, the Purkinje potential preceded the QRS complex by a mean of 66 ms during PVCs. In two patients (Patient' Nos. 2 and 4), RF currents were applied at successive points with surviving Purkinje potential on the infarction zone resulted in non-inducibility of the sustained VT which was reproducibly inducible before the ablation. In the remaining five patients, the ablation procedures led to the PVC elimination

Sup superior axis, *Inf* inferior axis, *AS* anteroseptal, *MS* mid septal, *PS* posteroseptal, *LVOT* left ventricular outflow tract, *NA* not applied, *RF* radiofrequency current delivery, *CA* catheter ablation

Fig. 40.4). It may imply that the surviving Purkinje fibers may play a role in the initiation of VT/VF and at least in a part in the perpetuation of tachycardia. It was clearly shown by a novel computer simulation study that a random reentry involving Purkinje network, multiple Purkinje-muscle connections, and ventricular muscle tissues can be induced by a programmed pacing, expressing as polymorphic VT in a simulated ECG [38].

A similar mechanism of pVT/VF is also shown to underlie the ES in the patients with acute heart failure associated with non-ischemic cardiomyopathy, in which catheter ablation targeting Purkinje fibers along the scar border is effective in the suppression of the ES [39].

40.3.2 Idiopathic Ventricular Fibrillation (IVF)

A pioneer work in this field was reported by Haissaguerre et al. [40]. Twenty seven patients with IVF in which catecholaminergic polymorphic ventricular tachycardia (CPVT), long QT syndrome (LQTS), and Brugada syndrome were all excluded, underwent catheter ablation targeting the triggering VPCs. Out of them, 19 patients underwent the catheter ablation emergently to suppress the ES. Two groups of VPC origins were distinguished, that is, the myocardium of right ventricular outflow tract (RVOT: four patients) and various locations in the Purkinje system (the remaining 23 patients). The VPC origin in the Purkinje system was widely distributed in both anterior right ventricle and lower half of septum of the left ventricle. Regarding the Purkinje origin, premature beats of left and right ventricular origins were equally observed. The VPCs from Purkinje fibers had relatively narrow QRS configuration (126 ± 18 ms) and short coupling intervals (280 ± 26 ms). Interestingly, the local earliest Purkinje potential preceded the local muscle activation with a greater degree in the left than in the right ventricle (46 ms vs 19 ms). During the follow-up of average 24 months, 24 patients (89%) have been free of the recurrence of VF. The remaining three patients who did not show VPCs during mapping had late recurrence

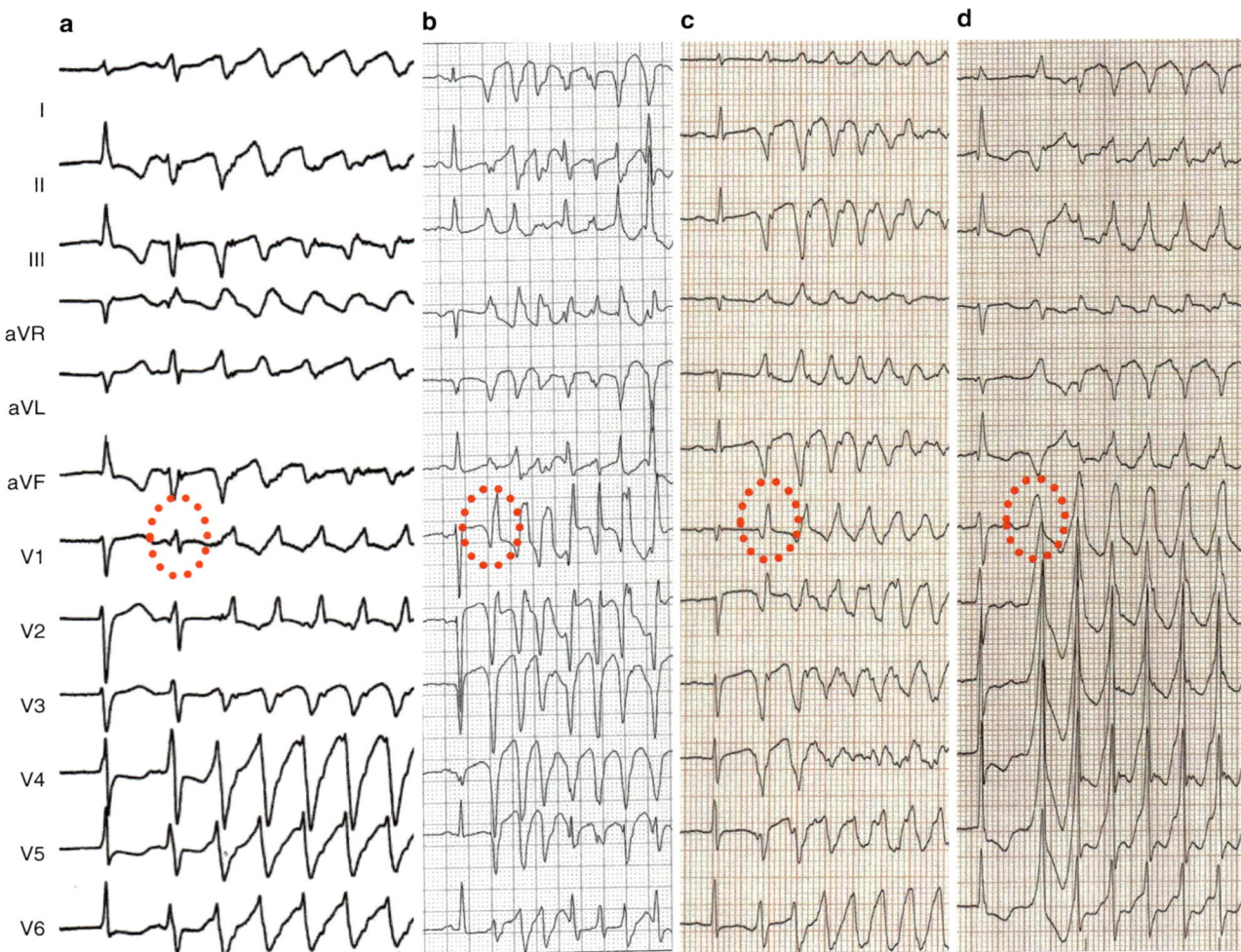

Fig. 40.2 Representative 12-leads ECG records during pVT induction by single VPC (panel **a–d**) in patients with ischemic heart disease. The QRS morphology of the triggering VPCs is right bundle branch block (RBBB) pattern with either superior or inferior axis (*dotted circles*). Most of VPCs show relatively narrow QRS complex except panel **d**

of VPCs, and consequently VF was documented in two patients and non-sustained pVT in one patient, respectively. Thus, catheter ablation targeting on the triggers has been shown to be effective in this category of patients [40–42]. Since, as it was pointed out [40], the occurrence of VPCs triggering VF is capricious, VPCs as well as VF tend to be clustered within a few days, resulting in the ES. Therefore the number of patients who can receive the merit of the catheter ablation is inferred to be small.

In Brugada syndrome and LQTS, the VPCs originating in the Purkinje fibers and RVOT also have some role in initiating pVT/VF; however, its importance seems to be less in these clinical entities as compared to the IVF of non-Brugada type. To date, there have been few reports on the trigger catheter ablation in congenital LQTS [43, 44]. Similarly, we can find only a few case reports on the trigger ablation in Brugada syndrome [43, 45]. Recently, the interests for the EP specialists have shifted to the sub-

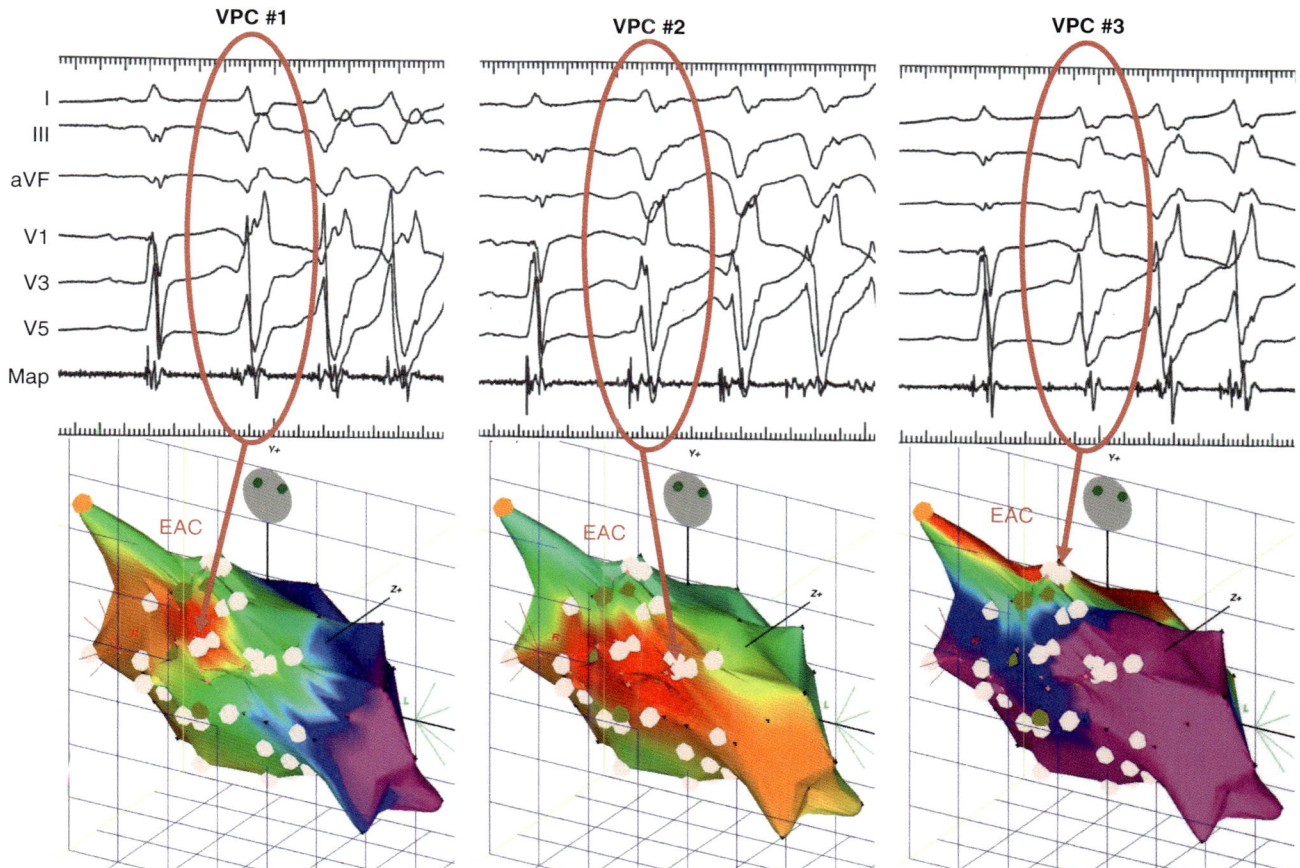

Fig. 40.3 The local electrogram of the earliest activation site for each VPC which initiated pVT in the patient #2 (see Tables 40.1 and 40.2). (*Upper panels*) and each corresponding 3-D activation mapping of LV for VPCs using CARTO mapping system (*lower panels*: projection RAO 30-Caudal). EAC: Earliest activation site, Map: mapping catheter. All the VPCs showed RBBB morphology and the intermediate axis in VPC#1, superior axis in VPC #2, and inferior axis in VPC #3. Accordingly, the earliest activation site was mid-septum, posterior-septum, and anterior-septum, respectively. Note that the local Purkinje potential preceded QRS complex in all the VPCs (Map). *White dots* represent the points at which local Purkinje potential preceding QRS complex was recorded

strate ablation in Brugada syndrome. The first study on the substrate ablation was reported by Nademanee et al. [46]. They searched arrhythmogenic substrate such as low voltage area with prolonged duration and fractionated potentials, and delayed potentials from both endocardial and epicardial approach. The successive RF deliveries targeting the abnormal potentials around RVOT, resulted in the normalization of Brugada ECG patterns and then completely suppressed recurrence of VF in the majority of patients. Another report from Asia [47] showed that the endocardial ablation targeting on the late activation zone defined as local electrical activity recognized during J point + 60 ms, abolished the ES in all four patients applied.

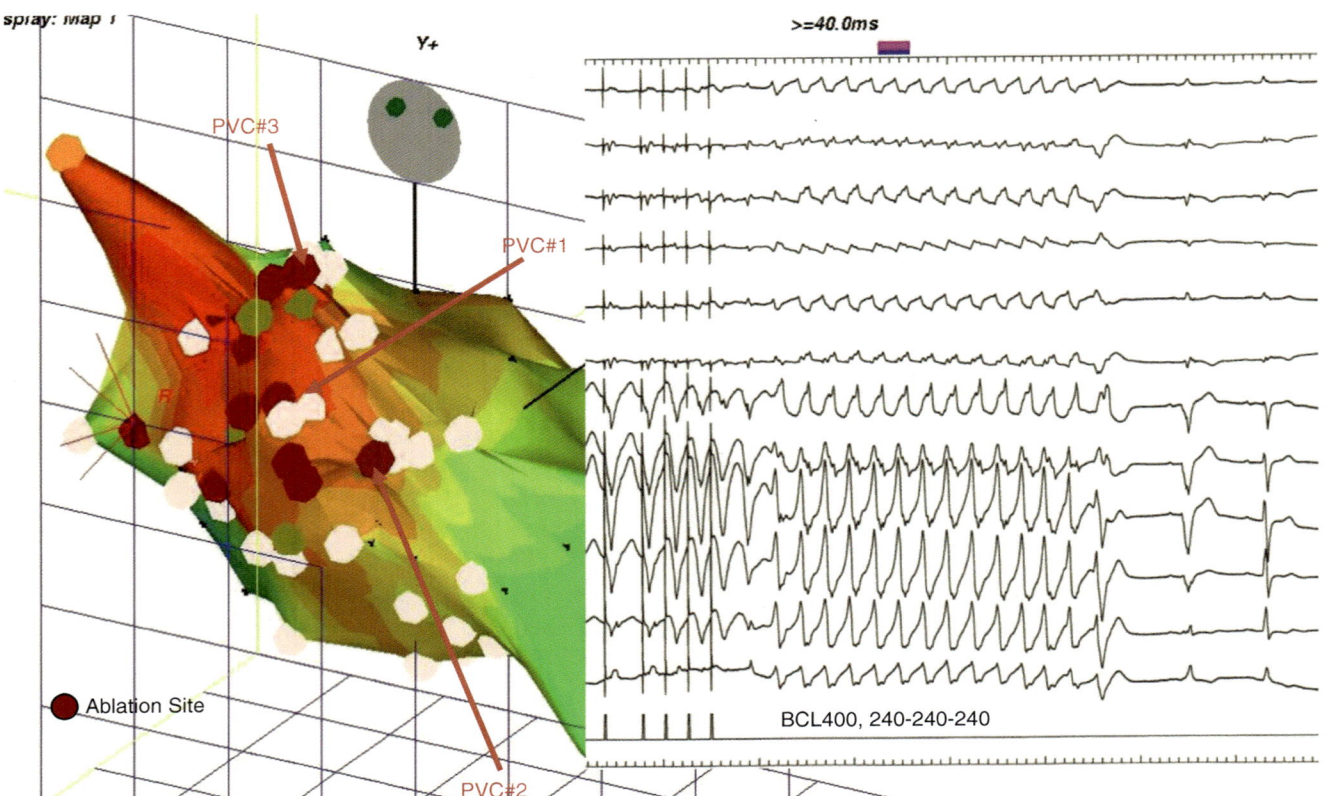

Fig. 40.4 A 3-D voltage map of the same patient as Fig. 40.3. The voltage map revealed that low voltage area (<0.50 mV) was widely distributed over LV septum, suggesting infarction lesion (*left panel*). The Purkinje potential which may reflect the activation of survived Purkinje network could be detected from almost entire part of the septum (*white* and *brown dots*). After the successful ablation of three triggering VPCs at the earliest activation site, spontaneous VPCs disappeared. However, the sustained pVT remained still easily inducible by the programmed pacing at that time, then we applied a total of 24 times RF deliveries on the surrounding survived Purkinje fiber (indicated by *brown dots*). Finally, the clinical sustained pVT was rendered non-inducible by the aggressive programmed pacing (*Right panel*). Only a non-sustained monomorphic VT could be inducible

40.4 Electrophysiology and Catheter Ablation in the ES of Monomorphic VT(mVT)

The strategies of the catheter ablation for mVT storm associated with the structural heart disease including both IHD and NICM are not particularly different from those commonly applied for the ablation of mVT of non-storm type [4, 18–22]. For the scar-related reentry and focal mechanism, the slow conduction channel or isthmus and tachycardia foci are searched utilizing the sophisticated 3-dimensional electro-anatomical mapping systems. For the patients with un-mappable mVT due to hemodynamic intolerance, non-inducibility, or multiple mVTs (pleomorphic VT), the substrate mapping and pace mapping are mainly used to estimate the localization of the channel and isthmus of the reentry. It should be advised that the culprit lesions of the tachycardia may exist deep inside from endocardium or epicardium, and the therapeutic option including bipolar ablation and epicardial ablation should be prepared. Also it should be noted that some mechanism of the His-Purkinje system related tachycardia have been shown to emerge in the patients with structural heart disease. In these cases, the lower specialized conduction tissues become the ablation target (see the reference) [48, 49].

Conclusion

The electrical storm is a life-threatening condition and an ominous predictor of the poor prognosis. The VT/VF storm occurs in a variety of cardiac disease with a variety of mechanism depending on the patients' background. The catheter ablation has now become a potent therapeutic modality to prevent the repeated applications of cardioversion. The indication and strategies of ablation have recently been extended. Therefore, we should be well versed in the disease-specific mechanism of VT/VF and the most susceptible target to the catheter ablation to prepare the emergent application of the catheter ablation.

References

1. Kowey PR. An overview of antiarrhythmic drug management of electrical storm. Can J Cardiol. 1996;12(Supple-B):3B–8B.
2. Maruyama M. Management of electrical storm: the mechanism matters. J Arrhythm. 2014;30:242–9.
3. Conti S, Pala S, Biagioli V, et al. Electrical storm: a clinical and electrophysiological overview. World J Cardiol. 2015;7:555–61.
4. Kautzner J, Peichi P. Catheter ablation of polymorphic ventricular tachycardia and ventricular fibrillation. Arrhythm Electrophysiol Rev. 2013;2:135–40.
5. Hansen EC, Levine FH, Kay HR, et al. Control of postinfarction ventricular irritability with the intraaortic balloon pump. Circulation. 1980;62(2pt2):I130–7.
6. Hoffmann BA, Steven D, Willems S, Sydow K. Renal sympathetic denervation as an adjunct to catheter ablation for the treatment of ventricular electrical storm in the setting of acute myocardial infarction. J Cardiovasc Electrophysiol. 2013;24:1175–8.
7. Ueno A, Kobayashi Y, Murata H et al. Incidence and clinical characteristics of electrical storm in hospitalized patients complicating acute myocardial infarction: a report from Tokyo CCU Network Registry. Annual scientific meeting 2016, Japan Circulation Society.
8. Credner SC, Klingenheben T, Mauss O, et al. Electrical storm in patients with transvenous implantable cardioverter-defibrillators. Incidence, management and prognostic implications. J Am Coll Cardiol. 1998;32:1909–15.
9. Exner DV, Pinski SL, Wyse G, et al. Electrical storm presages nonsudden death. The antiarrhythmics versus implantable defibrillators (AVID) trial. Circulation. 2001;103:2066–71.
10. Verma A, Kilicaslan F, Marrouche NF, et al. Prevalence, predictors, and mortality significance of the causative arrhythmia in patients with electrical storm. J Cardiovasc Electrophysiol. 2004;15:1265–70.
11. Gatzoulis KA, Andrikopoulos G, Apostolopoulos T, et al. Electricla storm is an independent predictor of adverse long-term outcome in the era of implantable defibrillator therapy. Europace. 2005;7:184–92.
12. Hohnloser SH, Al-Khalidi HR, Pratt CM, et al. Electrical storm in patients with an implantable defibrillator: incidence, features, and preventive therapy: insight from a randomized trial. Eur Heart J. 2006;27:3027–32.
13. Brigadeau F, Kouakam C, Klug D, et al. Clinical predictors and prognostic significance of electrical storm in patients with implantable cardioverter defibrillators. Eur Heart J. 2006;27:700–7.
14. Sesselberg HW, Moss AJ, McNitt S, et al. Ventricular arrhythmia storms in postinfarction patients with implantable defibrillators for primary prevention indications: a MADIT-II substudy. Heart Rhythm. 2007;4:1395–402.
15. Washizuka T, Chinushi M, Watanabe H, et al. Nifekalant hydrochloride suppresses severe electrical storm in patients with malignant ventricular tachyarrhythmias. Circ J. 2005;69:1508–13.
16. Murata H, Miyauchi Y, Hayashi M, et al. Clinical and electrophysiologic characteristics of electrical storms due to monomorphic ventricular tachycardia refractory to intravenous amiodarone. Circ J. 2015;79:2130–7.
17. Guerra F, Shkoza M, Flori M, Capucci A. Role of electrical storm as a mortality and morbidity risk factor and its clinical predictors: a meta-analysis. Europace. 2014;16:347–53.
18. Schreieck J, Zrenner B, Deisenhofer I, Schmitt C. Rescue ablation of electrical storm in patients with ischemic cardiomyopathy: a potential-guided ablation approach by modifying substrate of intractable unmappable ventricular tachycardia. Heart Rhythm. 2005;2:10–4.
19. Carbucicchio C, Santamaria M, Trevisi N, Maccabelli G, Giraldi F, Fassini G, Riva S, Moltrasio M, Cireddu M, Veglia F, Della Bella P. Catheter ablation for the treatment of electrical storm in patients with implantable cardioverter-defibrillators. Short- and long-term outcome in a prospective single-center study. Circulation. 2008;117:462–9.
20. Arya A, Bode K, Piorkowski C, Bollmann A, Sommer P, Gaspar T, Wetzel U, Husser D, Kottkamp H, Hindricks G. Catheter ablation of electrical storm due to monomorphic ventricular tachycardia in patients with nonischemic cardiomyopathy: acute results and its effect on long-term survival. Pacing Clin Electrophysiol. 2010;33:1504–9.
21. M K, Peichl P, Cihak R, Wichterle D, Vancura V, Bytesnik J, Kautzner J. Catheter ablation of electrical storm in patients with structural heart disease. Europace. 2011;13:109–13.
22. Kumar S, Fujii A, Kapur S, Romero J, Mehta NK, Tanigawa S, Epstein LM, Koplan BA, Michaud GF, John RM, Stevenson WG, Tedrow UB. Beyond the storm: comparison of clinical factors, arrhythmogenic substrate, and catheter ablation outcomes in structural heart disease patients with versus those without a history of ventricular tachycardia storm. J Cardiovasc Electrophysiol. 2016;28(1):56–67. https://doi.org/10.1111/jce.13117.
23. Maury P, Hocini M, haissaguerre M. Electrical storm in Brugada syndrome: review of pharmachologic and ablative therapeutic options. Indian Pacing Electrophysiol J. 2005;5:25–34.
24. Kaneko Y, Horie M, Niwano S, Kusano KF, Takatsuki S, Kurita T, Mitsuhashi T, Nakajima T, Irie T, Hasegawa K, Noda T, Kamakura S, Aizawa Y, Yasuoka R, Torigoe K, Suzuki H, Ohe T, Shimizu A, Fukuda K, Kurabayashi M, Aizawa Y. Electrical storm in patients with brugada syndrome is associated with early repolarization. Circ Arrhythm Electrophysiol. 2014;7:1122–8.
25. Kawata H, Morita H, Yamada Y, Noda T, Satomi K, Aiba T, Isobe M, Nagase S, Nakamura K, Fukushima Kusano K, Ito H, Kamakura S, Shimizu W. Prognostic significance of early repolarization in inferolateral leads in Brugada patients with documented ventricular fibrillation: a novel risk factor for Brugada syndrome with ventricular fibrillation. Heart Rhythm. 2013;10(8):1161.
26. Takagi M, Aonuma K, Sekiguchi Y, Yokoyama Y, Aihara N, Hiraoka M. Japan Idiopathic Ventricular Fibrillation Study (J-IVFS) Investigators. The prognostic value of early repolarization (J wave) and ST-segment morphology after J wave in Brugada syndrome: multicenter study in Japan. Heart Rhythm. 2013;10:533–9.
27. Aizawa Y, Sato M, Ohno S, Horie M, Takatsuki S, Fukuda K, Chinushi M, Usui T, Aonuma K, Hosaka Y, Haissaguerre M, Aizawa Y. Circadian pattern of fibrillatory events in non-Brugada-type idiopathic ventricular fibrillation with a focus on J waves. Heart Rhythm. 2014;11:2261–6.
28. Makita N, Yagihara N, Crotti L, Johnson CN, Beckmann BM, Roh MS, Shigemizu D, Lichtner P, Ishikawa T, Aiba T, Homfray T, Behr ER, Klug D, Denjoy I, Mastantuono E, Theisen D, Tsunoda T, Satake W, Toda T, Nakagawa H, Tsuji Y, Tsuchiya T, Yamamoto H, Miyamoto Y, Endo N, Kimura A, Ozaki K, Motomura H, Suda K, Tanaka T, Schwartz PJ, Meitinger T, Kääb S, Guicheney P, Shimizu W, Bhuiyan ZA, Watanabe H, Chazin WJ, George AL Jr. Novel calmodulin mutations associated with congenital arrhythmia susceptibility. Circ Cardiovasc Genet. 2014;7(4):466–74.
29. Murphy LL, Moon-Grady AJ, Cuneo BF, Wakai RT, Yu S, Kunic JD, Benson DW, George AL Jr. Developmentally regulated SCN5A splice variant potentiates dysfunction of a novel mutation associated with severe fetal arrhythmia. Heart Rhythm. 2012;9(4):590–7.
30. Janson CM, Poelzing S, Shah MJ. Combined inhibition of Na^+ and Ca^{2+} channels: a novel paradigm for the treatment of incessant ventricular arrhythmias in Andersen-Tawil syndrome. Heart Rhythm. 2014;11(2):318–20.

31. Clausen H, Pelaumer A, Kamberi S, et al. Electrical storm in children. PACE. 2013;36:391–401.
32. Bänsch D, Oyang F, Antz M, et al. Successful catheter ablation of electrical storm after myocardial infarction. Circulation. 2003;108:3011–6.
33. Szumowski L, Sanders P, Walczak F, et al. Mapping and ablation of polymorphic ventricular tachycardia after myocardial infarction. J Am Coll Cardiol. 2004;44:1700–6.
34. Kobayashi Y, Iwasaki Y, Miyauchi Y, Hayashi M, Ohno N, Yodogawa K, Morita N, Tanaka K, Kyoichi M. The role of Purkinje fibers in the emergence of an incessant form of polymorphic ventricular tachycardia or ventricular fibrillation associated with ischemic heart disease. J Arrhythm. 2008;24:200–8.
35. Fenoglio JJ, Pham TD, Harken AH, et al. Recurrent sustained ventricular tachycardia: structure and ultrastructure of subendocardial regions in which tachycardia originates. Circulation. 1983;68:518–33.
36. Sugi K, Karagueuzian HS, Fishbein MC, Mandel WJ, Peter T. Celular electrophysiologic characteristics of surviving subendocardial fibers in chronically infarcted right ventricular myocardium susceptible to inducible sustained ventricular tachycardia. Am Heart J. 1987;114:559–69.
37. Myers W, Honig CR. Amount and distribution of Rb86 transported into myocardium from ventricular lumen. Am J Physiol. 1966;211:739–45.
38. Berenfeld O, Jalife J. Purkinje-muscle reentry as a mechanism of polymorphic ventricular arrhythmias in a 3-dimensional model of the ventricles. Circ Res. 1998;82:1063–77.
39. Tan VH, Yap J, Hsu LF, et al. Catheeter ablation of ventricular fibrillation triggers and electrical storm. Europace. 2012;14:1687–95.
40. Haïssaguerre M, Shoda M, Jaïs P, Nogami A, Shah DC, Kautzner J, Arentz T, Kalushe D, Lamaison D, Griffith M, Cruz F, de Paola A, Gaïta F, Hocini M, Garrigue S, Macle L, Weerasooriya R, Clémenty J. Mapping and ablation of idiopathic ventricular fibrillation. Circulation. 2002 20;106(8):962–7.
41. Kneckt S, Sacher F, Wright M, et al. Long term follow up of idiopathic ventricular fibrillation ablation: a multicenter study. J Am Coll Cardiol. 2009;54:522–8.
42. Nogami A, Sugiyasu A, Kubota S, et al. mapping and ablation of idiopathic ventricular fibrillation from the Purkinje system. Heart Rhythm. 2005;2:646–9.
43. Haiisaguerre M, Extramiana F, Hocini M, et al. Mpping and ablation of ventricular fibrillation associated with long-QT and Brugada syndromes. Circulation. 2003;108:925–8.
44. Srivathsan K, Gami AS, Ackerman MJ, Asirvatham SJ. Treatment of ventricular fibrillation in a patient with prior diagnosis of long QT syndrome: importance of precise electrophysiologic diagnosis to successfully ablate the trigger. Heart Rhytjm. 2007;4:1090–3.
45. Nakagawa N, Takagi M, Tatsumi H, Yoshiyama M. Successful radiofrequency catheter ablation for electrical storm of ventricular fibrillation in a patient with Brugada syndrome. Circ J. 2008;72:1025–9.
46. Nademanee K, Veerakul G, Chandanamattha P, Chaothawee L, Ariyachaipanich A, Jirasirirojanakorn K, Likittanasombat K, Bhuripanyo K, Ngarmukos T. Prevention of ventricular fibrillation episodes in Brugada syndrome by catheter ablation over the anterior right ventricular outflow tract epicardium. Circulation. 2011;123:1270–9.
47. Sunsaneewitayakul B, Yao Y, Thamaree S, Zhang S. Endocardial mapping and catheter ablation for ventricular fibrillation prevention in Brugada syndrome. J Cardiovasc Electrophysiol. 2012;23(Suppl 1):S10–6.
48. Hayashi M, Kobayashi Y, Iwasaki YK, Morita N, Miyauchi Y, Kato T, Takano T. Novel mechanism of postinfarction ventricular tachycardia originating in surviving left posterior Purkinje fibers. Heart Rhythm. 2006;3:908–18.
49. Sakata T, Tanner H, Stuber T, Delacrétaz E. His-Purkinje system reentry in patients with clustering ventricular tachycardia episodes. Europace. 2008;10:289–93.

Printed by Printforce, the Netherlands